Pharmaceuticals: Clinical Research

Pharmaceuticals: Clinical Research

Edited by Sean Boyd

hayle
medical

New York

Hayle Medical,
750 Third Avenue, 9th Floor,
New York, NY 10017, USA

Visit us on the World Wide Web at:
www.haylemedical.com

ISBN: 978-1-63241-469-4

The publisher's policy is to use permanent paper from mills that operate a sustainable forestry policy. Furthermore, the publisher ensures that the text paper and cover boards used have met acceptable environmental accreditation standards.

Trademark Notice: Registered trademark of products or corporate names are used only for explanation and identification without intent to infringe.

Printed in the United States of America.

Cataloging-in-Publication Data

Pharmaceuticals : clinical research / edited by Sean Boyd.
    p. cm.
Includes bibliographical references and index.
ISBN 978-1-63241-469-4
1. Clinical pharmacology. 2. Drugs--Research. 3. Pharmacology. I. Boyd, Sean.
RM301.28 .P43 2017
615.1--dc23

Table of Contents

Preface

This book has been an outcome of determined endeavour from a group of educationists in the field. The primary objective was to involve a broad spectrum of professionals from diverse cultural background involved in the field for developing new researches. The book not only targets students but also scholars pursuing higher research for further enhancement of the theoretical and practical applications of the subject.

This book on pharmaceuticals deals with the study of pharmaceutical drug design and development. Drugs are usually classified according to mode of action, route of administering and the therapeutic effects of the same. Contents included in this book present the advanced topics of pharmaceutical research. The various studies that are constantly contributing towards advancing technologies and evolution this field are examined in detail. This book is a vital tool for all researching or studying pharmaceuticals as it gives incredible insights into emerging trends and concepts. With state-of-the-art inputs by acclaimed experts of this field, this book targets students and professionals.

It was an honour to edit such a profound book and also a challenging task to compile and examine all the relevant data for accuracy and originality. I wish to acknowledge the efforts of the contributors for submitting such brilliant and diverse chapters in the field and for endlessly working for the completion of the book. Last, but not the least; I thank my family for being a constant source of support in all my research endeavours.

Editor

Design and characterization of diclofenac diethylamine transdermal patch using silicone and acrylic adhesives combination

Dandigi M Panchaxari[1], Sowjanya Pampana[1*], Tapas Pal[2], Bhavana Devabhaktuni[2] and Anil Kumar Aravapalli[1]

Abstract

Background and purpose of the study: The objective of the study was to develop and characterize Diclofenac Diethylamine (DDEA) transdermal patch using Silicone and acrylic adhesives combination.

Methods: Modified solvent evaporation method was employed for casting of film over Fluoropolymer coated polyester release liner. Initial studies included solubilization of drug in the polymers using solubilizers. The formulations with combination of adhesives were attempted to combine the desirable features of both the adhesives. The effect of the permeation enhancers on the drug permeation were studied using pig ear skin. All the optimized patches were subjected to adhesion, dissolution and stability studies. A 7-day skin irritancy test on albino rabbits and an in vivo anti-inflammatory study on wistar rats by carrageenan induced paw edema method were also performed.

Results: The results indicated the high percent drug permeation (% CDP-23.582) and low solubility nature (1%) of Silicone adhesive and high solubility (20%) and low% CDP (10.72%) of acrylic adhesive. The combination of adhesives showed desirable characteristics for DDEA permeation with adequate % CDP and sufficient solubility. Release profiles were found to be dependent on proportion of polymer and type of permeation enhancer. The anti-inflammatory study revealed the sustaining effect and high percentage inhibition of edema of C4/OLA (99.68%). The acute skin irritancy studies advocated the non-irritant nature of the adhesives used.

Conclusion: It was concluded that an ideal of combination of adhesives would serve as the best choice, for fabrication of DDEA patches, for sustained effect of DDEA with better enhancement in permeation characteristics and robustness.

Keywords: Transdermal drug delivery system, Silicone adhesive, Acrylic adhesive, Permeation study, Dissolution, Skin irritancy and anti-inflammatory

Introduction

Drugs can be delivered across the skin to have an effect on the tissues adjacent to the site of application (topical delivery) or to have an effect after distribution through the circulatory system (systemic delivery). While there are many advantages for delivering drugs through the skin the barrier properties of the skin provide a significant challenge. By understanding the mechanisms by which compounds cross the skin it will be possible to devise means for improving drug delivery [1]. In the last decades, transdermal

dosage forms have been introduced for providing a controlled delivery via the skin into the circulation system.

A transdermal patch or skin patch is a medicated adhesive patch that is placed on the skin to deliver a specific dose of medication through the skin and into the blood stream. Drug-in-adhesive-type patches have been gaining increasing popularity as effective transdermal delivery systems during the last two decades [2] due to various advantages over other systems namely, they are easy to construct, less chances of dose dumping and patches with less thicknesses can be prepared.

Diclofenac is a well-established non-steroidal anti-inflammatory agent, widely used in musculoskeletal

* Correspondence: soujanya.pampana@gmail.com
[1]Department of Pharmaceutics, KLEU's college of Pharmacy, Nehru Nagar, Belgaum, Karnataka 590010, India
Full list of author information is available at the end of the article

disorders, arthritis, toothache, dysmenorrhea, etc., for symptomatic relief of pain and inflammation [3]. Diethylammonium salt of Diclofenac (Diclofenac Diethylamine) is reportedly used for topical applications. Diclofenac Diethylamine (DDEA) gel (1.16%; Voltaren® Emulgel®, Novartis, Nyon, Switzerland) has been used extensively in Europe since 1985 to relieve the symptoms of OA of the knee, as well as other painful, inflammatory tendon, ligament, muscle, and joint conditions [4]. However, all NSAIDs include a boxed warning highlighting the potential for increased risk of cardiovascular events as well as serious potential life-threatening gastrointestinal bleeding. The drug undergoes substantial hepatic first-pass metabolism and thus only about 50% of the administered dose reaches systemic circulation [3,5]. This originates the need of an alternative route of administration, which can bypass the hepatic first-pass metabolism. Transdermal route is an alternative choice of route of administration for such drugs. The drug, Diclofenac Diethylamine also possesses the ideal characteristics, such as poor bioavailability (40 to 60%), short biological half-life (2 to 3 h), smaller dose (25 to 50 mg), etc., to be formulated into a transdermal patch. Transdermal patches offer added advantages, such as maintenance of constant and prolonged drug level, reduced frequency of dosing, minimization of inter and intra patient variability, self-administration and easy termination of medication, leading to patient compliance [6].

It has been postulated that Diclofenac transdermal exerts its pharmacological effects through localized accumulation at the site of application rather than from the systemic absorption. The bioavailability of Diclofenac transdermal is approximately 1% that of oral Diclofenac, with an elimination half-life of 12 h compared with 1.2 to 2 h with oral Diclofenac [7].

The present study aimed at developing TDDS drug-in-adhesive patches of DDEA using Silicone adhesives, Acrylic adhesives and blend of Silicone and Acrylic adhesives.

Material and methods
Materials
The Silicone polymers (S_1 to S_6) were purchased from Dow Corning Corporation, (midland, MIA, USA), Acrylic polymer (A) was purchased from National Starch and Chemical company (Bridge Water, NJ, USA). Fluoropolymer coated polyester release liner and Polyester Backing laminate was purchased from 3 M Scotchpak (st. paul, USA). The drug Diclofenac Diethylamine B.P (DDEA) was obtained from Sparsha Pharma International Pvt Ltd (Hyd, India). Methanol and Acetonnitrile were of HPLC grade and purchased from Sigma-Aldrich corporation, India. All other reagents used were of highest reagent grade available.

Preparation of patches containing silicone adhesives
Preparation of placebo silicone patches
Transdermal patches were prepared by modified solvent evaporation method. It is similar to conventional method except, that the drug-polymeric solution was spread over the release liner with the help of manual coater over release liner. Transdermal patches using different silicone polymers (Table 1) without drug were prepared. For preparing transdermal patches, an adequate amount of polymeric solution was taken and then spread over the release liner with the help of a manual coater. The polymeric solution coated liner was dried at 80°C in an oven for 10 min. The patches were then finally laminated with polyester backing membrane. The obtained sheets were punched using suitable dyes (3, 10 and 50 cm²) to get patches of appropriate sizes, packed in aluminum foil and stored in a desiccator for further studies. Patches were prepared using different grades of silicone adhesives.

Physical evaluation of placebo patches
The tack of the patches – ball tack test
Tack is the ability of a pressure-sensitive adhesive to bond under conditions of light contact pressure and a

Table 1 Details of silicone and acrylic polymers used in the study

Code	Functional group	Solvent	Solid content (%)	Viscosity (Mpa.s)
Silicone Polymer				
S1	Amine compatible	Ethyl acetate	60	350
S2	Amine compatible	Ethyl acetate	60	800
S3	Amine compatible	Ethyl acetate	60	1200
S4	-	Ethyl acetate	60	650
S5	-	Ethyl acetate	65	2500
S6	-	Ethyl acetate	60	2600
Acrylic polymer				
A, Polyacrylate	COOH	Ethylacetae and Hexane	43.2	7000-19000

short contact time. The tack of the skin contact adhesive was measured by the rolling ball tack test using primary adhesive tester (Labthink Instruments Co. Ltd., China). The patch with a size of 50 cm^2 was fixed on a plate. Different diameter steel balls were released from the top of the inclined plate (angle 45°C). The number of the largest ball (0 – 9) which did not roll down was reported as the tack value [8].

Peel strength of patches

Peel strength measures the force required to peel away a pressure-sensitive adhesive once it has been attached to a surface. The test was performed with a Digital Peel tester with a load capacity up to 5 kg (Make: International Equipments, Model: CO). A piece of the patch which has a width of 10 mm and length of 25 mm was prepared, applied quickly to the end of the stainless steel plate and left the apparatus for 10 min.

The cello tape was affixed on the product. The free end of this tape was bending back 180° and it was attached firmly to the upper part of a peel testing machine with a clamp. The instrument was started with a speed of 300 mm/min and the values were recorded. Five patches form each batch were used measuring strength and their values were averaged [8].

Preparation of drug loaded silicone patches
Solubility of drug in adhesives

The solubility of drug in adhesive was tested in silicone adhesives (S$_3$ and S$_6$). Different concentrations of drug (5% w/w, 3% w/w, 2% w/w and 1% w/w of final patch formulation) were added to the adhesives under constant stirring with the help of magnetic stirrer. The stirring was continued for a period of 4 h in order to ensure complete mixing. The solution was kept aside overnight for visual observation. The solutions that showed turbidity were discarded and solutions that remained clear were coated over release liner and finally laminated with backing layer as described in the section 2.2.1.

Solubility enhancement techniques

Various solubility enhancements used to increase the solubility of Diclofenac Diethylamine in silicone adhesives include

Addition of solubilizers

Polyethylene glycol – 400 (PEG 400) and Propylene glycol (PG) in different concentrations (% w/w of final patch formulation) were used [9]. The adhesive polymeric solution, drug and solubilizer in required quantities were weighed and mixed with the aid of magnetic stirrer for a period of about 4–5 h. The solutions were monitored visually for appearance of turbidity/sedimentation. The formulations that showed

clear solution after 24 h were coated over release liner and laminated with polyester backing laminate. The patches were packed in aluminum foil, kept aside for 10 days for appearence of crystals visually and microscopically. The patches which did not show crystals after 10 days were selected for further study.

Addition of oils

Four oils were slected based on preliminary study to improve the solubility of Diclofenac Diethylamine [10]. The oils, Oleic acid (OLA), Iso stearic acid (ISA), Pharamasolve (PS) and Iso propyl myristate (IPM) in different ratios of drug: solubilizer were mixed with polymeric solution and then monitored visually for turbidity. The clear solutions were used for preparation of patches which were kept aside for 10 days for appearance of crystals.

Ex vivo skin permeation studies
Preparation of skin barrier

Fresh full-thickness (75–80 mm) pig ear skin was used for the study. The experiment was carried out according to the guidelines of the Committee for the Purpose of Control and Supervision of Experiments on Animals and approved by Animal Ethical Committee of Department of Genetics, Osmania University, Hyderabad, India (approval no.380/01/a/CPCSEA). Fresh pig ears were obtained from a local abattoir; to ensure integrity of the skin barrier, ears were removed post-sacrifice. The skin was dermatomed (Zimmer electric Dermatome Handset) to remove dermis [11,12]. The isolated epidermis (100 μm) was rapidly rinsed with hexane to remove surface lipids and then rinsed with water and used immediately.

The *ex vivo* skin permeation from the prepared drug polymeric patches across the porcine ear skin barrier was studied using Franz diffusion cell (Orchid Scientifics & Innovative India Pvt Ltd.), [13,14]. Twenty - five milliliters of phosphate buffer of pH 7.4 was used as an elution medium. The diameter of the donor compartment cell provided an effective constant area of 3.4 cm^2. The dermatomed pig ear skin was mounted between the two compartments of Franz diffusion cell with stratum corneum facing towards the donor compartment. A 3 cm^2 patch was used for the study. The release liner was removed. The patches to be studied were placed in between the donor and the receptor compartment in such a way that the drug releasing surface faced toward the receptor compartment. After securely clamping the donor and receptor compartments together, the elution medium was magnetically stirred for uniform drug distribution at a speed of 60 rpm. The temperature of the whole assembly was maintained at 32 ± 0.5°C by thermostatic arrangements. An aliquot of 0.5 mL was withdrawn at preset time intervals for a period of 24 h and an equivalent volume of fresh buffer was replaced. The samples removed were analysed by HPLC described below.

Preparation of patches containing acrylic adhesive
The formulations containing different concentrations of drug with acrylic adhesive were prepared by the method described under section 2.2. The patches prepared were monitered for appearance of crystals visually for 10 days. The properties of acrylic adhesive were mentioned in the Table 1. The patches which showed stability were subjected to peel test, ball test (described under 2.2) and permeation study (described in section 2.3).

Preparation of patches containing combination of silicone and arylic adhesives
Placebo patches containing combination of silicone and acrylate adhesives in different ratios and drug containing combinational patches were prepared by the following method:

In First step, required amount of drug (% w/w of final patch formulation) was made to dissolve completely in appropriate amount of acrylate adhesive by continuous stirring. Second step involves addition of silicone polymeric solution to clear solution formed in step 1 and then continuing mixing for a period of 12 h. The formulations that showed drug solubility after 24 h were laminated into patches. The patches which showed stability were subjected to peel test, ball test (described under 2.2) and permeation study (described in section 2.3).

Effect of permeation enhancers on drug loaded combinational patches
The incorporation of a permeation enhancer is indispensable for achieving the desired permeation rate for almost all drugs with the limited size of the patch. The permeation enhancers Oleic acid (OLA), Iso Stearic acid (ISA) and Isopropyl Myristate (IPM) at concentraions of 5% each were chosen to study their effect on permeation of Diclofenac Diethylamine across the skin. The solubilized combinational patches (C_4 and C_5) along with different permeation enhancers (5% concentration) were formulated and subjected for permeation study as described under 2.3.

Characterization of optimized patches
Various physicochemical tests employed for optimized transdermal patches were as shown

Thickness
Patch thickness was measured using digital micrometer screw gauge (Mitutoyo, Japan) at five different places. The average and standard deviation of five readings were calculated for each batch of the drug-loaded films.

Table 2 Draize evaluation of dermal reaction

Scoring	Reaction	
	Erythema	Edema
0	No erythema	No edema
1	Very slight erythema	Very slight edema
2	Well-defined erythema	Slight edema
3	Moderate to severe erythema	Moderate edema
4	Severe erythema	Severe edema

Weight uniformity
Five different films from individual batches were weighed individuall, and the average weight was calculated the individual weight should not deviate significantly from the weight was calculated, the individual weight should not deviate significantly from the average weight, so the standard deviation was calculated [15].

Drug content
Assay of Diclofenac Diethylamine was done with the help of HPLC. All the solvents used were of HPLC grade [16].

Sample solution
For determination of drug content one patch of 50 cm^2 was taken, dissolved in HPLC grade methanol and sonicated for 15 min. From above solution 1 mL was taken into a 50 mL volumetric flask, diluted up to the mark with methanol, filtered through Nylon membrane filters of 0.45 μ size (Pall Pharmalab Filtration Pvt. Ltd.) and injected (20 mL) into the HPLC column.

Standard solution
For preparing standard solution, 50 mg of Diclofenac Diethylamine was dissolved in 50 mL methanol (HPLC grade). From the above solution, 1 mL was taken and diluted to 50 mL with methanol which was finally filtered through a Nylon membrane filters of 0.45 μ size (Whatman GF/C) and injected (20 mL) into the HPLC column.

HPLC conditions
The HPLC system consisted of L-7110 pump (Shimadzu Corporation, Japan) with L-7420 variable-wavelength ultraviolet absorbance detector (Shimadzu Corporation, Japan) set at 274 nm. Analysis was performed on a reversed-phase column made of silica

Table 3 Adhesive mass values, ball test and peel test values for placebo silicone patches

Parameter and thickness	Polymer type				
	S_2	S_3	S_4	S_5	S_6
Ball tack test [a]	4	8	0	5	8
Peel test (Kg/cm) [b]	0.384	0.646	0.0938	0.495	0.645

(S_2, S_3, S_4, S_5 and S_6 represents different Silicone polymers used; a = 3 and b = 5).

Table 4 Solubilization summary of drug loaded silicone polymers

Formulation code	Drug concentration	Solubilizer concentration	Observation
DS_3	5%	-	Clear solution was not formed.
DS_3	3%	-	Clear solution was not formed.
DS_3	2%	-	Clear solution was not formed.
DS_3	1%	-	Clear solution indicating solubilization of drug
DS_3	0.5%	-	Clear solution indicating solubilization of drug.
DS_6	1%	-	Clear solution was not formed.
DS_3E_1	5%	5% PEG-400	Clear solution was not formed.
DS_3E_2	3%	5% PEG-400	Clear solution was not formed.
DS_3E_3	2%	3% PEG-400	Clear solution was formed.
DS_6E_4	1%	3% PEG-400	Clear solution was formed.
DS_6E_5	2%	3% PEG-400	Clear solution was not formed.
DS_3G_1	5%	5% PG	Clear solution was not formed.
DS_3G_2	2%	5% PG	Clear solution was formed.
DS_3G_3	1%	2% PG	Clear solution was formed.
DS_3O_1	3%	2% OLA	Clear solution was not formed
DS_3O_2	2%	2% OLA	Clear solution was not formed
DS_3O_3	1%	2% OLA	Clear solution was formed
DS_3I_1	4%	2% ISA	Clear solution was not formed
DS_3I_2	3%	2% ISA	Clear solution was not formed
DS_3I_3	1%	2% ISA	Clear solution was formed
DS_3M_1	1%	2% IPM	Clear solution was not formed
DS_3P_1	1%	2% Pharmasolve	Clear solution was not formed
$DS_3O_4I_4$	3%	5% OLA & 5% ISA	Clear solution was formed.

DS: drug with silicone polymer; S_3: Silicone polymer grade, S_3; S_6: Silicone polymer grade S_6; OLA: oleic acid; ISA: Iso stearic acid; IPM: Isopalmitic acid; PEG 400: Polyethylene glycol –400; PG: Propylene glycol.

(150 mm × 4.6 mm i.d., 5 µm, Chemsil BDS C18, Beijing China), operated at 40°C. The mobile phase consisted of 45: 55 ratio of 0.5% Glacial acetic acid in water and Acetonitrile. HPLC grade water was used for the preparation of 0.5% Glacial acetic acid solution. The flow rate of mobile phase was set at 0.8 mL/min, was used. The injection volume is 20 µL.

In vitro release – dissolution studies
The release-rate determination is one of the most important studies to be conducted for all controlled release delivery systems. The dissolution studies of patches are very crucial, because one needs to maintain the drug concentration on the surface of stratum corneum consistently and substantially greater than the drug concentration in the body, to achieve a constant rate of drug permeation [17].

A Paddle over disc assembly (USP 23, Apparatus 5) was used for the assessment of release of DDEA. The TDDS patch was mounted on the disc and placed at the bottom of the dissolution vessel. The dissolution medium, 900 ml degassed distilled water at pH 7.0. The apparatus was equilibrated to 32 ± 0.5°C and operated at 50 rpm [18] during the entire study period (24 h). The dissolution medium was degassed by a combination of heating up to 45°C and vacuum filtration followed by vigorous stirring of media under vacuum.

Stability study
The optimized formulations were subjected to stability study by storing patches at 40 ± 2°C and 75% RH in stability chamber for three months. Two parameters namely, peel strength and drug content were analyzed.

Surface morphology
The surface morphology of formulated transdermal patches (both stable and unstable) were investigated by using Scanning electron microscope (model: SEM JSM-6610) at 15 kV under different magnifications (950x, 1000x and 1500x). In order to make the samples electrically conductive the samples were gold coated prior to the study.

Acute skin irritancy test
The study was conducted on the basis of the approval of institutional animal ethical committee. Albino rabbits of either sex, each weighing 1.5 to 2.0 kg, divided into two groups, were used in this study (n = 4 in each group) [14]. They were housed in cages in the animal house under controlled temperature and light conditions. They were fed a standard laboratory diet and had access to water *ad libitum*. The dorsal surface of the rabbits was cleared and the hair was removed by shaving. The skin was cleared with rectified spirit. The experimental patch

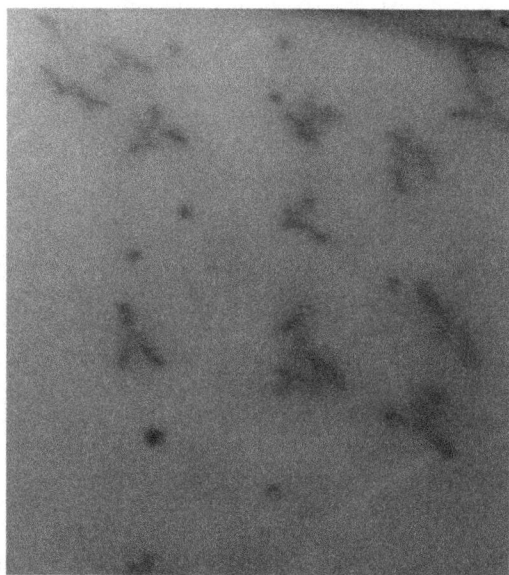

Figure 1 Photograph of Silicone patch, DS_3O_1, showing crystal formation.

(A1, group II), one patch per day, were applied to the shaved skin of rabbits and secured using USP adhesive tape (Johnson & Johnson limited, Mumbai). A 0.8% (v/v) aqueous solution of formaldehyde was applied as a standard irritant (group I). Its effect was compared with the test [19]. The animals were observed for any sign of

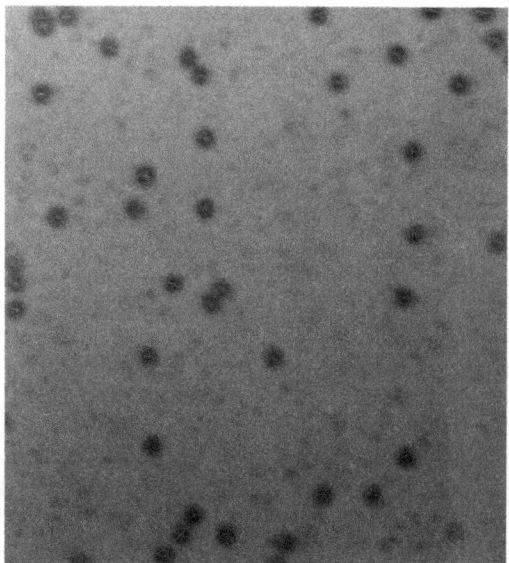

Figure 2 Photograph of Silicone patch, DS_3I_3, showing crystal formation.

erythema and edema for a period of 7 days and scored as reported by Draize et al. (1944) [20]. The Draize method of scoring was shown in Table 2.

Anti-inflammatory study

The study was conducted in accordance with the Ethical Guide- lines for Investigations in Laboratory Animals and was approved by the Ethics Review Committee for Animal Experimentation of Osmania University. The anti-inflammatory activity and sustaining action of the drug-loaded drug in adhesive patches were evaluated using "carrageenan-induced hind paw edema" method developed by Winter et al. (1965) [21]. Wistar rats were used after being allowed to acclimatize for 1 week. Before the day of administration, rats were fasted overnight but were allowed access to water ad libitum. Eight rats weighing 180–220 g (6–8 weeks old) divided into two groups were used for the study. The backsides of rats were shaved 12 h before starting the experiments.

Group – I (Control group): Paw edema was induced by injecting 0.1 mL of a 1% w/v homogeneous suspension of carrageenan in double-distilled water [21] The volume of injected paw was measured immediately (0 h) and at 0.5, 0.75, 1, 2, 3, 4, 5, 6, 8, 10, 12, 16 and 24 h after injection using a IMCORP plethysmometer [22]. The amount of paw swelling with respect to initial volume was determined time to time. It is obtained by subtracting volume of injected paw at time '0' from volume of injected paw at time 't' divided by volume of injected paw at time '0'.

Group – II (Test): Treated similar to control group except that patches were applied half an hour before subplantar injection of carrageenan. Percent (%) inhibition of edema produced by each patch- treated group was calculated against the respective control group using the following formula

$$\% \ Inhibition = \% \ edema(control) - \% \ edema(drug)$$
$$/\% \ edema(control) \times 100$$

(1)

Results and discussion
Evaluation of placebo silicone patches

The placebo patches using six grades of silicone polymer were prepared. The patches were smooth, flexible and uniform. The S_1 patches were ruled out because during preparation of patches after drying the polymer completely lost its adhesive property.

An ideal adhesive polymer for drug-in-adhesive system is one that exhibit greater adhesion value. The initial screening of the silicone adhesives was done by ball tack test and peel strength of patches. The peel test, ball test and adhesive mass test values of all placebo silicone

Table 5 Crystallization summary of drug loaded silicone patches with or without solubilizers

Formulation code	Drug concentration	Solubilizers concentration	Patch Observation after 10 days	Solution observation after 10 days
DS_3	0.5%	-	No sign of crystallization	Same as first day
DS_3	1%	-	No sign of crystallization	Same as first day
DS_3E_3	2%	3% PEG-400	No sign of crystallization	Oil globules were formed and the solution turned oily
DS_6E_4	1%	3% PEG-400	No sign of crystallization	Oil globules were formed and the solution turned oily
DS_3G_2	2%	5% PG	No sign of crystallization.	Oil globules were formed and the solution turned oily
DS_3G_3	1%	2% PG	No sign of crystallization.	Oil globules were formed and the solution turned oily
DS_3O_3	1%	2% OLA	Crystallization was seen.	Same as first day
DS_3I_3	1%	2% ISA	Crystallization was seen.	Same as first day
$DS_3O_4I_4$	3%	5% OLA & 5% ISA	Crystallization was seen.	Same as first day

patches of different thicknesses were as shown in Table 3. The ball test and peel test values for different formulations of thickness 200 μm were in the following order: S3 > S6 > S5 > S2 > S4. Hence, S_6 and S_3 polymers showed better peel adhesion and ball test values hence, selected for further study.

Evaluation of drug loaded silicone patches
Solubility of drug in pure silicone adhesives
The solubility of Diclofenac Diethylamine in S_3 and S_6 was tested. The solutions that remained clear after 24 h were coated over the release liner. Results were shown in (Table 4). The Polymeric adhesive S_3 only showed clear solution with 1% drug concentration. The results indicated low solubility of Diclofenac Diethylamine in Silicone adhesives and stresses on the need for the solubilizers for solubilization of drug.

Solubility enhancement techniques
Solubility of Drug in Silicone adhesives in the presence of solubilizers
Two solubilizers namely PEG - 400 and PG were tested to increase the solubility of Diclofenac Diethylamine in

Table 6 Permeation study of formulation DS₃ and DA

S. No	TIME (h)	DS₃ CDP (μg/cm²)	% CDP	DA CDP (μg/cm²)	% CDP
1.	0	0	0	0	0
2.	2	1.185	1.405138	5.934	0.84051
3.	4	2.6843	3.182964	12.847	1.819688
4.	6	4.2813	5.07664	19.131	2.709773
5.	8	5.9842	7.095889	25.819	3.657082
6.	10	7.7583	9.199565	31.824	4.507649
7.	12	9.3142	11.04451	38.119	5.399292
8.	14	11.042	13.09328	45.248	6.409065
9.	24	19.573	23.20909	75.692	10.72125

CDP: Cumulative drug permeated; % CDP: percent cumulative drug permeated; DA: drug with Acrylic polymer alone.

Silicone adhesives. Though PEG - 400 and PG increased Diclofenac Diethylamine solubility in water [9], their role to solubilize the drug in Silicone adhesive was abortive. Table 4 shows the drug concentration and solubilizer concentration used. Except few, all the solutions showed turbidity. In case of DS_3E_3 a clear solution was formed with 2% drug and 3% PEG - 400 while, in formulations containing S_6 polymer (DS_6E_5) a clear solution was not formed with 2% drug and 3% PEG - 400. Similar to PEG - 400, PG showed slight improvement in solubility of drug in S_3 polymer.

From solubility studies, it can be concluded that compared to S_6, S_3 polymer showed solubilization of DDEA to some extent. So, S_3 polymer was chosen for further study.

Solubility of Drug in Silicone adhesives in the presence of oils
As formulations with PEG - 400 and PG showed little/no improvement in solubility, various oils namely oleic acid (OLA), IsoStearic acid (ISA), Pharmsolve® and Isopropyl Myristate (IPM) were tested for their ability to improve solubility of drug using the method described in experimental section. The formulations which remained clear after 24 h were coated over release liner. Among various oils tested, OLA and ISA were promising. However, only

Table 7 Solubilization summary, peel test, ball test and adhesive mass value for acrylic adhesive patches

Polymer	Drug concentration	Observation
A	10%	Clear solution formed
A	15%	Clear solution formed
A	20%	Clear solution formed
A	25%	Clear solution was not formed
Parameter evaluated		**DA**
Peel test (Kg/cm)		0.9306
Ball test		8

(n is equal to 5 and 3 for Peel test and Ball test respectively).

Table 8 Solubility of drug in combinational patches

Formulation code	Ratio of Silicone: Acrylic	Targeted drug concentration	Solubility observation
C_1	10: 90	10%	YES
C_2	20: 80	10%	YES
C_3	30: 70	10%	YES
C_4	40: 60	10%	YES
C_5	50: 50	10%	YES
C_6	60: 40	10%	NO
C_7	70: 30	10%	NO
C_8	80: 20	10%	NO
C_9	90: 10	10%	NO

C: combination patches with Acrylic and Silicone adhesives.

1% drug was solubilized in both the cases (DS_3O_3 and DS_3I_3) While, IPM and Pharmsolve® did not even solubilize 1% drug. Combination of solubilizers was also tested but, only 3% drug solubilization was achieved in S_3 polymeric adhesive at 10% solubilizer concentration (OLA and ISA, 5% each).

The prepared patches (DS_3 with 1% drug, DS_3E_3, DS_6E_4, DS_3G_2, DS_3G_3, DS_3O_3, DS_3I_3 and $DS_3O_4I_4$) were uniform. However, after 10 days patches with additives OLA and ISA (DS_3O_3, DS_3I_3 and $DS_3O_4I_4$) ended up with formation of crystal growth. Figure 1 and Figure 2 shows crystallization in patches DS_3O_3 and DS_3I_3, respectively.

In case of formulations containing PEG - 400 and PG as additives, though the patches showed no crystallization, the solutions after 10 days took oil like consistency due to formation of oil globules in the solution resulting in loss of adhesion (Table 5).

The patches which did not contain any additives remained clear even after 10 days hence considered stable. Among various formulations prepared, DS_3 containing 1% drug was chosen for further study.

Ex vivo **skin permeation study**

The DS_3 patch containing 1% drug was chosen for conducting permeation study. The cumulative amount of drug permeated (CPD) at the end of 24 h was found to be 19.573 mcg/cm^2 (Table 6). Though the amount of drug permeated was low, the percentage cumulative amount of drug permeated was 23.209%. The low CPD value might be due to less amount of drug (1%) in the patch.

Evaluation of drug loaded acrylic patches

The extensive solubilization study conducted revealed that the silicone polymer is unsuitable for achieving very high concentrations of DDEA. Hence, solubility of drug in acrylic adhesive was tested by method described under experimental section I of IIIA. It was noticed that drug concentrations up to 20% was solubilized without use of any additives. The prepared patches were also stable after 10 days and did not showed crystal formation. While 25% of drug polymeric solution resulted in turbidity (Table 7). This might be because of drug loading greater than the saturation solubility of the drug in the adhesive used. However, the concentration of drug was fixed at 10% for further study since the formulation being studied is intended for topical use. The Ball test and peel strength values for DA were shown in Table 7.

Ex vivo **skin permeation study**

Skin permeation of Diclofenac Diethylamine was studied using DA patch containing 10% drug. Study was conducted for 24 h without using permeation enhancer. The cumulative amount of drug permeated into the receptor compartment was 75.692 mcg/cm^2 after 24 h (Table 6) that represents 10.72% of the total drug placed in the donor compartment.

Though the CDP of DA was significantly greater than CDP of DS_3 the percent drug permeated was high in case of DS_3 (23.209%). The CDP of DA was found to be

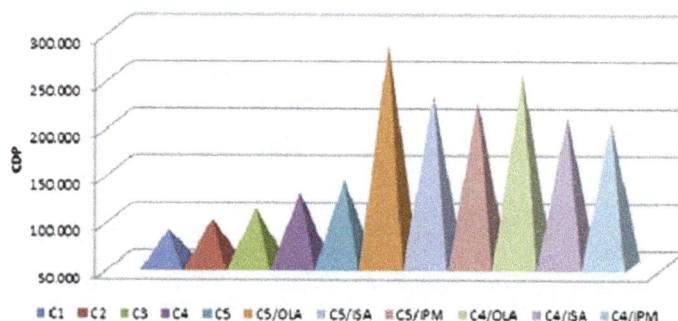

Figure 3 Graph showing cumulative amount of drug permeated (CDP) at the end of 24 h with and without permeation enhancers for combinational patches (C_4/OLA, C_4/ISA and C_4/IPM reprsents C_4 patch with oleic acid (OLA), Isostearic acid and Isopalmitic Myristate as permeation enhancers, respectively. Similar in case of C_5 combinational patches).

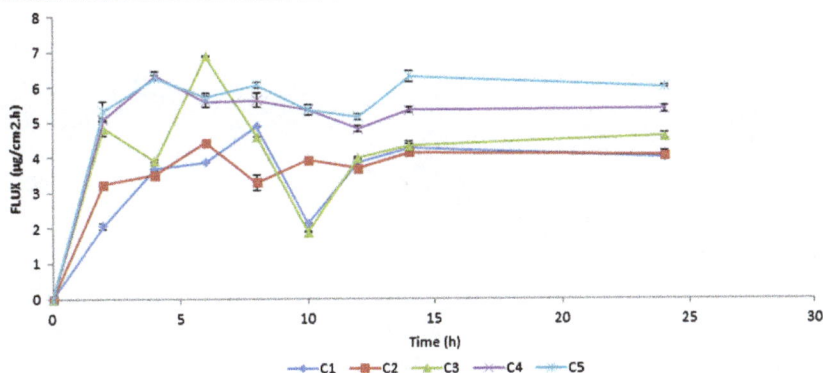

Figure 4 Graph showing the plot between Flux ($\mu g/cm^2.h$) and time (h) for C_1, C_2, C_3, C_4 and C_5 patches (data represented as mean ± S.D).

significantly high because the drug concentration in DA was 10 times greater than that of DS_3.

Evaluation of drug loaded combinational patches

Studies on Silicone adhesives revealed poor solubilization capacity and high percent cumulative drug permeation (%CDP) value whereas; acrylic polymers solubilized higher concentrations of drug but exhibited less%CDP. Hence an attempt was made to combine high%CDP property of Silicone and greater drug solubilization property of acrylic polymer by fabricating a drug formulation with combination of adhesives.

The placebo solutions containing different proportions of Silicone and Acrylic adhesives were prepared and used as reference for checking the solubility of drug in combination of adhesives. The combinations from C_1 to C_5 showed similar consistency as compared to respective

placebo patches after addition of drug. Table 8 shows the Solubility data of different combinations of Silicone and acrylic with 10% drug. The results indicated that minimum 50% acrylic polymer is required in the formulation to achieve 10% drug solubility (As acrylic polymer alone can solubilize 20% drug without any solubilizer as mentioned earlier, it is evident that 50% acrylic polymer is sufficient to solubilize 10% drug). Hence, formulations C_1, C_2, C_3, C_4 and C_5 were used for further study.

Ex vivo skin permeation experiment

In all the combinational patches, the CDP of combinational patches was higher than that DA patches which contains Acrylic polymer alone. Figure 3 shows the amount of drug permeated at the end of 24 h with and without combinational patches. The CDP of different combinational patches were in the following order:

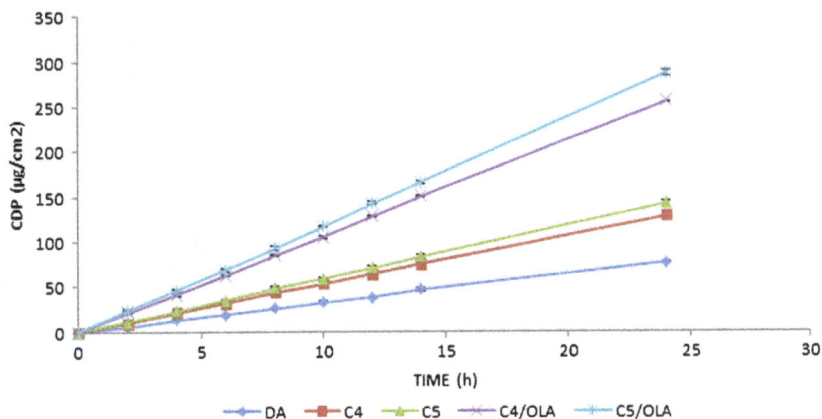

Figure 5 Graph showing the plot between cumulative amount of drug permeated (CDP, $\mu g/cm^2$) and time (h) for DA, C_4, C_5, C_5/OLA and C_4/OLA (data represented as mean ± S.D).

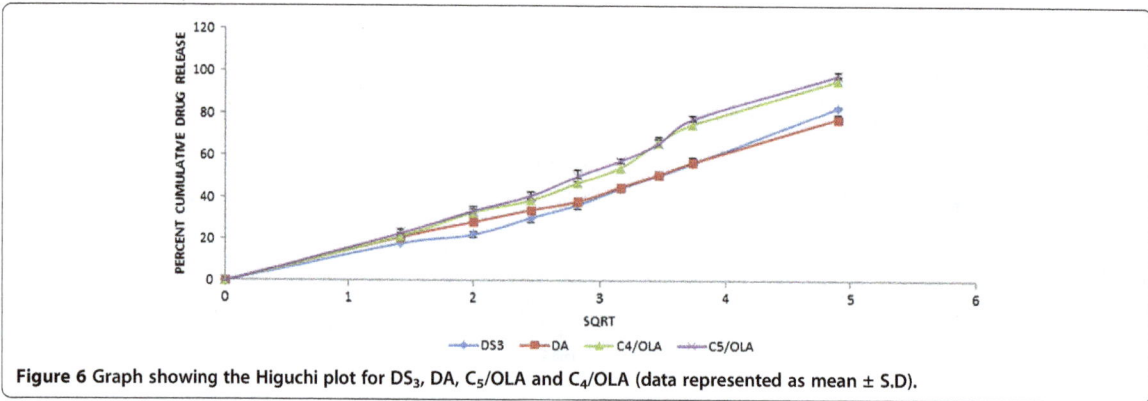

Figure 6 Graph showing the Higuchi plot for DS_3, DA, C_5/OLA and C_4/OLA (data represented as mean ± S.D).

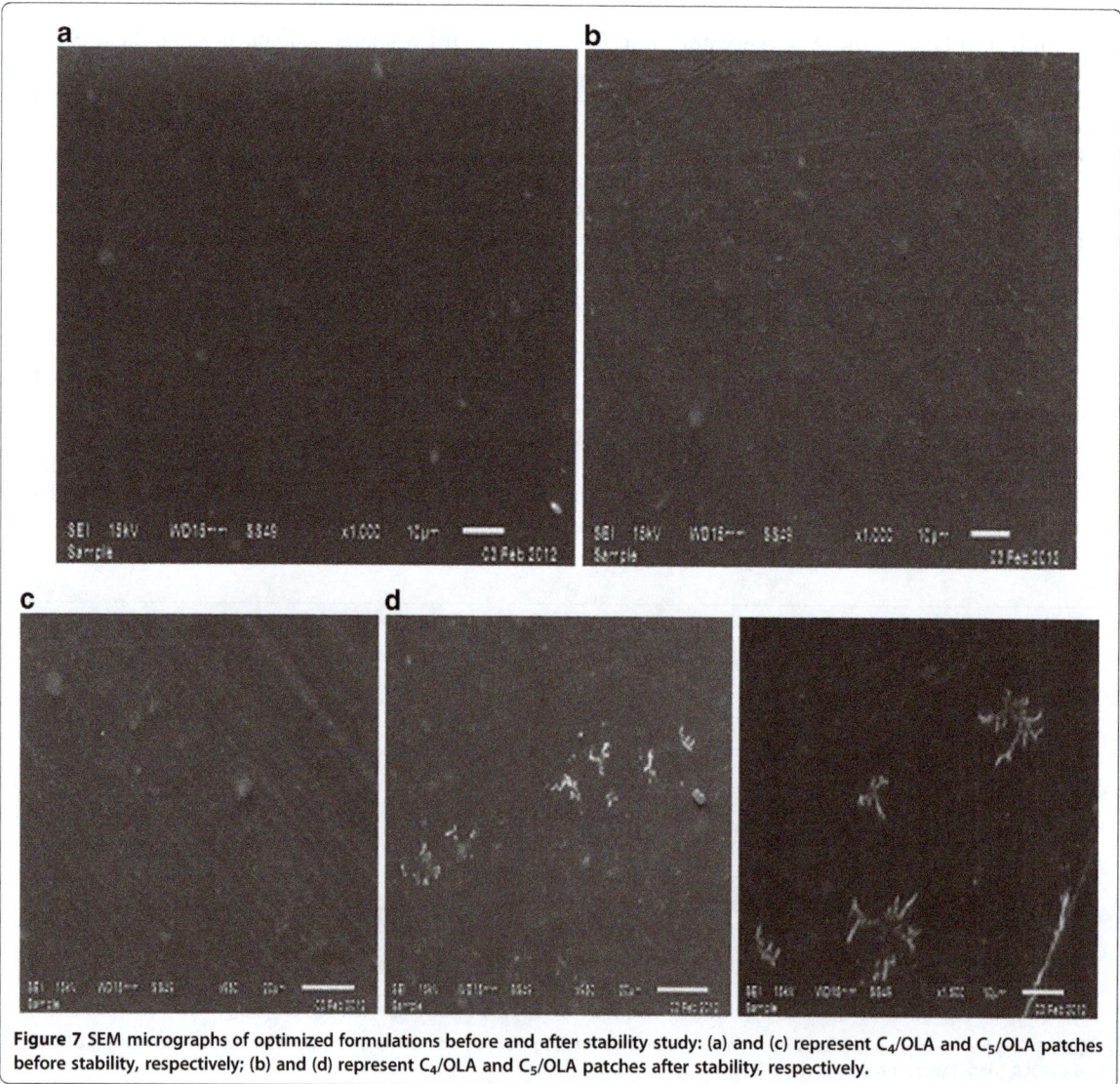

Figure 7 SEM micrographs of optimized formulations before and after stability study: (a) and (c) represent C_4/OLA and C_5/OLA patches before stability, respectively; (b) and (d) represent C_4/OLA and C_5/OLA patches after stability, respectively.

Table 9 Stability data for formulation C_4/OLA and C_5/OLA

Tested parameters	0 days	45 days	90 days
C_4/OLA			
Peel Strength (Kg/cm)	0.663	0.646	0.659
Drug content (%)	104.6	103.6	104.1
C_5/OLA			
Peel Strength (Kg/cm)	0.654	0.649	0.652
Drug content (%)	101.64	98.86	94.38

(C_4/OLA: C_4 combination patch with oleic acid, OLA, as permeation enhancer; C_5/OLA: C_5 combination patch with oleic acid, OLA, as permeation enhancer; n=3 for Drug content and n=5 for Peel strength).

Figure 9 Photograph of the patches C_5/OLA after stability.

$$C_5 > C_4 > C_3 > C_2 > C_1.$$

The above order once again reflected the previous results i.e. with increase in amount of Silicone polymer the amount of CDP increased. Among all five formulations C_5 displayed high CDP value due to its high Silicone content (50% of the total polymer).

Figure 4 shows plot between flux and time for all the five combinations. The graph showed little/less variation in the flux between different time intervals for C_4 and C_5. Moreover, the CDP was found to be relatively high for these two formulations. Hence, the formulations C_4 and C_5 were chosen for further study.

Effect of permeation enhancers on the permeation of DDEA

Three permeation enhancers namely, OLA, ISA and IPM were used at 5% concentration. The cumulative amount of drug permeated at the end of 24 h was represented in Figure 3. The permeation data revealed greater penetration enhancing capability of OLA than ISA and IPM. This is in line with the result reported where OLA increased the permeation of DDEA by 7–9 folds (Hussain Shah et al. 2012) [10]. Thus, it can be concluded that vehicles used here were predominantly influencing the partition of the drug into the skin. Hence, C_4/OLA and C_5/OLA which exhibited greater CDP among all were chosen as optimized formulations.

Figure 5 shows the plot between CDP and time for different formulations. From the graph, it can be predicted

that C_4 and C_5 showed high CDP compared to DA indicating more drug permeation capacity compared to individual Acrylic formulations. OLA application as a permeation enhancer was well justified as significant increase in CDP value was observed compared to patches without enhancers.

Dissolution study of patches

In vitro release profile is an important tool that predicts in advance how the drug will behave in vivo. Thus, we can eliminate the risk of hazards during experimentation in living system. Five patches, DS_3, DA, C_4/OLA and C_5/OLA were studied for drug release. The study was conducted for a period of 24 h. The percent drug release (Figure 6) was found to be in the following order:

$$C_5/OLA > C_4/OLA > DS_3 > DA$$

The dissolution values revealed that formulations containing OLA exhibited greater percent cumulative drug release (%CDR) than DS_3 and DA. This might be due to increased solubility of poorly soluble drug, DDEA, in water due to OLA. Among C_5/OLA and C_4/OLA the formulation containing greater portion of silicone polymer, C_5/OLA, showed greater %CDR.

Release kinetics

The dissolution data of C_4/OLA and C_5/OLA was put forth for release kinetic studies. Based on high R^2 value it was shown that drug release from the formulations followed Higuchi pattern of drug release, with R^2 value 0.978 for C_4/OLA and 0.981 for C_5/OLA, (Figure 6) where drug diffusion through the polymeric system was the main mechanism. The 'n' value from the korsemeyer-peppas plot revealed non-fickian/anomalous diffusion pattern (n>0.5).

Stability study

The formulations C_5/OLA and C_4/OLA were kept for 3 month stability study. During stability study in case of

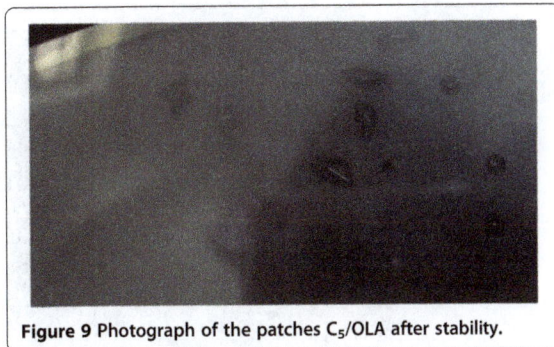

Figure 8 Photograph of the patches C_4/OLA after stability.

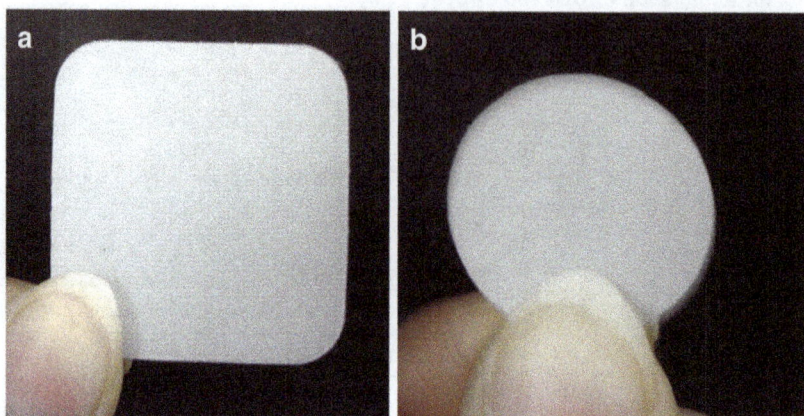

Figure 10 Photograph of optimized C$_4$/OLA patches both 10 cm^2 (a) and 3 cm^2 (b) patches.

C$_5$/OLA, crystallization (Figure 7) was observed which might be due to saturation of drug solubility which resulted in slow precipitation of drug. This is also reflected in its drug content shown in Table 9 where the percent drug content of the formulation kept on decreasing. Such a saturated matrix is unstable and the drug will recrystallize in such systems over time [23-25]. Recrystallization may however not be apparent immediately after manufacture because of the relatively low diffusion coefficients of drug in such highly viscous systems and the requirement of nucleation for the initiation of crystallization. Figure 8 shows the photograph of the C$_4$/OLA after stability with no crystals and Figure 9 shows photograph of the C$_5$/OLA after stability with crystal formation.

The peel test of both the formulations showed no significant change during stability study indicating the sustainability of adhesive property of the polymeric combination.

However, in case of C$_4$/OLA crystallization was not found and moreover the drug content remained stable representing robustness of the formulation during 3 month stability. Hence, the formulation C$_4$/OLA was found to be the optimized formulation.

Physical evaluation of optimized patches
Figure 10(a) and 10(b) shows the original patch C$_4$/OLA of sizes 10 cm^2 and 3 cm^2, respectively. The optimized formulation C$_4$/OLA was tested for various physical parameters. The thickness (n = 5) of C$_4$/OLA patches was found to be 181.63 ± 0.03 µm. Good weight uniformity among the batches was observed for all formulations and ranged from 214.33 – 216.35 mg. The results indicate that the process which was employed to prepare patches in this study was capable to produce patches with uniform drug content and minimal patch variability.

Acute skin irritancy study
The 7 day skin irritancy study revealed that the test formulation showed a skin irritation score (erythema and edema) of less than 1 (Table 10 & Figure 11). From the Draize method of scoring, the control animals showed severe erythema and moderate to slight edema whereas the test animals showed only very slight erythema and no edema on the site of application. According to Draize et al. (1944) [20] compounds producing scores of 2 or less are considered non-irritant [14]. Hence from the study, we can conclude that formulations are non-irritable to skin and safer for therapeutic use.

In vivo anti-inflammatory studies
The result of carrageenan induced paw edema test was shown in the Table 11. The table shows the data for the percent increase in edema with respect to initial volume and percentage inhibition of edema with respect to control during 24 h study for the test formulation. As shown in the table in case of control group animals, the mean percent increase in edema with respect to initial volume (Group –I) was 114.3 ± 15.0 at the end of 24 h which is because of swelling nature of carrageenan. While in case of test group animals the value is 0.37 ± 0.54 at the end of 24 h indicating that test patches, C$_4$/OLA, are

Table 10 Acute skin irritancy data for C$_5$/OLA (n = 4)

Day	Parameter	Standard				Test			
		1	2	3	4	1	2	3	4
Day 0	Erythema	0	0	0	0	0	0	0	0
	Edema	0	0	0	0	0	0	0	0
Day 7	Erythema	4	4	3	4	0	1	1	1
	Edema	3	2	2	3	0	0	0	0

(C$_4$/OLA: C$_4$combination patch with oleic acid, OLA, as permeation enhancer).

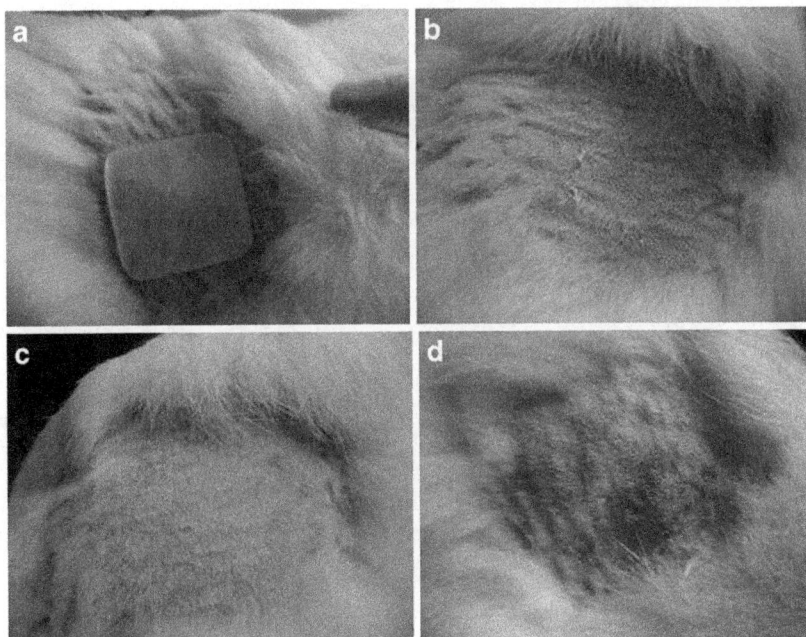

Figure 11 Images of skin irritancy study: (a) patch application to shaved area; (b) skin of rabbit at 0 day; (c) skin of test group rabbit after 7 days of patch application; (d) skin of standard group rabbit after 7 days.

effective in inhibiting carrageenan induced inflammation. Moreover, the test group animals showed 99.68% inhibition of edema with respect to control after 24 h indicating the efficacy of the formulation during the period. The initial percent increase in edema with respect to initial volume in case of test group half an hour after the carrageenan induction was 0.4 ± 0.54 as opposed to Control group (3.57 ±1.08) indicating that the test patch, C_4/OLA showed action from the first hour without any appreciable lag time. Throughout the study the percent increase in edema value with respect to initial volume for test group remained well below than the control group indicating the sustaining effect of the drug against carrageenan challenge.

Conclusion

The extensive solubilization study conducted on Silicone adhesive polymers revealed their unsuitability in fabrication of DDEA transdermal patches alone as not more than 1% drug was solubilized even with high concentration of solubilizer. On the other hand, Acrylic polymer showed high drug loading and greater control releasing capacity hence, alone can be used for fabricating transdermal patches of DDEA. However, use of Acrylic alone requires greater amount of drug incorporation due to its low value of percent cumulative drug permitted (10.72%). Hence, the combinations of adhesives were tested with the objective combining the greater permeation capacity of Silicone polymer and greater drug loading capacity of

Table 11 Paw edema data obtained on carrageenan induced rats half an hour after the patch application (data represented as mean ± S.D, n = 4)

	0.5	0.75	1	2	3	4	5	6	7	8	10	12	16	24
							Time (h)							
					% Edema with respect to initial volume									
Control	3.57 ±1.08	14.28 ± 2.05	35.71 ± 7.06	42.8 ±9.64	50.0 ± 12.95	60.7 ± 20.82	71.5 ± 19.72	83.0 ± 21.85	92.8 ± 11.05	100.0 ± 15.1	111.1 ± 18.6	121.4 ± 11.76	121.4 ±15.9	114.3 ± 15.0
Test (C_4/OLA)	0.4 ± 0.54	5.6 ± 2.91	11.3 ± 5.83	18.5 ± 0.97	39.4 ± 4.16	54.1 ± 0.31	62.6 ± 1.44	52.7 ± 9.29	42.6 ± 0.39	36.2 ± 4.39	21.2 ± 2.68	15.6 ± 0.82	2.5 ± 2.49	0.37 ± 0.54
					% inhibition of Edema with respect to control									
Test (C_4/OLA)	88.80	60.78	68.36	56.78	21.20	10.87	12.45	36.51	54.09	63.80	80.92	87.15	97.94	99.68

(C_4/OLA: C_4combination patch with oleic acid, OLA, as permeation enhancer).

Acrylic polymer. The combinational patches incorporating the both the desired properties were successfully prepared. Among various permeation enhancers tested OLA proved to be a good permeation enhancer as compared to ISA and IPM for DDEA. C_4/OLA was found to be optimized formulation displaying robustness in stability. The skin irritancy study revealed the non-irritant nature of the C_4/OLA patches and sustaining action of the patches were confirmed by anti-inflammatory test by carrageenan induced paw edema model. Thus, it can be concluded that an ideal of combination of adhesives would serve as the best choice, for fabrication of DDEA patches, for sustained effect of DDEA with better enhancement in permeation characteristics and robustness.

Competing interests
The manuscript has no conflict of interest and there are no financial sources for many organizations and the work is purely part of student thesis work.

Authors' contributions
The author DPM helped in conceptual design of entire work, the author SP was responsible for the entire practical work, TP contributed to the interpretation of data obtained at various steps, the author BD helped in carrying out the studies involving animals and AKA helped in the calculation part and in preparation and follow up of the manuscript. All authors read and approved the final manuscript.

Acknowledgement
The authors are grateful to Sparsha Pharma International Pvt. Ltd., Hyderabad, India for extending their timely help and full co-operation for carrying out the entire research work under their guidance.

Author details
[1]Department of Pharmaceutics, KLEU's college of Pharmacy, Nehru Nagar, Belgaum, Karnataka 590010, India. [2]Research Scientist, R&D divison, Sparsha Pharma International Pvt. Ltd., Hyderabad, India.

References
1. Debjit B, Chiranjib, Chandira M, Jayakar B, Sampath KP: Recent advances in transdermal drug delivery system. *Int. J Pharm Tech Res* 2010, **2**(1):68–77.
2. Jain P, Banga AK: Inhibition of crystallization in drug-in-adheisve-type transdermal therapeutic patches. *Int J Pharm* 2010, **394**:68–74.
3. John VA: The pharmacokinetics and metabolism of diclofenac sodium (Voltarol™) in animals and man. *Rheumatol Rehabil* 1979, Suppl 2:22–37.
4. Fritz UN, Morris SG, Gail SS, Jiun-min L, Markus U, Helmut HA, Francois E: Efficacy of topical diclofenac diethylamine gel in osteoarthritis of the knee. *J Rheumatol* 2005, **32**:2384–2392.
5. Keith AD: Polymer matrix consideration for transdermal devices. *Drug Dev Ind Pharm* 1983, **9**:605–621.
6. Nauman Rahim K, Gul Majid K, Abdur Rahim K, Abdul W, Muhammad Junaid A, Muhammad A, Abid H: Formulation, physical, *in vitro* and *ex vivo* evaluation ofdiclofenac diethylamine matrix patches containing turpentine oil as penetration enhancer. *Afr J Pharm Pharmaco* 2012, **6**(6):434–439.
7. Haroutinaian S, Drennan DA, Lipman AG: Topical NSAID therapy for musculoskeletal pain. *Pain Med* 2010, **11**(4):535–549.
8. Changshun R, Liang F, Lei L, Qiang W, Sihai L, LiGang Z, Zhonggui H: Design and evaluation of Indipamide transdermal patch. *Int J Pharm* 2009, **370**(1–2):129–135.
9. Khalil E, Najjar S, Sallam A: Aqueous solubility of diclofenac diethylamine in the presence of pharmaceutical additives: a comparative study with diclofenac sodium. *Drug Dev Ind Pharm* 2000, **26**(4):375–381.
10. Hussain Shah SN, Salman M, Ahmad M, Rabbani M, Badshah A: Effect of oleic acid on the permeation kinetics of Diclofenac Diethylamine. *J Chem Soc Pak* 2012, **34**(1):1–8.
11. Atrux-Tallau N, Pirot F, Falson F, Roberts MS, Maibach HI: Qualitative and quantitative comparison of heat separated epidermis and dermatomed skin in percutaneous absorption studies. *Arch Dermatol Res* 2007, **299**(10):507–511.
12. Kaidi Z, Singh J: *In vitro* percutaneous absorption enhancement of propranolol hydrochloride through porcine epidermis by terpenes/ethanol. *J Control Rel* 1999, **62**(3):359–366.
13. Bonferoni M, Rossi S, Ferrari F, caramella C: A modified Franz diffusion cell for simulataneous assessment of drug release and washability of mucoadhesive gels. *Pharm Dev Technol* 1999, **4**(1):45–53.
14. Mamatha T, venkateswara rao J, Mukkanti K, Ramesh G: Development of matrix type transdermal patches of lercanidipine hydrochloride: physicochemical and in-vitro characterization. *DARU* 2010, **18**(1):9–16.
15. Verma PR, Iyer SS: Transdermal delivery of propranolol using mixed grades of Eudragit: design and in-vitro and in-vivo evaluation. *Drug Dev Ind Pharm* 2000, **26**(4):471–476.
16. Vijaya Bhanu P, Shanmugam V, Lakshmi PK: Development and evaluation of Diclofenac Emulgel for topical drug delivery. *Pharmacie Globale IJCP* 2011, **9**(10):1–4.
17. Sood A, Panchagnula R: Role of dissolution studies in controlled release drug delivery system. *STP Pharma Sci* 1999, **9**:157–168.
18. Mohamed A, Yamin S, Asgar A: Matrix type transdermal drug delivery systems of metoprolol tartrate: in vitro characterization. *Acta Pharm* 2003, **53**(2):119–125.
19. Shinde AJ, Shinde AL, More HN: Design and evaluation transdermal drug delivery system of gliclazide. *Asian J Pharm* 2010, **4**(2):121–129.
20. Draize JH, Woodword G, Calvery HO: Methods for the study of irritation and toxicity of substances applied topically to the skin and mucous membranes. *J Pharmacol Exp Ther* 1944, **0**:377–379.
21. Winter CA: Antiinflammatory testing methods: Comparative evaluation of indomethacin and other agents. In *Nonsteroidal antiinflammatory drugs*. Edited by Garattini S, Dukes MNG. Amsterdam: Excerpta Medica Foundation; 1965:190–202. series no. 82.
22. Priyanka A, Biswajit M: Design, development, physicochemical, and in vitro and *In Vivo* evaluation of transdermal patches containing diclofenac diethylammonium salt. *J Pharm Sci* 2002, **91**(9):2076–2089.
23. Hadgraft J: Passive enhancement strategies in topical and transdermal drug delivery. *Int J Pharm* 1999, **184**(1):1–6.
24. Latsch S, Selzer T, Fink L, Kreuter J: Determination of the physical state of norethindrone acetate containing transdermal drug delivery systems by isothermal microcalorimetry, X-ray diffraction, and optical microscopy. *Eur J Pharm Biopharm* 2004, **57**(2):383–395.
25. Cilurzo F, Minghetti P, Casiraghi A, Tosi L, Pagani S, Montanari L: Polymethacrylates as crystallization inhibitors in monolayer transdermal patches containing ibuprofen. *Eur J Pharm Biopharm* 2005, **60**(1):61–66.

2

Effect of myrtle fruit syrup on abnormal uterine bleeding

Marzieh Qaraaty[1], Seyed Hamid Kamali[2*], Fataneh Hashem Dabaghian[3], Nafiseh Zafarghandi[4*],
Roshanak Mokaberinejad[5], Masumeh Mobli[6], Gholamreza Amin[6], Mohsen Naseri[1], Mohammad Kamalinejad[7],
Mohsen Amin[8], Azizeh Ghaseminejad[9], Seyedeh jihan HosseiniKhabiri[10] and Daryush Talei[11]

Abstract

Background: Myrtle (*Myrtus communis* L.) has been used in the Iranian Traditional Medicine as a treatment for abnormal uterine bleeding-menometrorrhagia. The main aim of this study is to evaluate the effect of myrtle fruit syrup on abnormal uterine bleeding-menometrorrhagia.

Methods: A randomized, double-blind, placebo-controlled pilot study was conducted on 30 women suffering from abnormal uterine bleeding-menometrorrhagia. Treatment comprised of giving 15 ml oral myrtle syrup daily (5 ml three times a day) for 7 days starting from the onset of bleeding. The myrtle syrup along with placebo was repeated for 3 consecutive menstrual periods. Menstrual duration and number of used pads were recorded by the Pictorial Blood loss Assessment Chart at the end of each menstrual period. The quality of life was also evaluated using the menorrhagia questionnaire.

Results: The mean number of bleeding days significantly declined from 10.6 ± 2.7 days to 8.2 ± 1.9 days after 3 months treatment with the syrup ($p = 0.01$) and consequently the participants in the intervention group used fewer pads after 3 months (16.4 ± 10.7) compared with the number of pads used at the beginning of the treatment (22.7 ± 12.0, $p = 0.01$). Bleeding days and number of pads used by the participants in the placebo group did not change significantly. Also significant changes of quality of life scores were observed in the intervention group after 3 months compared to the baseline.

Conclusion: Myrtle syrup is introduced as a potential remedy for abnormal uterine bleeding-menometrorrhagia.

Keywords: Abnormal uterine bleeding-menometrorrhagia, Effrat-e-tams, Iranian traditional medicine, *Myrtus communis* L, Myrtle, Myrtaceae

Introduction

Abnormal uterine bleeding (AUB) is one of the main reasons of visiting gynecologists [1]. AUB affects up to one-third of sexually active women [2] and the overall prevalence of this abnormality is 11%-13%, reaching 24% at the age of 36–40 [3]. AUB has a considerable high morbidity rate among women of childbearing age and imposes major medical, social and financial burdens on women, their families and health services [4]. Different types of AUB include a range of dysfunctional conditions affecting regularity, frequency, duration or volume of menstrual flow [5,6]. Menorrhagia or hypermenorrhea is defined as menstrual blood loss of more than 80 ml per cycle or longer than 7 days or both of them [7], while polymenorrhea is defined as having menstruations about every 21 days and occasionally at even shorter intervals causing irregular ovulation. Metrorrhagia is uterine bleeding at irregular intervals, particularly between the expected menstrual periods [8]. Abnormal uterine bleeding-Menometrorrhagia (AUB-MM) is defined as prolonged and excessive uterine bleeding in irregular intervals [9]. The most common

* Correspondence: kamaliseyyedhamid@yahoo.com; nafis_zafar@ymail.com
[2]Department of Traditional Medicine, Faculty of Traditional Medicine, Shahid Beheshti University of Medical Sciences, Tehran, Iran
[4]Department of Gynecology and Obstetrics, Faculty of Medical Sciences, Shahed University, Tehran, Iran
Full list of author information is available at the end of the article

causes of AUB may be pregnancy, genital tract diseases, certain medical conditions such as thyroid dysfunctions and hypothalamic suppressions including stress, weight loss, excessive exercise, and even coagulopathies [1,10]. AUB treatment includes administration of non-steroidal anti-inflammatory drugs (NSAIDs), antifibrinolytics such as tranexamic acid, cyclic oral progestins, oral contraceptives and levonorgestrel-releasing intra-uterine system [1,5,11]. Hormone therapies have many side effects [12] and the common complication of tranexamic acid is gastrointestinal disturbances [13]. AUB involves two-thirds of all hysterectomies leading to several complications [14,15].

Iranian Traditional Medicine (ITM) practitioners such as Ibn Sina (Avicenna, 980–1037 A.D) believed that the normal menstruation is a good sign of healthy status of a woman which results in chastity and modesty [16-18]. In ITM literature, AUB is described under the title of "Effrat-e-Tams" or "Kasrat-e-Tams" [7,18]. Menometrorrhagia is more compatible with Effrat-e-Tams in ITM [17-20].

Based on ITM literature, particularly Avicenna's book (Al-Qanun fit-teb or Canon of medicine, 1025 A.D), myrtle is known as "*mourd*" or "aa*ss*" (مورد یا آس) and its fruit that called *Habbol- aass*, is one of the effective medicinal herbs for decreasing the menstrual bleeding [18]. Myrtle is a fragrant evergreen shrub belonging to *myrtaceae* family, growing wild in Iran [21,22] and the Mediterranean area. The fruits have sweet-spicy tastes that are very astringent [23]. Myrtle has been used as antiviral, antifungal, antiseptic and antioxidant agent [24,25]. Myrtle berries extract has ulcer-protective properties [26] and anti-inflammatory effects [27]. The essential oils obtained from leaves, flowers and fruits have been used in flavor and fragrance industries [28]. Its biological effect in menstrual disturbances has been described in ITM which may be novel in modern medicine [18].

There is a lack of detailed trials on the effects of myrtle syrup on menstruation. The main objective of the present study was to investigate the effects of myrtle syrup on reducing AUB-MM in a pilot placebo-controlled clinical trial.

Materials and methods
Study design and target group
In this randomized, double-blinded, placebo-controlled pilot study, 30 patients were randomly assigned into two groups of placebo (n = 15) and myrtle treatment (n = 15). Participants were treated with either 15 ml of myrtle fruit syrup or placebo, 3 times a day for seven days starting from the onset of bleeding. The treatment was performed for 3 consecutive menstrual periods. Randomization of equal number of subjects to placebo or treated group was achieved using a simple random allocation strategy, using block randomization method. The participants

were selected according to the defined inclusion criteria: 20 to 55 years old, married women, not disposed toward hormone therapy, not pregnant, not lactating, normal gynecological observations, normal pap smear, endometrial thickness less than 12 mm, menstrual period more than 7 days in duration and/or less than 21 days from the start of one period until the start of the next menstrual period and/or clot excretion, use of more than 10 sanitary product items in a cycle. Sexually active women were required to use a suitable non-hormonal birth control. Initially, 92 patients were interviewed from which, 35 patients were recruited and randomized in two groups of placebo and extract treatment. 30 participants completed the study, 15 in each group (Figure 1). Two participants in the placebo group discontinued their therapy because of increasing bleeding during first cycle. One subject in the intervention group did not use the syrup completely and two persons discontinued the study because of personal reasons.

Women were excluded from the study if they had a history of significant medical problems (coagulopathies, diabetes mellitus, chronic inflammatory disease, thyroid dysfunctions); had a history of endometrial abnormalities (such as hyperplasia), cervical carcinoma, uterine or ovary malignancy; sub-mucosal or intramural fibroids more than 5 cm; needed surgery and emergency procedure because of increasing bleeding during the study. All of the subjects were free to withdraw at any time during the course of study.

Participants were not permitted to use mefenamic acid, tranexamic acid, any hormonal therapy, herbal medicine and medicinal herb during the study. Use of acetaminophen, oral iron therapy and analgesic opioids was permitted throughout the study.

All participants signed a written informed consent before recruiting in the study. The Ethics Committee of Shahed University approved the protocol (approval number: 41/138342). In addition, the trial was registered in the Iranian Registry of Clinical Trials under the number IRCT 201109077511 N1.

Plant material
Myrtle dried berries were collected from Manjil on road to Gilan (North of Iran) in 2011 and its identity was authenticated by Professor Gholamreza Amin. A voucher specimen of the plant has been deposited in Herbarium Tehran University of Medical Sciences, Faculty of Pharmacy under the voucher No 6632-TEH.

Preparation of syrup and placebo
Traditional decoction was prepared as described in "Qarabadin" (Ghayeni, Qarabadin-e-Salehi, 1765 AD; Aghili, Qarabadin-e-Kabir, 1781 AD) [29,30] texts belonging to ITM pharmaceutical discipline. 63 g of the

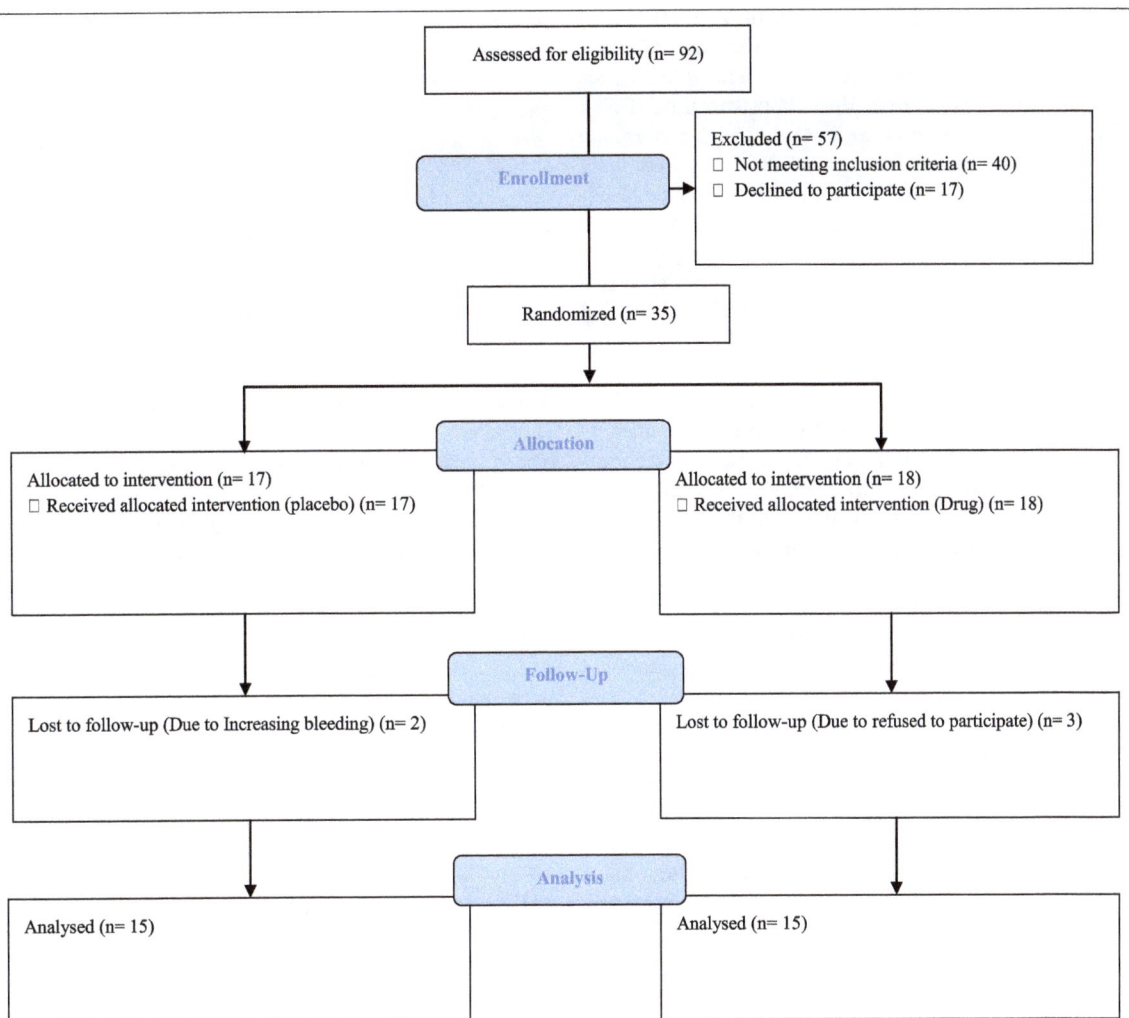

Figure 1 Study flow chart.

pulverized samples of myrtle fruits were macerated for 24 hours with 200 ml of distilled water, filtered and boiled for 15 min. 108 g sucrose was added to the extract in order to prepare the syrup. The medication was supplied in bottles of 120 ml, containing either drug or placebo.

Placebo was prepared based on pharmacopoeia simple syrup formula including approved color additives and looked the same as the myrtle syrup.

Myrtle syrup is standardized based on total phenols (Folin-Ciocalteau method) and gallic acid (Rhodanine assay) content. Each 5 ml of syrup contains 0.05 ± 0.03 g dry residue and 41 mg total phenols as gallic acid equivalents.

The participants were given either 5 ml of prepared syrup or placebo three times a day, 30 minute after each meal for seven days starting from the onset of bleeding.

This treatment was repeated for three consecutive menstruation cycle.

The myrtle syrup and placebo were identical in the same physical form, packaging and labeling and divided to groups 1 and 2. Physician prescribed syrups to the patients according to the label numbers. Physician and presenter of the myrtle syrup or placebo were blind for the contents. The pharmacist was the only person who was aware of the numbers assigned to the myrtle syrup or placebo.

Bleeding measurements

All the participants were evaluated based on a complete medical history and gynecological examination. Menstrual blood loss was assessed with Pictorial Blood loss Assessment Chart (PBAC). The quality of life was evaluated with menorrhagia questionnaire (MQ-Iranian Version) [31,32] before treatment and at the end of the study. Certain blood test including complete blood count (CBC), prothrombin time (PT), partial thromboplastin time (PTT), follicle-stimulating hormone (FSH), luteinizing hormone (LH) and thyroid stimulating hormone (TSH) were done before the study. PT and PTT were done to exclude bleeding disorders. TSH, FSH and LH were done to exclude thyroid dysfunction and hypothalamic pituitary dysfunction, respectively. CBC was performed to determine hemoglobin (Hb) and hematocrit (Hct). Trans-vaginal ultra sonography was also performed to find out if the subject had any pelvic pathological disorders and to determine the endometrial thickness. Cervical cytology (Pap smear) was done to rule out other abnormalities.

Menstrual blood loss and menstrual duration were measured using PBAC chart during three consecutive treatment cycles and was compared with the ones at the beginning of the treatment (baseline). The participants were requested to report the details of their menstrual cycle i.e., the start date, duration of menstruation, the number of sanitary pads used (considered as the intensity of bleeding) and any adverse effects. The information was recorded at the beginning of the treatment and at the end of each menstrual cycle. The PBAC chart had a sensitivity of 80% and specificity of 88% in diagnosing menorrhagia (as defined in the alkaline hematin method) [33].

Statistical analysis

The primary outcome measures included the duration of menstrual period, number of pads used during menstruation. The MQ score and the side effects were the secondary outcome measures.

Normal probability plot was used to test for normality of data in GraphPad Prism version 5. The data points appeared linear on the plot and the data were considered as normal distribution. Repeated-measures ANOVA function in the program GraphPad Prism version 5 was used to test for differences of primary outcomes within the groups. Repeated-measures ANOVA compares the means of more than two matched groups in a longitudinal study in which change over time is assessed. Student's t-test was used to compare the MQ scores before and after the treatment.

Results

Baseline characteristics

The baseline characteristics of the subjects are described on Table 1. There were no statistically significant differences in baseline characteristics between the groups. Hence, the groups were homogenous with respect to age, level of education and investigations. Age of the patients ranged from 20 to 55 years with the mean age 41.2 ± 6.9 years.

Table 1 Baseline characteristics of study subjects

Parameter	Intervention group	Placebo group	P value
Age	41.33 ± 7.228	41.13 ± 6.978	0.5
BMI	28.86 ± 4.68	31.99 ± 6.29	0.2
MQ score	47.8 ± 15.7	41.2 ± 15.3	0.2
Duration of abnormality (month)	53.93 ± 61.46	72.33 ± 69.92	0.3

Effects of myrtle fruit syrup on duration and intensity of bleeding

The average number of bleeding days and number of pads used during the study are summarized on Table 2. There was not statistically significant difference between the groups in terms of bleeding days and number of pads at the beginning of the study.

The number of bleeding days and consequently number of pads used by the participants significantly decreased in the intervention group after 3 months (P = 0.01), while changes of these variables were not significant in the placebo group.

Significant changes of MQ score was observed in the intervention group after 3 months compared to the baseline (P = 0.02).

Discussion

To the best of our knowledge, the present study is the first randomized placebo-controlled trial on the effects of myrtle fruit in women with AUB-MM. The results of this study showed that myrtle syrup had notable advantages over placebo in women with AUB-MM. Also, the quality of life was significantly improved in the intervention group with minor side effects.

During luteal phase in menstrual cycle, some inflammatory processes lead to tissue edema in endometrium and continue with excessive menstrual bleeding (EMB). Unusual secretion of local pro-inflammatory cytokines responsible in the vascular tone has been observed [2,4]. In these women, endometrium synthesizes much more prostaglandin E_2 (PGE$_2$) than it does with vasoconstrictor PGF$_{2\alpha}$. A noticeable increased PGE$_2$/PGF$_{2\alpha}$ ratio happens during luteal phase in women with menstrual blood loss (>90 ml). Endometrial synthesis of PGs and signaling in women with profuse menstruation is greater than women with normal menstrual bleeding [4]. These inflammatory molecules can be targeted to treat the disturbances in women suffering from AUB.

Myrtle berries aqueous extract contains phenolic-like tannins (galllic acid derivatives), anthocyanins and flavonoids [34]. Tannin-containing medications have been used traditionally as styptics [35]. Anti-inflammatory activities of anthocyanins have been proven in some studies [36]. Some studies have demonstrated that flavonoids can

Table 2 The effect of myrtle fruit syrup in bleeding at baseline and post treatment

Variable	Group	Title	Mean(±SD)	Mean difference (±SE) compared with baseline	95% CI*	P values**
Menstrual duration (day)	Intervention (n = 15)	Baseline	10.6(2.7)			
		After 1st cycle	8.8(2.3)	1.7(0.6)	−0.3– 3.8	0.08
		After 2nd cycle	8.9(3.8)	1.6(0.9)	−1.3– 4.7	0.08
		After 3rd cycle	8.2(1.9)	2.3(0.6)	0.3– 4.3	0.01
	Placebo (n = 15)	Baseline	9.8(3.5)			
		After 1st cycle	8.8(3.2)	1(0.5)	−0.7– 2.7	0.6
		After 2nd cycle	8.7(2.6)	1.1(0.6)	−0.8– 3.1	0.5
		After 3rd cycle	8.6(3.2)	1.2(0.4)	−0.08– 2.6	0.5
Number of pads used	Intervention (n = 15)	Baseline	22.7(12)			
		After 1st cycle	20(14)	2.6(1.6)	−2.4–−7.7	0.5
		After 2nd cycle	21.4(17.9)	1.3(2.7)	−7.1– 9.7	0.8
		After 3rd cycle	16.4(10.7)	6.3(1.5)	1.6– 11	0.01
	Placebo (n = 15)	Baseline	15.4(9.8)			
		After 1st cycle	13.9(7.2)	1.5(1.7)	−3.7– 6.8	0.6
		After 2nd cycle	11.6(7.8)	3.8(1.5)	−0.7– 8.4	01
		After 3rd cycle	15(8.7)	0.4(2)	−5.9– 6.7	0.9
MQ score	Intervention (n = 15)	Baseline	47.8(15.7)			
		After 3 months	39.4(16.7)	8.4(3.7)	0.4-16.4	0.02
	Placebo (n = 15)	Baseline	41.2(15.3)			
		After 3 months	39.2(14.5)	2(2.03)	−2.3– 6.4	0.7

*One-way analysis of variance (ANOVA) was used to compare the groups before and after each treatment with either placebo or extract. There was statistically significant difference between groups before and after three rounds of treatment with myrtle syrup, while the difference between groups before and after placebo treatment was not statistically significant.
**P values <0.05 are significant.

inhibit inflammatory mediators [37]. According to a preliminary study, micronized flavonoids suppressed endometrial prostaglandins and were safe and effective in AUB [38]. Another phytochemical compound in myrtle that suppresses prostaglandin E_2 formation efficiently is myrtucommulon [39]. Therefore, the presence of the effective anti-inflammatory components in the myrtle extract can render the myrtle syrup a potential source to reduce prostaglandin secretion and to cure AUB subsequently. Further mechanistic studies are suggested to prove the anti-inflammatory effects of the components in the myrtle extract.

This study had some potential limitations which are usually part of the nature of human studies. Firstly, ITM has two groups of principal variables: one is part of human nature, *mezaj* (temperament), racial/ethnic, sex, age, season, zone, profession [40], and the second factor is the composition of the herbal preparations which may vary based on the geographical habitat of the plant, the climate, and the time of reaping [41]. These factors have not been considered in our study.

In the present study, the subjects received syrup only for three cycles; therefore we cannot comment on any long-term efficacy of myrtle syrup. Also, the subjects were not followed up after finishing the study and the long-lasting effects are not clear to us.

Conclusion

The outcomes of this study showed that myrtle syrup is an effective drug as a short-term treatment of AUB-MM. Women in the test group experienced significant reductions of bleeding duration, as well as a significant decline of the intensity of bleeding while placebo did not affect the variables significantly. The quality of life improved among the subjects in the syrup-treated group. Based on the current novel results, a therapeutic role of myrtle syrup is suggested for women with AUB-MM, which is accessible and cost-effective therapy. Larger and longer randomized trials are being planned in our research group to confirm the long-term effects of myrtle on bleeding reduction in AUB-MM.

Abbreviations
AUB-MM: Abnormal uterine bleeding-menometrorrhagia; CBC: Complete blood count; EMB: Excessive menstrual bleeding; FSH: Follicle- stimulating hormone; Hb: Hemoglobin; Hct: Hematocrit; HMB: Heavy menstrual bleeding; ITM: Iranian traditional medicine; LH: Luteinizing hormone; MQ: Menorrhagia questionnaire; PG: Prostaglandin; PT: Prothrombin time; PTT: Partial thomboplastin time; TSH: Thyroid stimulating hormone.

Competing interests
The authors do not have any financial/ commercial competing interest in the study presented here.

Authors' contributions
MQ has made substantial contribution in designing, acquisition of data, and drafting the manuscript and has given the final approval of the version to be published. SHK participated involved in design, and revising, have given the final approval of the version to be published. FHD analyzed and interpreted the data. NZ the supervisor of conduction of the study, participated involved in design, and revising, have given the final approval of the version to be published. RM participated involved in revising. MM participated involved in revising. GHA participated in the identification of the plants, plant extraction and made substantial contributions in the study. MN co- study designer. MK participated involved in revising. MA participated involved in revising and analyzing the data of the manuscript. AGH participated involved in recruitment. SJHK participated involved in randomization procedure. DT participated involved in revising. All authors read and approved the final manuscript.

Acknowledgements
The authors thank all the study participants for their participation. The authors gratefully acknowledge the help of the following individuals: Dr Jale aliasl Mamaghani for editing the data and revising; Dr Zahra Ghorbanifar for editing and Dr. Maliheh Tabarrai for revising. This was supported by a research grant provided by Shahed University.

Author details
[1]Traditional Medicine Clinical Trial Research Center, Shahed University, Tehran, Iran. [2]Department of Traditional Medicine, Faculty of Traditional Medicine, Shahid Beheshti University of Medical Sciences, Tehran, Iran. [3]Research Institute for Islamic and Complementary Medicine, Iran University of Medical Sciences, Tehran, Iran. [4]Department of Gynecology and Obstetrics, Faculty of Medical Sciences, Shahed University, Tehran, Iran. [5]Department of Traditional Medicine, School of Traditional Medicine, Shahid Beheshti University of Medical Sciences, Tehran, Iran. [6]Department of Traditional Pharmacy, Faculty of Traditional Medicine, Tehran University of Medical Sciences, Tehran, Iran. [7]Department of Pharmacognosy, School of Pharmacy Shahid Beheshti University of Medical Sciences, Tehran, Iran. [8]Department of Drug and Food control, Faculty of Pharmacy, Tehran University of Medical Sciences, Tehran, Iran. [9]Department of Gynecology and Obstetrics, Tehran University of Medical Sciences, Tehran, Iran. [10]Khatam Hospital, Tehran, Iran. [11]Medicinal Plant Research Centre, Shahed University, Tehran, Iran.

References
1. Gibbs R, Karlan B, Haney A, Nygaard I: *Danforth's obstetrics and gynecology.* 10th edition. Philadelphia: Lippincott Williams & Wilkins; 2008:664–671.
2. Livingstone M, Fraser IS: Mechanisms of abnormal uterine bleeding. *Hum Reprod Update* 2002, 8(1):60–67.
3. Marret H, Fauconnier A, Chabbert-Buffet N, Cravello L, Golfier F, Gondry J, Agostini A, Bazot M, Brailly-Tabard S, Brun JL: Clinical practice guidelines on menorrhagia: management of abnormal uterine bleeding before menopause. *Eur J Obstet Gynecol Reprod Biol* 2010, 152(2):133–137.
4. Critchley HO, Maybin JA: Molecular and cellular causes of abnormal uterine bleeding of endometrial origin. *Semin Reprod Med; Thieme Med Pub* 2011, 29(5):400–409. doi: 10.1055/s-0031-1287664.
5. Shobeiri S, Sharei S, Heidari A, Kianbakht S: Portulaca oleracea L. in the treatment of patients with abnormal uterine bleeding: a pilot clinical trial. *Phytother Res* 2009, 23(10):1411–1414.
6. Telner DE, Jakubovicz D: Approach to diagnosis and management of abnormal uterine bleeding. *Can Fam Physician* 2007, 53(1):58–64.
7. Fathima A, Sultana A: Clinical efficacy of a Unani formulation 'Safoof Habis' in menorrhagia:A randomized controlled trial. *Eur J Integr Med* 2012, 4(3):e315–e322.
8. Speroff I, Glass R, Kase N: *Clinical gynecology endocrinology and infertility.* 8th edition. Philadelphia, USA: lippincott williams and wilkins; 2011:592–617.
9. Bereak SJ: *Break and Novaks Gynecology.* 15th edition. Philadelphia, USA: lippincott williams and wilkins; 2012:403–409.
10. JANET RA, Sharon K, Robert M: Abnormal uterine bleeding. *Am Fam Physician* 2004, 69(8):1915–1926.
11. Leminen H, Hurskainen R: Tranexamic acid for the treatment of heavy menstrual bleeding: efficacy and safety. *Int J Womens Health* 2012, 4:413–421.
12. Canonico M, Oger E, Plu-Bureau G, Conard J, Meyer G, Lévesque H, Trillot N, Barrellier MT, Wahl D, Emmerich J, the ESTHER study: Hormone therapy and venous thromboembolism among postmenopausal women impact of the route of estrogen administration and progestogens. *Circulation* 2007, 115(7):840–845.
13. Muoukkah S, Mazari Z, Ghoshtasbi A, Moayed Mohseni S: The effect of tranexamic acid on the quality of life and blood loss of woman with menorrhagia: A clinical trial. *Arak Med Uni J* 2012, 15(3):75–84.
14. Zafarghandi N, Torkestani F, Hadavand S, Zaeri F, Jalilinejad H: Evaluation of libido in post hystrectomy patients. *Tehran Uni Med J* 2006, 64(11):77–80.
15. Jensen JT, Parke S, Mellinger U, Machlitt A, Fraser IS: Effective treatment of heavy menstrual bleeding with estradiol valerate and dienogest: a randomized controlled trial. *Obstet Gynecol* 2011, 117(4):777–787.
16. Jorjani SE: *Al- Aghraz al- Tibbia val Mabohess al- Alaiia.* Iran, Tehran: Tehran university press; 2005:761–764.
17. Zafarghandi N, Jafari F, Moradi F, Alizade F, Karimi M, Alizade M: A study on the frequency of signs and symptoms of dystemperament in hypermenorrhea from viewpoint of Traditional Iranian Medicine. *IJOGI* 2012, 15(24):8–16.
18. Ibn-e-sina AH: *Al-Qanun fit-tib [The Canon of Medicine].* Beirut, Lebanon: Alaalami Beirut library Press (research of shamsedine); 2005:442–443.
19. Aqili khorasani SMHIMH: *Moalejate Aqili (medicine).* Iran, Qom: Jalaleddin; 2008:771–773.
20. Arzani MA: *Tebbe Akbari 2.* 1st edition. Iran, Qom: Jalaleddin; 2008:961–964.
21. Mozaffarian V: *Trees and Shrubs of Iran.* 1st edition. Tehran: Farhang Moaser Publishers; 2005:357.
22. Amin G: *Popular Medicinal plants of Iran.* 2nd edition. Tehran: Vice-chancellorship of Research, Tehran University of Medical sciences; 2005:254.
23. Fleming T: *PDR for herbal medicine.* 4th edition. Montvale: THomson; 2007:596–597.
24. Zanetti S, Cannas S, Molicotti P, Bua A, Cubeddu M, Porcedda S, Marongiu B, Sechi LA: Evaluation of the Antimicrobial Properties of the Essential Oil of Myrtus communis L. against Clinical Strains of Mycobacterium spp. *Interdiscip Perspect Infect Dis* 2010. doi: 10.1155/2010/931530.
25. Jorsaraei SG, Moghadamnia AA, Firoozjahi AR, Miri SM, Omranirad A, Saghebi R, Hashemi SF: A comparison on histopathological effects on Myrtle extract and silver sulfadiazine 1% on healing of second degree burn wound in rats. *J Qazvin Univ Med Sci* 2006, 10(1):6–15.
26. Sumbul S, Ahmad MA, Asif M, Saud I, Akhtar M: Evaluation of Myrtus communis Linn. berries (common myrtle) in experimental ulcer models in rats. *Hum Exp Toxicol* 2010, 29(11):935–944.
27. Zaidi SF, Muhammad JS, Shahryar S, Usmanghani K, Gilani A, Jafri W, Sugiyama T: Anti-inflammatory and cytoprotective effects of selected Pakistani medicinal plants in Helicobacter pylori-infected gastric epithelial cells. *J Ethnopharmacol* 2012, 141(1):403–410.
28. Serce S, Ercisli S, Sengul M, Gunduz K, Orhan E: Antioxidant activities and fatty acid composition of wild grown myrtle (Myrtus communis L.) fruits. *Pharmacogn Mag* 2010, 6(21):9.
29. Ghayeni M: *Salehi Garabadin.* Tehran: Islamic medicine and complementary medicine institute press; 2004:156.
30. Aghili M: *Kabir Garabadin.* Tehran: Islamic medicine and complementary medicine institute press; 2004:571–576.
31. Mazari Z, Ghoshtasbi A, Muoukkah S, Saki F: Translation of Iranian version of Menorrhagia questionaire. *Payesh* 2011, 11(1):83–88.
32. Ruta D, Garratt A, Chadha Y, Flett G, Hall M, Russell I: Assessment of patients with menorrhagia: how valid is a structured clinical history as a measure of health status? *Qual Life Res* 1995, 4(1):33–40.
33. Wyatt KM, Dimmock PW, Walker TJ, O'Brien P: Determination of total menstrual blood loss. *Fertil Steril* 2001, 76(1):125–131.
34. Tuberoso CIG, Rosa A, Bifulco E, Melis MP, Atzeri A, Pirisi FM, Dessi MA: Chemical composition and antioxidant activities of Myrtus communis L. berries extracts. *Food Chem* 2010, 123(4):1242–1251.
35. Evans WC: *Trease and evans pharmacognosy.* United Kingdom: Saunders; 2009:228.
36. Wang H, Nair MG, Strasburg GM, Chang Y-C, Booren AM, Gray JI, DeWitt DL: Antioxidant and antiinflammatory activities of anthocyanins and their aglycon, cyanidin, from tart cherries. *J Nat Prod* 1999, 62(2):294–296.

37. Gonzalez-Gallego J, Sánchez-Campos S, Tunon M: **Anti-inflammatory properties of dietary flavonoids.** *Nutr Hosp* 2007, **22**(3):287–293.
38. Mukherjeea GG, Gajarajb AJ, Mathiasc J, Marya D: **Treatment of abnormal uterine bleeding with micronized flavonoids.** *Int J Gynecol Obstet* 2005, **89**(2):156–157.
39. Koeberle A, Pollastro F, Northoff H, Werz O: **Myrtucommulone, a natural acylphloroglucinol, inhibits microsomal prostaglandin E2 synthase 1.** *Br J Pharmacol* 2009, **156**(6):952–961.
40. Mokaberinejad R, Zafarghandi N, Bioos S, Dabaghian FH, Naseri M, Kamalinejad M, Amin G, Ghobadi A, Tansaz M, Akhbari A: **Mentha longifolia syrup in secondary amenorrhea: a double-blind, placebo-controlled, randomized trials.** *DARU J Pharm Sci* 2012, **20**(1):1–8.
41. Kamali SH, Khalaj AR, Hasani-Ranjbar S, Esfehani MM, Kamalinejad M, Omidmalayeri S, Kamali SA: **Efficacy of 'Itrifal Saghir', a combination of three medicinal plants in the treatment of obesity; A randomized controlled trial.** *DARU J Pharm Sci* 2012, **20**:33.

3

Antiproliferative activity of methanolic extracts from two green algae, *Enteromorpha intestinalis* and *Rizoclonium riparium* on HeLa cells

Subhabrata Paul and Rita Kundu*

Abstract

Background: Natural compounds can be alternative sources for finding new lead anti-cancer molecules. Marine algae have been a traditional source for bioactive compounds. *Enteromorpha intestinalis* and *Rhizoclonium riparium* are two well distributed saline/brackish water algae from Sundarbans. There's no previous report of these two for their anti-proliferative activities.

Methods: Cytotoxicity of the algal methanolic extracts (AMEs) on HeLa cells were assayed by 3-(4, 5-dimethylthiazol-2-yl)-2, 5- diphenyltetrazolium bromide (MTT) reduction assay. Morphological examinations were done by Haematoxylin, Hoechst 33258 and Acridine orange staining. DNA fragmentation was checked. Gene expressions of Cysteine aspartate protease (Caspase) 3, Tumor protein (TP) 53, Bcl-2 associated protein X (Bax) were studied by Reverse transcription- polymerase chain reaction (RT-PCR) keeping Glyceraldehyde 3-phosphate dehydrogenase (GAPDH) as internal control. Protein expressions were studied for Caspase 3, phospho-p53, Bax, Microtubule associated proteins-1/ light chain B (MAP1/LC3B) by western blot.

Results: The AMEs were found to be cytotoxic with Inhibitory concentration 50 (IC50) values 309.048 ± 3.083 µg/ml and 506.081 ± 3.714 µg/ml for *E. intestinalis* and *R. riparium* extracts respectively. Treated cells became round with blebbings with condensed nuclei. Acidic lysosomal vacuoles formation occurred in treated cells. Expression of apoptotic genes in both mRNA and protein level was lowered. Expression of LC3B-II suggested occurrence of autophagy in treated cells.

Conclusions: These two algae can be potent candidates for isolating new lead anticancer molecules. So they need further characterization at both molecular and structural levels.

Keywords: *Enteromorpha intestinalis*, *Rhizoclonium riparium*, HeLa, MTT, Acridine orange, LC3B

Background

Cancer is considered to be the second leading cause of death [1]. An estimated 12.7 million new cases are registered each year with 7.6 million deaths and 24.6 million persons living with cancer worldwide [2]. According to a recent report of World Health Organization (WHO), cervical cancer ranks as the most frequent cancer among women between 15–44 years age group in India and all over the world. Currently a population of more than 366 million women of India (age group of 15 or more), are at a risk of developing cervical cancer. Every year 529828 women are diagnosed with the disease and 275128 die from this cancer throughout the world. The scenario is not very different in India also. Here, each year, the estimated number of new cases is 134420 and number of mortality is 72825. Considering the growth rate of population, the projected new cases of cervical cancer by 2025 will be 720060 and projected number of death will be 395095 in the global context, whereas , in India, the projected new cases will be 115171 which is very alarming [3,4].

Chemotherapy is still the standard treatment method along with surgery and radiation therapy. Most of the available treatments cause severe side effects such as bleeding, cognitive impairment, sensory abnormalities, infertility, damage to hoemopoetic tissue, hair-loss due to their non-

* Correspondence: kundu_rita@yahoo.co.in
Department of Botany, University of Calcutta, 35, Ballygunge Circular Road, Kolkata 700019, India

selective cytotoxicity. Emerging cancer drug resistance is another serious problem regarding chemotherapy [5]. Search for a new anticancer drug with lesser side effects and selective cytotoxicity has been one of the main thrust of cancer research worldwide. In this context, natural products, derived from plants, marine organisms and microorganisms, have drawn attentions of many scientists. According to WHO; 80% of world's population, especially in developing countries rely on plant derived medicines [6]. In the few decades natural products from higher plants were explored in great extent for possible anticancer activities, while other groups (algae, fungi) were not given proper attention. But, there is a tremendous scope to obtain novel bioactive compounds from the algae. Algae are a promising group to furnish various bioactive compounds as they are a group of diverse (unicellular to multicellular, prokaryotic to eukaryotic) members with diverse (freshwater to brakish/marine) habitats. They have been traditionally used as food and medicine in India, China, Japan, Korea, Ireland and Wales. Brown seaweeds (macroalgae) like *Laminaria, Undaria* are utilized as sources of iodine [7]. Alginate produced by brown algae (seaweeds) is used in food and pharmaceutical industries due to its ability to chelate metal ions. Carrageenans (water soluble sulfated galactans with an alternating backbone of $\alpha(1-4)$-3,6 anhydro- D-galactose and ß$(1-3)$ D galactose used as emulsifier/ stabilizers in milk based food products (icecream, pudding, desert gels, jams) are also obtained from macro algae (*Kappaphycus alvarezii*) [8]. Though, marine algae are rich source of pharmacologically active metabolites [9-13], having antimicrobial, antineoplastic, antiviral, anti-inflammatory and immunostimulant [14-16] activities, they were not exploited so far for their antiproliferating properties till today. Only few reports are available regarding the anticancer activities of algae. *Spirulina, Anabaena* and *Aphanizomenon*, members of Cyanophyceae (blue green algae) were reported to induce apoptosis in HL-60 and MCF7 cell lines [17-19]. But reports regarding the anticancer properties of Chlorophyta (green algae) are sparse. Extracts of *Udotea flabellum* was reported to have antiproliferative activity on HeLa, SiHa and KB cell lines [20].

In the present study, we have evaluated the cytotoxic potential of methanolic extracts of two green algae *Enteromorpha intestinalis* and *Rhizoclonium riparium*, using MTT assay on cervical cancer cell line (HeLa) followed by DNA fragmentation assay. Role of Caspase 3, p53 and Bax were studied in transcriptional and translational level to investigate their role in inducing cell death. Role of LC3B was studied at the translational level.

Methods
Chemicals and reagents
Methanol (Merck) was used to extract the algal materials. Dulbecco's Modified Eagle Medium (DMEM), Fetal Bovine Serum (FBS) and antibiotic-antimycotic solution [Penicillin, Streptomycin & Amphotericin], Sodium bicarbonate (NaHCO$_3$) (Himedia) were used in cell culture. 3-(4, 5-dimethylthiazol-2-yl)-2, 4-diphenyltetrazolium bromide (MTT) (Sigma) and Dimethyl sulfoxide (DMSO) (Merck) were used in cell viability assays. Haematoxylin (Gurr), Hoechst 33258 (Sigma), Paraformaldehyde (PFA)(HiMedia) were used in cellular and nuclear morphology study. Acridine orange (Sigma) was used in acidic vacuole staining. Non idet P-40 (NP40) (Sigma) was used in DNA isolation. Tris(hydroxymethyl)aminomethane (Tris), Ethylenediaminetetraacetic acid (EDTA), Acetic acid (Merck); Agarose, Ethidium bromide (EtBr) (Sigma) were used in Agarose gel electrophoresis. TRI reagent, Chloroform and Isopropanol (Sigma) were used for total RNA isolation. Sodium hypochlorite (NaClO) (Merck) used in RNA gel electrophoresis. First strand cDNA synthesis kit [MuLv RT kit] (Fermentas); Taq Polymerase, dNTPs (Chromus Biotech) were used in semi quantitative RT-PCR reactions. 100× protease inhibitor cocktail (G-Biosciences) was used at the time of protein isolation. Sodium hydroxide (NaOH), Sodium carbonate (Na$_2$CO$_3$), Sodium potassium tartrate (C$_4$H$_4$KNaO$_6$. 4H$_2$O), Copper sulfate (CuSO$_4$.5H$_2$O) (Merck); Bovine serum albumin (BSA), Folin phenol reagent (Sigma) were used in protein quantification. Acrylamide, Bis-acrylamide, Ammonium persulfate (APS), Sodium dodecyl sulfate (SDS) (Merck) and Tetramethylethylenediamine (TEMED) (Sigma) were used in polyacrylamide gel electrophoresis (PAGE). Caspase3 (Imgenex); LC3B, ß-tubulin (Sigma); IgG-AP (Santa Cruz Biotechnology); Bax, phospho-p53 (Cell Signalling Technology); nitro-blue tetrazolium/5-bromo-4-chloro-3'-indolyphosphate (NBT/BCIP) (Sigma) and nitrocellulose paper (NC) (Schleicher & Schuell) were used in western blot analysis.

Algal material
Two green algae, *Rhizoclonium riparium* (Roth) Harvey and *Enteromorpha intestinalis* (Linnaeus) [21] were collected during January 2012, from different blocks (Sandeshkhali and Jharkhali) of Sundarbans mangrove ecosystem (Indian part). Collected samples were properly identified and voucher specimens were deposited in the Calcutta University Herbarium (CUH). Accession numbers issued by CUH against *R. riparium* was CUH/AL/MW-48 and for *E. intestinalis* was CUH/AL/MW-50.

Preparation of algal extracts
10 gm of algal samples were excised to small pieces and extracted with methanol (3 times) for 72 hours at room temperature. The extract was concentrated and dried with freeze dryer (Eyela). The dried mass was weighed and again dissolved in appropriate volume of methanol to make the concentration of the AMEs as 20 µg/µl. The

extract was further filtered through a 0.22 μm sterile filter (Pall) and stored at –20°C for future use.

Cell line

For the *in vitro* assay HeLa cell line was used. HeLa cells are Human Papilloma virus (HPV) 18 positive human cervical cancer cell line, expressing high risk E6 and E7 oncoproteins [22] and low level of p53. 293 T cells are normal human embryonic kidney (HEK) cell line expressing large T antigen of Simian virus 40 (SV-40), often used as transfection host.

Cell culture

HeLa and 293 T cells were maintained in monolayer cultures in DMEM supplemented with 0.15% NaHCO3, 5% FBS, 2 mM L-glutamine, 0.45% L-glucose, 100units/ml penicillin, 100 μg/ml streptomycin and 250 ng/ml Amphotericin B at 37°C in a humidified incubator having 5% Carbon dioxide (CO_2).

MTT assay

Cytotoxicity of the AMEs was evaluated by standard MTT assay [23]. 2×10^4 HeLa and 293 T cells /well were seeded in 96 well flat bottom culture plates along with negative control sets (without cells). After overnight incubation cells were treated with different concentrations (in a range of 0–500 μg/ml) of the AMEs in triplicate along with a vehicle control set (2.5% of the growth medium). After 24 hours, the medium with treatments were removed and replaced with fresh medium along with 100 μg of MTT in each well and incubated for another 4 hours. Then the medium was removed and the formazan crystals were dissolved in 100 μl DMSO and absorbance was taken at 490 nm [24] in an Elisa reader (BioRad). The extent of cytotoxicity was determined using the following formula:

$$\%inhibition = [1-(Absorbance_{treated}/Absorbance_{non-treated})] \times 100$$

IC50 values were calculated subsequently. All the experiments were done with this IC50 doses.

Morphological studies

AMEs treated HeLa cells were stained with Haematoxylin and Hoechst 33258 to study cellular and nuclear morphology. Treated and control cells were stained with supravital stain Acridine orange to study the formation of acidic vacuoles. 5×10^4 HeLa cells/ coverslip were seeded and after overnight incubation, treated with IC50 values of the AMEs for 24 hours along with a non-treated set. Then fixed in 4% PFA and subsequently Haematoxylin and Hoechst staining were done.

For cellular morphology study, the fixed cells were stained with 1% acidic Mayer's Haematoxylin for 5 minutes at room temperature. For nuclear morphology, 2 μg/ml of Hoechst 33258 was used to stain the nuclei for 15 minutes in dark at room temperature. For Acridine orange staining, after 24 hours of AME treatment, cells were additionally incubated in fresh media containing Acridine orange (1 μg/ml) for 15 minutes without fixation.

After the staining procedures were over, extra stain was drained out, washed briefly in phosphate buffered saline (PBS) and mounted in PBS containing 10% glycerol, 2% N-propyl gallate. Cells were visualized under both bright field and fluorescence {excitation 356 nm, emission 465 nm for Hoechst and excitation 488 nm, emission 530(green) 650 (red) for Acridine orange} in an epi-fluorescence microscope (Olympus).

DNA fragmentation

10^7 HeLa cells were seeded in T25 flask. After overnight incubation, medium was replaced and fresh medium was added along with IC50 doses of AMEs. After 24 hours of treatment, cells were harvested and lysed with lysis buffer containing 20 mM EDTA, 50 mM Tris, 1%SDS and 1% NP-40 for 2 hours in ice. Then the total genomic DNA was purified and treated with RNase treatment (20 μg/ml) at 37°C for 1 hour. DNA was then precipitated, washed with 75% ethanol, briefly air-dried, dissolved in Tris-EDTA buffer (pH8) and electrophoresed in 1.5% agarose gel containing EtBr (0.5 μg/ml), Tris acetate EDTA (TAE) buffer at 4 V/cm, and subsequently visualized under ultra violet (UV) trans-illuminator and photographed in gel documentation system (UVP Multidoc-It).

Gene and protein expression studies

10^7 HeLa cells were seeded in T25 flask. After overnight incubation, medium was replaced and fresh medium was added along with IC50 doses of AMEs. After 24 hours of treatment, cells were harvested and RT-PCRs and Western blots were done.

Semi quantitative RT-PCR

Total RNA was isolated from the cells using TRI reagent following manufacturer's protocol. RNA integrity was checked in 1.5% agarose gel containing 0.3% NaClO [25], EtBr (0.5 μg/ml), TAE buffer at 4 V/cm with subsequent visualization under UV.

First strand cDNA synthesis was carried out taking 2 μg RNA using 1st strand cDNA synthesis kit [MuLv RT kit] following manufacturer's protocol. Taking 2 μl of cDNA as template, PCRs were conducted for Caspase-3, Bax and TP53 gene while GAPDH serves as an internal control. The PCR products were subsequently subjected to agarose gel electrophoresis (AGE), visualized under ultra violet (UV) trans-illuminator and photographed in gel documentation system (UVP Multidoc-It). Densitometric analysis of the bands was done using UVP Doc-ItLS image analysis software.

The primers used were designed by Primer-3 software using FASTA sequences from NCBI-Nucleotide. The forward and reverse primer sequences along with their respective PCR profiles are listed in Table 1.

Western blot

Total protein was isolated by lysing HeLa cells using 1xSDS gel loading buffer (50 mM Tris-Cl pH 6.8, 2% SDS, 10% 2-Mercaptoethanol, 0.01% Bromophenol blue, 10% Glycerol) along with 1× protease inhibitor (with EDTA) followed by incubation in boiling water bath for 10 min. Then the lysates were centrifuged at 14000 g for 15 minutes at 4°C. Supernatants stored at −20°C for further uses.

Extracted protein samples were quantified following micro-Lowry method with slight modifications. To 2 μl of lysates 200 μl of 10% TCA was added and incubated 30 minutes at −20°C and the centrifuged at 15000 g for 15 minutes at 4°C. The precipitated protein pellets then re-dissolved in 100 μl of 1(N) NaOH and subsequently incubated in 1 ml Lowry reagent (2% Na_2CO_3:2% $C_4H_4KNaO_6.4H_2O$: 1% $CuSO_4.5H_2O$ = 100:1:1) for 10 minutes at room temperature. Then 100 μl of Folin phenol reagent (diluted 1:1 with milli Q grade water) added to the samples and further incubated in dark at room temperature for 30 minutes. O.D of the samples was taken at 750 nm in a double beam spectrophotometer (Hitachi) and concentration of the samples was determined using a standard curve prepared with BSA.

100 μg of each protein samples were separated in 12% polyacrylamide gels. Semi dry transfer of the protein samples were done using 0.45 μm nitrocellulose paper,

incubated in blocking buffer (5% BSA) for 2 hours at room temperature. Then the membrane was incubated at 4°C with appropriate dilutions of primary antibodies (1:2000 for anti ß-tubulin, 1:1000 for anti Bax, 1:500 for anti phospho-p53 and anti LC3B, 1:250 for anti Caspase 3) for overnight. After subsequent incubation of 2 hours with AP conjugated IgG (1:5000) at room temperature, NBT-BCIP solution was added and incubated until bands appeared. Pictures of the membranes were taken in gel documentation system (UVP Multidoc-It). Densitometry analysis of the bands was done using UVP Doc-ItLS image analysis software.

Statistical analysis

All the experiments were carried out thrice in triplicates. All numerical data were expressed as mean of triplicates ± standard error (SE). Statistical analysis and generation of histograms were performed using Graphpad Prism 5.02 software. All datasets obtained from the experiments were subjected to grouped analysis by two-way analysis of variance (ANOVA) followed by Bonferroni post tests keeping $p < 0.05$ in all cases.

Results

MTT assay

To study the antiproliferative potential of the methanolic extract of these two algae on Hela cells and 293 T cells, MTT assays were done. Reduction of the substrate (MTT) by cellular dehydrogenase to form water insoluble formazan is the basis of the cytotoxicity test. Reduction in colour intensity in the treated sets than the non treated ones clearly indicated cytoxicity of the AME's on HeLa cells. From the experiment it was observed that cell death was concentration dependent, number of nonviable cells increased with increased concentration of AMEs.

Table 1 Primer sequences and PCR profiles for the genes Caspase 3, Bax, TP53 and GAPDH

A	Primer sequence (5′ → 3′)	
Gene	Forward	Reverse
Caspase 3	ATTGTGGAATTGATGCGTGA	GGCAGGCCTGAATAATGAAA
TP53	ATGGCCATCTACAAGCAG	ACAGTCAAGAGCCAACCTCAG
Bax	GTGGCAGCTGACATGTTTTC	GGAGGAAGTCCAATGTCCAG
GAPDH	CAAGGTCATCCATGACAACTTTG	GTCCACCACCCTGTTGCTGTAG

B			PCR profile				
PCR steps Gene	Initial denaturation	Denaturation	Annealing	Extension	No. of cycles	Final extension	Product length (bp)
Caspase 3		94°C – 60s	52°C – 45 s	72°C – 60s			205
TP53	94°C – 4 m	94°C – 30s	58°C – 30s	72°C – 45 s	35	72°C – 7 m	210
Bax		94°C – 60s	57°C – 30s	72°C – 45 s			151
GAPDH		94°C – 30s	58°C – 30s	72°C – 45 s			496

(A) Primer sequences, designed by Primer3 software tabulated.
(B) PCR profiles after optimization for single band for a target.

We have observed that the IC50 doses of the AMEs in HeLa cells were 309.048 ± 3.083 µg/ml and 506.081 ± 3.714 µg/ml for *E. intestinalis* and *R. riparium* extracts respectively. For 293 T cells, the IC50 doses were 651.183 ± 1.198 µg/ml and 905.727 ± 4.034 µg/ml. The vehicle control set showed 4.345 ± 0.594 percent inhibition. From the study it was observed that methanolic extract of *E. intestinalis* was more cytotoxic than *R. riparium* (Figure 1a & b).

Cell and nuclear morphology

Both the AMEs treated HeLa cells showed distinct differences in their cellular and nuclear morphology in

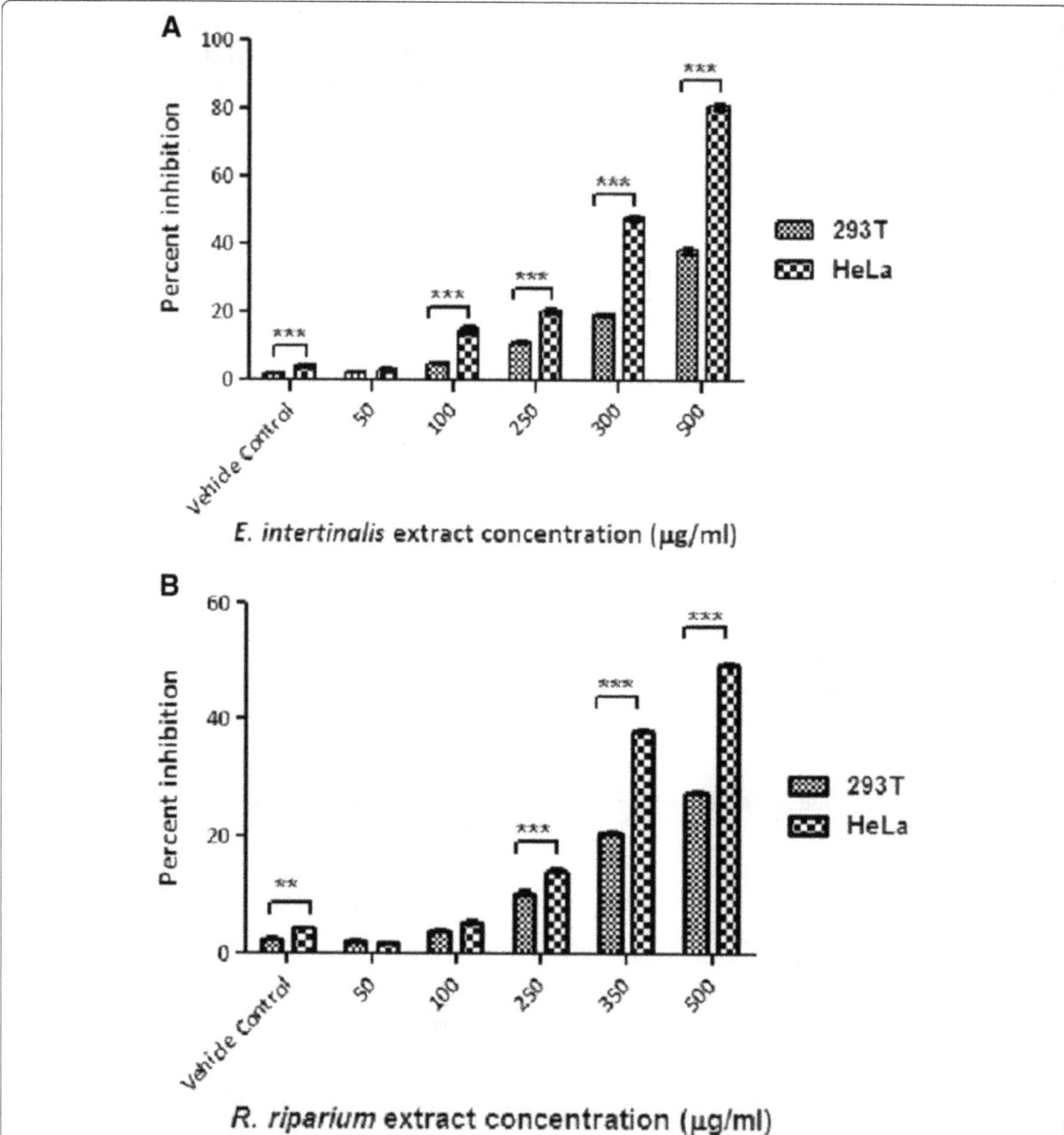

Figure 1 Histograms showing the antiproliferative effects of the AMEs on HeLa and 293 T cell lines. The cells were treated with increasing concentration of AMEs for 24 hours. Cytotoxicity of the AMEs was evaluated by MTT assay. Results showed percent inhibition of cell growth against increasing concentration of the extracts. **(A)** *E. intestinalis* extract treated, **(B)** *R. riparium* extract treated.Columns with bars represent mean ± SE of triplicates. Percent inhibitions of the AMES at each concentration point were compared between the two cells lines. According to the significance levels found, they were further categorized using various symbols as follows, **: $p < 0.01$; ***: $p < 0.001$.

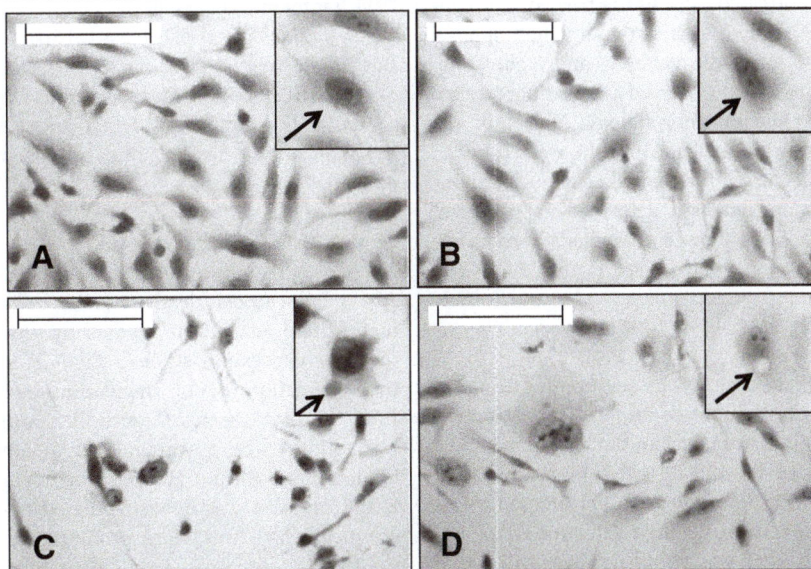

Figure 2 HeLa cells grown on sterile cover slips were treated with IC50 doses of the AMEs for 24 hours. Then they were stained with Haematoxylin to study the cellular morphology. Scale indicates 50 μm. Inset shows magnified view. **A)** Non-treated cells, the arrow shows normal cellular morphology **B)** Vehicle control cells, the arrow shows normal cellular morphology **C)** Cells treated with *E. intestinalis* extract, the arrow shows cytoplasmic blebbings **(D)** Cells treated with *R. riparium* extract, the arrow shows cytoplasmic vacuolation.

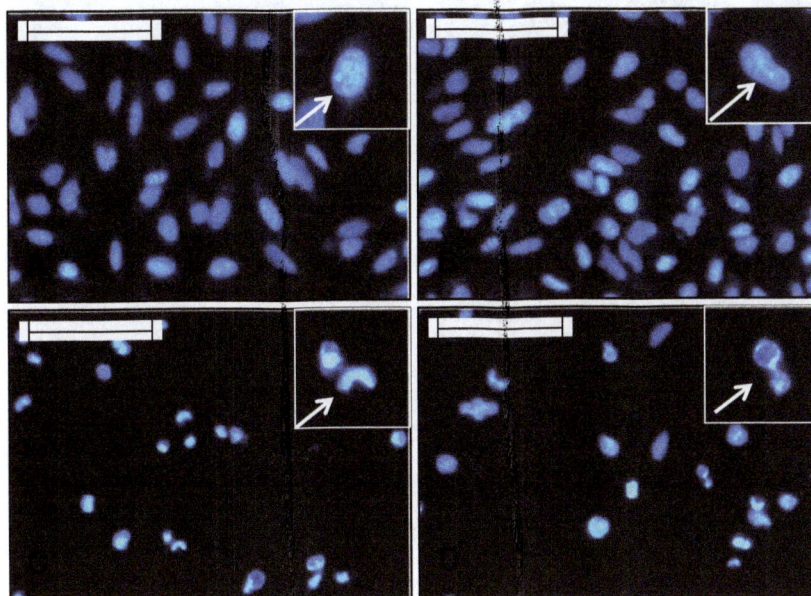

Figure 3 HeLa cells grown on sterile cover slips were treated with IC50 doses of the AMEs for 24 hours. Then they were stained with Hoechst 33258 to study the nuclear morphology. Scale indicates 50 μm. Inset shows magnified view. **(A)** Non-treated cells, the arrow shows normal looking nucleus; **(B)** Vehicle control cells, the arrow shows normal elliptical nucleus; **(C)** *E. intestinalis* extract treated sets, the arrow shows nuclei with deformity; **(D)** *R. riparium* treated cells, the arrow shows highly condensed nuclei.

comparison to the untreated cells. In the treated sets, cells became round, lost their characteristic stretched appearance, showed clear cytoplasmic blebbings and vacuolation. Cells stained with Hoechst, observed under fluorescence microscope showed nuclear morphology. Nuclei of the control sets were elliptical in shape, but the treated nuclei were somewhat different. In the treated cells nuclear condensation was pronounced with deformed appearances. Vehicle sets in both cases showed characteristic morphological features as the non-treated ones (Figures 2 and 3).

Acidic vacuole localization

Acridine orange in uncharged form, stain both cytoplasm and nucleic acids which fluoresce bright green. Whereas in protonated form it accumulates in the lysosomal acidic vacuoles, form aggregates and fluoresce bright red [26]. When studied under a fluorescence microscope, it was observed that in the non-treated and vehicle control sets minimal red fluorescence was found, whereas, increased red fluorescence were observed in the treated cells. In *R. riparium* extract treated cells almost the whole cytoplasm became red (Figure 4) indicating the merging of all the acidic vacuoles.

DNA fragmentation assay

DNA fragmentation is a classical hallmark of apoptosis. But in the treated cells no sign of DNA laddering was observed (Figure 5). Intact genomic DNA was found in all the cells which implied that apoptosis might not be the mechanism for inducing cell death in the treated ones.

Semi-Q RT-PCR

To investigate the role of Caspase 3, Bax and p53 in AMEs induced cell death in HeLa cells, expression profile of these genes were studied by semi q RT-PCR. For the gene expression studies, RT-PCR gave us a qualitative estimation of up regulation/down regulation of some apoptotic genes (Figure 6). Caspase 3 expression was found to be downregulated in both *E. intestinalis* treated (75.45%) and *R. riparium* treated (85.54%) cells. Bax expression was down regulated in both the treated samples, which was more pronounced in *E. intestinalis* (58.13%) extract treated cells than *R. riparium* (46.34%) treated cells. TP53 expression also decreased in both the samples, slightly higher in *E. intestinalis* (58.22%) extract treated cells than *R. riparium* (53.22%) treated cells. The down regulated expression profiles of caspase 3 and Bax

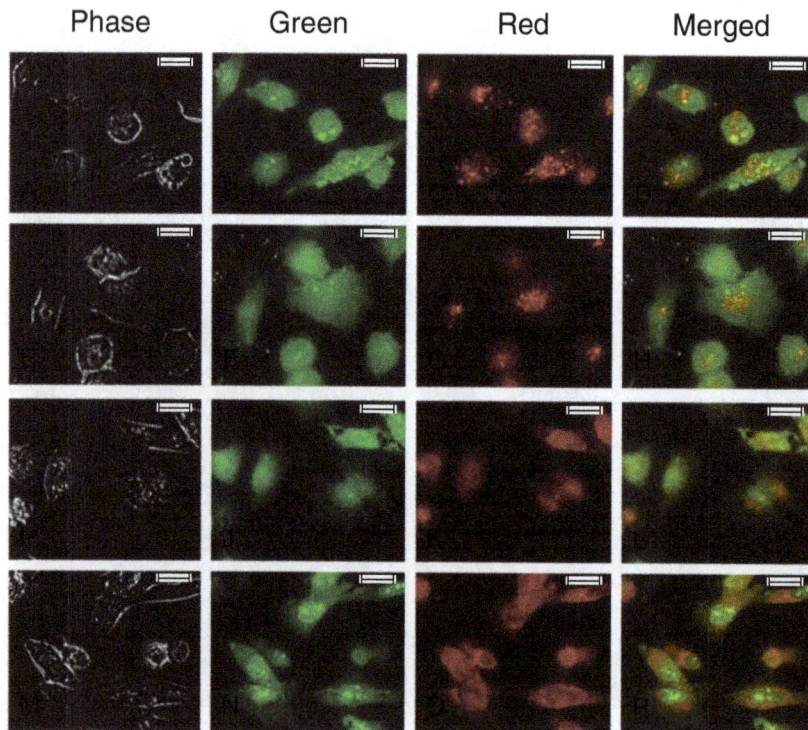

Figure 4 HeLa cells grown on sterile cover slips were treated with IC50 doses of AMEs for 24 hours. Then they were stained with Acridine orange (1 μg/ml) to study the formation of acidic vacuoles. Scale indicates 50 μm. **A-D)** Non-treated, **E-H)** Vehicle control, **I-L)** *E. intestinalis* extract treated, **M-P)** *R. riparium* treated HeLa cells.

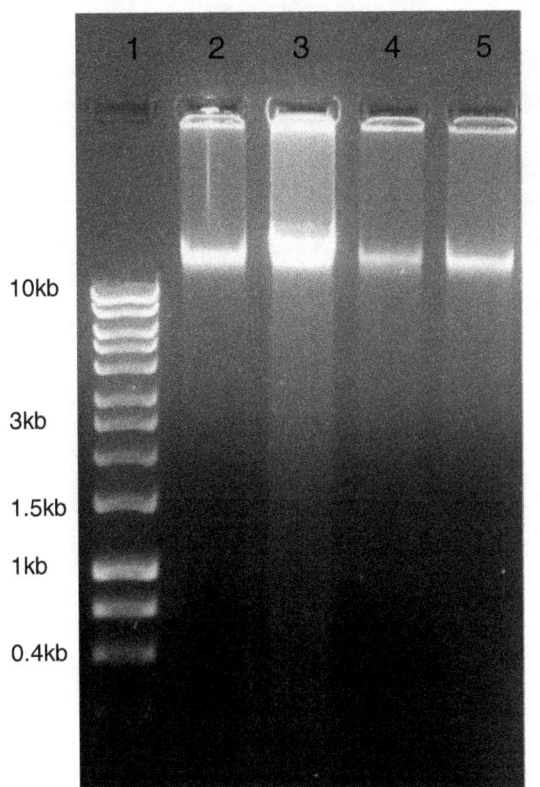

Figure 5 HeLa cells grown in T25 flask were treated with IC50 doses of AMEs for 24 hours along with a control set.
Genomic DNA was isolated from all the sets and electrophorased in 1.5% agarose gel. Lane **1)** Molecular marker (0.4-10 kb, Lane **2)** Non-treated, Lane **3)** Vehicle control, Lane **4)** *E. intestinalis* extract treated, Lane **5)** *R. riparium* extract treated.

in the treated cells indicate that cell death was not mediated by Bax and caspase3.

Immunoblotting
Expression level of some apoptotic and autophagic proteins were monitored at the translational level (Figure 7). In all the samples cleaved caspase3 expression was absent while Pro-Caspase 3 expression was less down regulated in *E. intestinalis* (17.35%) than *R. riparium* (26.85%) treated cells. Bax expression on the other hand was found to be more down regulated in *E. intestinalis* (27.83%) than *R. riparium* (18.86%) treated cells. Expression of phospho-p53 was absent in all the samples. Expression of LC3B-I and LC3B-II was found in both the treated samples while absent in non-treated and vehicle control sets. LC3B-I and LC3B-II expressions were higher (8.07% and 19.79% respectively) in *R. riparium* extract treated cells than the *E. intestinalis* treated cells.

Discussion
In this study, we have evaluated the methanolic extracts of two green algae, *E. intestinalis* and *R. riparium* for their antiproliferative activity in human cervical cancer cell line HeLa. These two green algae are found widely in the water bodies of Sundarbans mangrove ecosystem and commonly used as fish feed. There were no previous reports about their antiproliferative property on cervical cancer cell lines. An alkali extracted polysachharide (DAEB) from *E. intestinalis*is was found to be capable of preventing formation of Sarcoma 180 tumor and had some antitumor activity which was mediated by immunoenhancement of immune system instead of direct cytotoxicity [27].

To determine the IC50 doses of these two AMEs, MTT assays were done. Along with HeLa cells, a non-cancerous cell line, 293 T (human embryonic kidney cell line) were treated with the AMEs. From the results, it was observed that IC50 doses of the AMEs were significantly much higher for the 293 T cell line that the HeLa cell line. Which indicates that the AMEs were less cytotoxic to the non-cancerous cell line. Grouped analysis using Two-way ANOVA followed by Bonferroni posttests revealed that with respect to the control 293 T cells cytotoxicity of the AMEs in HeLa cells were significant above 50 µg/ml for *E. intestinalis* extract and above 100 µg/ml for *R.riparium* extract. This implies that *E.intestinalis* extract is more potent than *R.riparium* extract.

Cellular and nuclear morphology observed in the treated cells showed clear indication of cytotoxicity. But the responses were different for the two extracts. In *E. intestinalis* extract treated cells, cytoplasmic blebbings were observed along with deformed nuclei, while cytoplasmic vacuolation with condensed nuclei was observed in *R. riparium* treated cells. Chromatin condensations into compact figures, which are often globular or crescent shaped, are defined as stage II chromatin condensation, and occurs in apoptosis. Cytoplasmic blebbings are generally associated with apoptosis where cells undergoing apoptosis breaks down into apotosomes/apoptotic bodies, which were further absorbed by macrophages (*in vivo*), whereas cytoplasmic vacuolation is associated with autophagic cell death, a type II programmed cell death. During autophagy, portions of the cytoplasm and subcellular organelles are sequestered by endoplasmic reticulum, resulting in vesicular bodies which acted as autophagosomes. They are further fused with the lysosomes to form autophagosomal vesicles where the contents are enzymatically degraded [28]. For detecting the acidic compartments, lysosomotropic agent acridine orange was used for staining. Cells treated with *R. riparium* extract showed higher amount of acidic vacuole formation. On the other hand cells treated with *E. intestinalis* extract showed lesser number of acidic vacuole formation. In *R. riparium* treated cells,

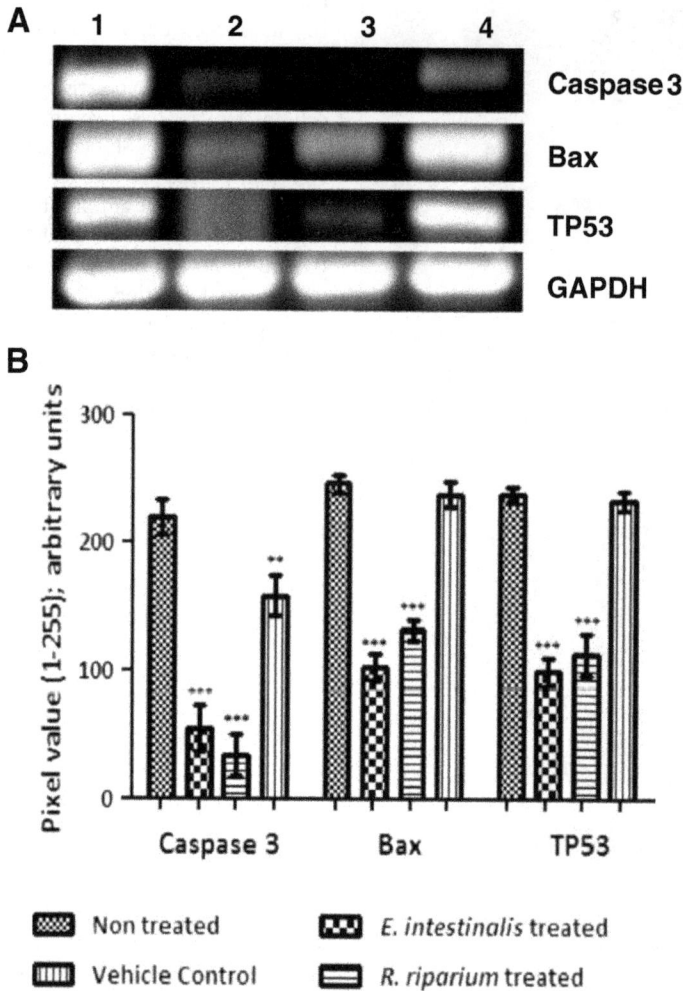

Figure 6 Gene expression profiles of Caspase 3, Bax, TP53, GAPDH in HeLa cells treated with AMEs (IC50 doses) by semi quantitative RT-PCR. (A) Representative pictures of three independent experiments. Lane 1) Non-treated, Lane 2) *E. intestinalis* extract treated, Lane 3) *R. riparium* treated, 4) Vehicle control. **(B)** Relative levels of gene expressions after normalization for GAPDH were determined by densitometry analysis of the bands, represented by histogram. Columns with bars represent mean ± SE of triplicate pixel values for the bands. Intensity for each band in the treated sets was compared with that of in non treated sets. According to the significance levels found, they were further categorized using various symbols as follows, **: $p < 0.01$; ***: $p < 0.001$.

all most the whole cell became red, due to merging of all the acidic vacuoles. The observation was further validated by immunoblot results.

DNA fragmentation is a classical hallmark of apoptosis. In response to apoptotic signals (DNA damage/ stress) proapoptotic Bcl2 family protein Bax becomes activated resulting in mitochondrial membrane permeabilization. As a result cytochrome C and APAF-1 (apoptotic protease activating factor 1) are released from the inter-membrane space and activate caspase 9 through cleavage. Caspase 9 generates a signaling cascade of caspase cleavage that results in DNA fragmentation into 180 basepairs and multiples of it. The effecter caspase is caspase 3. p53 has a

major role in cell survival . In healthy cells the nuclear amount of p53 is very low. Due to binding of adapter protein MDM2, p53 is subsequently exported to cytosol and degraded. Whereas in the cells with damaged DNA, p53 becomes phosphorylated. As MDM2 cannot recognize phosphorylated p53, the nuclear p53 is stabilized and induce pro-apoptotic proteins (Bax, Puma and Noxa etc.). We have found some signs of apoptotic features (nuclear and cellular) in the AMEs treated cells, so we have undertaken the DNA fragmentation assay and the same time assessed the expressions of caspase 3, Bax and p53 at the transcriptional level. From our observation we found that DNA fragmentation was

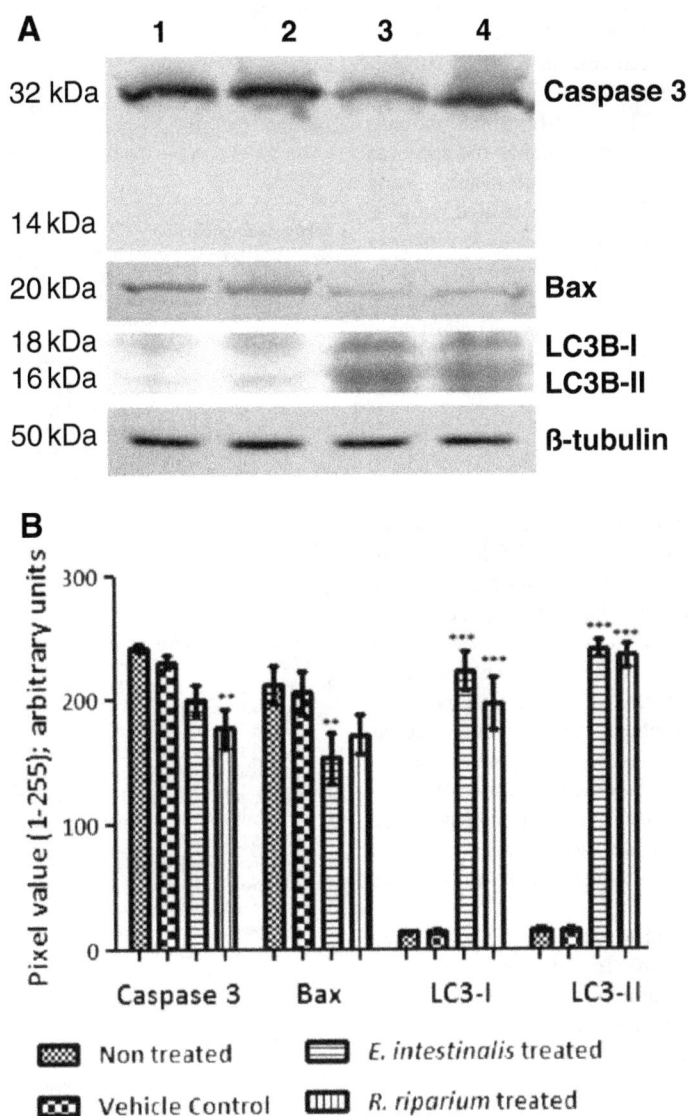

Figure 7 Protein expression profiles of Caspase 3, Bax, LC3B-I & II and ß-tubulin in HeLa cells treated with AMEs (IC50 doses) by Western blot. (A) Representative pictures of three independent experiments. Lane 1) Non-treated, Lane 2) Vehicle control 3) *E. intestinalis* extract treated, Lane 4) *R. riparium* treated. **(B)** Relative levels of gene expressions after normalization for ß-tubulin were determined by densitometry analysis of the bands, represented by histogram. Columns with bars represent mean ± SE of triplicate pixel values for the bands. Intensity for each band in the treated sets was compared with that of in non treated sets. According to the significance levels found, they were further categorized using various symbols as follows, ******: p < 0.01; *******: p < 0.001.

absent indicating a cell death process not mediated by caspase 3 or Bax.

RT-PCR observation also validates the findings. Here Bax and caspase 3 expressions were found to be less in comparison to the controlled cells and expression of p53 was down regulated in all the samples. In translational levels, the expression of cleaved pro-caspase 3 and Bax were found to be down regulated in both the samples whereas no expressions of cleaved caspase 3 and phospho-

p53 (data not shown) were observed. Absence of DNA fragmentation, down regulation of Bax, p53 and absence of cleaved caspase 3 strongly indicated a cell death pathway other than apoptosis or type I cell death.

As the AMEs treated samples showed some signs positive (vacuolation in cytosol) for autophagy or type-II cell death, role of LC3 was studied by western blot. LC3 (MAP1) is a mammalian homolog of the yeast ATG8 protein, a ubiquitin like protein that becomes lipidated and tightly associated with autophagosomal membranes. LC3 proteins are specifically cleaved at their carboxy terminal to form LC3-I, which has an exposed carboxy terminal glycine that is conjugated to phosphatidylethanolamine to form LC3-II. This LC3-II protein bounds tightly with the autophagosomal membranes and serves as an autophagic marker protein [29]. Our results clearly showed the presence of LC3-I in both the treated samples, while the presence of LC3-II was distinct in *R. riparium* treated samples. All these observations strongly suggest that these two algal extracts are capable of inducing cell death by autophagy. Previously autophagy was considered as a pro-survival mechanism of the cell. But recent studies suggest that autophagy result in cell deaths and sometimes activates apoptosis.

Conclusions

From the results it was quite evident that, both the AMEs had potent cytotoxicity on HeLa cells. With the lesser IC50 value, *E. intestinalis* extract was found to be more antiproliferative (usage of Methanol as vehicle exert negligible amount of cytotoxicity to the cells). The cellular morphological examinations revealed presence of vacuoles which may be due to formation of auto lysosomal vacuoles. In case of nuclear morphology study, though nuclear condensation was observed, absence of fragmented nuclei along with absence of DNA laddering indicated that any other mechanism than apoptosis is responsible for the cell death. Whereas increase in acidic vacuoles and expression of LC3B-II had suggested autophagic cell death in the treated samples.

Both the *E. intestinalis* and *R. riparium* methanolic extracts were found to be cytotoxic to HeLa cells, most probably by the involvement of autophagy. So they were potent candidates for further characterization of their chemical constituents and the molecular pathway by which they worked.

Abbreviations

AGE: Agarose gel electrophoresis; AME: Algal methanolic extract; APS: Ammonium persulfate; Bax: Bcl-2 associated protein X; BSA: Bovine serum albumin; $C_4H_4KNaO_6.4H_2O$: Sodium potassium tartrate; Caspase 3: Cysteine aspartate protease 3; CUH: Calcutta university herbarium; $CuSO_4.5H_2O$: Copper sulfate; DMEM: Dulbecco's modified eagle medium; DMSO: Dimethyl sulfoxide; EDTA: Ethylenediaminetetraacetic acid; EtBr: Ethidium bromide; FBS: Fetal bovine serum; GAPDH: Glyceraldehyde 3-phosphate dehydrogenase; HPV: Human papilloma virus; IC50: Inhibitory concentration 50; MAP1/LC3B: Microtubule associated proteins-1/ light chain B; MTT: 3-(4, 5-dimethylthiazol-2-yl)-2, 5- diphenyltetrazolium bromide; Na_2CO_3: Sodium bicarbonate; NaClO: Sodium hypochlorite; NaHCO3: Sodium bicarbonate; NaOH: Sodium hydroxide; NBT/BCIP: Nitro-blue tetrazolium/5-bromo-4-chloro-3'-indolyphosphate; NC: Nitrocellulose; NP-40: Non idet P40; PAGE: Polyacrylamide gel electrophoresis; PBS: Phosphate buffered saline; PFA: Paraformaldehyde; RT-PCR: Reverse transcription- polymerase chain reaction; SE: Standard error; SDS: Sodium dodecyl sulfate; TAE: Tris acetate EDTA buffer; TCA: Trichloro acetic acid; TEMED: Tetramethylethylenediamine; TP53: Tumor protein 53; Tris: Tris(hydroxymethyl)aminomethane; WHO: World health organization.

Competing interest
The authors declare that they have no competing interest.

Author's contributions
SP: Collected algae, prepared extracts and performed all the experiments; RK: conceived the experiment, and participated in its design and coordination and helped to draft the manuscript. All authors read and approved the final manuscript.

Acknowledgements
The research was supported by Centre of Advance Study (CAS) - Department of Botany, University of Calcutta. SP is thankful to University Grant Commission (UGC), Government of India for his fellowship. Authors are thankful to Department of Biotechnology & Department of Biochemistry, University of Calcutta for the instrumentation facilities. HeLa and 293 T cells were kind gifts from Dr. R. N. Baral, Chittaranjan National Cancer Institute, Kolkata. Authors would like to express their sincere gratitude to Dr.Ruma Pal, Associate Professor, Department of Botany, University of Calcutta for identifying the algal specimens. Authors are also thankful to Mr. Chinmoy Saha and Mr. Gour Gopal Satpati for their help in statistical analysis and algal voucher specimen preparation respectively.

References
1. Xu H, Yao L, Sung H, Wu L: Chemical composition and antitumor activity of different polysaccharides from the roots Actinidia eriantha. Carbohydr Pol 2009, 78:316–322.
2. Jemal A, Bray F, Center MM, Ferlay J, Ward E, Forman D: Global cancer statistics. Ca Cancer J Clin 2011, 60:69–90.
3. WHO/ICO Information Centre on HPV and Cervical Cancer (HPV Information Centre). Human Papillomavirus and Related Cancers in India. Summary Report 2010. www.hpvcentre.net/statistics/reports/IND.pdf.
4. Globocan 2008. globocan.iarc.fr/pages/fact_sheets_cancer.aspx.
5. Gottesman MM: Mechanisms of cancer drug resistance. Annu Rev Med 2002, 53:615–627.
6. Gurib-Fakim A: Medicinal plants: traditions of yesterday and drugs of tomorrow. Mol Aspects Med 2006, 27(1):1–93.
7. Boopathy NS, Kathiresan K: Anticancer drugs from marine flora: an overview. J Oncol 2010, 2010:1–18.
8. Cardazo KHM, Guaratini T, Barros MP, Falcao VR, Tonon AP, Lopes NP, Campos S, Torres MA, Souza AO, Colepicolo P, Pinto E: Metabolites from algae with economic impact. Comparative Biochemistry and Physiology Part C 2007, 146:60–78.
9. Cannell JPR: Algae as a source of biologically active products. Pestic Sci 1993, 39:147–153.
10. Nekhoroshev MV: The black sea algae are potential source of antitumor drugs. Al'-gologiya 1996, 6(1):86–90.
11. Mayer A, Lehmann V: Marine pharmacology in 1999: antitumor and cytotoxic compounds. Anticancer Res 2001, 21:2489–2500.
12. Mayer AMS, Gustafson KR: Marine pharmacology in: antitumor and cytotoxic compounds. Int J Cancer 2000, 2003(105):291–299.
13. Faulkner DJ: Marine natural products. Nat Prod Rep 2000, 17:7–55.
14. Rinehart KL Jr, Shaw PD, Shield LS, Gloer JB, Harbour GC, Koker MES, Samain D, Schwartz RE, Tymiak AA, Weller DL, Carter GT, Munro MHG: Marine natural products as sources of antiviral, antimicrobial, and antineoplastic agents. Pure and Appl Chem 1981, 53:795–871.
15. Tziveleka LA, Vagias C, Roussis V: Natural products with anti-HIV activity from marine organisms. Curr Top Med Chem 2003, 3(13):1512–1535.
16. Konig GM, Wright AD: Marine natural products research. Current directions and future potential. Planta Med 1995, 62:193–211.
17. Bechelli J, Coppage M, Rosell K, Liesveld J: Cytotoxicity of algae extracts on normal and malignant cells. Leuk Res Treatment 2011, 2011:Article ID 373519, 7 pages.
18. Li B, Chu X, Gao M, Li W: Apoptotic mechanism of MCF-7 breast cells in vivo and in vitro induced by photodynamic therapy with C-phycocyanin. Acta Biochim Biophys Sin 2010, 42:80–89.
19. Oftedal L, Selheim F, Wahlsten M, Sivonen K, Døskeland SO, Herfindal L: Marine benthic cyanobacteria contain apoptosis-inducing activity

synergizing with daunorubicin to kill leukemia cells, but not cardiomyocytes. *Mar Drugs* 2010, **8**:2659–2672.

20. Moo-puck R, Robledo D, Fredle-Pelegrin Y: **In vitro cytotoxic and antiproliferative activities of marine macroalgae from Yucatan, Maxico.** *Ciencias Marinas* 2009, **35**(4):345–358.
21. *Algaebase.* http://www.algaebase.org.
22. DeFilippis RA, Goodwin EC, Wu L, DiMaio D: **Endogenous human papillomavirus E6 and E7 proteins differentially regulate proliferation, senescence, and apoptosis in HeLa cervical carcinoma cells.** *J Virol* 2003, **77**:1551–1563.
23. Carmicheal J, DeGraff WG, Gazder AF: **Evaluation of a tetrazolium-based semiautomated colorimetric assay: assessment of chemosensitivity testing.** *Cancer Res* 1987, **47**:936–942.
24. Pang M, Gao Wu Z, Lv N, Wang Z, Tang X, Qu P: **Apoptosis induced by yessotoxins in Hela human cervical cancer cells in vitro.** *Molecular Medicine Reports* 2010, **3**:629–634.
25. Aranda PS, LaJoie DM, Jorcyk CL: **Bleach gel: a simple agarose gel for analyzing RNA quality.** *Electrophoresis* 2002, **33**:366–369.
26. Paglin S, Hollister T, Delohery T, Hackett N, McMahill M, Sphicas E, Domingo D, Yahalom J: **A novel response of cancer cells to radiation involves autophagy and formation of acidic vacicles.** *Cancer Res* 2001, **61**:439–444.
27. Jiao L, Li X, Li T, Jiang P, Wu M, Zhang L: **Characterization and anti-tumor activity of alkali-extracted polysaccharide from *Enteromorpha intestinalis*.** *Int Immunopharmacol* 2009, **9**:324–329.
28. Yang Y, Liang Z, Gu Z, Qin Z: **Molecular mechanism and regulation of autophagy.** *Acta Pharmacol Sin* 2005, **26**(12):1421–1434.
29. Hansen TE, Johansen T: **Following autophagy step by step.** *BMC Biol* 2011, **9**:39.

4

Synthesis and cytotoxic evaluation of some new [1,3]dioxolo[4,5-g]chromen-8-one derivatives

Eskandar Alipour[1], Zinatsadat Mousavi[1], Zahra Safaei[1], Mahboobeh Pordeli[2], Maliheh Safavi[3], Loghman Firoozpour[4], Negar Mohammadhosseini[5], Mina Saeedi[5], Sussan Kabudanian Ardestani[2], Abbas Shafiee[5] and Alireza Foroumadi[5*]

Abstract

Background: Homoisoflavonoids are naturally occurring compounds belong to flavonoid classes possessing various biological properties such as cytotoxicity. In this work, an efficient strategy for the synthesis of novel homoisoflavonoids, [1,3]dioxolo[4,5-g]chromen-8-ones, was developed and all compounds were evaluated for their cytotoxic activities on three breast cancer cell lines.

Methods: Our synthetic route started from benzo[d][1,3]dioxol-5-ol which was reacted with 3-bromopropanoic acid followed by the reaction of oxalyl chloride to afford 6,7-dihydro-8H-[1,3]dioxolo[4,5-g]chromen-8-one. The aldol condensation of the later compound with aromatic aldehydes led to the formation of the title compounds. Five novel derivatives **4a-e** were tested for their cytotoxic activity against three human breast cancer cell lines including MCF-7, T47D, and MDA-MB-231 using the MTT assay.

Results: Among the synthesized compounds, 7-benzylidene-6,7-dihydro-8H-[1,3]dioxolo[4,5-g]chromen-8-one (**4a**) exhibited the highest activity against three cell lines. Also the analysis of acridine orange/ethidium bromide staining results revealed that 7-benzylidene-6,7-dihydro-8H-[1,3]dioxolo[4,5-g]chromen-8-one (**4a**) and 7-(2-methoxybenzylidene)-6,7-dihydro-8H-[1,3]dioxolo[4,5-g]chromen-8-one (**4b**) induced apoptosis in T47D cell line.

Conclusion: Finally, the effect of methoxy group on the cytotoxicity of compounds **4b-4d** was investigated in and it was revealed that it did not improve the activity of [1,3]dioxolo[4,5-g]chromen-8-ones against MCF-7, T47D, and MDA-MB-231.

Keyword: Homoisoflavonoids, [1,3]dioxolo[4,5-g]chromen-8-one, Cancer, Cytotoxic activity

Background

Homoisoflavonoids, naturally occurring compounds belong to flavonoid classes and possess a wide spectrum of biological properties such as anti-inflammatory [1], antioxidant [2], antiproliferative [3], antifungal [4], antiviral [5], and antimutagenic activities [6]. They mainly include a chromanone, chromone, or chromane skeleton and are ubiquitous in plants such as *Ophiopogon* [7], *Polygonatum* [8], *Scilla* [9], *Eucomis* [10], and *Muscari* [11]. Recently, several homoisoflavonoids have been successfully isolated from plants and evaluated for their bioactivities [12,13].

Chalcones have been the center of attention owing to their significant biological activities [14-18]. Also they are the most important precursors for the formation of α, β-unsaturated carbonyl system in flavonoid classes. Homoisoflavonoids including chalcone system have shown selective biological activities [19]. The isolated natural homoisoflavonoids having 3-benzylidenechroman-4-one skeleton were found to be potent and selective MAO-B inhibitors. Compounds involving benzylidene chromanone have depicted significant medicinal properties such as antioxidant [20], anticancer [21], anti-inflammatory [22], anti-human-immune deficiency virus (HIV-I) activities [23].

Two naturally occurring homoisoflavonoids, bonducellin [24] **1** and eucomin [25] **2** (Figure 1), isolated from *Caesalpiniabonducella* and *Eucomis bicolor* BAK (Liliaceae) were

---

* Correspondence: aforoumadi@yahoo.com
[5]Department of Medicinal Chemistry, Faculty of Pharmacy and Pharmaceutical Sciences Research Center, Tehran University of Medical Sciences, Tehran, Iran
Full list of author information is available at the end of the article

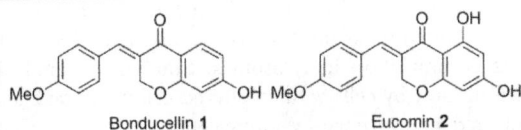
Figure 1 Bonducellin 1 and Eucomin 2.

considered. These compounds and their synthetic analogues have shown important biological properties such as anti-tuberculosis activity [26] and inhibition of protein tyrosine kinase (PTK) [27].

On the synthesis of bioactiveheterocycles containing oxygen specially chalcones and homoisoflavonoids [9,21,28,29]; herein, we focused on new substituted [1,3]dioxolo[4,5-g] chromen-8-one derivatives **4** to profit from both chalcones and homoisoflavonoids (Scheme 1). Then, we evaluated their cytotoxic activities against three human breast cancer cell lines; MCF-7, T47D, and MDA-MB-231 using the MTT assay.

Methods
Chemistry
All starting materials, reagents, and solvents were prepared from Merck (Germany). Melting points were determined on a Kofler hot stage apparatus (Vienna, Austria) and are uncorrected. ^{1}H-NMR spectra were recorded using a Bruker 400 spectrometer (Bruker, Rheinstatten, Germany), and chemical shifts are expressed as δ (ppm) with tetramethylsilane (TMS) as internal standard. The IR spectra were obtained on a Nicolet Magna FT-IR 550 spectrophotometer (potassium bromide disks).

General procedure for the synthesis of [1,3]dioxolo[4,5-g] chromen-8-one derivatives 4
3-(Benzo[d][1,3]dioxol-5-yloxy)propanoic acid **2** and 6,7-dihydro-8H-[1,3]dioxolo[4,5-g]chromen-8-one **3** prepared according to [30] (Scheme 1).

Dry hydrogen chloride gas was passed through an ice-cold solution of 6,7-dihydro-8H-[1,3]dioxolo[4,5-g]chromen-8-one **3** (0.5 mmol) and benzaldehyde derivative (0.7 mol) in absolute EtOH (3 mL) for 2 min. The reaction mixture was allowed to stand at room temperature for 48 h. The precipitated product was filtered off, dried, and recrystallized from ethanol and water.

7-Benzylidene-6,7-dihydro-8H-[1,3]dioxolo[4,5-g]chromen-8-one (4a)
Yield: 48%, mp 141–144°C. IR (KBr): 1664 (C = O) cm^{-1}. ^{1}H-NMR (CDCl$_3$, 400 MHz) δ: 7.83 (s, 1H, benzylidene), 7.43 (s, 1H, H$_9$), 7.42-7.25 (m, 5H, Ph), 6.41 (s, 1H, H$_4$), 6.00 (s, 2H, H$_1$, CH$_2$), 5.29 (s, 2H, CH$_2$). Anal. Calcd. for C$_{17}$H$_{12}$O$_4$: C, 72.85; H, 4.32. Found: C, 72.68; H, 4.18.

7-(2-Methoxybenzylidene)-6,7-dihydro-8H-[1,3]dioxolo[4,5-g] chromen-8-one (4b)
Yield: 31%, mp 160–163°C. IR (KBr): 1660 (C = O) cm^{-1}. ^{1}H-NMR (CDCl$_3$, 400 MHz) δ: 7.961 (s, 1H, benzylidene), 7.39 (s, 1H, H$_9$), 7.04-6.94 (m, 4H, H$_{3'}$, H$_{4'}$, H$_{5'}$, H$_{6'}$), 6.40 (s, 1H, H$_4$), 6.00 (s, 2H, H$_1$, CH$_2$), 5.17 (s, 2H, CH$_2$), 3.86 (s, 3H, OCH$_3$). Anal. Calcd. for C$_{18}$H$_{14}$O$_5$: C, 69.67; H, 4.55. Found: C, 69.52; H, 4.41.

7-(3-Methoxybenzylidene)-6,7-dihydro-8H-[1,3]dioxolo[4,5-g] chromen-8-one (4c)
Yield: 42%, mp 161–163°C. IR (KBr): 1662 (C = O) cm^{-1}. ^{1}H-NMR (CDCl$_3$, 400 MHz) δ: 7.79 (s, 1H, benzylidene), 7.38 (s, 1H, H$_9$), 7.04-6.93 (m, 4H, H$_{2'}$, H$_{4'}$, H$_{5'}$, H$_{6'}$), 6.41 (s, 1H, H$_4$), 6.00 (s, 2H, H$_1$, CH$_2$), 5.29 (s, 2H, CH$_2$), 3.84 (s, 3H, OCH$_3$). Anal. Calcd. for C$_{18}$H$_{14}$O$_5$: C, 69.67; H, 4.55. Found: C, 69.83; H, 4.72.

7-(4-Methoxybenzylidene)-6,7-dihydro-8H-[1,3]dioxolo[4,5-g] chromen-8-one (4d)
Yield: 31%, mp 169–172°C. IR (KBr): 1665 (C = O) cm^{-1}. ^{1}H-NMR (CDCl$_3$, 400 MHz) δ: 7.79 (s, 1H, benzylidene), 7.38 (s, 1H, H$_9$), 7.26 (d, J = 8.4 Hz, 2H, H$_{2'}$, H$_{6'}$), 6.96 (d, J = 8.4 Hz, 2H, H$_{3'}$, H$_{5'}$), 6.42 (s, 1H, H$_4$), 6.00 (s, 2H, H$_1$, CH$_2$), 5.32 (s, 2H, CH$_2$), 3.86 (s, 3H, OCH$_3$). Anal. Calcd. for C$_{18}$H$_{14}$O$_5$: C, 69.67; H, 4.55. Found: C, 69.53; H, 4.82.

7-(Benzo[d][1,3]dioxol-5-ylmethylene)-6,7-dihydro-8H-[1,3] dioxolo[4,5-g]chromen-8-one (4e)
Yield: 42%, mp 198–200°C. IR (KBr): 1667 (C = O) cm^{-1}. ^{1}H-NMR (CDCl$_3$, 400 MHz) δ: 7.73 (s, 1H, benzylidene), 7.37 (s, 1H, H$_9$), 6.86-6.67 (m, 3H, H$_{3'}$, H$_{4'}$, H$_{6'}$), 6.41 (s, 1H, H$_4$), 6.03 (s, 2H, H$_1$,CH$_2$), 6.00 (s, 2H, H$_1$, CH$_2$), 5.29 (s, 2H, CH$_2$). Anal. Calcd. for C$_{18}$H$_{12}$O$_6$: C, 66.67; H, 3.73. Found: C, 66.48; H, 3.55.

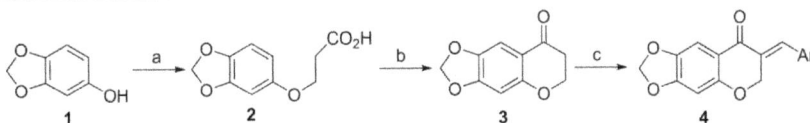
Scheme 1 Synthesis of [1,3]dioxolo[4,5-g]chromen-8-ones 4. (a) NaOH, Na$_2$CO$_3$, Br(CH$_2$)$_2$COOH, H$_2$O, reflux, **(b)** oxalyl chloride, SnCl$_4$, benzene, **(c)** aromatic aldehydes, HCl (g), 0°C.

Biological assay

Cell lines and cell culture

Human breast cancer cell lines including MDA-MB231, MCF-7 and T47D cells were obtained from the National Cell Bank of Iran, Pasteur Institute, Tehran, Iran. Cancer cell lines were grown in RPMI-1640 medium supplemented with 10% heat-inactivated fetal calf serum, 100 μg/ml streptomycin and 100 U/ml penicillin at 37°C in a humidified atmosphere with 5% CO_2.

In vitro cytotoxicity assay

The in vitro cytotoxic activity of [1,3]dioxolo[4,5-g]chromen-8-ones **4a-e** was achieved using MTT colorimetric assay. The *in-vitro* cytotoxic activity of all synthesized compounds were evaluated against three human breast cancer cell lines including MCF-7, T47D and MDA-MB-231 using MTT colorimetric assay according to the method of Mosman [31]. Cancer cell lines were grown in RPMI-1640 medium supplemented with 10% heat-inactivated fetal calf serum (Gibco BRL), 100 μg/ml streptomycin and 100 U/ml penicillin at 37°C in a humidified atmosphere with 5% CO_2.

Briefly, cultures in the exponential growth phase were trypsinized and diluted in complete growth medium to give a total cell count of 5×10^4 cells/ml. 195 μl of the cell suspension was seeded into the wells of 96-well plates (Nunc, Denmark). The plates were incubated overnight in a humidified air atmosphere at 37°C with 5% CO_2. After overnight incubation, 5 μl of the media containing various concentrations of the compounds was added per well in triplicate (final concentration 1, 5, 10 and 20 μg/ml). The plates were incubated for further 72 h. The final concentration of DMSO in the highest concentration of the applied compounds was 0.1%. In each plate, there were three control wells (cells without test compounds) and three blank wells (the medium with 0.1% DMSO) for cell viability. Etoposide and doxorubicine were used as positive controls for cytotoxicity. After treatment, the medium was removed and 200 μl phenol red-free medium containing MTT (1 mg/ml), was added to wells, followed by 4 h incubation. After incubation, the culture medium was then replaced with 100 μl of DMSO and the absorbance of each well was measured by using a microplate reader at 492 nm. For each compound, the concentration causing 50% cell growth inhibition (IC_{50}) compared with the control was calculated from concentration response curves by regression analysis.

Fluorescence microscopy evaluation

Acridine orange/ethidium bromide (AO/EB) double staining [32] was applied to observe the morphological changes in cell death induced by the most potent compounds **4a** and **4b**. Acridine orange is taken up by both viable and dead cells and emitting green fluorescence if intercalated into double stranded nucleic acid (DNA) or red fluorescence if bound to single stranded nucleic acid (RNA) due to its accumulation in lysosomes. Ethidium bromide is taken up only by cells with an altered cell membrane and emits red fluorescence by intercalation into DNA. Cells were seeded in 6-well plates (4×10^5 cell/well) for 24 h. Then, cells were treated with IC_{50} concentration of test compounds for 24 h at 37°C with 5% CO_2. After treatment, cells were washed twice with phosphate buffer saline (PBS) and then 1 μl of dye mixture (100 μg/ml AO and 100 μg/ml EB in PBS) were mixed with 25 μl of cell suspension (0.4×10^6 cells/well) on a clean microscope slide. The suspension was immediately examined by Axoscope 2 plus fluorescence micro- scope from Zeiss (Germany) at 40× magnification.

Results and discussions

Benzo[*d*][1,3]dioxol-5-ol **1** (Scheme 1) was converted to 3-(benzo[d][1,3]dioxol-5-yloxy)propanoic acid **2** and subsequently to 6,7-dihydro-8*H*-[1,3]dioxolo[4,5-g]chromen-8-one **3** according to the procedure [30]. In the next step, we investigated the reaction of 6,7-dihydro-8*H*-[1,3]dioxolo[4,5-g]chromen-8-one **3** and 4-methoxybenzaldehyde to obtain the corresponding product, 7-(4-methoxybenzylidene)-6,7-dihydro-8*H*-[1,3]dioxolo[4,5-g]chromen-8-one (**4d**) (Table 1).

To run successful aldol condensation reaction, acid-catalyzed and base-catalyzed approaches were investigated using various conventional acids and base in different solvents. It was found that the aldol condensation was conducted in better yield in the presence of HCl (g).

Then, various derivatives including 7-(2-methoxybenzylidene)-6,7-dihydro-8*H*-[1,3]dioxolo[4,5-g]chromen-8-one (**4b**) and 7-(3-methoxybenzylidene)-6,7-dihydro-8*H*-[1,3]dioxolo[4,5-g]chromen-8-one (**4c**) possessing methoxy (OMe) group at ortho and meta positions were prepared to compare their bioactivities against the studied cell lines with that of the control. Also other two derivatives, 7-benzylidene-6,7-dihydro-8*H*-[1,3]dioxolo[4,5-*g*]

Table 1 Chemical structures and *in vitro* cytotoxic activity (IC_{50}, μg/ml)[a] of compounds 4a-4e against breast cancer cell lines

Entry	Compound	MCF-7	T47D	MDA-MB-231
1		6.2 ± 0.1	4.6 ± 0.1	9.3 ± 2.1
2		>100	5.7 ± 0.07	27.3 ± 7.1
3		>100	18.8 ± 2.3	29.05 ± 1.7
4		>100	9.2 ± 2.9	>100
5		>100	>100	>100
6	Doxorubicin	0.002 ± 0.002	0.03 ± 0.002	0.006 ± 0.004
7	Etoposide	7.5 ± 0.32	7.9 ± 0.45	11.9 ± 0.87

[a]The IC_{50} values represent an average of three independent experiments (mean ± SD).

chromen-8-one (**4a**) and 7-(benzo[*d*][1,3]dioxol-5-ylmethylene)-6,7-dihydro-8*H*-[1,3]dioxolo[4,5-*g*]chromen-8-one (**4e**) were prepared to investigate the effect of methxoy substituent on the cytotoxicity (Table 1).

The *in vitro* cytotoxic activity of [1,3]dioxolo[4,5-*g*] chromen-8-one derivatives **4**, were tested against three human breast cancer cell lines including MCF-7, T47D, and MDA-MB-231. The 50% growth inhibitory concentration (IC_{50}) for all derivatives were calculated and depicted in Table 1.

According to MTT assay results in Table 1, 7-benzylidene-6,7-dihydro-8*H*-[1,3]dioxolo[4,5-*g*]chromen-8-one (**4a**) showed the highest activity against MCF-7, T47D, and MDA-MB-231 cell lines with IC_{50} values of 6.2 ± 0.1, 4.6 ± 0.1, and 9.3 ± 2.1 µg/ml, respectively. In contrast, 7-(benzo[*d*][1,3]dioxol-5-ylmethylene)-6,7-dihydro-8*H*-[1,3]dioxolo[4,5-*g*]chromen-8-one (**4e**) did not show any cytotoxicity at the concentrations used. It seems that the presence of benzo[*d*][1,3]dioxole in benzylidene moiety decreases the cytotoxic activity of the corresponding compound. As can be seen in Table 1 (Entries 2–4), by introduction of OMe into the ortho, meta or para positions of benzylidenemoiety (compounds **4b**, **4c**, and **4d**), different results were observed. All of them were inactive against MCF-7 cell line ($IC_{50} > 100$ µg/ml), whereas they exhibited good activity against T47D cell line with IC_{50} values of 5.7 ± 0.07, 18.8 ± 2.3, and 9.2 ± 2.9 µg/ml,

respectively. It should be noted that compounds **4b** and **4c** were active against MDA-MB-231 cell line and **4d** did not show any activity in this cell line. Presence of OMe in benzylidene moiety did not play crucial role on the improvement of cytotoxicity effects.

To study the effect of our synthetic compounds on cell lines, acridine orange/ethidium bromide double staining technique was used to evaluate the occurrence of apoptosis in cells. Analysis of the acridine orange/ethidium bromide staining results showed that 7-benzylidene-6,7-dihydro-8*H*-[1,3]dioxolo[4,5-*g*]chromen-8-one (**4a**) and 7-(2-methoxybenzylidene)-6,7-dihydro-8*H*-[1,3]dioxolo [4,5-*g*]chromen-8-one (**4b**) induced apoptosis in T47D cell line (Figure 2). The cells treated with the most potent compounds increased the extent of apoptosis relative to untreated control cells. As shown in Figure 2, the non-apoptotic control cells were stained green and the apoptotic cells had orange particles in their nuclei due to nuclear DNA fragmentation.

Conclusion

In conclusion, novel [1,3]dioxolo[4,5-*g*]chromen-8-one derivatives were synthesized and tested for their cytotoxic activity against three human breast cancer cell lines including MCF-7, T47D, and MDA-MB-231 using the MTT assay. 7-Benzylidene-6,7-dihydro-8*H*-[1,3]dioxolo [4,5-*g*]chromen-8-one (**4a**) showed the highest activity

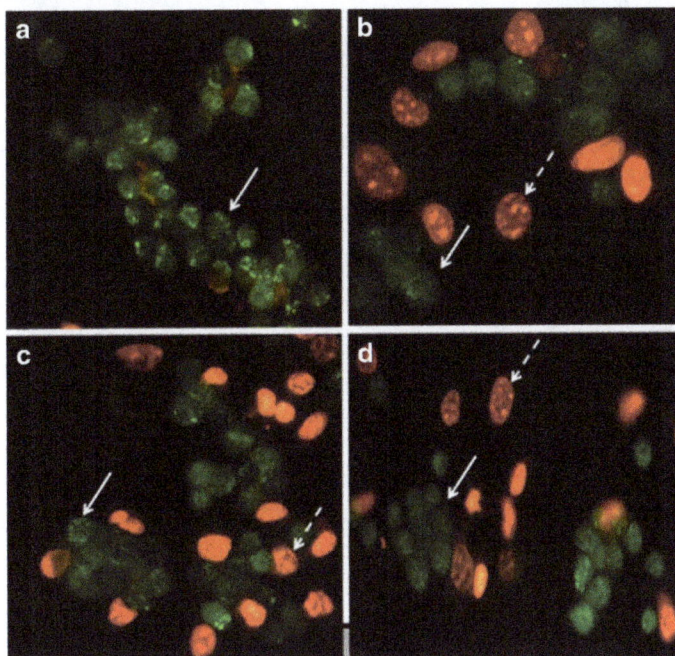

Figure 2 Morphological analysis of T47D cells treated with 4a and 4b by acridine orange/ethidium bromide double staining method.
a) DMSO 1% as control, **b)** etoposide as positive control, **c)** cells treatedwith 4a for 24 h. **d)** cells treatedwith 4b for 24 h. White arrow indicates live cells, dashed arrow shows apoptotic cells. The images of cells were taken with a fluorescence microscope at 400 × magnification.

against the three studied cell lines. Also the analysis of acridine orange/ethidium bromide staining results revealed that the cytotoxic effect of 7-benzylidene-6,7-dihydro-8H-[1,3]dioxolo[4,5-g]chromen-8-one (**4a**) and 7-(2-methoxybenzylidene)-6,7-dihydro-8H-[1,3]dioxolo[4,5-g]chromen-8-one (**4b**) may be due to inducing apoptosis in cancer cell lines.

Competing interests
The authors declare that they have no competing interests.

Authors' contributions
EA: Supervision of the synthetic part. ZM: Synthesis of the title compounds. ZS: Synthesis of the title compounds. MP: Performed the cytotoxic tests. MS: Performed the cytotoxic tests and collaborated in manuscript preparation. LF: Design of target compounds. NM: Synthesis of the title compounds. MS: collaborated in manuscript preparation. SKA: Supervision of the cytotoxic tests. AS: Collaboration in identifying the structures of target compounds. AF: Design of target compounds and supervision of the synthetic and pharmacological parts. All authors read and approved the final manuscript.

Acknowledgements
The authors are thankful for financial support from the Research Council of Islamic Azad University and Iran National Elite Foundation (INEF).

Author details
[1]Department of Chemistry, Islamic Azad University, Tehran-North Branch, Zafar St, Tehran, Iran. [2]Department of Biochemistry, Institute of Biochemistry and Biophysics, University of Tehran, Tehran, Iran. [3]Biotechnology Department, Iranian Research Organization for Science and Technology, Tehran, Iran. [4]Drug Design and Development Research Center, Tehran University of Medicinal Sciences, Tehran, Iran. [5]Department of Medicinal Chemistry, Faculty of Pharmacy and Pharmaceutical Sciences Research Center, Tehran University of Medical Sciences, Tehran, Iran.

References
1. Hung TM, Thu CV, Dat NT, Ryoo SW, Lee JH, Kim JC, Na M, Jung HJ, Bae K, Min BS: Homoisoflavonoid derivatives from the roots of Ophiopogon japonicus and their in vitro anti-inflammation activity. Bioorg Med Chem Lett 2010, 20:2412–2416.
2. Siddaiah V, Maheswara M, Rao CV, Venkateswarlu S, Subbaraju GV: Synthesis, structural revision, and antioxidant activities of antimutagenic homoisoflavonoids from Hoffmanosseggiaintricata. Bioorg Med Chem Lett 2007, 17:1288–1290.
3. Perjési P, Das U, De Clercq E, Balzarini J, Kawase M, Sakagami H, Stables JP, Lorand T, Rozmer Z, Dimmock JR: Design, synthesis and antiproliferative activity of some 3-benzylidene-2,3-dihydro-1-benzopyran-4-ones which display selective toxicity for malignant cells. Eur J Med Chem 2008, 43:839–845.
4. Al Nakib T, Bezjak V, Meegan MJ, Chandy R: Synthesis and antifungal activity of some 3-benzylidenechroman-4-ones, 3-benzylidenethiochroman-4-ones and 2-benzylidene-1-tetralones. Eur J Med Chem 1990, 25:455–462.
5. Tait S, Salvati AL, Desideri N, Fiore L: Antiviral activity of substituted homoisoflavonoids on enteroviruses. Antiviral Res 2006, 72:252–255.
6. Miadokova E, Masterova I, Vlckova V, Duhova V, Toth J: Antimutagenic potential of homoisoflavonoids from Muscari racemosum. J Ethnopharmacol 2002, 81:381–386.
7. Li N, Zhang JY, Zeng KW, Zhang L, Che YY, Tu PF: Anti-inflammatory homoisoflavonoids from the tuberous roots of Ophiopogon japonicus. Fitoterapia 2012, 83:1042–10455.
8. Guo H, Zhao H, Kanno Y, Li W, Mu Y, Kuang X, Inouye Y, Koike K, Jiang H, Bai H: A dihydrochalcone and several homoisoflavonoids from Polygonatum odoratum are activators of adenosine monophosphate-activated protein kinase. Bioorg Med Chem Lett 2013, 23:3137–3139.
9. Bezabih M, Famuyiwa SO, Abegaz BM: HPLC analysis and NMR identification of homoisoflavonoids and stilbenoids from the inter-bulb surfaces of Scilla nervosa. Nat Prod Commun 2009, 4:1367–1370.
10. Koorbanally C, Crouch NR, Langlois A, Du Toit K, Mulholland DA, Drewes SE: Homoisoflavanones and spirocyclic nortriterpenoids from three Eucomis species: E. comosa, E. schijffii and E. pallidiflora subsp. pole-evansii (Hyacinthaceae). S Afr J Bot 2006, 72:428–433.
11. Urbancíková M, Masterová I, Tóth J: Estrogenic/antiestrogenic activity of homoisoflavonoids from bulbs of Muscari racemosum (L.) Miller. Fitoterapia 2002, 73:724–726.
12. Mutanyatta J, Matapa BG, Shushu DD, Abegaz BM: Homoisoflavonoids and xanthones from the tubers of wild and in vitro regenerated Ledebouria graminifolia and cytotoxic activities of some of the homoisoflavonoids. Phytochemistry 2003, 62:797–804.
13. Qi J, Xu D, Zhou YF, Qin MJ, Yu BY: New features on the fragmentation patterns of homoisoflavonoids in Ophiopogon japonicus by high-performance liquid chromatography/diode-array detection/electrospray ionization with multi-stage tandem mass spectrometry. Rapid Commun Mass Spectrum 2010, 24:2193–2206.
14. Hsieh HK, Tsao LT, Wang JP, Lin CN: Synthesis and anti-inflammatory effect of chalcones. J Pharm Pharmacol 2000, 52:163–171.
15. Domínguez JN, León C, Rodrigues J, de Domínguez NG, Gut J, Rosenthal PJ: Synthesis and evaluation of new antimalarial phenylurenylchalcone derivatives. J Med Chem 2005, 48:3654–3658.
16. Nielsen SF, Larsen M, Boesen T, Schønning K, Kromann H: Cationic chalcone antibiotics. design, synthesis, and mechanism of action. J Med Chem 2005, 48:2667–2677.
17. Qiao S, Wang Q, Zhang F, Wang Z, Bowling T, Nare B, Jacobs RT, Zhang J, Ding D, Liu Y, Zhou H: Chalcone–Benzoxaborole hybrid molecules as potent antitrypanosomal agents. J Med Chem 2012, 55:3553–3557.
18. Lorenzo P, Alvarez R, Ortiz MA, Alvarez S, Piedrafita FJ, de Lera AR: Inhibition of IκB kinase-β and anticancer activities of novel chalcone adamantyl arotinoids. J MedChem 2008, 51:5431–5440.
19. Desideri N, Bolasco A, Fioravanti R, Monaco LP, Orallo F, Yáñez M, Ortuso F, Alcaro S: Homoisoflavonoids: natural scaffolds with potent and selective monoamine oxidase-B inhibition properties. J Med Chem 2011, 54:2155–2164.
20. Foroumadi A, Samzadeh-Kermani A, Emami S, Dehghan G, Sorkhi M, Arabsorkhi F, Heidari MR, Abdollahi M, Shafiee A: Synthesis and antioxidant properties of substituted 3-benzylidene-7-alkoxychroman-4-ones. Bioorg Med Chem Lett 2007, 17:6764–6769.
21. Noushini S, Alipour E, Emami S, Safavi M, Ardestani SK, Gohari AR, Shafiee A, Foroumadi A: Synthesis and cytotoxic properties of novel (E)-3-benzylidene-7-methoxychroman-4-one derivatives. DARU J Pharm Sci 2013, 21:31.
22. Shaikh MM, Kruger HG, Bodenstein J, Smith P, du Toit K: Anti-inflammatory activities of selected synthetic homoisoflavanones. Nat Prod Res 2012, 26:1473–1482.
23. Xu ZQ, Bucheit RW, Stup TL, Flavin MT, Khilevich A, Rezzo JD, Lin L, Zembower DE: In vitro anti-human immunodeficiency virus (HIV) activity of the chromanone derivative, 12-oxocalanolide A, a novel NNRTI. Bioorg Med Chem Lett 1998, 8:2179–2184.
24. Purushothaman KK, Kalyani K, Subramaniam K: Structure of bonducellin: a new homoisoflavonoids from Caesalpinia bonducella. India J Chem Sect B: Org Chem Incl Med Chem 1982, 21:383–386.
25. Heller W, Andermatt P, Schaad WA, Tamm E: Homoisoflavonone IV. Neue inhaltsstoffe der eucomin-reihe von Eucomis bicolor. Helv Chim Acta 1976, 59:2048–2058.
26. Yempala T, Sriram D, Yogeeswari P, Kantevari S: Molecular hybridization of bioactives: synthesis and antitubercular evaluation of novel dibenzofuran embodied homoisoflavonoids via Baylis–Hillman reaction. Bioorg Med ChemLett 2012, 22:7426–7430.
27. Lin LG, Xie H, Li HL, Tong LJ, Tang CP, Ke CQ, Liu QF, Lin LP, Geng MY, Jiang H, Zhao WM, Ding J, Ye Y: Naturally occurring homoisoflavonoids function as potent protein tyrosine kinase inhibitors by c-Src-based high-throughput screening. J Med Chem 2008, 51:4419–4429.
28. Nakhjiri M, Safavi M, Alipour E, Emami S, Atash AF, Jafari-Zavareh M, Ardestani SK, Khoshneviszadeh M, Foroumadi A, Shafiee A: Asymmetrical 2,6-bis (benzylidene)cyclohexanones: synthesis, cytotoxic activity and QSAR study. Eur J Med Chem 2012, 50:113–123.

29. Vosooghi M, Yahyavi H, Divsalar K, Shamsa H, Kheirollahi A, Safavi M, Ardestani SK, Sadeghi-Neshat S, Mohammadhosseini N, Edraki N, Khoshneviszadeh M, Shafiee A, Foroumadi A: **Synthesis and In vitro cytotoxic activity evaluation of (E)-16-(substituted benzylidene) derivatives of dehydroepiandrosterone.** *DARU J Pharm Sci* 2013, **21**:34.

30. Cueva JP, Giorgioni G, Grubbs RA, Chemel RB, Watts VJ, Nichols DE: **Trans-2,3-Dihydroxy-6a,7,8,12b-tetrahydro-6H-chromeno[3,4-c] isoquinoline: synthesis, resolution, and preliminary pharmacological characterization of a new dopamine D1 receptor full agonist.** *J Med Chem* 2006, **49**:6848–6857.

31. Mosmann T: **Rapid colorimetric assay for cellular growth and survival: application to proliferation and cytotoxicity assays.** *J Immunol Methods* 1983, **65**:55–63.

32. Baskic D, Popovic S, Ristic P, Arsenijevic NN: **Analysis of cycloheximide-induced apoptosis in human leukocytes: fluorescence microscopy using annexin V/propidium iodide versus acridin orange/ethidium bromide.** *Cell BiolInt* 2006, **30**:924–932.

5

Effect of *Linum usitatissimum* L. (linseed) oil on mild and moderate carpal tunnel syndrome

Mohammad Hashem Hashempur[1,2], Kaynoosh Homayouni[3,4], Alireza Ashraf[5,3*], Alireza Salehi[1], Mohsen Taghizadeh[6] and Mojtaba Heydari[2]

Abstract

Background: Carpal tunnel syndrome is known as the most common entrapment neuropathy. Conservative treatments cannot reduce the symptomatic severity satisfactorily; therefore, effectiveness of *Linum usitatissimum* L. (linseed) oil on carpal tunnel syndrome, as a complementary treatment, was evaluated in the current study. Linseed oil is a well-known preparation in Iranian traditional medicine and its analgesic, anti-inflammatory and anti-oxidative effects have been shown in previous studies.

Methods: A randomized, double-blind, placebo-controlled clinical trial was conducted. One hundred patients (155 hands) with idiopathic mild to moderate carpal tunnel syndrome aged between 18 and 65 years old were randomized in two parallel groups. These two groups were treated during 4 weeks with topical placebo and linseed oil. In addition, a night wrist splint was prescribed for both groups. Symptomatic severity and functional status were measured using Boston Carpal Tunnel Questionnaire. In addition, median sensory nerve conduction velocity, motor distal latency, sensory distal latency and compound latency as electrodiagnostic parameters were measured at baseline and after the intervention period.

Results: After the intervention, significant improvement was observed regarding Boston Carpal Tunnel Questionnaire symptomatic severity and functional status mean differences ($p < 0.001$) in the linseed oil group compared with those in the placebo group. Also, regarding the mean differences of both groups, significant improvement of nerve conduction velocity of the median nerve was seen in the linseed oil group by a value of 2.38 m/sec ($p < 0.05$). However, motor distal latency and sensory distal latency of the median nerve showed no between-group significant changes ($p = 0.14$ for both items). Finally, compound latency was improved slightly in the case group, comparing mean differences between the groups ($p < 0.05$). No significant adverse events were reported from using linseed oil.

Conclusions: It seems that linseed oil could be effective in the management of mild and moderate carpal tunnel syndrome, especially in improving the severity of symptoms and functional status. In addition, its effect on electerodiagnostic parameters, especially on the nerve conduction velocity, can be considered as a valuable point.

Keywords: Carpal tunnel syndrome, *Linum usitatissimum*, Linseed oil, Iranian traditional medicine, Randomized controlled trial, Herbal medicine, Complementary therapies

* Correspondence: sbahar7@gmail.com
[5]Shiraz Burn Research Center, Shiraz University of Medical Sciences, Shiraz, Iran
[3]Department of Physical Medicine and Rehabilitation, Shiraz University of Medical Sciences, Shiraz, Iran
Full list of author information is available at the end of the article

Background

Carpal tunnel syndrome (CTS), a condition in which the median nerve compression occurs, is known as the most common entrapment neuropathy [1]. Various treatment options, as surgical and non-surgical, have been suggested for CTS. Surgery is usually considered for patients with an experience of conservative treatment failure and those who have severe CTS [2,3], while non-surgical treatments are usually prescribed as an initial option for the patients who do not have any evidence of denervation in electromyography, cannot undergo surgery, or suffer from non-constant symptoms of mild to moderate CTS [4,5]. Standard non-surgical treatments vary from exercise and activity modification to wrist splinting (as the most frequently reported treatment [6]), use of oral medications like NSAIDs and corticosteroids, and even locally injected steroids [7,8]. However, conservative treatments cannot reduce symptomatic severity satisfactorily [9-11]; therefore, new conservative treatments are needed to be evaluated in randomized controlled trials.

Nowadays, complementary and alternative medicine (CAM) is welcomed by general population, governments and World Health Organization. Easy accessibility, lower costs and origination of them from nature are the main causes of this worldwide popularity [12]. Therefore, CAM treatments can play an important role as new conservative treatments for CTS.

Linum usitatissimum L. (from the family Linaceae), commonly known as flax or linseed, is a herb that is native to Europe, Asia and Mediterranean regions [13]. Linseed oil or flaxseed oil is obtained from its dried ripe seeds. In addition to edible uses of this oil, it is known as an anti-inflammatory [14,15] antioxidant [16,17] and analgesic [18] oil. Therefore, due to the mentioned beneficial properties, it is used in several studies on a variety of subjects such as arthritis [15], dermatologic complaints [19], breast cancer [20] and even keratoconjunctivitis [21].

The topical use of linseed oil has been approved for a variety of skin disorders [22]. For instance, the Brazilian national pharmacopoeia has approved its topical administration in cases with pruritus, and in patients of burn [13]. In addition, some studies examined the topical usage of this compound in animal model of skin wound healing, and in the prevention of peri-ileostomy skin excoriation. No toxicity was reported in such studies [23].

Linseed oil could play an anti-inflammatory role when used by different routes of administration in animal models. In fact, its inhibition on prostaglandin E_2, leukotriene B_4, histamine and bradykinin can make it a potent anti-inflammatory agent against distinct phases of inflammation, comparable with standard aspirin [24]. In addition, it seems that analgesic activity of linseed oil is peripherally mediated [18]. Analgesic activity of linseed oil may be due to a combination of its inhibitory effect of prostaglandin, histamine, bradykinin and acetylcholine [25].

In addition, linseed oil is a well-known and frequently-used medicine in Iranian traditional medicine (ITM). According to the most famous and reliable ITM books, i.e. Avicenna's Canon of Medicine and Liber Continens of Rhazes, linseed oil can be used as an analgesic and anti-fibrosis drug [26,27].

Therefore, according to ITM concepts and some unpublished experiences by experts about potential effect of linseed oil on CTS and also supporting data about some properties of linseed oil (e.g. analgesic, antioxidant and anti-inflammatory), we hypothesized its possible effect for CTS. Therefore, the current study aimed to assess the effectiveness of topical flaxseed oil in patients with mild and moderate CTS.

Materials and methods

Study design

The study was designed as a two-arm, randomized, placebo-controlled, double- blind clinical trial using a parallel design.

Ethical considerations

The study protocol was in compliance with the Declaration of Helsinki (1989 revision) and approved by the Local Medical Ethics Committee of Shiraz University of Medical Sciences (SUMS) with reference number: CT-92-6709. The trial was registered in Iranian Registry of Clinical Trials (registration ID: IRCT2012103111341N1). A written informed consent was signed by all of the enrolled participants.

Preparation of test drug, placebo and wrist splint

Seeds of the test drug were purchased from the local market and authenticated by a botanist at Kashan University of Medical Sciences. A voucher specimen was preserved for future reference.

The seeds were coarsely ground in an environment of mild heat, and then cold-pressed (35°C). The extracted oil was subjected to gas chromatographic (GC) analysis. The findings revealed the presence of major components as linolenic acid (54.2%), oleic acid (20.39%), linoleic acid (12.26%), palmitic acid (5.99%), and stearic acid (5.7%). Nitrogen purging was carried out to avoid oxidation. In addition, the bottles had no head space (the oil was filled to the bottle brim).

Pharmaceutical graded paraffin was considered as the placebo. In addition, standard coloring agent in a little amount and standard range was used to make paraffin's color similar to that of the linseed oil.

A wrist splint (Dr. K. H.*) immobilized the wrist in an extension position (external angle: 20° and internal angle: 5°). The splint was made of 5-mm medical foam, lined internally with fabric and externally with thin leather. In addition, it had three adjustable Velcro fastenings on its dorsal side (Figure 1).

Inclusion and exclusion criteria

Patients (from the Outpatient Clinic of Shahid Faghihi Hospital, an academic teaching center, affiliated with SUMS) with suspected CTS (according to history and physical examination) were selected after electrophysiologic confirmation study.

Detailed inclusion and exclusion criteria are shown in Table 1. The eligibility criteria included briefly: patients of both sexes aged between 18 and 65 years old, with idiopathic mild and moderate CTS. Some of the most important exclusion criteria were: coexisting serious illness, rheumatoid arthritis, CTS related to systemic diseases and pregnancy. In addition, the patients were excluded if they had previous surgery for CTS or intracarpal steroid injections.

Electrodiagnosis

The electrophysiologic assessments were performed by a "MEDLEC SYNERGY VIASIS" electromyography device with two 6 mm felt tips bar electrodes as the stimulators and recorders (diameter of pads 23 mm apart). Median distal motor latency was measured by a bipolar stimulating electrode at the wrist and a bipolar surface-recording located on the abductor pollicis brevis muscle (8 cm from stimulus electrodes at the wrist). Antidromic sensory nerve action potentials evoked at the wrist were recorded from the middle finger. Standard distances (7 cm from recorder, at mid palm and 14 cm from recorder at wrist) were kept between the stimulator and recorder electrodes. For recording the compound nerve action potential, stimulation at mid palm and recording at wrist (7 cm apart) was performed. In addition, using a

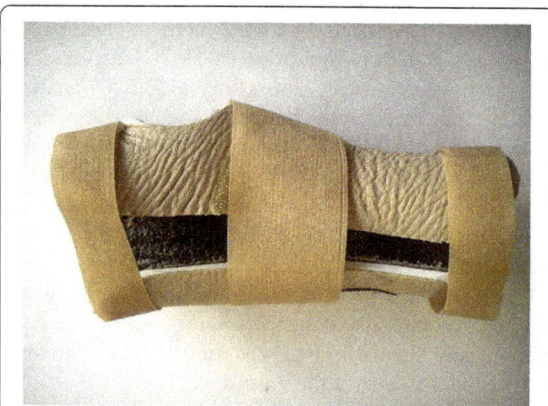

Figure 1 A photograph of fabricated wrist splint that was prescribed for all of the participants (dorsal view).

concentric needle electrode, electromyography was performed on the abductor pollicis brevis muscle. We defined denervation as sustained, abnormal spontaneous activity. This ranged from 0 to 4+, in the form of positive waves or fibrillations. The skin temperature during all of the electrodiagnostic studies was at least 31°C and all of the assessments were carried out in a similar constant room temperature between 23°C and 25°C. In addition, due to the possibility of diurnal variation in clinical and electrophysiologic assessments [28], all of the patients were assessed at the follow up visit at a similar time of the day as the first session. In addition, the patients were assessed on their visits by the same authors (K.H and A.A) who performed clinical examinations and electrodiagnostic assessments and were blinded about each patient's allocation.

Intervention

Splint

All of the patients were prescribed to use the wrist splint during the study period. In fact, the test drug and placebo were added to this standard treatment. The wrist splint prescription was night-only because of symptoms usually worsening at night, in addition to obtaining a higher compliance, considering the patient's concern about splint's interference with his/her daily activities.

Placebo and test drug

Both of the drug and placebo were prescribed to be used in the morning and evening time for a period of 4 weeks, 5 drops per use, topically on the palmar wrist territory. The patients were advised not to massage the mentioned zone.

Outcome assessment

Boston Carpal Tunnel Questionnaire (BCTQ), as a self-administered, validated measurement, was the primary outcome measure. The BCTQ assesses symptom severity score (BCTQ SYMPT) and functional status score (BCTQ FUNCT). These scores are evaluated by an eleven-item scale and an eight-item scale, respectively [29]. The items of each scale consist of multiple-choice responses from 1 (as the mildest) to 5 (as the most severe). The BCTQ SYMPT and FUNCT are calculated as the mean of the scores for the individual items.

We used the Persian version of BCTQ that was validated previously, showing to have a reasonable reliability, sensitivity and internal consistency [30].

Secondary outcome measures were median nerve sensory distal latency (SDL), sensory nerve conduction velocity (NCV), motor distal latency (MDL) and compound latency (CL).

At the beginning of the enrollment and after 4 weeks of intervention, the data related to both primary and

Table 1 Inclusion and exclusion criteria

Inclusion criteria	Patients of both sexes aged between 18 and 65 years old willing to sign the informed consent form
	Clinical symptoms and signs of CTS (at least 2 symptoms or 1 sign plus 1 symptom[37]), including:
	- Pain
	- Paraesthesia
	- Hypoesthesia
	- Numbness
	- Tingling
	- Positive Phalen test
	- Positive Tinnel test
	Electrodiagnostic evidence of mild and moderate idiopathic CTS, including:
	• SDL > 3.7 m Sec
	• SNCV < 40 m/Sec
	• MDL > 4.2 m Sec
	• CL > 2.4 m Sec
Exclusion criteria	Positive history of hypersensitivity to linseed oil
	Inability of data gathering forms completion (such as cognitive impairment or language problem)
	Patients with severe CTS, clinical and electrodiagnostic evidence including (if any of these evidences was found):
	– Thenar atrophy
	–Fibrillation potentials or reinnervation on needle EMG of APB muscle
	–Electrophisiologic study:
	• SDL > 5.3 m Sec OR Absent
	• SNCV < 28 m/Sec
	• MDL > 6.5 m Sec OR Absent
	• CL > 3.2 m Sec
	Coexisting cervical radiculopathies, brachial plexopathies or more proximal median mononeuropathies
	Clinical and electrophysiological signs of polyneuropathy
	Rheumatologic diseases, like RA, systemic sclerosis, SLE and amyloidosis
	Endocrinologic diseases, such as DM and hypothyroidism
	Conditions that can mimic CTS such as multiple sclerosis
	Pregnancy
	Coexisting serious illness, such as renal and heart failure
	Recent or ongoing inevitable use of corticosteroids or analgesics
	Previous surgery for CTS
	Intra-articular injection within the previous 6 months
	Positive history of severe trauma or fracture of wrist bones

SDL: sensory distal latency; SNCV: sensory nerve conduction velocity; MDL: motor distal latency; CL: compound latency; EMG: electromyography; APB: abductor policis brevis; RA: rheumatoid arthritis; SLE: systemic lupus erythematosus; DM: diabetes mellitus.

secondary outcome measures were obtained and recorded on the patient's data form. We excluded the patients who had recent or ongoing inevitable use of corticosteroids or analgesics; however, the included patients were asked to record their use of analgesics as the rescue drug.

Randomization, blinding and concealment of allocation

The eligible patients were randomly allocated to two parallel groups, the drug and placebo groups, by the secretary of the clinic. She was trained and instructed to use a block-randomization list (non-stratified, with the same block lengths, generated by computer) sequentially. In the case of patients affected by CTS bilaterally, both wrists were allocated to the same intervention (i.e. drug or placebo). The physicians, researchers, and statisticians were blind to the allocation of patients. Moreover, due to the same shape and size of the drug and placebo containers and similarity in color, the patients were blind to their allocation.

Statistical analysis

The intention-to-treat population used in all of the analyses included all randomized patients who completed their follow up, whether adhering completely to the clinical trial protocol or not.

Demographic and clinical characteristics of the participants were shown as the mean ± standard deviation (SD) for continuous variables. Differences of pre- and post-treatment were reported as mean and 95% confidence intervals.

Normality for continuous variables was checked using Kolmogorov-Smirnov test. Data were analyzed using Chi-square test, independent and paired samples t-test, and Mann–Whitney test. P values less than 0.05 were considered statistically significant.

Results

The first enrollment was done in October 2013 and the last patient's follow-up was completed in January 2014. A total of 119 patients (183 hands) were assessed for eligibility, and finally 100 patients (155 hands) who were eligible and gave their written informed consent were randomly assigned to drug and placebo groups (79 and 76 hands for placebo and drug, respectively). Sixty four hands in the linseed oil group and 68 hands in the placebo group completed the study. Detailed description of the patients' enrolment, randomization and outcomes are outlined in Figure 2.

The baseline demographic and clinical characteristics of the patients are shown in Table 2. No significant differences with regard to age, gender, duration of symptoms and BMI were observed between two arms. Additionally,

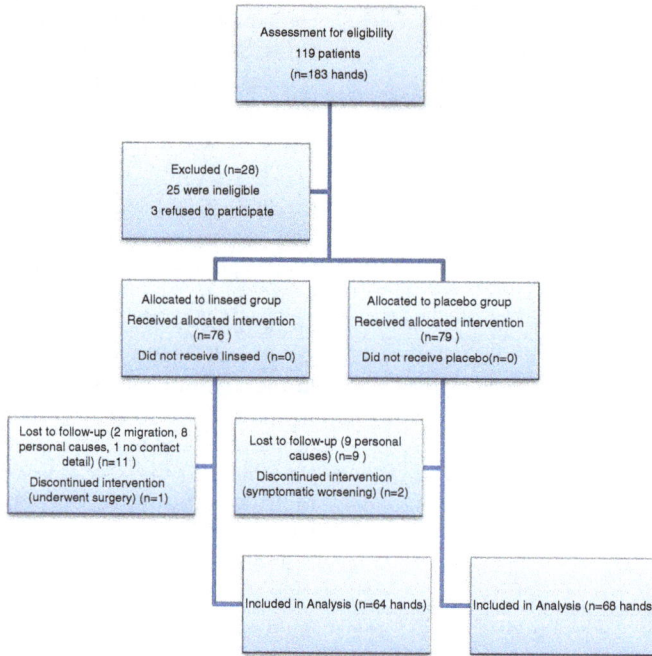

Figure 2 The trail flowchart.

baseline measures for all of the outcome assessments were similar in both groups.

The patients were asked about their adherence to the study protocol at the follow-up visit. In the linseed oil group, only 3 patients reported some missing doses of oil and 2 patients had not used the splint as it was prescribed. In addition, in the placebo group 4 and 2 patients reported some forgotten doses of oil and inappropriate use of splint, respectively. However, all of them were analyzed in

the predetermined groups. Additionally, according to the patients' report, no rescue drug was used by them in each group.

Table 3 shows a full description of each outcome measurement changes, considering before and after trial, as well as mean differences in each group. Comparison of the mean differences between the groups showed a significant improvement in BCTQ SYMPT and FUNCT of the linseed oil group, after a 4 week period of

Table 2 Baseline demographic and clinical characteristics of participants in the two groups of linseed oil and placebo

Variable	Placebo group (n = 79)	Linseed oil group (n = 76)	p value	Statistical test
Age (years), Mean(±SD)	45.01(±8.71)	42.95(±10.63)	0.227	t-test
Male/female (n)	4/64	10/54	0.069	Chi-Square
Duration(months), Mean(±SD)	13.66(±13.45)	13.56(±13.78)	0.912	Mann–Whitney
BMI (kg/m^2), Mean(±SD)	27.03(±3.25)	25.99(±5.22)	0.173	t-test
BCTQ SYMPT (pts), Mean(±SD)	2.75(±0.62)	2.74(±0.75)	0.921	t-test
BCTQ FUNCT (pts), Mean(±SD)	2.41(±0.74)	2.61(±0.71)	0.120	t-test
Median NCV (m/sec), Mean(±SD)	36.27(±4.29)	35.54(±3.81)	0.303	t-test
Median MDL (msec), Mean(±SD)	4.16(±0.20)	4.20(±0.34)	0.384	t-test
Median CL (msec), Mean(±SD)	2.533(±0.17)	2.52(±0.14)	0.872	t-test
Median SDL (msec), Mean(±SD)	3.99(±0.26)	3.95(±0.43)	0.519	t-test

SD: standard deviation, BMI: body mass index, BCTQ: Boston Carpal Tunnel Questionnaire, SYMPT: symptom severity, FUNCT: functional status, pts: points, NCV: nerve conduction velocity, MDL: motor distal latency, CL: compound latency, SDL: sensory distal latency.

Table 3 Changes in BCTQ symptoms, BCTQ function and electrophysiologic measurements, comparing mean values before and after trial within groups, and mean differences between groups

	Study groups	Before (Mean ± SD)	After (Mean ± SD)	p-value	Statistical test	Mean difference	p-value	Statistical test
BCTQ SYMPT	Linseed oil	2.74 ± 0.75	1.90 ± 0.54	<0.0001	Paired t-test	0.83 ± 0.59 (CI 95% 0.69–0.99)	<0.001	Independent t-test
	Placebo	2.75 ± 0.62	2.59 ± 0.75	<0.0001	Paired t-test	0.16 ± 0.48 (CI95% 0.05–0.28)		
BCTQ FUNCT	Linseed oil	2.61 ± 0.71	2.17 ± 0.71	<0.0001	Paired t-test	0.44 ± 0.5 (CI 95% 0.32–0.56)	<0.001	Independent t-test
	Placebo	2.41 ± 0.74	2.59 ± 0.80	0.024	Paired t-test	- 0.18 ± 0.5 (CI 95% -0.31- -0.07)		
Median NCV	Linseed oil	35.54 ± 3.81	37.92 ± 6.23	0.007	Paired t-test	2.38 ± 6.78 (CI 95% 0.72–4.04)	0.034	Independent t-test
	Placebo	36.27 ± 4.29	36.22 ± 6.07	0.57	Paired t-test	0.04 ± 6.21 (CI 95% -1.52–1.43)		
Median MDL	Linseed oil	4.20 ± 0.34	4.06 ± 0.33	<0.0001	Paired t-test	0.14 ± 0.29 (CI 95% 0.07–0.21)	0.140	Independent t-test
	Placebo	4.16 ± 0.20	4.10 ± 0.35	<0.0001	Paired t-test	0.06 ± 0.32 (CI 95% -0.02–0.14)		
Median CL	Linseed oil	2.52 ± 0.14	2.43 ± 0.23	0.004	Paired t-test	0.09 ± 0.21 (CI 95% 0.03–0.15)	0.044	Independent t-test
	Placebo	2.53 ± 0.17	2.54 ± 0.32	0.145	Paired t-test	−0.008 ± 0.28 (CI 95% -0.08–0.06)		
Median SDL	Linseed oil	3.95 ± 0.43	3.82 ± 0.34	0.032	Paired t-test	0.12 ± 0.45 (CI 95% 0.01–0.24)	0.144	Independent t-test
	Placebo	3.99 ± 0.26	3.97 ± 0.36	0.053	Paired t-test	0.02 ± 0.36 (CI 95% -0.07–0.11)		

SD: standard deviation, BCTQ: Boston Carpal Tunnel Questionnaire, SYMPT: symptom severity, FUNCT: functional status, NCV: nerve conduction velocity, MDL: motor distal latency, CL: compound latency, SDL: sensory distal latency, CI 95%: 95%confidence interval

treatment (p <0.001). Mean differences of these measures were 0.83 (CI 95% 0.69 – 0.99) and 0.44 (CI 95% 0.32 – 0.56), respectively.

In addition, regarding mean differences of both groups, a significant improvement of NCV of the median nerve was seen in the linseed oil group by a difference of 2.38 m/sec (CI 95% 0.72 – 4.04, $p = 0.034$). However, mean differences of the median nerve's MDL and SDL in the linseed oil group showed no significant differences as compared with the placebo group ($p = 0.14$ for both items). Finally, comparison of the mean differences between the groups revealed a slight improvement in the CL of the linseed oil group (CI 95% 0.03 – 0.15, $p = 0.044$).

Safety and tolerability

The patients in both groups were asked about positive history of dermal reactions to any topical products and if it was positive, they were instructed to test the prescribed oil on their arm for the first use.

Linseed oil was well tolerated by patients. No serious adverse effects, neither local nor systemic, were reported in the treated group. Likewise, no additional neuropathy or local neural injury was noted in electrophysiologic tests on the follow-up visit.

Discussion

To the best of our knowledge, the present study is the first research to evaluate the effects of linseed oil on CTS. However, this herbal preparation has an ancient history of administration for different disorders, dating back to more than 10 centuries ago in ITM [22,23]. Linseed oil is a rich source of α-linolenic acid that has been proved to possess noticeable anti-inflammatory activity

[31]. In addition, further studies have confirmed its anti-inflammatory [14,15], antioxidant [16,17], and analgesic [18] properties.

Different mechanisms for its anti-inflammatory effects are explained. The linseed oil inhibits prostaglandin E_2, leukotriene B_4, histamine and bradykinin-induced inflammation. The oil also inhibits arachidonic acid-induced inflammation. It shows inhibition of both cyclooxygenase and lipoxygenase pathways of arachidonate metabolism [18]. Similar to other multiple herbal formulations, anesthetic properties of topical use of linseed is also shown in animal models [32]. According to the important role of inflammatory and oxidative processes in the pathophysiology of CTS [33,34], its significant effect on improving symptomatic and functional status of our patients, and slightly but statistically significant improving effect on NCV and CL can be explained partially.

Although no previous study on the efficacy of linseed oil on CTS was found, some studies evaluated other herbal preparations in the management of CTS. In a study by Zhang et al. on the efficacy of Chinese herbal therapy on CTS comparing with two other groups, 22 patients who received this therapy had a superior benefit on their visual analogue scale (VAS) score than the splint group and no significant changes of electromyography was shown [35]. Our results are in compliance with symptomatic relief of their patients with a common aspect about the presence of oleic and linoleic acid in some of these used herbs. However, this study was not blind and had a small sample size. Furthermore, they did not assess the effects of a specific herb with determined constituents and they used an uncommon drug delivery system (steaming and washing). Also, Branco et al. published an open protocol study in which CTS patients, who experienced standard treatments failure, were treated by a two-stage protocol. They were treated primarily with a specific laser acupuncture and microamps transcutaneous electrical nerve stimulation and secondarily with herbal formulas and supplements in a case-by-case manner [36]. Similar to our trial, this small size study (only 36 patients) showed a significant effect on symptomatic improvement (91.6%). However, the complexity of their management can result in practical difficulties during usage.

Another notable study, which was conducted by Eftekharsadat et al. on two groups of 30 patients, evaluated the efficacy of topical *Eremostachys laciniata* on CTS. This medicinal herb has been shown to have anti-inflammatory and antioxidant properties, like linseed oil. They showed significant improvement on palmar prehension and VAS of pain, compared with placebo. However, this plant had a local popularity, and no significant effect on electrodiagnostic criterion was reported [37].

There is also a case-series carried out by Jung et al. that assessed the usefulness of Jackyakamcho-tang on muscle spasm and pain on 81 patients complaining about these symptoms. The usefulness was reported as 72.8% for treating CTS (where only 11 CTS patients had been included). But, unlike the safety of linseed oil, they reported adverse effects in 11.1% of the total patients, 3.7% of which were severe [38].

In regard of the topical treatment for CTS, few studies were found. Of those, Jazayeri et al. published a clinical trial evaluating EMLA cream which had some beneficial effects [39]. However, this trial was not blind and EMLA cream was not as cheap and available as linseed oil.

According to ITM, patient's temperament can affect some herbal medicine effects [40]. Therefore, as a minor assessment we evaluated the participant's temperament. However, no relationship was found between the participant's temperament and outcome measures. It could be explained in some ways. The used questionnaire was not designed for our target population [41] and the drug effects are possibly independent of the patient's temperament.

Linseed oil has some important advantages as feasibility of use as a topical drug and no disturbance of ordinary daily activities (comparable with treatments such as wrist splint), conservative and noninvasive nature (regarding some invasive options such as surgery), price of the oil (1 $ for a 40 cc bottle that is adequate for a one month use), worldwide availability, and its acceptable and significant effects, especially on symptomatic and functional status and even on some electrodiagnostic parameters.

Study limitations

Here we should highlight some limitations that we have faced with in this trial. First, insufficient number of male participants (only about 10.5% of our patients), which can affect the generalizability of our findings. In fact, according to previous epidemiologic studies, about 30% of CTS encounters were attributable to males [42]. Indeed, this is a common problem in several trials on CTS, even with male samples as small as 0-10% [43-45].

Second, as regards to reliable and valid assessment by BCTQ about subjective functional status of patients, objective functional outcome measures such as dynamometer findings could offer more reliable results.

The other important issue is to determine the transdermal penetration of the linseed oil. In this respect, the measurement of transdermal permeation of the oil and its consequent absorption into the systemic circulation can be the subject of the future studies.

And finally, the short term follow-up is another limitation. However, this is partially related to our aim as evaluation of efficacy and safety of topical linseed oil as a new complementary treatment for the management of CTS. It is also considerable that herbal medicaments might show delayed pharmacological activity. Thus, long term assessment possibly leads to better results. On the other side, unwanted effects may also be revealed in long term evaluation.

Conclusion

It seems that linseed oil could be effective as an adjunctive therapy in the management of mild and moderate CTS, especially in improving the severity of symptoms and functional status. In addition, its effect on electerodiagnostic parameters, especially on NCV, can be considered as a valuable point.

It is, therefore, suggested that further trials of longer follow-up and larger sample size, including appropriate male/female ratio and objective functional status outcome measures are needed to confirm the value of linseed oil as a good choice for CTS and for evaluation of the involved mechanisms. Moreover, other easily applicable pharmaceutical dosage forms (such as ointment, cream, gel and patch form) can be considered in future studies.

Abbreviations
CTS: Carpal tunnel syndrome; ITM: Iranian traditional medicine; BCTQ: Boston carpal tunnel questionnaire; NCV: Nerve conduction velocity; MDL: Motor distal latency; SDL: Sensory distal latency; CL: Compound latency; CAM: Complementary and alternative medicine; BMI: Body mass index; SUMS: Shiraz University of Medical Sciences; GC: Gas chromatography; SYMPT: Symptom severity; FUNCT: Functional status; SD: Standard deviation; VAS: Visual analogue scale.

Competing interests
The authors declare no competing interests.

Authors' contributions
MHH has made substantial contributions in conception, designing, acquisition of data and drafted the manuscript. KH had contribution in designing and preformed electrodiagnostic assessments. AA had

contribution in designing, preformed electrodiagnostic assessments and revised the manuscript critically for important intellectual content. AS had contribution in designing and analyzing of data. MT produced the linseed oil and performed its standardization. MH had contribution in conception and designing and revised the manuscript critically for important intellectual content. All authors read and approved the final manuscript.

Acknowledgments
This study was a part of a PhD thesis by Dr. Mohammad Hashem Hashempur that was supported by Shiraz University of Medical Sciences (grant number: 92–6709). The authors would like to thank the Vice Chancellery of Technology and Research of the University, all the study participants for their participation, the University's Research Consultation Center for editing the final manuscript.

Author details
[1]Research Center for Traditional Medicine and History of Medicine, Shiraz University of Medical Sciences, Shiraz, Iran. [2]Essence of Parsiyan Wisdom Institute, Traditional Medicine and Medicinal Plant Incubator, Shiraz University of Medical Sciences, Shiraz, Iran. [3]Department of Physical Medicine and Rehabilitation, Shiraz University of Medical Sciences, Shiraz, Iran. [4]Shiraz Geriatric Research Center, Shiraz University of Medical Sciences, Shiraz, Iran. [5]Shiraz Burn Research Center, Shiraz University of Medical Sciences, Shiraz, Iran. [6]Research Center for Biochemistry and Nutrition in Metabolic Disease, Kashan University of Medical Sciences, Kashan, Iran.

References
1. Ashraf A, Daghaghzadeh A, Naseri M, Nasiri A, Fakheri M: A study of interpolation method in diagnosis of carpal tunnel syndrome. Ann Indian Acad Neurol 2013, 16:623–626.
2. Bleecker ML: Splinting vs surgery for carpal tunnel syndrome. JAMA 2003, 289:420.
3. Di Geronimo G, Caccese AF, Caruso L, Soldati A, Passaretti U: Treatment of carpal tunnel syndrome with alpha-lipoic acid. Eur Rev Med Pharmacol Sci 2009, 13:133–139.
4. Page MJ, Massy-Westropp N, O'Connor D, Pitt V: Splinting for carpal tunnel syndrome. Cochrane Database Syst Rev 2012, 7:CD010003.
5. Ashraf A, Moghtaderi A, Yazdani A, Mirshams S: Evaluation of effectiveness of local insulin injection in none insulin dependent diabetic patient with carpal tunnel syndrome. Electromyogr Clin Neurophysiol 2008, 49:161–166.
6. Miller RS, Iverson DC, Fried RA, Green LA, Nutting PA: Carpal tunnel syndrome in primary care: a report from ASPN. Ambulatory Sentinel Practice Network. J Fam Pract 1994, 38:337–344.
7. Bland JD: Carpal tunnel syndrome. BMJ 2007, 335:343–346.
8. Piazzini DB, Aprile I, Ferrara PE, Bertolini C, Tonali P, Maggi L, Rabini A, Piantelli S, Padua L: A systematic review of conservative treatment of carpal tunnel syndrome. Clin Rehabil 2007, 21:299–314.
9. Marshall S, Tardif G, Ashworth N: Local corticosteroid injection for carpal tunnel syndrome. Cochrane Database Syst Rev 2002, 4:CD001554.
10. O'Connor D, Marshall S, Massy-Westropp N: Non-surgical treatment (other than steroid injection) for carpal tunnel syndrome. Cochrane Database Syst Rev 2003, 1:CD003219.
11. Scholten RJ, Mink van der Molen A, Uitdehaag BM, Bouter LM, de Vet HC: Surgical treatment options for carpal tunnel syndrome. Cochrane Database Syst Rev 2007, 4:CD003905.
12. World Health Organization: WHO traditional medicines strategy 2002–2005. Geneva: World Health Organization; 2002.
13. de Souza FE, de Aquino CM, de Medeiros PL, Evencio LB, da Silva Goes AJ, de Souza Maia MB: Effect of a Semisolid Formulation of Linum usitatissimum L (Linseed) Oil on the Repair of Skin Wounds. Evid Based Complement Alternat Med 2012, 2012:270752.
14. Kaithwas G, Majumdar DK: Therapeutic effect of linum usitatissimum (flaxseed/linseed) fixed oil on acute and chronic arthritic models in albino rats. Inflammopharmacology 2010, 18:127–136.
15. Singh S, Nair V, Gupta YK: Linseed oil: an investigation of its antiarthritic activity in experimental models. Phytother Res 2012, 26:246–252.
16. Shahidi F: Antioxidant factors in plant foods and selected oilseeds. Biofactors 2000, 13:179–185.
17. Kinniry P, Amrani Y, Vachani A, Solomides CC, Arguiri E, Workman A, Carter J, Christofidou-Solomidou M: Dietary flaxseed supplementation ameliorates inflammation and oxidative tissue damage in experimental models of acute lung injury in mice. J Nutr 2006, 136:1545–1551.
18. Kaithwas G, Mukherjee A, Chaurasia AK, Majumdar DK: Anti-inflammatory, analgesic and antipyretic activities of Linum usitatissimum L. (flaxseed/linseed) fixed oil. Indian J Exp Biol 2011, 49:932–938.
19. Rahman M, Alam K, Ahmad MZ, Gupta G, Afzal M, Akhter S, Kazmi I, Jyoti, Ahmad FJ, Anwar F: Classical to current approach for treatment of psoriasis: a review. Endocr Metab Immune Disord Drug Targets 2012, 12:287–302.
20. Thompson LU, Chen JM, Li T, Strasser-Weippl K, Goss PE: Dietary flaxseed alters tumor biological markers in postmenopausal breast cancer. Clin Cancer Res 2005, 11:3828–3835.
21. Neves ML, Yamasaki L, Sanches Ode C, Do Amaral MS, Stevanin H, Giuffrida R, Candido ER, Goes JE, Zulim LF, Schweigert A, Fukui RM, Meirelles CC, Sasaki CA, Andrade SF: Use of linseed oil to treat experimentally induced keratoconjunctivitis sicca in rabbits. J Ophthalmic Inflamm Infect 2013, 3:4.
22. 2559: In Martindale: The Complete Drug Reference: Supplementary Drugs and Other Substances, Volume 3. 37th edition. Edited by Sweetman SC. London: Pharmaceutical Press; 2011:2559.
23. Saxena S, Suryawanshi S, Somashekar U, Sharma D: Use of linseed oil in preventing peri-ileostomy skin excoriation. Indian J Gastroenterol 2009, 28:190–191.
24. Kaithwas G, Majumdar DK: Effect of L. usitatissimum (flaxseed/linseed) fixed oil against distinct phases of inflammation. ISRN Inflamm 2013, 2013:735158.
25. Kaithwas G, Majumdar DK: Evaluation of antiulcer and antisecretory potential of Linum usitatissimum fixed oil and possible mechanism of action. Inflammopharmacology 2010, 18:137–145.
26. Ibn-e-sina (Avicenna Husain): Al-Qanun fit-tib [The Canon of Medicine], (research of ebrahim shamsedine). Beirut, Lebanon: Alaalami Beirut library Press; 2005 [in Arabic].
27. Razi Mohammad ibn-e-Zakarya: Alhavi al-kabir [Liber Continens]. Tehran: The Institute for Medical History- Islamic and Complementary Medicine, Tehran University of Medical Sciences; 2010. in Arabic.
28. Sozay S, Sarfakoglu AB, Ayas S, Cetin N: Diurnal variation in clinical and electrophysiologic parameters associated with carpal tunnel syndrome. Am J Phys Med Rehabil 2011, 90:731–737.
29. Levine DW, Simmons BP, Koris MJ, Daltroy LH, Hohl GG, Fossel AH, Katz JN: A self-administered questionnaire for the assessment of severity of symptoms and functional status in carpal tunnel syndrome. J Bone Joint Surg Am 1993, 75:1585–1592.
30. Afshar A, Yekta Z, Etemadi A, Mirzatoloee F: Outcome measurement questionnaires for carpal tunnel syndrome. Iranian Orthopaedic Surg 2005, 3:46–50.
31. Nykter M, Kymäläinen H-R, Gates F, Sjöberg A-M: Quality characteristics of edible linseed oil. Agric Food Sci 2006, 15:402–413.
32. Heydari M, Shams M, Homayouni K, Borhani-Haghighi A, Salehi A, Hashempur MH: An option for painful diabetic neuropathy with simultaneous 'antioxidative' and 'anesthetic' properties: topical citrullus colocynthis. J Exp Integr Med 2014, 4:9–12.
33. Kim JK, Koh YD, Kim JS, Hann HJ, Kim MJ: Oxidative stress in subsynovial connective tissue of idiopathic carpal tunnel syndrome. J Orthop Res 2010, 28:1463–1468.
34. Werner RA, Andary M: Carpal tunnel syndrome: pathophysiology and clinical neurophysiology. Clin Neurophysiol 2002, 113:1373–1381.
35. Zhang CY, Wang YX: Observation on therapeutic effects of acupuncture combined with TDP irradiation and chinese herbal steaming and washing therapy for treatment of carpal tunnel syndrome in early stage. Zhongguo Zhen Jiu 2009, 29:708–710.
36. Branco K, Naeser MA: Carpal tunnel syndrome: clinical outcome after low-level laser acupuncture, microamps transcutaneous electrical nerve stimulation, and other alternative therapies–an open protocol study. J Altern Complement Med 1999, 5:5–26.
37. Eftekharsadat B, Kazem Shakouri S, Shimia M, Rahbar M, Ghojazadeh M, Reza Rashidi M, Hadi Faraji M: Effect of E. laciniata (L) ointment on mild and moderate carpal tunnel syndrome: a double-blind, randomized clinical trial. Phytother Res 2011, 25:290–295.
38. Jung WS, Moon SK, Park SU, Ko CN, Cho KH: Clinical assessment of usefulness, effectiveness and safety of jackyakamcho-tang

(shaoyaogancao-tang) on muscle spasm and pain: a case series. *Am J Chin Med* 2004, **32:**611–620.

39. Moghtaderi A, Jazayeri S, Azizi S: **EMLA cream for carpal tunnel syndrome: how it compares with steroid injection.** *Electromyogr Clin Neurophysiol* 2008, **49:**287–289.

40. Mokaberinejad R, Zafarghandi N, Bioos S, Dabaghian FH, Naseri M, Kamalinejad M, Amin G, Ghobadi A, Tansaz M, Akhbari A, Hamiditabar M: **Mentha longifolia syrup in secondary amenorrhea: a double-blind, placebo-controlled, randomized trials.** *Daru* 2012, **20:**97.

41. Mojahedi M, Naseri M, Majdzadeh R, Keshavarz M, Ebadini M, Nazem E, Isfeedvajani M: **Reliability and validity assessment of Mizaj questionnaire: a novel self-report scale in Iranian traditional medicine.** *Iran Red Crescent Med J.* in press.

42. Charles J, Fahridin S, Britt H: **Carpal tunnel syndrome.** *Aust Fam Physician* 2009, **38:**665.

43. Bye R, Hajiaqai B, Frorough B: **Comparison between efficacy of manu splint and cock-up splint in carpal tunnel syndrome treatment.** *J Babol Univ Med Sci* 2011, **13:**51–57.

44. Çeliker R, Arslan S, Inanc F: **Corticosteroid injection vs. nonsteroidal antiinflammatory drug and splinting in carpal tunnel syndrome.** *Am J Phys Med Rehabil* 2002, **81:**182–186.

45. Kumnerddee W, Kaewtong A: **Efficacy of acupuncture versus night splinting for carpal tunnel syndrome: a randomized clinical trial.** *J Med Assoc Thai* 2010, **93:**1463–1469.

6

Cost-effectiveness of different interferon beta products for relapsing-remitting and secondary progressive multiple sclerosis: Decision analysis based on long-term clinical data and switchable treatments

Shekoufeh Nikfar[1,2], Abbas Kebriaeezadeh[1], Rassoul Dinarvand[1], Mohammad Abdollahi[1,3], Mohammad-Ali Sahraian[4], David Henry[5] and Ali Akbari Sari[1,6*]

Abstract

Background: Multiple sclerosis (MS) is a highly debilitating immune mediated disorder and the second most common cause of neurological disability in young and middle-aged adults. Iran is amongst high MS prevalence countries (50/100,000). Economic burden of MS is a topic of important deliberation in economic evaluations study. Therefore determining of cost-effectiveness interferon beta (INF β) and their copied biopharmaceuticals (CBPs) and biosimilars products is significant issue for assessment of affordability in Lower-middle-income countries (LMICs).

Methods: A literature-based Markov model was developed to assess the cost-effectiveness of three INF βs products compared with placebo for managing a hypothetical cohort of patients diagnosed with relapsing remitting MS (RRMS) in Iran from a societal perspective. Health states were based on the Kurtzke Expanded Disability Status Scale (EDSS). Disease progression transition probabilities for symptom management and INF β therapies were obtained from natural history studies and multicenter randomized controlled trials and their long term follow up for RRMS and secondary progressive MS (SPMS). A cross sectional study has been developed to evaluate cost and utility. Transitions among health states occurred in 2-years cycles for fifteen cycles and switching to other therapies was allowed. Calculations of costs and utilities were established by attachment of decision trees to the overall model. The incremental cost effectiveness ratio (ICER) of cost/quality adjusted life year (QALY) for all available INF β products (brands, biosimilars and CBPs) were considered. Both costs and utilities were discounted. Sensitivity analyses were done to assess robustness of model.

Results: ICER for Avonex, Rebif and Betaferon was 18712, 11832, 15768 US Dollars ($) respectively when utility attained from literature review has been considered. ICER for available CBPs and biosimilars in Iran was $847, $6964 and $11913.

(Continued on next page)

* Correspondence: akbarisari@tums.ac.ir
[1]Department of Pharmacoeconomics and Pharmaceutical Administration, Faculty of Pharmacy, Tehran University of Medical Sciences, Tehran, Iran
[6]Department of Health Management and Economics, School of Public Health, Tehran University of Medical Sciences, Tehran, Iran
Full list of author information is available at the end of the article

(Continued from previous page)

Conclusions: The Markov pharmacoeconomics model determined that according to suggested threshold for developing countries by world health organization, all brand INF β products are cost effective in Iran except Avonex. The best strategy among INF β therapies is CBP intramuscular INF β-1a (Cinnovex). Results showed that a policy of encouraging accessibility to CBPs and biosimilars could make even high technology products cost-effective in LMICs.

Keywords: Cost-Effectiveness, Decision analysis, Economic evaluation, Interferon beta, Markov model, Modeling, Switching

Multiple sclerosis (MS) is a highly debilitating immune mediated disorder of the central nervous system [1]. Since MS is a complicated illness to diagnose accurately, the worldwide variation in prevalence and incidence is not precisely known. The best estimate is that around 2.5 million people in the world suffer from MS [2]. The range of prevalence estimates of MS in different countries and regions differs from 5 to 189 per 100,000 [3,4]. In a report published in 2000, Iran as a Middle Eastern country was listed among low to medium zone incidence of MS based on the theory of geographical epidemiology [4]. The prevalence rate of MS is estimated to be 50 per 100,000, translating to around 35,000 cases (Table 1) [5-17]. Therefore, Iran can be considered to be amongst high MS prevalence countries [4]. The onset of MS usually occurs during early adulthood (age 15–45 years) [18] making MS the second most common cause of neurological disability in young and middle-aged adults [19]. In Iran, the mean age for incidence and prevalence of MS are 27 and 32, respectively with a 2.8 times higher incidence in women than that of men. The most recent census of the Iranian population (2011) shows a youth bulge in the age range of 20 to 29 years old [20]. This means that health providers have to be ready to face the MS burden and its economic consequences.

Several immunomodulatory treatments including interferon beta (INF β), glatiramer acetate and natalizumab and one immunosuppressive treatment (mitoxantrone) have been approved for MS patients with a relapsing course [21]. Three preparations of recombinant IFN β have been approved for use in MS, subcutaneous IFN β-1a (SC IFN β-1a), intramuscular IFN β-1a (IM IFN β-1a), and subcutaneous IFN β-1b (SC IFN β-1b). IFN β is indicated for the treatment of relapsing-remitting form of MS to reduce the frequency of clinical exacerbations and delay the development of physical disability [22]. According to a previous meta-analysis, INF β's effectiveness in MS varies with the different kinds of INF β and the types of MS. Generally, IFN β can control remission in MS but its effectiveness in secondary progressive multiple sclerosis (SPMS) and relapsing remitting multiple sclerosis (RRMS) is questionable [22,23]. On other hand, the use of the immunomodulatory therapies in clinical practice has been a topic of substantial debate concerning clinical and cost-effectiveness. Although interferon has not been recommended formally by The National Institute for Clinical Excellence (NICE) in the UK many clinical practice guidelines have recommended the immunomodulatory therapies for the treatment of MS [18].

Based on the experience of using INF β in treatment of patients with MS for about 20 years in the Europe and United States, it is considered expensive but modestly effective in terms of reduction of morbidity and improving the quality of life [24-26]. However, it is a challenge for most countries to afford new expensive therapies for MS within limited public resources [27]. Although studies have shown considerable differences between high-income and low- or middle-income countries in capacity to afford the flow of costly new therapies, INFs β have been in use in Iran since 1995, starting with SC INF β-1b and there has been an exponential increase in use. Since 2009, the 'copied biopharmaceuticals' (CBPs) and biosimilars versions of INF β with lower and more affordable prices have been registered and have become accessible in Iran [28,29].

Iran as an Asian country located in the Eastern Mediterranean region and a middle-income country has some specific demographic, economic and health indicators that are presented in Table 2 [30]. Iran is one of the oldest countries in the region that adopted a National Drug Policy (NDP) many years ago [31]. On the basis of the NDP, a specific National Drug List was established to regulate strategies and to ensure registration of only high-quality effective drugs for Iranian citizens at the lowest possible price, mostly by use of subsidization [32,33]. To implement this goal, the Iranian Food and Drug Organization has the mission to control the price of medicines and balance their usage on the basis of the established NDP [34] by considering cost efficacy and equity of access [35].

Cost-effectiveness and cost-utility analyses (CEA/CUAs) have been used increasingly in the last two decades by funders to judge the balance between the added expenses of new drugs and their incremental benefits (e.g., improved patient outcomes). The majority of published CEA/CUA reports on INF β therapies for MS

Table 1 Epidemiologic details of published studies of multiple sclerosis (MS) in Iran

Study	Number of patients	Location	Prevalence/ 100000	Incidence rate/ 100000	Female/ Male ratio	Age (mean ± SD)	Age of onset (mean ± SD)	Education (High school graduated & University education %)	Occupational State (Employed %)
Yousefi Pour et al., 2002 [5]	142	Fars	5.3	-	1.2:1	32.7±6.5	-	-	-
Kalani et al., 2003 [6]	200	Tehran, (Loghman hospital)	-	-	2.5:1	-	27±7.4	95%	-
Saadatnia et al., 2007 [7]	1718	Isfahan	43.8	3.64	-	-	25.36±8.6	-	-
Hashemilar et al., 2011 [8]	1000	East Azarbayjan	27.7	-	2.7:1	33.4	-	-	-
Abedini et al., 2008 [9]	582	Mazandaran	20.1	-	2.6:1	34.4±9.4	26.9±8.3	-	24.6%
Milo and Kahana, 2010 [10]	-	Iran	44	-	-	-	-	-	-
Sahraian et al., 2010 [11]	8146	Tehran	51.9	-	2.6:1	-	27.74±8.32	-	-
Etemadifar et al., 2006 [12]	1391	Isfahan	-	-	3.6:1	32.5	-	50.9%	30.8%
Elhami et al., 2011 [13]	7896	Tehran	50.57	2.93	3.11:1	-	-	-	-
Nabavi et al., 2006 [14]	203	Tehran (Shahid Mostafa Khomeini hospital)	-	-	1.5:1	35.6	-	-	30.2%
Ghandehari et al., 2010 [15]	800	Khorasan (Razavi, Northern, Southern)	9.86	-	1.6:1	-	-	-	-
Ghabaee et al., 2007 [16]	70	Tehran (Emam Khomeini hospital)	-	-	2:1	32.58±10.24	27.55±10.42	39.2%	-
Ale-Yasin et al., 2002 [17]	318	Iran	-	-	1.52	35.4±9.6	26.6±8.1	73.2%	-

Table 2 Demographic, economic and health indicators of Iran

Total Population	73,974,000
Gross national income per capita (PPP) ($)	11,490
GDP/capita ($)	5810
Life expectancy at birth male/female(years)	70/75
Total expenditure on health per capita ($, 2010)	836
Total expenditure on health as % of GDP (2010)	6.8
Distribution of years of life lost by causes (2008)	
Communicable/Noncommunicable/Injuries	% 28/49/23

$: International Dollars.

come from studies carried out in high income countries [18,19,36-41]. Economic evaluations based on decision analytic modeling are an alternative to trial-based economic evaluations. The use of decision analytic models in economic evaluations is the only framework that has the potential to meet all the requirements for economic evaluation for decision making and to ensure their applicability in countries of varying national wealth [42]. Markov models are particularly useful when the clinical setting involves a risk that is ongoing over time.

The cost-effectiveness of INF β treatments has been estimated by Markov models in previous studies, but these have ignored differences of effectiveness and tolerability of different INF β products. Previous studies done by us have highlighted the varying efficacy of different kinds of INF β in RRMS or SPMS [22,23]. When there is a probability of switching to other drugs in a decision analysis model, overhead costing may affect results and decision-making processes [35]. Thus in this study we consider results due to switching to other drugs.

The main goal of this study was to perform CEA/ CUA evaluations using a decision analysis model of INF β therapies for MS from the perspective of a low-middle-income countries (LMICs). We examined the cost-effectiveness of 4 treatment strategies in patients diagnosed with RRMS (symptom management alone and in combination with IM IFN β-1a, SC IFN β-1a, or SC IFN β-1b).

Methods
Description of the model
A new Markov model was set up to assess the cost-effectiveness of 4 treatment strategies to manage a hypothetical cohort of patients diagnosed with RRMS in Iran. A decision analysis approach was used to model the effects of switching treatments (Figure 1). The incremental cost-effectiveness analysis was the main analytical plan for the study, combining cumulative measures of costs over time with a cumulative measure of effectiveness. This approach evaluates the incremental costs per clinical benefit gained (expressed as cost per QALY gained). The analysis was performed for a hypothetical cohort of 30-year-old patients. The inclusion criteria used in the randomized controlled trials (RCTs) of INF β was taken into account and the effectiveness was noted as QALYs. The model embraced patterns of resource utilization in both outpatient and inpatient care. Also, both direct non-medical and indirect costs were included.

The treatment strategies were management of diseases symptoms alone and in combination with one of the following medicines: IM IFN β-1a, SC IFN β-1a, or SC IFN β-1b. The clinical course of RRMS (e.g., disease progression and transition to SPMS) was modeled in terms of the Kurtzke expanded disability status scale (EDSS) and withdrawal from treatment [43]. Specifically, 7 health states were modeled (Figure 1):

1. RRMS-EDSS 1–3.5: no or few limitations in mobility
2. RRMS-EDSS 4–6: moderate limitations in mobility

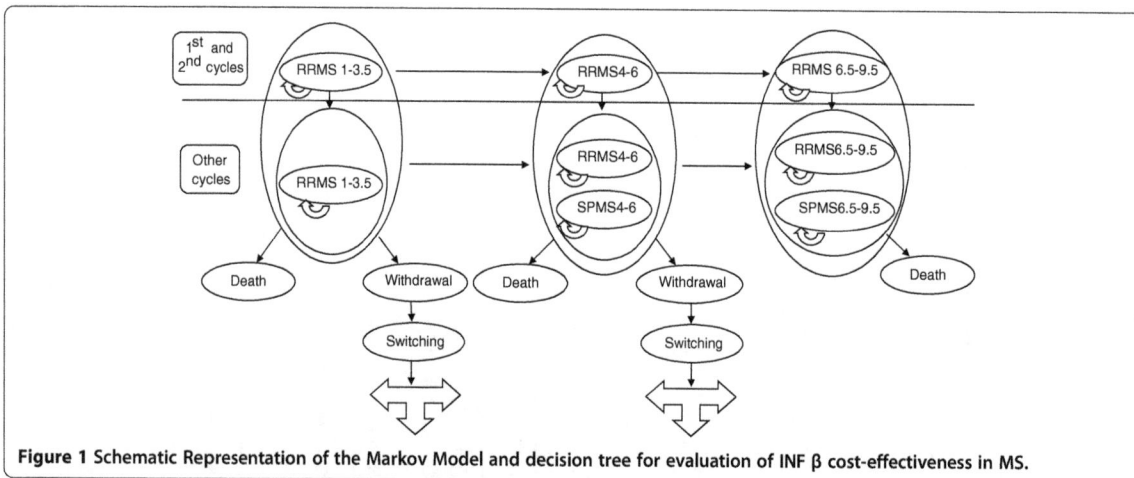

Figure 1 Schematic Representation of the Markov Model and decision tree for evaluation of INF β cost-effectiveness in MS.

3. RRMS-EDSS 6.5-9.5: walking aid or wheelchair required and restricted to bed
4. SPMS-EDSS 4–6: moderate limitations in mobility
5. SPMS-EDSS 6.5-9.5: walking aid or wheelchair required and restricted to bed
6. Death (natural causes or EDSS 10)
7. Withdrawal due to side effects and perceived lack of efficacy or other causes like pregnancy and financial problems

Transitions among the health states occurred in 2-years cycles. A 2-years cycle time was used, because this interval closely approximates the follow-up period of the IFN β RCTs for preventive treatment in RRMS. Most of information for SPMS was reported in 3 year intervals; thus they were calculated for 2 years to input to the model. The baseline time horizon of the model was assumed to be a lifetime in order to capture the full benefits of immunomodulatory therapy, which was assumed to be around 30 years after onset of the disease (15 cycles). Costs and outcomes were estimated from the societal perspective and were discounted at 7.2% per annum for cost [44] and 3% for quality of life [45]. The costs and QALYs were discounted from the end of first year. All the costs were reported in 2012 U.S. dollars and exchange rates of IRR to U.S. dollars of 12260. Data were obtained from literature covering RCTs of IFN β, official prices, and tariff lists (see below for details). To validate the methodology (model structure and assumptions), four expert opinion leaders were consulted.

The model calculated the following outcomes: numbers of patients remaining in lower EDSS; numbers of patients remaining in RRMS; numbers of patients remaining relapse free; QALYs; total costs and costs by component (i.e., IFN β therapy cost, MS-related medical costs [e.g., drugs for symptom management], and lost worker productivity costs; direct non-medical costs and incremental cost-effectiveness ratios (ICER) comparing symptom management alone with symptom management combined with each of the 3 IFN β therapies. Given that there is no accurate threshold calculated for Iran, the cost/QALY ICERs were compared with multiples of the gross domestic product (GDP) per capita according to recommendations of the World Health Organization (WHO) [46]. According to the WHO the treatments of MS with different IFN β would be considered "highly cost effective" if the cost/QALY is less than GDP per capita, "cost-effective" if the cost/QALY was between one to three times of GDP per capita and "not cost-effective" if it was more than three times of GDP per capita. The GDP per capita of Iran was considered as 5810 USD [30]. Model parameters were varied in sensitivity analyses.

A number of underlying assumptions were adopted for the base-case model:

1. In the model, all patients start in the health state stage of EDSS 1–3.5.
2. The point at which patients transitioned from RRMS to SPMS was assumed to be in the third cycle (approximately 5 years after diagnosis of illness) and the model assumed that this took place between EDSS 4–6 and EDSS 6.5-9.5 [47]. Corresponding to this assumption, the model assumed that relapses occurred in patients didn't change the state of EDSS [48].
3. The model assumed that as per product labeling and off-labeled prescriptions, only RRMS and SPMS patients in EDSS of 1–6 were eligible for and received IFN β therapies.
4. Switching among the IFN β therapies was permitted once in the model. Patients who withdrew IFN β therapy during the first three cycles were assigned the transition probabilities for relapse and disease progression used in the symptom management arm or other two IFN β arms. Patients who discontinued therapy were not permitted to reinitiate therapy. Switching between IFN β was acceptable within brands or biosimilar and CBPs only.
5. In case of withdrawal from IFN β therapy in cycles of 4 to 15, patients were allocated to the transition probabilities for relapse and disease progression used in the symptom management arm.
6. It was presumed that there was no variation in mortality between patients with or without preventive treatment [22] and there was no sex-related mortality risk factor in RRMS and SPMS [49].
7. Other direct medical and non-medical costs and indirect costs were calculated according to utilization in different status and stages of disease and the cycle of Markov model.
8. Medicinal treatments and laboratory tests for management of MS morbidity in different groups were deemed according to results of our previous meta-analysis [22]. Cost of antidepressants, anti-spasmodics, anti-fatigues, pain killers, and NSAIDs were considered in our model.
9. Weighted mean costs were considered for other medicines consumed by MS patients in both generic or brand forms. Frequency of use was based on survey data [28].
10. Calculations were performed for cost of hospitalization, physicians' visits, laboratory tests, imaging, psychotherapy and physiotherapy according to percentages of patients using governmental and private facilities or outpatient admission to daycare clinics.

Clinical and economic outcomes

The effectiveness measurement was based on the concept of utility, which measures the QALYs [50].

The cost assessment was based on the assignment of costs to the health states and interventions.

Data sources

Three different types of data can be distinguished in modeling studies:

1. Probabilities of clinical events: progress of disease, chance of an acute exacerbation, withdrawal, and death.
2. Utilities of different Markov health states.
3. Costing information derived from estimates of the units of resource utilization and their prices/tariffs (product of unit and price).
4. Probabilities of switching to other INF β or symptomatic treatments.

To design the strategy of retrieving data from PubMed, Scopus, Web of Science, and the Cochrane library, Iranmedex, SID, and MagIran were searched for studies reporting efficacy and/or tolerability of IFN β in multiple sclerosis, and epidemiology, natural history and costs of MS. Data were collected from 1966 to 2012 (up to December). The search terms were: "multiple sclerosis" or "MS" and "IFN beta" or "Interferon beta"; "multiple sclerosis" or "MS" and "Iran"; "multiple sclerosis" or "MS" and "IFN beta" or "Interferon beta" and "modeling" or "decision analysis", "cost". The language was restricted to English and Persian. The reference lists from retrieved articles were also reviewed to avoid missing any relevant studies (Figure 2).

The probabilities of clinical events, including disease progression, probability of an acute exacerbation, and withdrawal were based on IFN β clinical trial data and their long term data. A cross sectional study has been developed to evaluate cost and utility. An approved questionnaire was adopted and validated. Two-hundred MS patients were recruited consecutively in a random manner from three referral hospitals of two different cities and three private offices of MS specialists and members of Iranian society of MS through society's office in

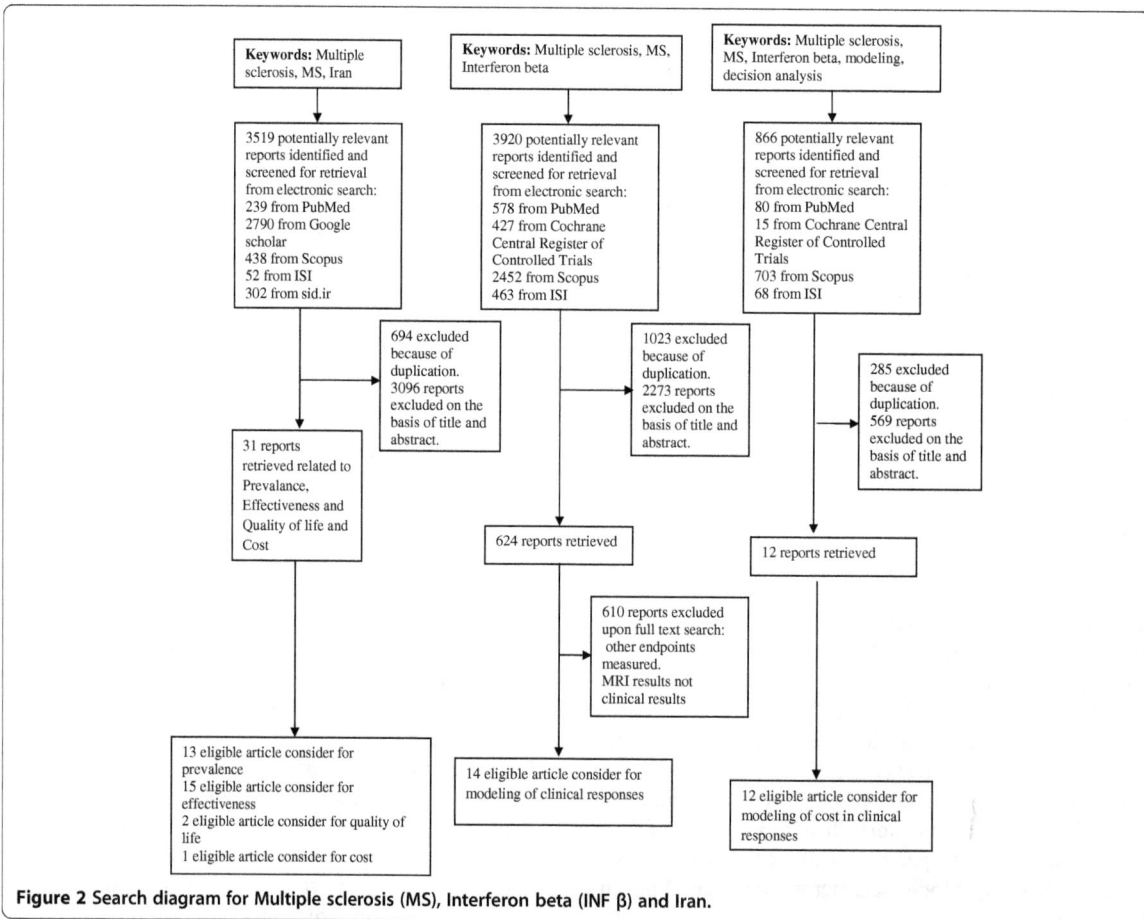

Figure 2 Search diagram for Multiple sclerosis (MS), Interferon beta (INF β) and Iran.

Table 3 Baseline characteristics of patients recruited to evaluate quality adjusted life years QALYs and Cost for multiple sclerosis (MS) in Iran (n = 200)

	Total recruited MS patients	RRMS EDSS			SPMS EDSS		Unknown or PPMS
		1-3.5	4-6	>6	4-6	>6	
Numbers of Patients	200	104	29	12	24	4	PPMS: 19 Unknown: 8
Age (mean±SD)	33.8±9.1	29±7.7	36±7.2	36.6±9.2	42.4±6.7	46±3.7	PPMS: 41.8±6.3 Unknown: 34.5±8.2
Sex (Female/Male)	148/52	80/24	24/5	10/2	16/8	2/2	PPMS:10/9 Unknown: 6/2
Urban/Rural	174/26	93/11	25/4	12/0	20/4	4/0	PPMS: 13/6 Unknown 4/4
Education (High school graduated & University education %)	83%	83%	79%	83%	83%	100%	PPMS: 53% Unknown: 75%
Occupational State (Employed %)	31%	37%	48%	0%	29%	0%	PPMS: 0% Unknown: 13%

MS multiple sclerosis, *RRMS* relapsing remitting multiple sclerosis, *SPMS* secondary progressive multiple sclerosis, *PPMS* primary progressive multiple sclerosis, *EDSS* expanded disability status scale.

Tehran and Arak and patients' email [51]. Evaluation of recruitment showed no bias (p>0.05) according to feature of MS retrieved through systematic review (Table 3). ANOVA statistical test for normal numerical variables was used to detect differences in the groups retrieved from literature search and recruited group corrected by Bonferroni post hoc test.

Age and sex-specific mortality rates assumed that MS alters life expectancy and increases the rate of death threefold across the different age or sex groups (Table 4) [49]. Age and sex-specific population mortality rates were derived from national statistics data [52].

Probabilities were derived from published literature (Table 5): Relapse and disease progression transition probabilities within the symptom management arm were obtained from published natural history studies [47,53,54].

Treatment Effects of the IFN β treatment effects were obtained from RCTs (IM IFN β-1a, SC IFN β-1a, SC IFN β-1b) and long-term follow-up studies [55-65].

The QALYs for the different health states were derived from a cross-sectional study as shown in Table 6. Utility estimates were based on direct elicitation methods of visual analogue scale (VAS) and generic preference-based measures of the EuroQol (EQ-5D) and the Health Utilities Index 3 (HUI3) by in-house translated and validated questionnaires. We also derived utility loss per EDSS and relapse from literatures [19,66,67].

Other necessary information were obtained indirectly by calculations that were done on the basis of long-term

follow up data, hazard rate, variances of Kaplan–Meier curves [68,69] and/or by solving multiple-step equations.

Probabilities of switching to other INF βs or no treatment in case of withdrawal due to side effects or lack of perceived efficacy were derived from the cross sectional study.

Costs

Data on costs were derived from cross sectional study (Table 7).

We used a backward-looking approach in which resource utilization and clinical data were gathered at a single point in time and covered the one-year period prior to the dates of inclusion. The cost of care of MS was calculated for patients in current clinical practice in Iran in 2012 for each state of disease. The costs due to relapses derived from the cost-of-care study in same cross sectional study and evaluating of patients files archived in the hospitals. All prices were extracted from official list of tariffs [70,71]. The friction cost method was used to evaluate workday's loss by on the go patients [72]. By use of this method, the significance of productivity loss was assumed to be 80% of the ordinary rate of employee's productivity during the "friction period." Thereafter, it was assumed that sick employees could be replaced. Time lost by inactive patients was considered as leisure time lost and was valued at 40% of the average wage, productivity and friction period in Iran [20,73,74].

Sensitivity analysis

Elementary effects sensitivity analyses were done according to basic clinical and economic assumptions and their changes in the clinical-outcome model. This was used to test the stability of the suppositions of the analysis over a range of assumptions, probability estimates, and value judgments. The first sensitivity analysis was performed to assess

Table 4 Age and sex adjusted mortality rate for multiple sclerosis (MS) patients

Age (range)	30-35	36-40	41-45	46-50	51-55	56-60	61-65	66-70
Mortality rate (%)	7.69	7.61	8.29	10.17	12.71	14.19	16.2	18.9

Table 5 Probability of related outcomes to multiple sclerosis (MS) and interferon beta (INF β) therapy

	Natural History		Interferon beta-1a (Avonex)		Interferon beta-1a 44 Mcg/0.5 ml (Rebif)		Interferon beta-1b (Betaferon)	
Probability of EDSS progression within RRMS								
RRMS 1-3 to RRMS 3.5-6	0.4		0.219		0.193		0.2	
RRMS 3.5-6 to RRMS 6≤	0.27		0.11		0.115		0.15	
Probability of progression from RRMS to SPMS (the same EDSS)								
RRMS 3.5-6 to SPMS 3.5-6	0.43		0.43		0.197		0.433	
RRMS 6≤ to SPMS 6≤	0.31		0.31		0.31		0.31	
Probability of EDSS progression within SPMS								
SPMS 3.5-6 to SPMS 6≤	0.5		0.3		0.5		0.4	
Relapse rate								
RRMS	Cycle 1	2.54	Cycle 1	1.34	Cycle 1	1.73	Cycle 1	1.68
	Other cycles	2.04	Other cycles	1.31	Other cycles	1.18	Other cycles	1.01
SPMS	0.7		0.47		0.5		0.35	
Withdrawal								
RRMS 1-3	-		Cycles1 &2	0.04	Cycles1 &2	0.078	Cycles1 &2	0.086
			Other cycles	0.04	Other cycles	0.05	Other cycles	0.09
RRMS 3.5-6	-		Cycle 2	0.26	Cycle 2	0.42	Cycle 2	0.247
			Other cycles	0.04	Other cycles	0.05	Other cycles	0.09
SPMS 3.5-6	-		0.19		0.357		0.25	

RRMS relapsing remitting multiple sclerosis, *SPMS* secondary progressive multiple sclerosis, *EDSS* expanded disability status scale, *Mcg* microgram, ml milliliter.

the impact of CBPs and biosimilars on the analysis. We performed the second analysis to assess the sensitivity of the model to different ways of QALYs assessments obtained from questionnaires and literatures' searches-based QALYs. The third sensitivity analysis was performed to evaluate the sensitivity of analysis to discount cost and QALYs.

Consent

The study was approved in the Institute Review Board with code number 91-10-24:1–1. Additionally, the study was approved by Iranian Society of MS. Written informed consent was obtained from the patient for the publication of this report and any accompanying images.

Results
ICER of symptom management combined with IFN β comparing to symptom management alone
ICER of adding IM IFNβ-1a (Avonex) to symptom management based on evaluation of utility by literatures search, VAS, EQ-5D, and HUI3 as measurement tools of QALYs was $18712, $19954, $17398 and $20045. Not cost-effective intervention except while evaluated by EQ-5D.

Table 6 Utility scores related to multiple sclerosis (MS) type and expanded disability status scale (EDSS) states in cost-effectiveness model

State	Utility score			
	Literature review	Visual Analog Scale (VAS)	European Quality of Life-5 Dimensions (EQ-5D)	Health Utility Index 3 (HUI 3)
RRMS EDSS 1-3.5	0.68	0.79	0.76	0.68
RRMS EDSS 4-6	0.52	0.62	0.57	0.41
SPMS EDSS 4-6	0.52	0.58	0.52	0.18
RRMS EDSS 6<	0.17	0.38	0.18	0.08
SPMS EDSS 6<	0.17	0.18	0.02	0.06
Relapse (Utility loss)	0.5	0.42	0.42	0.42
Death	0	0	0	0

All utility scores have been obtained from cross section study based on questionnaire.

Table 7 Cost of multiple sclerosis disease (MS) and interferon beta (INF β) therapy

Cost per patient per year ($)		RRMS 1-3.5	RRMS 4-6	RRMS 6<	SPMS 4-6	SPMS 6<
		Total costs for other medications is related to" Interferons-beta" administration and duration, EDSS and type of disease				
Total medical direct cost (Medicines)						
Interferon beta-1a (Avonex)*		9861	9861	0	9861	0
Interferon beta-1a (Rebif)*		7106	7106	0	7106	0
Interferon beta-1b (Betaferon)*		9176	9176	0	9176	0
Interferon beta-1a IM (CBPs)*		3762	3762	0	3762	0
Interferon beta-1a SC (CBPs)*		5873	5873	0	5873	0
Interferon beta-1b (CBPs & BS)*		7969	7969	0	7969	0
Antidepressant medications	The first 3 cycles	2.3	2.7	3.2	2.7	3.2
	Other Cycles	1.5	1.8	2.2	1.8	2.2
Anti-spasm medications		11.65	11.65	11.65	11.65	11.65
Anti-fatigue medications		1.36	1.36	1.36	1.36	1.36
Pain killer medications		4.7	6.6	9.8	23.5	29.9
NSAIDs (control SE)	for Interferon beta-1a IM	0.15	0.15	0	0.15	0
	for Interferon beta-1a SC	0.42	0.42	0	0.42	0
	for Interferon beta-1b	0.53	0.53	0	0.53	0
Other medical direct cost (total)		**167**	**316**	**1543**	**316**	**1543**
Laboratory tests		13	13	0	13	0
Imaging		103	103	0	103	0
Physicians visits		45	32	14	32	14
Physiotherapy		0	15	326	15	326
Psychotherapy		6	64	0	64	0
Nursing		0	41	816	41	816
Cane, walker, wheelchair, Medical bed, Medical wave mattress		0	48	387	48	387
Non-medical direct cost (total)		**266**	**1841**	**3037**	**1841**	**3037**
Transport		266	373	40	373	40
House reconstructions		0	0	1529	0	1529
Car rebuilding		0	1468	1468	1468	1468
Indirect cost (total)		**90**	**130**	**616**	**379**	**740**
Absence from work		71	120	0	65	0
Unemployment or early retirement		7	0	616	308	740
Mortality		12	10	0	6	0
Cost per patient per relapse (total)		**33**	**33**	**33**	**54**	**54**
Medical treatment		27	27	27	45	45
Hospitalization		6	6	6	9	9

$ US Dollars 2012, *IM* intramuscular, *SC* subcutaneous, *NSAIDs* non steroid anti- inflammatory drugs, *Cost of injection is included for interferons beta; *CBPs* Copied biopharmaceuticals including IM IFNβ-1a (Cinnovex, Actovex), SC IFNβ-1a (Recigen, Actorif) and SC IFNβ-1b (Ziferon, Actoferon), *BS* biosimilar including SC IFNβ-1b (Extavia).

ICER of adding SC IFNβ-1a (Rebif) to symptom management based on evaluation of utility by literatures search, VAS, EQ-5D, and HUI3 was $11832, $11850, $10433 and $11437 (cost-effective intervention).

ICER of adding SC IFNβ-1b (Betaferon) to symptom management based on evaluation of utility by literatures search, VAS, EQ-5D, and HUI3 was $15768, $16864, $15030 and $16314 (cost-effective intervention).

ICER of adding CBPs IM IFNβ-1a (Cinnovex, Actovex with 98 and 2 percent of market share among CBPs IM IFNβ-1a) to symptom management based on evaluation of utility by literatures search, VAS, EQ-5D, and HUI3 as a measurement tools of QALYs was $847, $904, $788 and $908 (highly cost-effective intervention).

ICER of adding CBPs SC IFNβ-1a (Recigen, Actorif with 87.5 and 12.5 percent of market share among CBPs SC IFNβ-1a) to symptom management based on evaluation of utility by literatures search, VAS, EQ-5D, and HUI3 was $6964, $6975, $6140 and $6731 (cost-effective intervention).

ICER of adding CBPs SC IFNβ-1b (Ziferon, Actoferon with both 12.5 percent and (biosimilar); Extavia with 75 percent of market share among CBPs and biosimilar SC IFNβ-1b) to symptom management based on evaluation of utility by literatures search, VAS, EQ-5D, and HUI3 was $11913, $12740, $11355, and $12325 (cost-effective intervention). All results have been provided in Table 8.

Discounted ICER of symptom management combined with IFNβ comparing to symptom management alone

Discounted ICER of adding IM IFNβ-1a (Avonex) to symptom management based on evaluation of utility by literatures search, VAS, EQ-5D, and HUI3 as a measurement tools of QALYs was $18873, $20370, $18050, and $20104 (not cost-effective intervention).

Discounted ICER of adding SC IFNβ-1a (Rebif) to symptom management based on evaluation of utility by literatures search, VAS, EQ-5D, and HUI3 as a measurement

tool of QALYs was $13482, $13885, $12347, and $13092 (cost-effective intervention).

Discounted ICER of adding SC IFNβ-1b (Betaferon) to symptom management based on evaluation of utility by literatures search, VAS, EQ-5D, and HUI3 was $15142, $16452, $14808, and $15663 (cost-effective intervention).

Discounted ICER of adding CBPs IM IFNβ-1a (Cinnovex, Actovex with 98 and 2 percent of market share among CBPs IM IFNβ-1a) to symptom management based on evaluation of utility by literatures search, VAS, EQ-5D, and HUI3 as a measurement tools of QALYs was $4026, $4345, $3850, and $4288(highly cost-effective intervention).

Discounted ICER of adding CBPs SC IFNβ-1a (Recigen, Actorif with 87.5 and 12.5 percent of market share among CBPs SC IFNβ-1a) to symptom management based on evaluation of utility by literatures search, VAS, EQ-5D, and HUI3 was $9553, $9838, $8749, and $9276 (cost-effective intervention).

Discounted ICER of adding CBPs SC IFNβ-1b (Ziferon, Actoferon with both 12.5 percent and (biosimilars) Extavia; with 75 percent of market share among CBPs and biosimilar SC IFNβ-1b) to symptom management based on evaluation of utility by literatures search, VAS, EQ-5D, and HUI3 was $11903, $12933, $11641 and $12312 (cost-effective intervention). All results have been provided in Table 9.

Table 8 ICER ($) of different Interferons-Beta in comparison to placebo therapy in MS patients according to different utility measurement methods

Therapy	Literature-based	VAS	EQ-5D	HUI 3
Interferon beta-1a (Intramuscular) (Avonex)	18712	19954	17398	20045
Interferon beta-1a (Subcutaneous) (Rebif)	11832	11850	10433	11437
Interferon beta-1b (Betaferon)	15768	16864	15030	16314
Interferon beta-1a (Intramuscular) (CBPs)	847	904	788	908
Interferon beta-1a (Subcutaneous) (CBPs)	6964	6975	6140	6731
Interferon beta-1b (CBPs and BS)	11913	12740	11355	12325

$ US dollars, *ICER* incremental cost effectiveness ratio, *VAS* visual analogue scale, *EQ-5D* EuroQol, *HUI3*: Health Utilities Index 3, *CBPs* Copied biopharmaceuticals including IM IFNβ-1a (Cinnovex, Actovex), SC IFNβ-1a (Recigen, Actorif) and SC IFNβ-1b (Ziferon, Actoferon), *BS* biosimilar including SC IFNβ-1b (Extavia).

Table 9 Discounted ICER ($) of different Interferons-Beta in comparison to placebo therapy in MS patients according to different utility measurement methods

Therapy	Literature-based	VAS	EQ-5D	HUI 3
Interferon beta-1a (Avonex)	18873	20370	18050	20104
Interferon beta-1a (Rebif)	13482	13885	12347	13092
Interferon beta-1b (Betaferon)	15142	16452	14808	15663
Interferon beta-1a (Intramuscular) (CBPs)	4026	4345	3850	4288
Interferon beta-1a (Subcutaneous) (CBPs)	9553	9838	8749	9276
Interferon beta-1b (CBPs & BS)	11903	12933	11641	12312

$ US dollars, *ICER* incremental cost effectiveness ratio, *VAS* visual analogue scale, *EQ-5D* EuroQol, *HUI 3* Health Utilities Index 3, *CBPs* Copied biopharmaceuticals including IM IFNβ-1a (Cinnovex, Actovex), SC IFNβ-1a (Recigen, Actorif) and SC IFNβ-1b (Ziferon, Actoferon), *BS* biosimilar including SC IFNβ-1b (Extavia).

Discussion

The results of these analysis showed that all kinds of available branded, CBPs or biosimilar IFN β in Iran are cost-effectiveness except Avonex. The analysis was based on Markov model and long-term data of effectiveness and tolerability and considering progress to SPMS. Switching is the noteworthy difference of this model that has been implemented for the first time for cost-effectiveness of IFN β in MS. WHO's recommendation about threshold of developing countries considers ICER less than triplet of GDP as a cost-effective intervention [46]. GDP of 2012 for Iran is 5810 USD, thus all ICER less than 17430 USD per QALYs could be considered cost-effective. Analysis showed ICER of 847 to 16864 USD per QALYs for CBPs and biosimilar of IM IFNβ-1a, SC IFNβ-1a and SC IFNβ-1b, Rebif and Betaferon. For Avonex, intervention is cost-effective only when EQ-5D has been applied for assessment of utility. The differences of QALYs assessment tools in calculation of utility in MS have been demonstrated before [75]. It seems that this difference happened because EQ-5D questionnaire is not capable to measure one of the important disutility of MS, cognition. However sensitivity analysis showed that our model was not sensitive to evaluation methods of utility or literature-based ones. The model is not sensitive to discounting either. Our model is sensitive to replacing CBPs and biosimilars that it is a dominated approach. Sensitivity in case of bivariate analysis of discounting and CBPs IM IFNβ-1a and SC IFNβ-1a have occurred. This may happen because of significant impact of IFN β in cost of MS treatment. Therefore, reducing the price of IFN β by replacement with CBPs will decrease the influence of this factor and may highlight other reasons that affect utility. It must be emphasized that the unit price of CBPs IM IFNβ-1a and SC IFNβ-1a are significantly lower than Avonex and Rebif in Iran. Overall sensitivity analysis in this study showed robustness of this model.

This is the first time that cost-effectiveness of IFN β have been analyzed in context of one of developing countries by applying decision analytic modeling. Markov model has been applied to assess the progression of disease and its prevention with adding IFN β to management protocol. Spreading on the concept of switching to other IFN β in case of withdrawal due to side effects or lack in perceived efficacy to model is novel. The idea for modifying the Markov model in case of switchable interventions has been established by Nikfar 2012 [35]. In case of probability of switching to other drugs in decision analysis model, overhead costing and utility may affect results and decision-making processes, thus, for the first time we consider switching to other IFN β in case of withdrawal from one of them. Therefore, to conclude the utility and cost of each intervention, decision tree model has been used as an additional decision analytic modeling.

Additional analysis showed that without considering switching to other IFN β, ICER will be beyond threshold and intervention will not be cost-effective.

In our Markov model, the probability of transition to SPMS is one of the transition states. Nuijten and Hutton have also considered SPMS in their Markov model [19]. Their analysis revealed that IFN β were much more cost-effective compared with the results of other cost-effectiveness study performed in patients with RRMS only. They believe that reduction in the cost-effectiveness ratio of IFN β may be in line for a longer follow-up period and continuation of treatment with IFN β in SPMS.

Our designed model is based on thirty-year that is kind of life-long follow up complying with life expectancy of MS patients that is almost 10 years less than healthy population [49]. Considering the rate of mortality in MS patients rather than general population [18,19,41], the reliability of study is increased. Seeing IFN β act in MS patients differently is in contrast with modeling of Bell et al., and Nuijten and Hutton [18,19] and robust the results of current cost-effectiveness study and may help decision makers accurately. It should be emphasized that assuming tolerability as an essential part of drug therapy that interferes with health-related outcomes [76] is another advantage of this study. Withdrawal due to side effects of medicines or lack of effectiveness in long-term treatments may have a great impact in cost-effectiveness analysis [77]. Chilcott et al. [41] didn't consider withdrawal in their decision analysis model, although Nuijten and Hutton [19] and Bell and his colleagues [18] have used withdrawal data in their model. The withdrawal data was retrieved from short-term trials and only due to side effects [19] or lack of efficacy [18] and just for one cycle of model. To be closer to reality, withdrawal is considered in all long of intervention in recent model. Availability of long-term follow-up data (effectiveness and withdrawal) of patients initially enrolled in clinical trials [63-65] helped us to not repeating the mistake of previous studies in use of extrapolated data from short-term trials to assess effectiveness and discontinuation of therapy [19,41].

However, our model is much more improved but always the results of modeling need to be treated with some degree of caution from a health-economic perspective. Amongst is the data for probabilities of preventive effects for IFN β. All such kinds of data in this analysis have been retrieved from RCTs and their long-term follow up data. Therefore, the fact of controversy between real effectiveness and efficacy obtained from protocol-restricted RCTs will remain. Usually, conducting meta-analysis can solve this problem, but in case of rare diseases like MS due to lack of variety of available trials, this method is even unlikely. The indirect cost in developing countries may be affected by low productivity of such regions. Furthermore, Iran has adapted generic based pharmaceutical policy.

These two reasons may consequence underestimation of the cost in this model and the low ICER than other cost-effectiveness studies [18,19,41,78] that reported approximately 50000 USD per QALYs, for prevention effect of IFN β. The utilities in our model were derived from a cross-sectional study based on EDSS and disease conditions. Adverse effects of therapeutics medicines have not been considered in assessment of utilities and this may also modify the results of ICERs. There are specific health related quality of life (HRQOL) questionnaires for MS like Hamburg Quality of Life Questionnaire in Multiple Sclerosis (HAQUAMS) or multiple sclerosis quality of life with 54 questions (MSQOL-54), moreover quality of life in MS can be also determined by generic HRQOL like EQ-5D or HUI-3. The problem of specific HRQOL is measurement of utility or preference-based measures by them that is impossible; on the other hand, utility or preference-based measures have the advantage of leading to a single number that balances gains in one domain against losses in another. The best known utility or preference-based measures according to reliability, validity and feasibility for MS are the HUI-3 and the EQ-5D index [79,80]. There are varieties in concepts and scores of utility measurement tools. It seems that HUI3 with potential of scoring cognitive problems of MS patients could act better than other tools like EQ-5D or VAS. Nevertheless, sensitivity analysis in our model didn't show differences between utilities obtained from different forms and literature reviews. The characteristics of patients related to age, sex, educational and employment status were taken from 200 patients in cross sectional filled questionnaires. According to prevalence of different kind of MS and EDSS state, in some states like higher EDSS or SPMS there are too few recruited patients. This problem may underweight the results and considering equal and sufficient amount of patients for each state, in future studies is recommended to vigorous results. Our model with 50% progression to SPMS after 10 years and 90% after 25 years [47] and life expectancy of thirty after incidence of illness corresponds with natural history of MS [49].

Our results showed that prescribing of all kind of IFN β except Avonex in context of Iran is cost-effective. Due to the fact that there is no difference among IFN β as regards of effectiveness and safety, thus the choice of them depends on clinicians in many cases. However, it seems that price is an important factor for prescription. Therefore CBP of IM IFNβ-1a (Cinnovex) is prescribed more than 50% in Iran [28]. As a pharmaceutical regulatory rule, clinical data for brands and CBPs and biosimilar of IFN β in this study considered to be the same [28,81]. If by availability of post marketing surveillance, we reach the same conclusion about ranking for ICERs, the most efficient way is to choose the most cost-effective IFN β with respect of compliance.

The results of this study demonstrated that generic based NDP is one of the strength of each country's policy to make medicines more accessible.

Competing interests
The authors declare that they have no competing interests. Since MA is Editor-in-Chief of DARU, all review process of the submission was handled by one of Section Editors.

Authors' contributions
SN made design of the study, acquisition of data, analysis and interpretation of data, drafted the article and revising it critically for important intellectual content, AK and RD reviewed all data and supervised whole study, MA supervised whole study and revised the paper critically for important intellectual content, MAS contributed in acquisition of data and interpretation of data, DH contributed in design of the study, AAS reviewed all data and design of study and supervised whole study. All authors approved final version for submission.

Acknowledgment
Authors thank Iranian Society of multiple sclerosis for their kind assistance in collecting information of patients. This paper is the outcome of a PhD thesis of the first author and was supported by Faculty of Pharmacy, Tehran University of Medical Sciences.

Author details
[1]Department of Pharmacoeconomics and Pharmaceutical Administration, Faculty of Pharmacy, Tehran University of Medical Sciences, Tehran, Iran. [2]Food & Drug Organization, Ministry of Health & Medical Education, Tehran, Iran. [3]Faculty of Pharmacy, and Pharmaceutical Sciences Research Center, Tehran University of Medical Sciences, Tehran, Iran. [4]Department of Neurology, Sina Hospital, Tehran University of Medical Sciences, Tehran, Iran. [5]Institute for Clinical Evaluative Sciences, Toronto, Canada. [6]Department of Health Management and Economics, School of Public Health, Tehran University of Medical Sciences, Tehran, Iran.

References
1. Disanto G, Morahan JM, Ramagopalan SV: **Multiple sclerosis: risk factors and their interactions.** *CNS Neurol Disord Drug Targets* 2012, **11**(5):545–555.
2. *Multiple sclerosis International federation.* http://www.msif.org
3. Ahlgren C, Odén A, Lycke J: **High nationwide prevalence of multiple sclerosis in Sweden.** *Mult Scler* 2011, **17**(8):901–908.
4. Kurtzke JF: **Multiple sclerosis in time and space-geographic clues to cause.** *J Neurovirol* 2000, **6**(2):S134–S140.
5. Yousefi Pour GA, Ali Reza Rasekhi AR: **Multiple sclerosis: a risk factor analysis Iran.** *Arch Iran Med* 2002, **5**(3):191–193.
6. Kalanie H, Gharagozli K, Kalanie AR: **Multiple sclerosis: report on 200 cases from Iran.** *Mult Scler* 2003, **9**:36–38.
7. Saadatnia M, Etemadifar M, Maghzi AH: **Multiple sclerosis in Isfahan, Iran.** *Int Rev Neurobiol* 2007, **79**:357–375.
8. Hashemilar M, Savadi Ouskui D, Farhoudi M, Ayromlou H, Asadollahi A: **Multiple sclerosis in East-Azerbaijan, north west Iran.** *Neurol Asia* 2011, **16**(2):127–131.
9. Abedini M, Habibi Saravi R, Zarvani A, Farahmand A: **Epidemiology of Multiple sclerosis in Mazandaran in 2007 (in Persian).** *J Mazand Univ Med Sci* 2008, **18**(66):82–87.
10. Milo R, Kahana E: **Multiple sclerosis: Geoepidemiology, genetics and the environment.** *Autoimmun Rev* 2010, **9**:A387–A394.
11. Sahraian MA, Khorramnia S, Ebrahim MM, Moinfar Z, Lotfi J, Pakdaman H: **Multiple sclerosis in Iran: a demographic study of 8,000 patients and changes over time.** *Eur Neurol* 2010, **64**:331–336.
12. Etemadifar M, Janghorbani M, Shaygannejad V, Ashtari F: **Prevalence of multiple sclerosis in Isfahan, Iran.** *Neuroepidemiology* 2006, **27**:39–44.
13. Elhami SR, Mohammad K, Sahraian MA, Eftekhar H: **A 20-year incidence trend (1989–2008) and point prevalence (March 20, 2009) of multiple sclerosis in Tehran, Iran: a population-based study.** *Neuroepidemiology* 2011, **36**(3):141–147.

14. Nabavi M, Poorfarzam S, Ghasemi H: Epidemiology, clinical trend and prognosis of multiple sclerosis in 203 patients of MS clinic in Shahid Mostafa Khomeini hospital in 2002 (in Persian). *Tehran Univ Med J* 2006, 64(7):90–97.

15. Ghandehari K, Riasi HR, Nourian A, Boroumand AR: Prevalence of multiple sclerosis in north east of Iran. *Mult Scler* 2010, 16(12):1525–1526.

16. Ghabaae M, Qelichnia Omrani H, Roostaeizadeh M: Epidemiology of multiple sclerosis in Tehran: a three year study. *Tehran Univ Med J* 2007, 65(5):74–77.

17. Ale-Yasin H, Sarai A, Alaeddini F, Ansarian E, Lotfi J, Sanati H: Multiple sclerosis: a study of 318 cases. *Arch Iran Med* 2002, 5(1):24–27.

18. Bell C, Graham J, Earnshaw S, Oleen-Burkey M, Castelli-Haley J, Johnson K: Cost-effectiveness of four immunomodulatory therapies for relapsing-remitting multiple sclerosis: a Markov model based on long-term clinical data. *J Manag Care Pharm* 2007, 13(3):245–261.

19. Nuijten MJ, Hutton J: Cost-effectiveness analysis of interferon beta in multiple sclerosis: a Markov process analysis. *Value Health* 2002, 5(1):44–54.

20. *Statistical center of Iran.* http://www.amar.org.ir

21. Nikfar S, Rahimi R, Rezaie A, Abdollahi M: A meta-analysis on the efficacy and tolerability of natalizumab in relapsing multiple sclerosis. *Arch Med Sci* 2010, 6(2):236–244.

22. Nikfar S, Rahimi R, Abdollahi M: A meta-analysis of the efficacy and tolerability of interferon-β in multiple sclerosis, overall and by drug and disease type. *Clin Ther* 2010, 2(11):1871–1888.

23. Nikfar S, Rahimi R, Abdollahi M: A systematic review on the efficacy of interferon beta in relapsing multiple sclerosis; comparison of different formulations. *Inter J Pharmacol* 2010, 6(5):638–644.

24. Packer C, Simpson S, Stevens A: International diffusion of new health technologies: a ten-country analysis of six health technologies. *Int J Technol Assess Health Care* 2006, 22(4):419–428.

25. *European medicines agency, EMEA.* http://www.erna.europa.eu/ema/index

26. *United States of America Food and drug administration, US-FDA.* http://www.accessdata.fda.gov/scripts/cder/drugsatfda/index

27. Palesh M, Jonsson PM, Jamshidi H, Wettermark B, Tomson G, Fredrikson S: Diffusion of interferon beta in Iran and its utilization in Tehran. *Pharmacoepidemiol Drug Saf* 2008, 17(9):934–941.

28. *Iranian Food and Drug Organization.* http://fdo.behdasht.gov.ir

29. Cheraghali AM: Biosimilars; a unique opportunity for Iran national health sector and national pharmaceutical industry. *Daru* 2012, 20(1):35.

30. World Health Organization, WHO (Ed): www.who.int

31. Nikfar S, Kebriaeezadeh A, Majdzadeh R, Abdollahi M: Monitoring of National Drug Policy (NDP) and its standardized indicators; conformity to decisions of the national drug selecting committee in Iran. *BMC Int Health Hum Rights* 2005, 5(1):5.

32. Abdollahiasl A, Nikfar S, Kebriaeezadeh A, Dinarvand R, Abdollahi M: A model for developing a decision support system to simulate national drug policy indicators. *Arch Med Sci* 2011, 7(5):744–746.

33. Cheraghali AM, Nikfar S, Behmanesh Y, Rahimi V, Habibipour F, Tirdad R, Asadi A, Bahrami A: Evaluation of availability, accessibility and prescribing pattern of medicines in the Islamic Republic of Iran. *East Mediterr Health J* 2004, 10(3):406–415.

34. Nikfar S, Khatibi M, Abdollahiasl A, Abdollahi M: Cost and utilization study of antidotes: An Iranian experience. *Int J Pharmacol* 2011, 7(1):46–49.

35. Nikfar S: A new model for decision analysis in economic evaluations of switchable health interventions. *J Med Hypotheses Ideas* 2012, 6:12–15.

36. Kobelt G, Jonsson L, Fredriksson S: Cost-utility of interferon beta1b in the treatment of patients with active relapsing-remitting or secondary progressive multiple sclerosis. *Eur J Health Econ* 2003, 4(1):50–59.

37. Iskedjian M, Walker JH, Gray T, Vicente C, Einarson TR, Gehshan A: Economic evaluation of Avonex (interferon beta-1a) in patients following a single demyelinating event. *Mult Scler* 2005, 11(5):542–551.

38. Bose U, Ladkani D, Burrell A, Sharief M: Cost-effectiveness analysis of glatiramer acetate in the treatment of relapsing-remitting multiple sclerosis: first estimates. *J Med Econ* 2001, 4:207–219.

39. Parkin D, McNamee P, Jacoby A, Miller P, Thomas S, Bates D: A cost-utility analysis of interferon beta for multiple sclerosis. *Health Technol Assess* 1998, 2(4):iii–54.

40. Phillips CJ, Gilmour L, Gale R, Palmer M: A cost utility model of beta-interferon in the treatment of relapsing-remitting multiple sclerosis. *J Med Econ* 2001, 4:35–50.

41. Chilcott J, McCabe C, Tappenden P, O'Hagan A, Cooper NJ, Abrams K, Claxton K, Miller DH, Cost Effectiveness of Multiple Sclerosis Therapies Study Group: Modelling the cost effectiveness of interferon beta and glatiramer acetate in

the management of multiple sclerosis. Commentary: evaluating disease modifying treatments in multiple sclerosis. *BMJ* 2003, 326(7388):522.

42. Briggs A, Claxton K, Sculpher M: Decision modelling for health economic evaluation. In *Handbooks in health economic evaluation*. vol. 1st edition. Oxford: Oxford University Press; 2006.

43. Kurtzke JF: Rating neurologic impairment in multiple sclerosis: an expanded disability status scale (EDSS). *Neurology* 1983, 33(11):1444–1452.

44. Abdoli G: Estimation of social discount rate for Iran. *Eco Res Rev* 2009, 10:135–156.

45. Robberstad B: Estimation of private and social time preferences for health in northern Tanzania. *Soc Sci Med* 2005, 61(7):1597–1607.

46. Baltussen R, Adam T, Tan Torres T, Hutubessy R, Acharya A, Evans DB, Murray CJL: Generalized cost-effectiveness analysis: a guide. In *World Health Organization. Global programme on evidence for health policy.* Geneva: World Health Organization (WHO); 2002.

47. Weinshenker BG, Bass B, Rice GP, Noseworthy J, Carriere W, Baskerville J, Ebers GC: The natural history of multiple sclerosis: a geographically-based study. I. Clinical course and disability. *Brain* 1989, 112:133–146.

48. Hirst C, Ingram G, Pearson O, Pickersgill T, Scolding N, Robertson N: Contribution of relapses to disability in multiple sclerosis. *J Neurol* 2008, 255(2):280–287.

49. Hirst C, Swingler R, Compston DA, Ben-Shlomo Y, Robertson NP: Survival and cause of death in multiple sclerosis: a prospective population-based study. *J Neurol Neurosurg Psychiatry* 2008, 79:1016–1021.

50. Whitehead SJ, Ali S: Health outcomes in economic evaluation: the QALY and utilities. *Br Med Bull* 2010, 96:5–21.

51. Tappenden P, Chilcott JB, Eggington S, Oakley J, McCabe C: Methods for expected value of information analysis in complex health economic models: developments on the health economics of interferon-β and glatiramer acetate for multiple sclerosis. *Health Technol Assess* 2004, 8(27). http://www.hta.ac.uk/fullmono/mon827.pdf

52. *National organization for civil registration: Survival data of Iran.* www.sabteahval.ir

53. Tremlett H, Zhao Y, Devonshire V: Natural history of secondary-progressive multiple sclerosis. *Mult Scler* 2008, 14:314–324.

54. Tremlett H, Zhao Y, Devonshire V: Natural history comparisons of primary and secondary progressive multiple sclerosis reveals differences and similarities. *J Neurol* 2009, 256:374–381.

55. European Study Group on interferon beta-1b in secondary progressive MS: Placebo-controlled multicentre andomized trial of interferon beta-1b in treatment of secondary progressive multiple sclerosis. *Lancet* 1998, 352(9139):1491–1497.

56. Secondary Progressive Efficacy Clinical Trial of Recombinant Interferon-beta-1a in MS (SPECTRIMS) Study Group: Randomized controlled trial of interferon-beta-1a in secondary progressive MS: clinical results. *Clinical results. Neurology* 2001, 56(11):1496–1504.

57. Jacobs LD, Cookfair DL, Rudick RA, Herndon RM, Richert JR, Salazar AM, Fischer JS, Goodkin DE, Granger CV, Simon JH, Alam JJ, Bartoszak DM, Bourdette DN, Braiman J, Brownscheidle CM, Coats ME, Cohan SL, Dougherty DS, Kinkel RP, Mass MK, Munschauer FE III, Priore RL, Pullicino PM, Scherokman BJ, Whitham RH, et al: Intramuscular interferon beta-1a for disease progression in relapsing multiple sclerosis. The Multiple Sclerosis Collaborative Research Group (MSCRG). *Ann Neurol* 1996, 39(3):285–294.

58. Panitch H, Miller A, Paty D, Weinshenker B, North American Study Group on Interferon beta-1b in Secondary Progressive MS: Interferon beta-1b in secondary progressive MS: results from a 3-year controlled study. *Neurology* 2004, 63(10):1788–1795.

59. PRISMS (Prevention of Relapses and Disability by Interferon beta-1a Subcutaneously in Multiple Sclerosis) Study Group: Randomised double-blind placebo-controlled study of interferon beta-1a in relapsing/remitting multiple sclerosis. *Lancet* 1998, 352(9139):1498–1504.

60. Andersen O, Elovaara I, Färkkilä M, Hansen HJ, Mellgren SI, Myhr KM, Sandberg-Wollheim M, Soelberg Sørensen P: Multicenter, randomized, double blind, placebo controlled, phase III study of weekly, low dose, subcutaneous interferon beta-1a in secondary progressive multiple sclerosis. *J Neurol Neurosurg Psychiatry* 2004, 75(5):706–710.

61. Leary SM, Miller DH, Stevenson VL, Brex PA, Chard DT, Thompson AJ: Interferon beta-1a in primary progressive MS: an exploratory, randomized, controlled trial. *Neurology* 2003, 60(1):44–51.

62. The IFN, β Multiple Sclerosis Study Group: Interferon beta-1b is effective in relapsing-remitting multiple sclerosis. I. Clinical results of a multicenter,

randomized, double-blind, placebo-controlled trial. *Neurology* 1993, **43**(4):655–661.

63. Kappos L, Traboulsee A, Constantinescu C, Erälinna JP, Forrestal F, Jongen P, Pollard J, Sandberg-Wollheim M, Sindic C, Stubinski B, Uitdehaag B, Li D: Long-term subcutaneous interferon beta-1a therapy in patients with relapsing-remitting MS. *Neurology* 2006, **67**:944–953.

64. Ebers GC, Traboulsee A, Li D, Langdon D, Reder AT, Goodin DS, Bogumil T, Beckmann K, Wolf C, Konieczny A, Investigators of the 16-year Long-Term Follow-Up Study: Analysis of clinical outcomes according to original treatment groups 16 years after the pivotal IFNB-1b trial. *J Neurol Neurosurg Psychiatry* 2010, **81**:907–912.

65. Rudick RA, Lee JC, Cutter GR, Miller DM, Bourdette D, Weinstock-Guttman B, Hyde R, Zhang H, You X: Disability progression in a clinical trial of relapsing-remitting multiple sclerosis: eight-year follow-up. *Arch Neurol* 2010, **67**(11):1329–1335.

66. Phillips CJ: The cost of multiple sclerosis and the cost effectiveness of disease-modifying agents in its treatment. *CNS Drugs* 2004, **18**(9):561–574.

67. O'Brien B: *Multiple sclerosis.* London: Office of Health Economics; 1987.

68. Tappenden P, Chilcott J, O'Hagan A, McCabe C: Cost effectiveness of beta interferons and glatiramer acetate in the management of multiple sclerosis. In *Final Report to the National Institute for Clinical Excellence.* London: National Institute for Clinical Excellence (NICE); 2001.

69. Gani R, Giovannoni G, Bates D, Kemball B, Hughes S, Kerrigan J: Cost-effectiveness analyses of natalizumab (Tysabri®) compared with other disease-modifying therapies for people with highly active relapsing-remitting multiple sclerosis in the UK. *PharmacoEconomics* 2008, **26**(7):617–627.

70. Iran ministry of health and medical education: *Tariff of healthcare services in public and private sectors in Iran (2012).* Tehran: Iran ministry of health and medical education press; 2012.

71. *National Organization of Transportation.* http://upto.ir

72. Koopmanschap MA, Rutten FFH, Van Ineveld BM, Van Roijen L: The friction cost method for measuring indirect costs of disease. *J Health Econ* 1995, **14**:171–189.

73. Ganjali M, Baghfalaki T: Bayesian analysis of unemployment duration data in presence of right and interval censoring. *JRSS* 2012, **5**(1):17–32.

74. Asian Productivity Organization: *APO productivity data book 2012.* Tokyo: Keio university press INC; 2012.

75. Fisk JD, Brown MG, Sketris IS, Metz LM, Murray TJ, Stadnyk KJ: A comparison of health utility measures for the evaluation of multiple sclerosis treatments. *J Neurol Neurosurg Psychiatry* 2005, **76**:58–63.

76. Strom BL, Kimmel SE: *Textbook of pharmacoepidemiology.* Chichester, West Sussex: John Willey & Sons; 2006.

77. Bobes J, Cañas F, Rejas J, Mackell J: Economic consequences of the adverse reactions related with antipsychotics: an economic model comparing tolerability of ziprasidone, olanzapine, risperidone, and haloperidol in Spain. *Prog Neuropsychopharmacol Biol Psychiatry* 2004, **28**:1287–1297.

78. Goldberg LD, Edwards NC, Fincher C, Doan QV, Al-Sabbagh A, Meletiche DM: Comparing the cost-effectiveness of disease-modifying drugs for the first-line treatment of relapsing-remitting multiple sclerosis. *J Manag Care Pharm* 2009, **15**(7):543–555.

79. Fisk JD, Brown MG, Sketris IS, Metz LM, Murray TJ, Stadnyk KJ: A comparison of health utility measures for the evaluation of multiple sclerosis treatments. *J Neurol Neurosurg Psychiatry* 2005, **76**(1):58–63.

80. Kuspinar A, Rodriguez AM, Mayo NE: The effects of clinical interventions on health-related quality of life in multiple sclerosis: a meta-analysis. *Mult Scler* 2012, **18**(12):1686–1704.

81. European Medicines Agency (EMEA): EMEA Guideline on Similar Biological Medicinal Products, CHMP/437/04. [http://www.emea.europa.eu/docs/en_GB/document_library/Scientific_guideline/2009/09/WC500003517.pdf]

7

Evaluation of antitumor activity of a TGF-beta receptor I inhibitor (SD-208) on human colon adenocarcinoma

Abolfazl Akbari[1], Saeid Amanpour[2], Samad Muhammadnejad[2], Mohammad Hossein Ghahremani[1,3], Seyed Hamidollah Ghaffari[4], Ahmad Reza Dehpour[5], Gholam Reza Mobini[1], Fatemeh Shidfar[1], Mahdi Abastabar[6], Ahad Khoshzaban[7], Ebrahim Faghihloo[9], Abbas Karimi[10] and Mansour Heidari[7,8*]

Abstract

Background: Transforming growth factor-β (TGF-β) pathway is involved in primary tumor progression and in promoting metastasis in a considerable proportion of human cancers such as colorectal cancer (CRC). Therefore, blockage of TGF-β pathway signaling via an inhibitor could be a valuable tool in CRC treatment.

Methods: To evaluate the efficacy of systemic targeting of the TGF-β pathway for therapeutic effects on CRC, we investigated the effects of a TGβRI (TGF-β receptor 1) or TβRI kinase inhibitor, SD-208, on SW-48, colon adenocarcinoma cells. In this work, *in vitro* cell proliferation was studied by methyl thiazolyl tetrazolium (MTT) and bromo-2′-deoxyuridine (BrdU) assays. Also, the histopathological and immunohistochemical evaluations were conducted by hematoxylin and eosin, and Ki-67 and CD34 markers were stained, respectively.

Results: Our results showed no significant reduction in cell proliferation and vessel formation (170 ± 70 and 165 ± 70, $P > 0.05$) in treated SW-48 cells with SD-208 compared to controls.

Conclusion: Our data suggested that SD-208 could not significantly reduce tumor growth and angiogenesis in human colorectal cancer model at least using SW-48 cells.

Keywords: SD-208, Colorectal cancer, SW-48, Immunohistochemistry staining

Background

Colorectal cancer (CRC) is the second leading cause of cancer death among adults, making it as an excellent and desirable area for clinicians and researchers to study [1,2]. It has been also found that a large proportion of cancers such as CRC display inactivation of the growth factors specially transforming growth factor-β (TGF-β) pathway but they are characterized by increasing the factor production. In man, three isoforms of TGF-β including TGF-β1, TGF-β2 and TGF-β3 have been well characterized [3,4]. The homology searching has revealed that these proteins share up to 75% amino acid sequences. In spite of the fact that they have demonstrated comparable signaling activities, they are differentially expressed in cell lineages and tissues. It has been also frequently reported that TGF-β is the most effective growth inhibitor for normal epithelial, hematopoietic and immune cells. Studies showed that TGF-β acts as a double-edged sword in the biological processes [3-6]. In addition, it plays important roles in primary tumor progression and in promoting metastasis and has become an attractive target for therapy [5-7]. TGF-β exerts its effects by acting on two types of transmembrane receptors: type I (TGβRI) and type II (TGβRII). These receptors are involved in signal transduction, triggers through interaction of the TGF-β with TGβRII. Once TGF-β binds to TGβRII leads to the recruitment, phosphosphorylation, and activation of TGβRI. Activation of the TGβRI invokes several TGF-β signaling pathway targets and downstream genes [7,8]. Based on the literature, targeting of TGF-β signaling could be a valuable tool to treatment of human cancers such as CRC, glioblastoma and breast cancer [6-10]. Several studies

* Correspondence: mheidari@sina.tums.ac.ir
[7]Stem Cells Preparation Uinte, Farabi Eye Hospital, Tehran University of Medical Sciences, Tehran, Iran
[8]Department of Medical Genetics, School of Medicine, Tehran University of Medical Sciences, Tehran, Iran
Full list of author information is available at the end of the article

reported that a series of pyridopyrimidine-based TGβRI kinase inhibitors such as SD-208 could be a powerful approach for the treatment of various cancers. SD-208 is a small-molecule kinase inhibitor that bind to the ATP-binding site of the TGβRI kinase and maintains the enzyme in its inactive configuration [11-13]. Despite advances in our understanding of the molecular and genetic basis of CRC, effective treatment of the disease remains a clinical challenge. As pointed out, TGF-β promotes cell proliferation, development, invasion and metastasis in several types of tumors. It is thought that TGβRI inhibitor may have a therapeutic benefit in CRC; therefore, pharmacological blockade of the TGF-β signaling pathway has been proposed as a benefit strategy for CRC therapy. In the current study, SW-48, colon adenocarcinoma cell line was treated with different doses of SD-208, an anti-cancer agent. We evaluated the effects of SD-208 on cell proliferation and differentiation *in vitro* and *in vivo*.

Methods

Cell culture

Human colorectal adenocarcinoma cell line with pathologic differentiation grade of the original tumors IV, SW-48, was obtained from National Cell Bank of Iran (NCBI) affiliated to Pasteur Institute (Tehran, Iran). The cell line was grown in RPMI-1640 medium (Gibco; Germany) containing 25 mM D-glucose, 4 mM L-glutamine and 1 mM sodium pyruvate and supplemented with 5% (v/v) heat inactivated fetal bovine serum (FBS) (Gibco; Germany), 2 mM glutamax (Gibco; Germany), 100 units/ml penicillin, 100 µg/ml streptomycin and 250 ng/ml amphoterycin (Gibco; Germany) in culture flask 25 cm^2 (SPL Life Sciences; South Korea). The cells were kept at 37°C in a humidified 95% atmosphere, 5% CO$_2$ atmosphere incubator designated as culture at a steady-state condition. Cell viability was assessed using trypan blue exclusion test and routinely found to all flasks contain more than 95% viable cells.

Chemical description and biological activity TGβRI kinase inhibitor, SD-208

SD-208 (Sigma Aldrich; Belgium) is a selective and orally active pyridopyrimidine type TGβRI kinase inhibitor with an IC50 of approximately 35 nmol/L against TβRI kinase activity *in vitro*. The drug was dissolved in 100% dimethylsulfoxide (DMSO; Sigma Aldrich; Belgium) and prepared as stock solutions of 5 mM in DMSO and kept at −20°C until use.

MTT assay

The *in vitro* growth inhibitory effect of SD-208 was measured by the MTT assay (Roche Applied Science; Germany). This assay is dependent on the ability of viable cells to reduce a yellow tetrazolium salt (MTT) metabolically to a purple formazan product. This reaction

takes place when the cell is viable and mitochondrial reductase enzymes are active. Briefly, monolayer cultures were trypsinized in exponential growth phase, and viable cell counts were assessed using trypan blue exclusion. Then, cells were seeded in 96-well flat-bottom microtitration plates (SPL Life Sciences; South Korea) at a density of 5×10^4 cells/well (200 µL media/well). After 24 h, once the cells reached ~85% confluence they were treated with different concentrations of SD-208 (0.5 µM, 1 µM and 2 µM). Following 24 h drug exposure, for the recovery period, the cells were washed two times with fresh and free-FBS medium and the culture continued (Figure 1). Subsequently, fresh medium containing FBS was replaced for removal of efflux and unbound drug. In all *in vitro* experiments, control cells were incubated with dimethylsulfoxide (DMSO) alone (with the final concentration 0.2%). Complete medium was replaced with 100 µl MTT after 48 h incubations. The cells were incubated for 3 h at 37°C then MTT was removed, and 300 µl DMSO were added to each well. Finally, the optical densitometry was measured at a wavelength of 490 nm with background subtraction at 630 nm using a spectrophotometric microplate reader (BioTek Elx 808). The growth inhibition rate was calculated using the following formula:

$$\text{Growth inhibition rate (\%)} = 1 - \left(OD_{\text{drug exposure}}/OD_{\text{control}}\right) \times 100$$

BrdU assay

The BrdU assay was performed using BrdU ELISA kit according to the manufacturer's instructions (Roche Applied

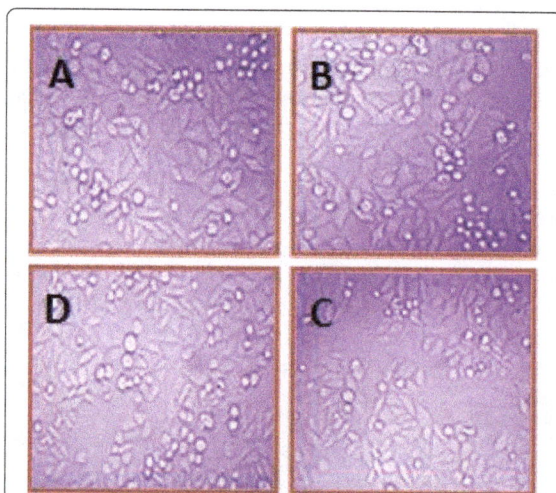

Figure 1 Continuous culture of SW-48 cells and treatment with SD-208. The cells were grown as monolayer epithelial-like morphology. SW-48 cells after treatment by DMSO alone as control (A), SD-208 concentrations 0.5 µM (B), 1 µM (C) and 2 µM (D).

Science; Germany) for the quantification of cell proliferation base on the measurement of BrdU incorporation during DNA synthesis. Briefly, the SW-48 cells were seeded in 96-well flat-bottom microtitration plates at a density of 5×10^4 cells/well (100 µl media/well). After 24 h at 37°C, the cells were treated with different concentrations of SD-208 (0.5 µM, 1 µM and 2 µM). Every well, except for the background controls, received 10 µl marker solution (1:100 dilution with a sterile medium) and the cells were further incubated for 5 h at 37°C under 5% CO_2. Removal of the medium from the wells was followed by incubation of the cells in 200 µl FixDenat for 30 min. The FixDenat was removed, and the cells were further incubated for 75 min with the antibody solution. The cells were then washed three times with 200 µl washing buffer (1:10 dilution) and then incubated in 100 µl substrate solution (tetramethylbenzidine) for 15 min. Absorbance was measured at a wavelength of 490 nm using a spectrophotometric microplate reader (BioTek Elx 808). Cells from the same population and treatment that were not BrdU-labeled were used as the background controls. The cell proliferation was calculated using the following formula:

$$\text{Cell proliferation } (\%) = \left(OD_{\text{drug exposure}} / OD_{\text{control}} \right) \times 100$$

Animal model implanted with adenocarcinoma cell line (SW-48) and treatment protocol

6–week–old female athymic C56BL/6 nude mice (n = 8 per group) were obtained from Omid Institute for Advanced Biomodels (Tehran, Iran). Animals were kept under optimized hygienic conditions in an individually ventilated cage system. The mice were fed with autoclaved commercial diet and water ad libitum. All animal experiments were carried out according to the Tehran University of Medical Sciences, Ethical Committee Acts and were approved by the TUMS Ethical Committee. In order to establish the xenograft model of SW-48 cell line, the cells were cultured in RPMI 1640 containing 10 percent FBS in 75 cm^2 cell culture flasks. The cells were trypsinized and harvested. After washing, totally 5×10^6 cells were resuspended and inoculated subcutaneously at a 200 µl volume of serum–free medium into the flank of the animals. Tumor growth was measured twice a week. The volume of tumors was calculated by standard formula (Length × width^2 × 0.52) and growth curve was drawn (Tomayko, 1989). Xenograft tumors were allowed to reach a size of 100 mm^3. Then, the animals were randomly divided into two groups of 8 to receive either SD-208 (50 mg/kg/d) or vehicle orally for three weeks. Control animals were received daily drug-free and DMSO-containing deionized water (vehicle). At the end of the treatment period, mice were killed by CO_2 inhalation and obtained tumors after

isolating from animal were fixed in 10% buffered formalin and were subjected to histopathological staining.

Histopathological diagnosis and immunohistochemistry

Hematoxylin and eosin (H&E) staining for SW-48 tumor confirmation and immunohistochemistry (IHC) staining for Ki-67 and CD34 markers were done. Then, five sections at routine thickness (5 µm) were prepared from the formalin-fixed paraffin-embedded tissue blocks and floated onto charged glass slides (Super-Frost Plus, Fisher Scientific). The slides then were dried overnight at 60°C. For the revision of the histopathological diagnosis and confirmation of developed the SW-48 cell-derived tumors, two hemotoxylin and eosin stained sections were obtained from tissue blocks. Immunohistochemistry carried out for the evaluation of SD-208 effects on proliferation and angiogenesis (Ki-67 and CD34 marker, respectively) in the tumor xenografts. For this, three sections were deparaffinized and hydrated using graded concentrations of ethanol to deionized water from each block. These sections were stained immunohistochemically using three steps-indirect streptavidin method for Monoclonal Mouse Anti-Human Ki-67 Antigen (MIB-1), clone M 7240 (Dako; Denmark) and Monoclonal Mouse Anti-Human CD34, clone QBEnd-10 (Dako; Denmark). Negative controls were obtained by omitting the primary antibody for aforementioned markers under identical test condition. Sections from a lymph node with follicular lymphoid hyperplasia known to be immunoreactive for Ki-67 and CD34 were used as a positive control (as recommended by the manufacturer).

Statistical analysis

Statistical analysis was performed, and statistical significance of differences between data was evaluated by independent sample Student's t-test for tumor markers (Ki-67 and CD34) and one-way analysis of variance (ANOVA) followed by Tukey's post tests for multiple comparisons of differences between treatment groups. Data were expressed as mean ± SEM (the standard error of the mean). P values less than 0.05 were considered to indicate statistically significant differences between data sets.

Results

In vitro effects of SD-208 on SW-48 cell line

In order to examine the growth inhibitory effect of SD-208 on CRC, the SW-48 cell line was cultured with different SD-208 concentrations (0.5 µM, 1 µM and 2 µM) for 48 h (Figure 1). As shown in Table 1, evaluation of *in vitro* growth inhibition by MTT (Figure 2A) and BrdU assays (Figure 2B) revealed no significant changes in treated versus untreated cells (P > 0.05).

Table 1 Effects of SD-208 on growth of SW-48 cell line

MTT assay			
Inhibition rate (IR)%	P value	OD value (mean ± SEM)	Concentration of SD-208 (μM)
		2.06 ± 0.085	Untreated
2.36	0.69	1.64 ± 0.098	Control (DMSO)
2.57	0.63	1.61 ± 0.093	0.5
3.4	0.6	1.54 ± 0.099	1
3.64	0.57	1.51 ± 0.098	2
BrdU assay			
		2.14 ± 0.079	Untreated
2.24	0.68	1.73 ± 0.081	Control (DMSO)
2.32	0.64	1.71 ± 0.087	0.5
2.6	0.63	1.69 ± 0.097	1
3.2	0.59	1.62 ± 0.098	2

Colon adenocarcinoma model

To determine the potential toxicity effects of SD-208, the appropriate numbers of SW-48 cells were injected into nude mice. Subsequently, animals were treated with or without SD-208 (as described in the Methods section). Following SD-208 treatment, we could not observe any changes in animal behavior, body weight and lifespan. These data suggest that SD-208 lacks toxic effects on mice bearing SW-48 tumor (data not shown).

Ten days after the subcutaneous inoculation, all 24 nude mice with an observed tumor growth survived with a balanced diet (Figure 3). Based on the standards of cancer-bearing models, 24 mice were selected for further experiments. The mice were sacrificed, and their tumor tissues were excised for pathological examinations.

The H&E staining demonstrates marked cellularity with profound hyperchromatism and pleomorphism (Figure 4). Pleomorphic malignant epithelial cells with the clearly nucleolus were visible. In tumor cells, the ratio of nucleus to the cytoplasm was 1/1. Also, high mitotic index and atypical areas were observed in both samples (treated versus controls). The pattern of adenocarcinoma was identical with the human origin in which the cancerous cells were poorly differentiated. Figure 4 indicates H&E staining of tumor tissues from studied animals. These results revealed no major differences in the sizes and the histology of the tumors ($P > 0.05$).

Immunohistochemistry

Immunohistochemical analysis was conducted using Ki-67 and CD34 antibodies. Immunoreactive SW-48 cells to anti- Ki-67 are brown nuclear with a diffuse pattern. It was scored by counting about 1000 cells in 10 different fields. Each brown stained nucleus was considered positive, regardless of intensity (Figure 5). Immunohistochemical staining of treated and untreated nude mice's

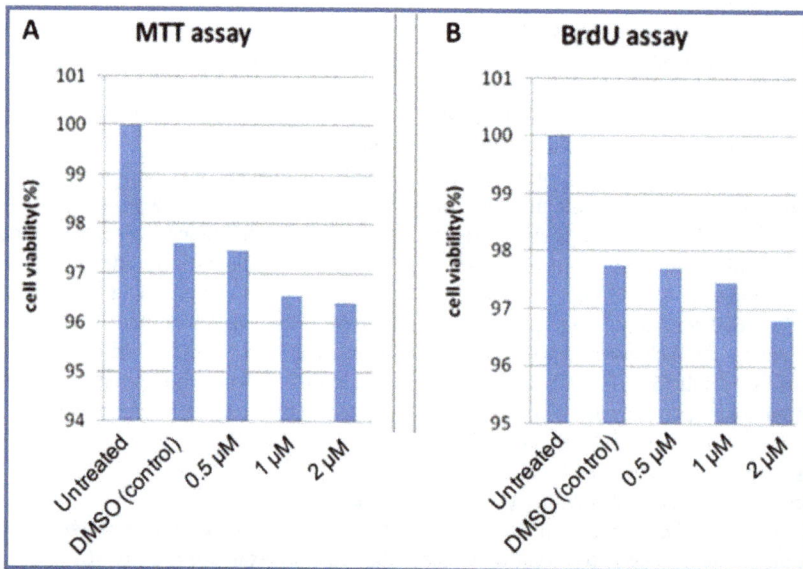

Figure 2 Effect of SD-208 on the cell growth and proliferation of the SW-48 cells. SW-48 cells were treated by 0.5, 1 and 2 μM for 48 h. Cell proliferation was examined by MTT and BrdU assays as described in methods. **A**: MTT assay of SW-48 cells after treatment with SD-208 in comparison with controls (untreated and treated with DMSO). **B**: BrdU assay of SW-48 cells after treatment with SD-208 comparison with controls (untreated and treated with DMSO). All data are reported as the percentage change in comparison with the controls, which were arbitrarily assigned 100% cell proliferation. Analysis of one-way ANOVA was used to compare the cell proliferation of SW-48 cells in different concentrations of SD-208 to control. P value < 0.05 was regarded as statistically significant. Results are expressed as the mean ± SEM from three independent experiments.

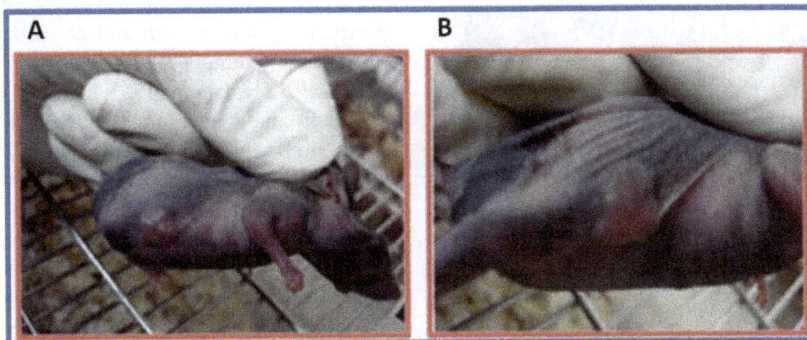

Figure 3 A representative of colorectal adenocarcinoma model. Tumor implantation; athymic nude mice implanted by SW-48 cell line, the cells were grown as tumor xenografts after 10 days. Cancer-bearing nude mice were treated with 50 mg/kg/day of SD-208 **(A)** or without SD-208 **(B)**.

tissues using anti-CD34 (as shown in the Figure 6) showed no significant changes among studied samples.

Ki-67 and CD34 expressions in the tumor xenografts

The results from the immunochemical assay indicated that Ki-67 was predominantly expressed in the nucleus. As already pointed out, the immunohistochemically stained tumors with anti-Ki-67 showed positively brown nuclear in the studied tissues (Figure 5). The Ki-67 expression levels between the test and control groups did not show significant changes (P > 0.05). Immunohistochemical staining using anti-CD34 antibody on tumor tissues from either treated or untreated nude mice with SD-208 showed cytoplasmic membrane of endothelial cells in brown color and marked microvessels proliferation (Figure 6).

Discussion

Despite aggressive surgery, radiotherapy and chemotherapy, treatment of malignant CRC remains formidable. Even though that TGF-β suppresses proliferation of certain carcinoma cells and is well-known to be a tumor suppressor, it promotes tumor development, progression and metastasis in human cancers including CRC, glioma, osteosarcoma, breast, lung and pancreatic cancers [14-16]. The insights into the role of the TGF-β signaling in carcinogenesis importantly have come due to experimental study on animal models. Understanding the mechanisms by which TGF-β signaling regulates tumor development and progression is critical for designing the beneficial therapeutic strategies for the cancers [14,16-18]. In the last few years, because of availability and easily drug delivery, the targeting of receptor kinases by small-molecule inhibitors has been a profound area of experimental cancer studies [16,17,19].

It is thought that pharmacological blockade of the TGF-β signaling pathway by TGβRI inhibitors may be as a potential strategy for cancer therapy [17-19]. For the first time, we evaluated the efficacy of systemic targeting of the TGF-β pathway by a TGβRI kinase inhibitor, SD-208, on a high-grade colon adenocarcinoma cell line, SW-48, *in vitro* and in developed heterotopic colon tumors in model that shares similarities with human colon cancer. Our findings using MTT and BrdU assays demonstrated that treatment of SW-48 cells with SD-208 using different doses had no significant inhibitory effects on cell growth and proliferation. Our *in vitro* results were consistent with one study revealing SD-208 can not reduce viability or proliferation of human malignant glioma cells [17]. However, this study showed that SD-208 regulates the growth of glioma in syngeneic mice without changes in proliferation, apoptosis or angiogenesis. Also, other investigators demonstrated that SD-208 failed to inhibit R3T tumor growth or metastasis in athymic nude mice [20]. On the other hand, some studies suggested that the various kinase inhibitors including SD-208, were able to inhibit TGF-β-evoked migration and invasion [20-22]. These results indicated that reduction of tumors was due to regulation of immune

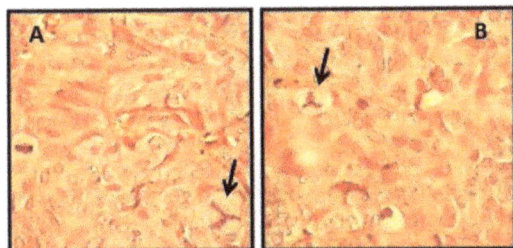

Figure 4 A representative results of pathological examinations of nude mice tumors with or without SD-208 treatment. A: tumors of nude mice treated with 50 mg/kg/day stained with H&E. **B**: H&E staining of tumor tissues of control. No significant difference histologically was observed (P > 0.05).

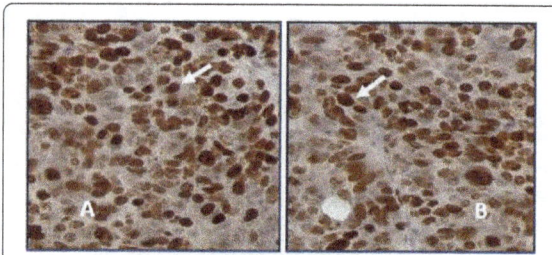

Figure 5 Colon adenocarcinoma (grade IV) stained immunohistochemically with anti-Ki-67. Positive immunoreactive showing brown nuclear expression of Ki-67 with a large number (~80%) of stained nuclei reflecting active cellular proliferation in the treated nude mice with SD-208 **(A)** and control **(B)**: Immunohischemical assay showed no significant difference between tests and controls in terms of cellular proliferation (P > 0.05).

surveillance and importantly correlated with tumor-reactive immune regulation and increased immune infiltration [21,22]. Thereby, it has been commented that SD-208 could be a promising agent for the treatment of human malignancy and other conditions associated with pathological TGF-β activity.

In addition, we revealed that when drinking water contains SD-208 daily, the drug could not inhibit the growth of established heterotopic SW-48 tumors and its progression in nude mice. Further histological analysis indicated that SD-208 had no significant effects on proliferation (Ki-67 positivity) or the number of blood vessels and angiogenesis (CD34 positivity). This is consistent with reports by others showing SD-208 had no effect on the growth of primary and metastatic R3T mammary tumors in athymic nude mice [18]. In the agreement with our results and previous studies, it has been shown that an inhibitor of TGF-β receptor 1 kinase, SM16, lost efficacy against the AB12 mesothelioma model in SCID mice [21].

Also, we found that SD-208 is not effective in limiting heterotopic tumor growth and not proper to treat established primary tumors settings at least in SW-48 colorectal cancer cells. The failure of SD-208 to inhibit SW-48 tumor growth in nude mice suggests that the suppression of angiogenesis and proliferation could be dependent on cell lineage and cell context [23]. Our results are not the first report suggesting the inability of SD-208 to inhibit angiogenesis and proliferation. Some researchers reported that SD-208 was unable to cause differences in microvessel density in gliomas [17]. Furthermore, a study of two TGF-βR1 inhibitors, SD-093 and SD-208, on two murine mammary carcinoma cell lines (R3T and 4 T1) revealed that SD-208 failed to inhibit R3T tumor growth or metastasis in athymic nude mice. However, SD-208 treatment led to a reduction in microvessel density in mammary tumors [20].

It is quite understandable that the efficacy of this kinase inhibitor is a controversial issue in cancer treatment [20]. In this regard, several scenarios could be proposed to elucidate the failure of SD-208 as an anti-tumor: (1) genetic alterations such as chromosomal abnormalities and (2) gene mutation in any TGF-β signaling pathway.

Conclusion

We have demonstrated that SD-208, a TGβRI kinase inhibitor, was not able to reduce tumor growth and angiogenesis in a heterotopic human colorectal cancer model. Our results also for the first time indicated that this anti-cancer agent could not potentially have a therapeutic benefit in at least proportion of CRC. To get more insight into the potential biological effects of SD-208 on CRC, different CRC cells with various differentiated status are required to treat with SD-208. Moreover, because of the complexity of TGF-β signaling role and crosstalk with other factors (such as immunochemotactic and angiogenic agents) in the derived

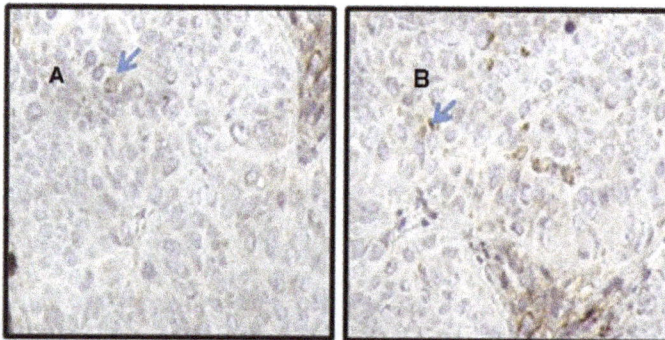

Figure 6 Colon adenocarcinoma (grade IV) stained immunohistochemically with anti-CD34. The paraffin embedded sections of tumor tissues were stained with anti-CD34 antibody and positive immunoreactive indicating brown cytoplasmic membrane of endothelial cells and marked microvessel's proliferation. Microvessel density (MVD) was ~40 microvessel/mm^2. SD-208-treated tumors **(A)** vs controls **(B)** revealed no significant immunohistologically differences (P > 0.05). Note the prominent vascularity. Arrows indicate CD34 staining of the cytoplasmic membrane.

tumor microenvironment, designing therapeutic intervention strategies for targeting tumors in this field, should be very carefully.

Abbreviations

TGF-β: Transforming growth factor-β; CRC: Colorectal cancer; TGβRI or TβRI: TGF-β receptor 1, TGβRII or TβRII, TGF-β receptor 2; SW-48: A colon adenocarcinoma cell line; SD-208: A TGF-β receptor I kinase inhibitor; MTT: Methyl thiazolyl tetrazolium; BrdU: Bromo-2'-deoxyuridine; H&E: Hematoxylin and Eosin; IHC: Immunohistochemistry.

Competing interests

The authors declare they have no competing interests.

Authors' contributions

MH and AA contributed to idea and study design; ARD contributed to the supervision of sections of the study. MHG, SHG, GRM and FS assisted with cell culture study and experimentation and provided scientific advice, MA assisted with analysis of the data. SM and SA assisted with IHC staining and data analysis. AA prepared the manuscript which SM, MH and AK significantly revised. All authors read and approved the final manuscript.

Acknowledgements

This study represents a part of a Ph.D. dissertation by Abolfazl Akbari. We wish to thank the School of Advanced Medical Technologies, the Tehran University of Medical Sciences (TUMS) for financially supporting this study.

Author details

[1]Department of Molecular Medicine, School of Advanced Medical Technologies, Tehran University of Medical Sciences, Tehran, Iran. [2]Cancer Research Center, Cancer Institute of Iran, Tehran University of Medical Sciences, Tehran, Iran. [3]Department of Pharmacology and Toxicology, Faculty of Pharmacy, Tehran University of Medical Sciences, Tehran, Iran. [4]Hematology, Oncology and Stem Cell Transplantation Research Center, Shariati Hospital, Tehran University of Medical Sciences, Tehran, Iran. [5]Department of Pharmacology, School of Medicine, Tehran University of Medical Sciences, Tehran, Iran. [6]Invasive Fungi Research Center, Department of Medical Mycology and Parasitology, School of Medicine, Mazandaran University of Medical Sciences, Sari, Iran. [7]Stem Cells Preparation Uinte, Farabi Eye Hospital, Tehran University of Medical Sciences, Tehran, Iran. [8]Department of Medical Genetics, School of Medicine, Tehran University of Medical Sciences, Tehran, Iran. [9]Department of Virology, School of Public Health, Tehran University of Medical Sciences, Tehran, Iran. [10]Department of Molecular Medicine, Faculty of Advanced Technologies in Medicine (FATiM), Iran University of Medical Sciences, Tehran, Iran.

References

1. Jemal A, Siegel R, Ward E, Hao Y, Xu J, Murray T, Thun MJ: Cancer statistics. *CA Cancer J Clin* 2008, **58:**71–96.
2. Kinzler KW, Vogelstein B: The Genetic Basis of Human Cancer. 2nd edition. New York: McGraw-Hill; 2002:583–612.
3. Luo K, Lodish HF: Signaling by chimeric erythropoietin-TGF-β receptors: homodimerization of the cytoplasmic domain of the type I TGF-β receptor and heterodimerization with the type II receptor are both required for intracellular signal transduction. *EMBO J* 1996, **15:**4485–4496.
4. Siegel PM, Massague J: Cytostatic and apoptotic actions of TGF-β in homeostasis and cancer. *Nature Rev Cancer* 2003, **3:**807–821.
5. Moustakas A, Heldin CH: Non-Smad TGF-β signals. *J Cell Sci* 2005, **118:**3573–3584.
6. Miriam Barrios R, Kevin R, Barish O, Rohit B, Zhong L, RS D, Fukiko SH, Yongmei L, Joanna D, Taylor IW, Valbona L, Mark R, Harukazu S, Yoshihide H, Igor J, Jeffrey LW: High-throughput mapping of a dynamic signaling network in mammalian cells. *Science* 2005, **307:**1621–1625.
7. Bierie B, Moses HL: TGF-β and cancer. *Cytokine Growth Factor Rev* 2006, **17:**29–40.
8. Levy L, Hill CS: Alterations in components of the TGF-β superfamily signaling pathways in human cancer. *Cytokine Growth Factor Rev* 2006, **17:**41–58.
9. Yingling JM, Blanchard KL, Sawyer JS: Development of TGF-β signaling inhibitors for cancer therapy. *Nature Rev Drug Discov* 2004, **3:**1011–1022.
10. Jean-Jacques L: The dual role of TGF in human cancer: from tumor suppression to cancer metastasis. *ISRN Molecular Biology* 2012, **7:**1–28.
11. Peng SB, Yan L, Xia X, Watkins SA, Brooks HB, Beight D, Herron DK, Jones ML, Lampe JW, McMillen WT, Mort N, Sawyer JS, Yingling JM: Kinetic characterization of novel pyrazole TGF-β receptor I kinase inhibitors and their blockade of the epithelial-mesenchymal transition. *Biochemistry* 2005, **44:**2293–2304.
12. Hill R, Song Y, Cardiff RD, Van Dyke T: Selective evolution of stromal mesenchyme with p53 loss in response to epithelial tumorigenesis. *Cell* 2005, **123:**1001–1011.
13. Inman GJ, Nicolás FJ, Callahan JF, Harling JD, Gaster LM, Reith AD, Laping NJ, Hill CS: SB-431542 is a potent and specific inhibitor of transforming growth factor-β superfamily type I activin receptor-like kinase (ALK) receptors ALK4, ALK5, and ALK7. *Mol Pharmacol* 2002, **62:**65–74.
14. Bruna A, Darken RS, Rojo F, Ocaña A, Peñuelas S, Arias A, Paris R, Tortosa A, Mora J, Baselga J, Seoane J: High TGFbeta-Smad activity confers poor prognosis in glioma patients and promotes cell proliferation depending on the methylation of the PDGF-B gene. *Cancer Res* 2003, **63:**7791–7798.
15. Qipeng F, Miao H, Tao S, Xiaoli Z, Mala S, Bruce L, Xingbo Z, Jing Wu X: Requirement of TGF Signaling for SMO-mediated Carcinogenesis. *J Biol Chem* 2010, **47:**36570–36576.
16. Bierie B, Harold LM: TGFβ: the molecular Jekyll and Hyde of cancer. *Nat Rev Cancer* 2006, **6:**506–520.
17. Uhl M, Steffen A, Jörg W, Markus W, Jing Ying M, Ramona A, Ruban M, Yu-Wang L, Michael P, Ulrich H, Alison M, Darren H, Wolfgang W, Higgins LS, Michael W: SD-208, a novel transforming growth factor-β receptor I kinase inhibitor, inhibits growth and invasiveness and enhances immunogenicity of murine and human glioma cells *in vitro* and *in vivo*. *Cancer Res* 2004, **64:**7954–7961.
18. Subramanian G, Schwarz RE, Linda H, Glenn M, Sarvajit C, Sundeep D, Michael R: Targeting endogenous transforming growth factor-β receptor signaling in SMAD4-deficient human pancreatic carcinoma cells inhibits their invasive phenotype1. *Cancer Res* 2004, **64:**5200–5211.
19. Leung SY, Niimi A, Noble A, Oates T, Williams AS, Medicherla S, Protter AA, Chung KF: Effect of transforming growth factor-beta receptor I kinase inhibitor 2,4-disubstituted pteridine (SD-208) in chronic allergic airway inflammation and remodeling. *J Pharmacol Exp Ther* 2006, **319:**586–594.
20. Ge R, Rajeev V, Ray P, Lattime E, Rittling S, Medicherla S, Protter A, Murphy A, Chakravarty J, Dugar S, Schreiner G, Barnard N, Reiss M: Inhibition of growth and metastasis of mouse mammary carcinoma by selective inhibitor of transforming growth factor-beta type I receptor kinase *in vivo*. *Clin Cancer Res* 2006, **12:**4315–4330.
21. Suzuki E, Kim S, Cheung HK, Corbley MJ, Zhang X, Sun L, Shan F, Singh J, Lee WC, Albelda SM, Ling LE: A novel small-molecule inhibitor of transforming growth factor β type I receptor kinase (SM16) inhibits murine mesothelioma tumor growth *in vivo* and prevents tumor recurrence after surgical resection. *Cancer Res* 2007, **67:**2351–2359.
22. Khalid SM, Delphine J, Pierrick GJ, Maria N, Ryan M, Xiang HP, Duong V, Lauren KD, Alain M, Theresa AG: TGF-β-RI kinase inhibitor SD-208 reduces the development and progression of melanoma bone metastases. *Cancer Res* 2011, **71:**175–184.
23. Medicherla S, Li L, Ma JY, Kapoun AM, Gaspar NJ, Liu YW, Mangadu R, O'Young G, Protter AA, Schreiner GF, Wong DH, Higgins LS: Antitumor activity of TGF-β inhibitor is dependent on the microenvironment. *Anticancer Res* 2007, **27:**4149–4158.

8

Adenosine deaminase activity modulation by some street drug: molecular docking simulation and experimental investigation

Massoud Amanlou[1*], Ali-akbar Saboury[2], Roya Bazl[2], Mohammad Reza Ganjali[2] and Shokoofeh Sheibani[3]

Abstract

Background: Adenosine deaminase (ADA) is an enzyme that plays important roles in proliferation, maturation, function and development of the immune system. ADA activity may be altered by variety of substances including synthetic or natural products. Morphine, cocaine and their analogs exert immune suppressive activities by decreasing immune system function. The purpose of this study is to confirm that this possible effect may be modulated by interaction of these substances with ADA activity by experimental and computational method.

Methods: The structural changes in ADA have been studied in presence of cocaine, ethylmorphine, homatropine, morphine and thebaine by determination of ADA hydrolytic activity, circular dichroism and fluorescence spectroscopy in different concentrations. Docking study was performed to evaluate interaction method of test compound with ADA active site using AutoDock4 software.

Results: According to in-vitro studies all compounds inhibited ADA with different potencies, however thebaine activated it at concentration below 50 μM, ethylmorphine inhibited ADA at 35 μM. Moreover, fluorescence spectra patterns were differed from compounds based on structural resemblance which were very considerable for cocaine and homatropine.

Conclusion: The results of this study confirms that opioids and some other stimulant drugs such as cocaine can alter immune function in illegal drug abusers. These findings may lead other investigators to develop a new class of ADA activators or inhibitors in the near future.

Keywords: Adenosine deaminase, Opioid, Cocaine, Immune system, Docking

Introduction

Adenosine deaminase (ADA) is an enzyme that irreversibly converts adenosine to inosine [1]. This enzyme exists in all human tissues, but the highest levels and activity are found in the lymphoid system such as lymph nodes, spleen, and thymus [2]. It is also essential for the proliferation, maturation and function of T lymphocyte cells. It is assumed that ADA plays a crucial role in development of the immune system, while its innate deficiency causes severe combined immunodeficiency (SCID) [3]. Moreover, ADA activity changes in a variety of other diseases including acquired immunodeficiency syndrome (AIDS), anemia, various lymphomas, tuberculosis, and leukemia [4,5]. On the other hand, ADA regulates the levels of endogenous adenosine which results in immune system suppression by inhibiting lymphoid or myeloid cells [6,7], including neutrophils [8], macrophages [9], lymphocytes [10,11] and platelets [12].

Two distinct isoenzymes of ADA, known as ADA_1 and ADA_2, are found in mammalian [13-15]; former has highest levels of activity in spleen, and thymus whereas latter is found in other parts of body [15]. As the most abundant type of white blood cells that responds to infection and attacks of foreign invaders, neutrophils might possess more than one type of adenosine receptor [16], and adenosine regulates neutrophil function in an opposing manner through the ligation of ADA_1 (immunostimulatory) and ADA_2 (immunosuppressive) receptors [17].

* Correspondence: amanlou@tums.ac.ir
[1]Department of Medicinal Chemistry, Faculty of Pharmacy, Pharmaceutical Sciences Research Center, Tehran University of Medical Sciences, Tehran, Iran
Full list of author information is available at the end of the article

A number of ADA inhibitors with various degrees of potency have been reported [18]. In one study, immunosuppressive and anti-inflammatory effects of FR234938, as a non-nucleoside inhibitor of ADA, were investigated [19]. Moreover, deoxycoformycin, another ADA inhibitor, has been investigated in treatment of colon carcinoma cells [20,21] and hematological neoplasms [22]. By contrast, ibuprofen [23] and medazepam [24] effects on immune deficiency have been reported. This revealed that purine compound may act as ADA activator; but still more experiments are needed to confirm this finding.

Opioids have variety of clinical applications. Naltrexone in low dosage can suppress human ovarian cancer and provides novel non-toxic therapies for the treatment of this lethal neoplasia [25]. The idea that opioids suppress the immune system and reduce resistance to infections is not new [26]. Several studies on animals and humans have illustrated that opioids can exert immunosuppressive effects by interfering B and T cell function [27-29]. In this regard, Sacerdote et al. have reported that immune function is affected by morphine and tramadol [30]. In other investigations, chronic treatment with morphine has been shown to affect the function of T cells and reduce immunity by directly interacting with cells of the immune system [28,30-34]. On the other hand, studies about heroin abusers showed that patients were suffering from a disease that diminishes their immunity, by affecting T-lymphocyte function and therefore cause (HIV) infection [33,34]. In addition, long term usage of cocaine and homatropine leads to a heart attack, tremors, and apnea, cardiac arrest respectively. The possible involvement of adenosine in opioid antinociception has been supported by Ho et al. [34]. Interaction between an opioid and an adenosine receptor has been proposed. Yet, binding efficiency of ADA1 is reduced in the presence of morphine [35,36]. Also, transferring of opioids to the pontine reticular formation (PRF) and substantia innominata (SI) causes adenosine to decrease in the PRF and SI [37].

Although the knowledge about effects of opioids on immune responses has been improved, there is relatively little information about these immunosuppressive effects. Therefore, the present investigation was conducted to find the effects of this group of opiates and two other alkaloid compounds on ADA activity; by means of computational and experimental methods to found new compounds for modulation of adenosine deaminase activity.

Material and methods
Materials
Adenosine deaminase (EC 3.5.4.4) extracted from bovine spleen was purchased from sigma, and all other used materials were of analytical grade and acquired from Merck. PBS that is used in assay was adjusted at 7.4, at

which, enzyme has optimal activity in [38,39]. All solutions were prepared in MilliQ (Millipore, USA) water.

Biological assays
Released ammonia resulted by enzyme activity was determined by specific Berthelot colorimetric method which was used for micro determination of ADA activity in serum [40]. Briefly, this method is based on the reaction of liberated ammonia with hypochlorite (OCl^-) to form a monochloramine and subsequent reaction of this intermediate with phenol to produce blue-colored indophenols that absorbance is measured at 625 nm. In this process sodium nitroprusside is used as the catalyst. The reaction was initiated by addition of adenosine as a substrate at 37°C to preincubated enzyme with different concentrations of tested compounds at different concentrations (5–300 μM). Finally, the enzymatic reaction was stopped at the end of 30 minutes of incubation by adding phenol nitroprusside solution. The mixture kept again for 30 minutes at 37°C before absorbance determination.

Obtained absorbance was normalized through blank sample, and IC_{50} values were calculated by Prism software (Ver. 5, GraphPad Software Inc., San Diego CA,).

Circular dichroism spectroscopy
CD spectra were measured in the far-UV (200–260 nm) region with JASCO J-715 spectropolarimeter (Japan). JASCO J-715 software not only gave us the possibility of data smoothing, but also used to predict the secondary structure changes of the protein according to the statical method [41]. Each scan was recorded in 1 nm increments at 37°C, repeated three times, and averaged. The protein was in 0.1 M PBS buffer, pH = 7.4, and its concentration was adjusted to 2 mg/ml in 1 cm path length cuvette. The results were expressed in molar ellipticity [θ] (deg cm^2.dmol^{-1}).

Fluorescence spectroscopy
Fluorescence spectroscopy was performed on a Hitachi fluorescence spectrophotometer model MPF-4 with 1 cm path length fluorescence cuvette and final volume of 400 μL. The excitation wavelength was adjusted in 290 nm, and the emission was scanned every 1 nm in the range of 300 to 400 nm. The final concentration of enzyme was 6 μM and different concentrations of tested compounds were changed from 1.7 to 73.4 μM.

Docking simulation
To have a better understanding about the inhibitory mechanism of the test compounds and clarification of type of interactions, docking were performed using the AutoDock 4.2 package [42]. The ability of software in next predictions was determined with re-docking of co-crystallized inhibitor of protein x-ray structure pdb ID:

1ADD and compared to inhibitor orientation in crystal structure. This crystal structure has been used since its > 80% similarity in structure with bovine spleen and active site amino acids conservation. The structure of all compound have sketched by Marvin sketch applet (Marvin package, Chemaxon Company). AutoDockTools (ADT) 1.5.6 was used for preparing input files using Autodock 4.2 atom types and calculating all needed charges [42].

Adding polar hydrogens and rotatable bonds were done with ADT; docking with a maximum number of 25×10^6 energy evaluations using the Lamarckian Genetic Algorithm (LGA) were performed. All other parameters were set to default values. The docked conformations of each ligand were ranked into clusters based on the binding energy. After clustering analysis, conformation with the most favourable binding energy was selected.

Table 1 IC$_{50}$ values and binding energies of test compounds in presence of 2 mg/ml adenosine deaminase enzyme

No.	Name	Structure	IC$_{50}$ (µM)	ΔG° binding (kcal/mol)
1	Thebaine		50*/163	−7.2
2	Morphine		43.7	−8.1
3	Ethylmorphine		35	−8.0
4	Cocaine		180	−6.8
5	Homatropine		96	−7.2

*Thebaine was activated ADA till this concentration.

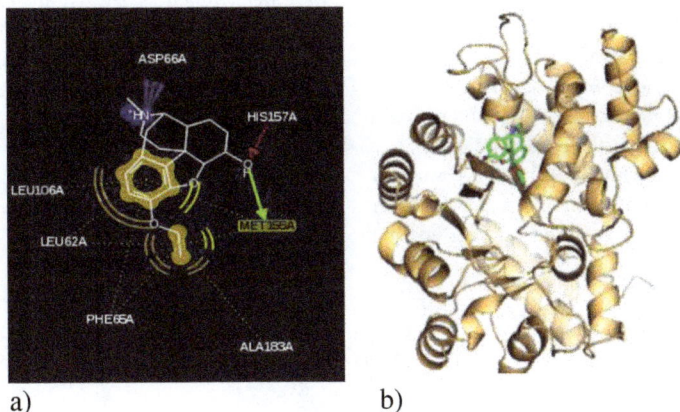

Figure 1 Ethylmorphine binding site of adenosine deaminase 2D (a) and 3D (b) demonstration.

Results and discussion
Determination of ADA activity

The target compounds were evaluated against ADA enzymatic activity in vitro and obtained IC_{50} values are summarized in Table 1. As shown in Table 1 all tested compounds inhibit ADA activity in micromolar range. In general, compounds in group1 (consisted of ethylmorphine, morphine and thebaine) showed better inhibitory activities than compounds in the other structurally related group (group 2: cocaine and homatropine). As shown, despite of partially closed binding energies, each compound inhibits the enzyme in variety of concentrations. Enhance in inhibition potency may be due to a decrease in conformational flexibility and better stabilization in inhibition site. In first group the order of inhibitory activities showed the potency of ethylmorphine > morphine > thebaine. This tendency is due to the presence of different substitute on A and C rings of perhydrophenanthrene structure. Ethylmorphine with ethoxy group on A ring shows better potency (IC_{50}: 35 μM) than those with hydroxyl and methoxy substitutes. Upon further modification on C-ring in thebaine, the activity further decreased.

This drop in inhibition activity may be due to inappropriate stabilization of compound to bind to target amino acids or inappropriate interactions which was confirmed by the molecular docking study. The binding energy of thebaine was calculated –7.2 kcal/mol compare to ethylmorphine ($\Delta G°$: –8 kcal/mol). Interestingly in this series, thebaine activated enzyme hydrolytic activity till 50 μM and up to this level showed inhibition effect with IC_{50}: 163 μM (Table 1). However, thebaine, cocaine and homatropine shows IC_{50} higher than other inhibitors (ethylmorphine and morphine), it can imply some immunity problem in the opioid consumers may result by ADA inhibition.

In another group hydroxyl substitution may be responsible for the homatropine inhibition efficiency which might build H-bond with adjacent residues at active site of ADA. In addition, cocaine showed weaker inhibitory activity which indicated the influence of position and size of the substitute on tropan ring on the inhibitory activity. For more insight to obtained IC_{50} values and interaction site recognition the docking study has been performed.

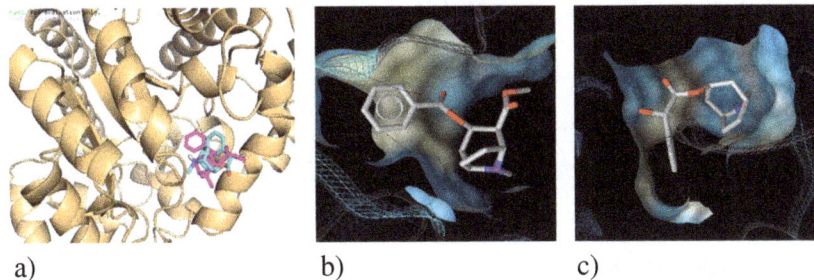

Figure 2 Docking pose of cocaine and homatropine in the adenosine deaminase binding pocket at their lowest energy of binding conformation: a) Overlay of cocaine and homatropine. b) Cocaine and c) Homatropine.

Docking experiments

Docking studies are used at different stages of drug discovery such as in the prediction of ligand-receptor interaction and also to rank the compounds based on the binding energies. Docking of co-crystallized inhibitor with ADA was performed to evaluate the efficacy of docking software and the reasonable RMSD of 0.39 Å was obtained. Docking of tested compounds with the ADA enzyme was performed, and corresponded binding energies

were determined as shown in Table 1. The interacting energies followed the order of the in vitro IC_{50} values with rational correlation (R^2: 0.84). All compounds posed in ADA active site entrance or partially penetrated in active site.

For the most potent inhibitor, ethylmorphine, the hydroxyl group of C-ring formed a hydrogen bond with Met155 and His157. Moreover, presence of ethoxy group in ring A resulted in hydrophobic interactions with Leu62,

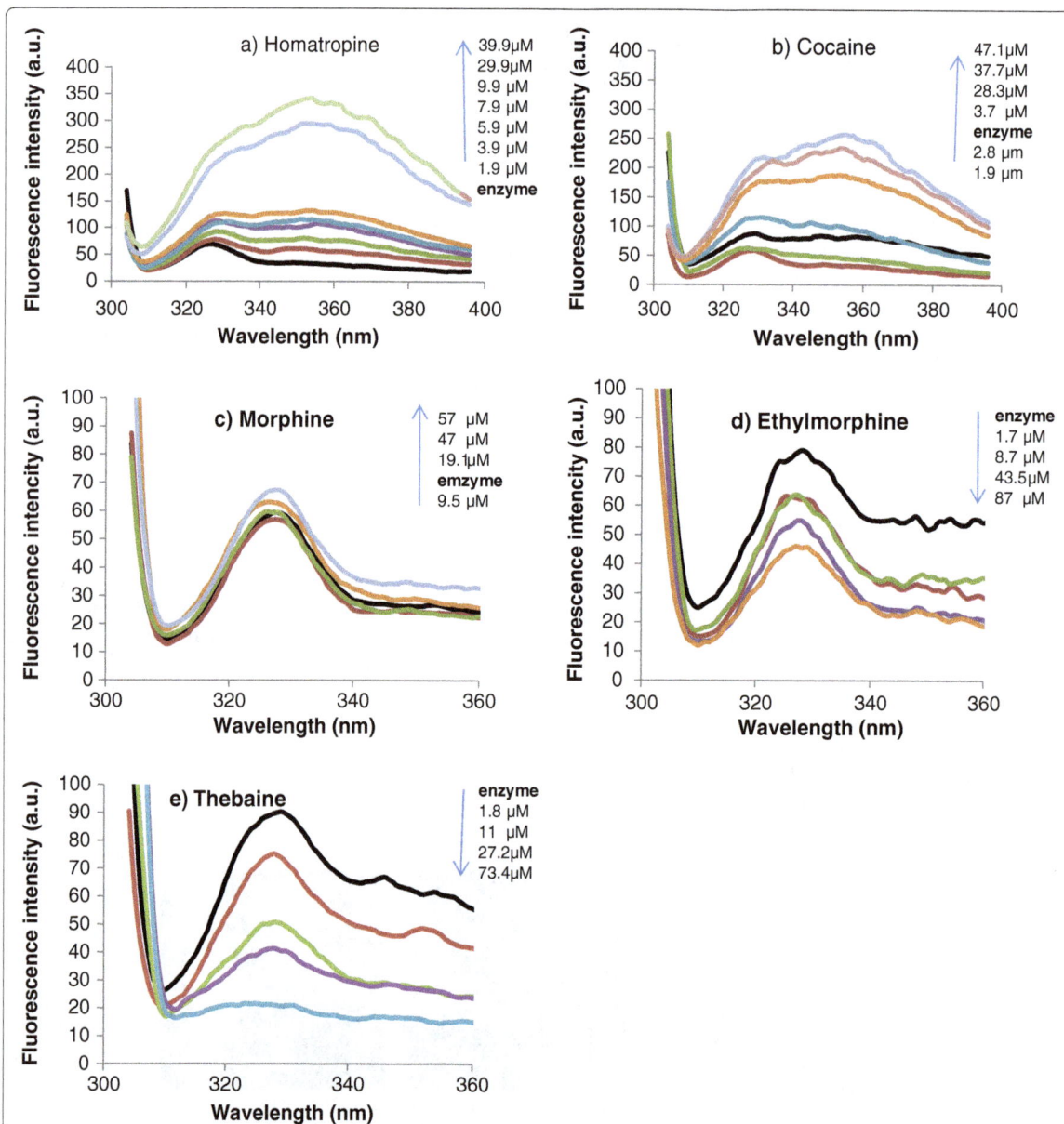

Figure 3 Change in fluorescence spectra of adenosine deaminase in presence of different concentration of a), Homatropine, b) Cocaine, c) Morphine, d) Ethylmorphine, and e) Thebaine in pH: 7.4.

Phe65, Leu106, Met155 and Ala183 as well as electrostatic interaction of nitrogen atom made it much more stabilized in binding site (Figure 1). Thebaine exhibited binding energy of "-7" kcal/mol which correlated with the experimentally observed activity due to flat T-shape structure which resulted in less penetration into active site. On the other hand, in comparison to morphine replacing of hydroxy with methoxy group on C-ring caused

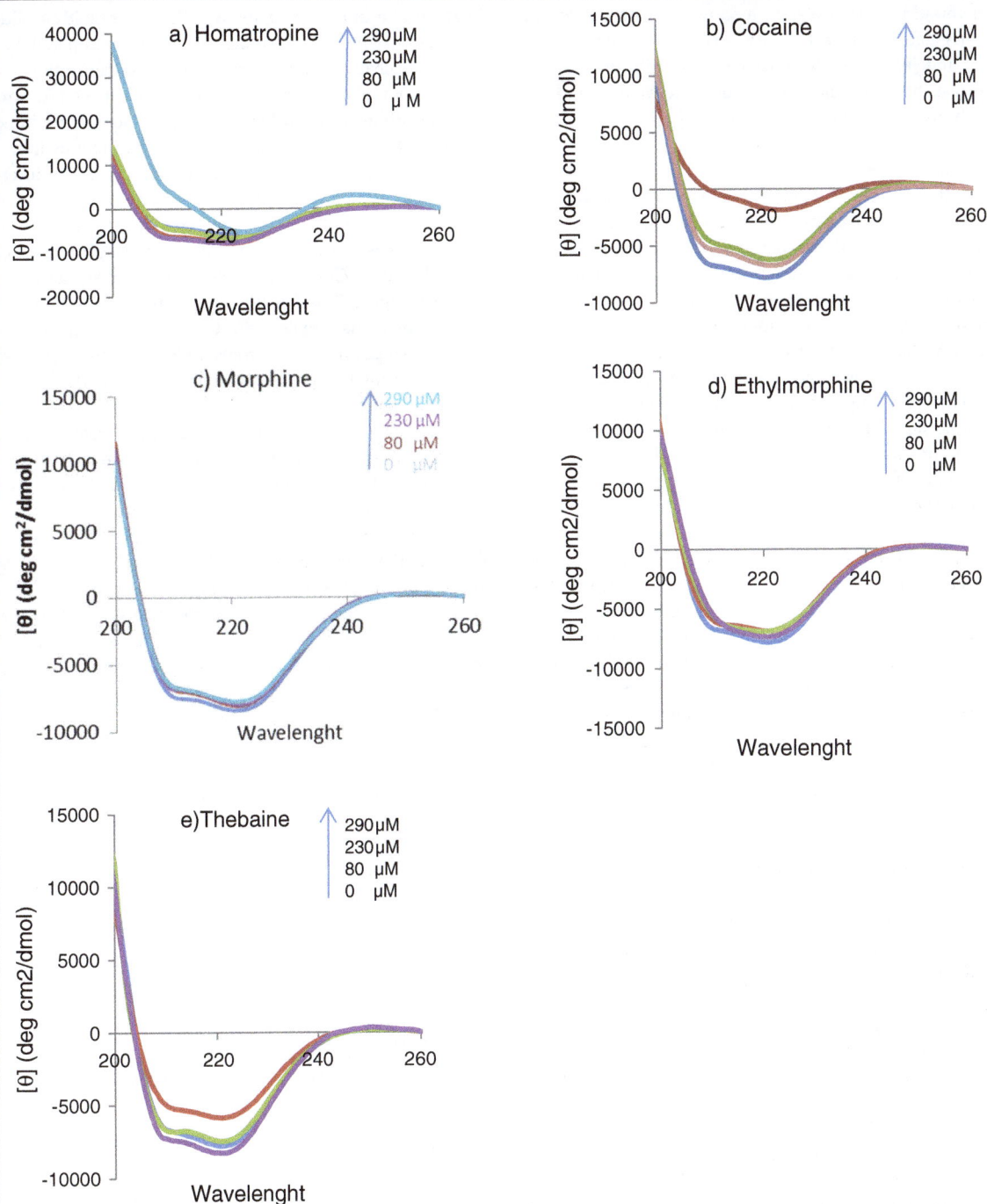

Figure 4 CD spectra of adenosine deaminase in presence of different concentration (0–300 μM) of a) Homatropine, b) Cocaine, c) Morphine, d) Ethylmorphine, e) Thebaine in pH: 7.4.

removing of H-bond with His157, consequently resulted in lower efficiency. This effect was illustrated in ethylmorphine which in existing H-bond made it more stabilized in binding site. In the other group, homatropine binds to ADA with lower binding energy than cocaine with IC_{50} 96 and 180 µM respectively. As it shown in Figure 2 cocaine doesn't diffuse into active site because of bulkier substitute, and just poses on enzyme active site entrance. In contrast, homatropine enters from phenyl part and OH group makes H-bond with Leu62.

Fluorescence spectroscopy

Interaction of tested compounds with Trp residues can be studied by change in emission spectra of ADA in 320-340 nm. In other words, any environmental alteration as well as three-dimensional structure changes in Trp amino acid and enzyme respectively, can change the innate spectrum of Trp residues in enzyme. As shown in Figure 3, there are two totally different patterns in interaction with Trp residues. In the first group, homatropine and cocaine in high concentrations, demonstrate bathochromic shift. This change may be probably due to severe change of three dimensional structure of the enzyme. In the other series: morphine, ethylmorphine and thebaine do not show noticeable change and shift in fluorescence spectra; indeed compounds with bulkier structure don't penetrate efficiently in binding pocket, and place in longer distance with Trp residues. Thebaine and ethylmorphine in this group decrease Trp emission as their concentration increase. This could be an indication that these compounds have bonded with the active sites or other sites of the ADA enzyme and therefore the Trp amino acid is out of access. According to the Berthelot test results, thebaine till 50 µM stimulates enzyme to break down faster, but above this concentration the activity of thebaine slows down and the concentration of 163 µM, results in 50% of inhibition.

Circular dichroism spectroscopy

CD spectra of ADA in the presence of different concentration of compounds have been illustrated in Figure 4. ADA showed two transitions in 210 and 222 nm which are attribute to $n \rightarrow \pi^*$ and $\pi \rightarrow \pi^*$ respectively. According to percent of different patterns of 2D structure of enzyme, among α-helix structure has been undergone sever changes, and mostly convert to random coil. This effect can be explained by compounds intercalation between helix residues and broken of H-bonds. According to the Figure 3 in high concentrations of cocaine, bathochromic shift in the fluorescence spectra was observed. On the other hand as it shown in Figure 4, in cocaine concentration around 180 µM drastic changes in CD spectra were observed. Also, based on in-vitro studies 50% of enzyme's activity has been diminished in 180 µM,

so it can infer from this point despite of strong alteration in overall ADA structure or active site remains much more intact.

Conclusion

Regarding to immunosuppressive effects of opioids, evaluation of enzyme activity studies was performed parallel to structural changes caused by different concentrations of test compounds. Thebaine activated ADA in certain low concentrations; while in higher concentrations it inhibited the enzyme. On the contrary, all other compounds inhibited the enzyme in studied range (0-300 µM). The interaction site as well as existing interactions in stabilization of each compound was obtained by docking studies. Finally, changes in two and three dimensional structures of ADA (based on Circular dichroism and fluorescence spectroscopy Figure 3 and 4) revealed that only cocaine and homatropine, had major effects on the enzyme (made drastic changes in the enzyme); while these changes were not significant for morphine, etylmorphine and thebaine in studied concentrations.

Regarding that the adenosine deaminase enzyme has a very important role in the immune system activity, so the inhibition of this enzyme's natural function in the human body can lead to debilitation of the immune system. Therefore, the results of this experiment support the idea that persons with addiction and regular drug abuse have a weaker immune system than others. This study can also help other researchers to develop a new class of ADA activators or inhibitors in the near future to manage malfunction of the immune system.

Competing interest
There are no other conflicts of interest related to this publication.

Authors' contributions
All authors contributed to the concept and design, making and analysis of data, drafting, revising and final approval. MA is responsible for the study registration, financial and administrative support. RB & SHSH are responsible for biological assays. RB & MA were involved for docking studies. AAS & MRG were responsible for experimental analysis. All authors were participated in data assembly and analysis, interpretation and manuscript writing. They read and approved the final manuscript.

Acknowledgments
This study was supported by a grant from the Research Council of Tehran University of Medical Sciences.

Author details
[1]Department of Medicinal Chemistry, Faculty of Pharmacy, Pharmaceutical Sciences Research Center, Tehran University of Medical Sciences, Tehran, Iran. [2]Institute of Biochemistry and Biophysics, University of Tehran, Tehran, Iran. [3]Center of Excellence in Electrochemistry, Faculty of Chemistry, University of Tehran, Tehran, Iran.

References
1. Brady T: **Adenosine deaminase.** *Biochem J* 1942, **36:**478–484.

2. Gorrell MD, Gysbers V, McCaughan GW: **CD26: a multifunctional integral membrane and secreted protein of activated lymphocytes.** *Scand J Immunol* 2001, **54**:249–264.

3. Resta R, Thompson LF: **SCID: the role of adenosine deaminase deficiency.** *Immunol Today* 1997, **18**:371–374.

4. Gakis C, Calia C, Naitana A, Pirino D, Semi G: **Serum adenosine deaminase activity in HIV positive subjects: a by pothesis on the significance of ADA-2.** *Panminerva Med* 1989, **31**:107–113.

5. Glader BE, Backer K, Diamond LK: **Elevated erythrocyte adenosine deaminase activity in congenital hypoplastic anemia.** *Eng J Med* 1983, **309**:1486–1490.

6. Ohta A, Sitkovsky M: **Role of G-protein-coupled adenosine receptors in down regulation of inflammation and protection from tissue damage.** *Nature* 2001, **414**:916–920.

7. Sitkovsky MV, Lukashev D, Apasov S, Kojima H, Koshiba M, Cald-well C, Ohta A, Thiel M: **Physiological control of immune response and inflammatory tissue damage by hypoxia-inducible factors and adenosine A2A receptors.** *Annu Rev Immunol* 2004, **22**:657–682.

8. Fredholm BB: **Purines and neutrophil leukocytes.** *Gen Pharmacol* 1997, **28**:345–350.

9. Murphree LJ, Sullivan GW, Marshall MA, Linden J: **Lipopolysac-charide rapidly modifies adenosine receptor transcripts in murine and human macrophages: role of NF-kappa B in A2A, adenosine receptor induction.** *Biochem* 2005, **391**:575–580.

10. Lappas CM, Rieger JM, Linden J: **A2A adenosine receptor induction inhibits IFN-gamma production in murine CD^{4+} T cells.** *J Immunol* 2005, **174**:1073–1080.

11. Koshiba M, Rosin DL, Hayashi N, Linden J, Sitkovsky MV: **Patterns of A2A extracellular adenosine receptor expression in different functional subsets of human peripheral T cells. Flow cytometry studies with anti-A2A receptor monoclonal antibodies.** *Mol Pharmacol* 1999, **55**:614–624.

12. Varani K, Gessi S, Dalpiaz A, Borea PA: **Pharmacological and biochemical characterization of purified A2a adenosine receptors in human platelet membranes by 3[H]-CGS 21680 binding.** *Br J Pharmacol* 1996, **117**:1693–1701.

13. Van Der Weyden MB, Kelly WN: **Human adenosine deaminase. Distribution and properties.** *J Biol Chem* 1976, **251**:5448–5456.

14. Hirschhorn R, Ratech H: **Isozymes of adenosine deaminase.** In *Current Topics in Biological and Medical Research*, Volume 1. Edited by Ratazzi MC, Scandalia JG, Whitt GS. New York: Alan R Liss; 1980:132–157.

15. Kurata N: **Adenosine deaminase.** *Nihon Rinsho* 1995, **53**:122–127.

16. Rose FR, Hirschhorn R, Weissmann G, Cronstein BN: **Adenosine promotes neutrophil chemotaxis.** *J Exp Med* 1988, **167**:1186–1194.

17. Haskó G, Cronstein BN: **Adenosine: an endogenous regulator of innate immunity.** *Trends Immunol* 2004, **25**:33–39.

18. Cristalli G, Costanzi S, Lambertucci C, Lupidi G, Vittori S, Volpini R, Camaioni E: **Adenosine deaminase: functional implication and different classes of inhibitors.** *Med Res Rev* 2001, **21**:105–128.

19. Kuno M, Seki N, Tsujimoto S, Nakanishi I, Kinoshita T, Nakamura K, Terasaka T, Nishio N, Sato A, Fujii T: **Anti-inflammatory activity of FR234938.** *Eur J Pharmacol* 2006, **534**:241–249.

20. Bemi V, Tazzini N, Banditelli S, Giorgelli F, Pesi R, Turchi G, Mattana A, Sgarrela F, Tozzi MG, Camici M: **Deoxyadenosine metabolism in a human colon-carcinoma cell line LoVo, in relation to its cytotoxic effect in combination with deoxycoformycin.** *Int J Cancer* 1998, **75**:713–720.

21. Camici M, Turriani M, Tozzi MG, Turchi G, Cos J, Alemany C, Miralles A, Noe V, Ciudad CJ: **Purine enzyme profile in human colon carcinoma cell lines and differential sensitivity to deoxycoformycin and 2'-deoxyadenosine in combination.** *Int J Cancer* 1995, **17**:176–183.

22. Pettitt AR: **Mechanism of action of purine analogues in chronic lymphocytic leukaemia.** *Br J Haematol* 2003, **121**:692–702.

23. Kalantari S, Rezaei-Tavirani M, Khodakarim S: **Effects of different therapeutical doses of ibuprofen on the adenosine deaminase activity at physiologic and pathologic temperatures.** *Koomesh* 2011, **13**:50–56.

24. Centelles JJ, Franco R, Bozal J: **Purification and partial characterization of brain adenosine deaminase: Inhibition by purine compounds and by drugs.** *J Neurosci Res* 1988, **19**:258–267.

25. Donahue RN, McLaughlin PJ, Zagon IS: **The opioid growth factor OGF, and low dose naltrexone LDN, suppress human ovarian cancer progression in mice.** *Gynecol Oncol* 2011, **122**:382–388.

26. Vallejo R, de Leon-Casasola O, Benyamin R: **Opioid therapy and immunosuppression.** *Am J Ther* 2004, **11**:354–365.

27. Peterson PK, Molitor TW, Chunc CC: **Mechanism of morphine induced immunomodulation.** *Biochem Pharmacol* 1993, **46**:343–348.

28. Sacerdote P, Manfredi B, Mantegazza P, Panerai AE: **Antinociceptive and immunosuppressive effects of opiate drugs: a structure-related activity study.** *Br J Pharmacol* 1997, **121**:834–840.

29. Eisenstein TK, Hilburger ME: **Opioid modulation of immune responses: effects on phagocyte and lymphoid cell populations.** *J Neuroimmunol* 1998, **83**:36–44.

30. Sacerdote P, Bianchi M, Gaspani L, Manfredi B, Maucione A, Terno G, Ammatuna M, Panerai AE: **The Effects of Tramadol and Morphine on Immune Responses and Pain After Surgery in Cancer Patients.** *Anesth Analg* 2000, **90**:1411–1414.

31. Zhang EY, Xiong J, Parker BL, Chen AY, Fields PE, Ma X: **Depletion and recovery of lymphoid subsets following morphine administration.** *Br J Pharmacol* 2011, **164**:1829–1844.

32. Ho IK, Loh HH, Way EL: **Cyclic adenosine monophosphate antagonism of morphine analgesia.** *J Pharmacol Exp Ther* 1973, **185**:336–346.

33. Risdahl JM, Khanna KV, Peterson PK, Molitor TW: **Opiates and infections.** *J Neuroimmunol* 1998, **83**:4–18.

34. Donahoe RM, Vlahov D: **Opiates as potential cofactors in progression of HIV-1 infections to AIDS.** *J Neuroimmunol* 1998, **83**:77–87.

35. Matthes HW, Maldonado R, Simonin F, Valverde O, Slowe S, Kitchen I, Befort K, Dierich A, Le Meur M, Dollé P, Tzavara E, Hanoune J, Roques BP, Kieffer BL: **Loss of morphine-induced analgesia, reward effect and withdrawal symptoms in mice lacking the mu-opioid-receptor gene.** *Nature* 1996, **383**:819–823.

36. Bailey A, Matthes H, Kieffer B, Slowe S, Hourani SM, Kitchen I: **Quantitative autoradiography of adenosine receptors and NBTI-sensitive adenosine transporters in the brains and spinal cords of mice deficient in the mu-opioid receptor gene.** *Brain Res* 2002, **943**:68–79.

37. Nelson AM, Battersby AS, Baghdoyan HA, Lydic R: **Opioid induced decreases in rat brain adenosine levels are reversed by inhibiting adenosine deaminase.** *Anesthesiology* 2009, **111**:1327–1333.

38. Brady TG, O'Connell W: **A purification of adenosine deaminase from the superficial mucosa of calf intestine.** *Biochim Biophys Acta* 1962, **62**:216–229.

39. Saboury AA, Divsalar A, Ataie G, Amanlou M, Moosavi-Movahedi AA, Hakimelahi GH: **Inhibition study of adenosine deaminase by caffeine using spectroscopy and isothermal titration calorimetry.** *Acta Biochim Pol* 2003, **50**:849–855.

40. Martinek RG: **Micromethod for estimation of serum adenosine deaminase.** *Clin Chem* 1963, **102**:620–625.

41. Yang JT, Wu CS, Martinez HM: **Calculation of protein conformation from circular dichroism.** *Meth Enzymol* 1986, **130**:208–269.

42. Morris GM, Huey R, Lindstrom W, Sanner MF, Belew RK, Goodsell DS, Olson AJ: **AutoDock4 and AutoDockTools4: Automated docking with selective receptor flexibility.** *J Comput Chem* 2009, **16**:2785–2791.

9

The antimicrobial effects of selenium nanoparticle-enriched probiotics and their fermented broth against *Candida albicans*

Erfan Kheradmand[1,2], Fatemeh Rafii[3], Mohammad Hossien Yazdi[1], Abas Akhavan Sepahi[2], Ahmad Reza Shahverdi[1,4*] and Mohammad Reza Oveisi[5]

Abstract

Background: Lactic acid bacteria are considered important probiotics for prevention of some infections. The aim of this work was to investigate the effect of selenium dioxide on the antifungal activity of *Lactobacillus plantarum* and *L. johnsonii* against *Candida albicans*.

Methods: *Lactobacillus plantarum* and *L. johnsonii* cells, grown in the presence and absence of selenium dioxide, and their cell-free spent culture media were tested for antifungal activity against *C. albicans* ATCC 14053 by a hole-plate diffusion method and a time-kill assay.

Results: Both *L. plantarum* and *L. johnsonii* reduced selenium dioxide to cell-associated elemental selenium nanoparticles. The cell-free spent culture media, from both *Lactobacillus* species that had been grown with selenium dioxide for 48 h, showed enhanced antifungal activity against *C. albicans*. Enhanced antifungal activity of cell biomass against *C. albicans* was also observed in cultures grown with selenium dioxide.

Conclusions: Selenium dioxide-treated *Lactobacillus* spp. or their cell-free spent broth inhibited the growth of *C. albicans* and should be investigated for possible use in anti-*Candida* probiotic formulations in future.

Keywords: *Candida albicans*, Secretory products, Selenium nanoparticles, Antimicrobial effect, *Lactobacillus plantarum*, *Lactobacillus johnsonii*

Introduction

Candida albicans, although it is a commensal yeast in the oral cavity, gastrointestinal tract and urogenital tract, can cause a variety of mild to serious infections. *C. albicans* usually infects immunocompromised patients or others who use antibiotics for a long time [1]. One reason for the overgrowth of *C. albicans* and infection is disequilibrium in the microbiota [2,3]. Probiotics are microorganisms which, when consumed in adequate amounts, can improve intestinal microbial balance and provide benefits for human health [4]. Lactic acid bacteria (LAB) are important probiotics and also part of the normal Gram-positive

microflora inhabiting the intestinal mucosa. They aid in prevention of colonization by pathogenic microorganisms [5]. In the vagina, normal *Lactobacillus* species have a critical role in protection against vaginal infections and the transmission of pathogens responsible for sexually transmitted diseases [4-8]. These bacteria produce lactic acid, acetic acid, hydrogen peroxide, and other antimicrobial substances, which allow them to prevent the colonization of pathogens [8,9]. Some LAB strains can protect the human vagina from candidiasis through the production of these exometabolites [10-14]. As yet uncharacterized metabolites from selenium-enriched probiotics have recently been shown to exert an antibacterial effect against *Escherichia coli* [15]. In the present work, we aimed to study the antimicrobial effect of two selenium-enriched *Lactobacillus spp.* cultures and their exometabolites against *C. albicans* ATCC 14053 and to compare these results with anti-*Candida* effects

* Correspondence: shahverd@tums.ac.ir
[1]Department of Pharmaceutical Biotechnology and Biotechnology Research Center, Faculty of Pharmacy, Tehran University of Medical Sciences, Tehran, Iran
[4]Department of Medical Biotechnology, School of Advanced Medical Technologies, Tehran University of Medical Sciences, Tehran, Iran
Full list of author information is available at the end of the article

of spent broth of non-selenium-enriched *Lactobacillus* cultures.

Materials and methods
Microbial strains
L. plantarum (ATCC 8014) and *C. albicans* (ATCC 14053) were obtained from the American Type Culture Collection (ATCC). The other *Lactobacillus* was a clinical isolate, which was identified as *L. johnsonii* during a previous study [16].

Effect of *Lactobacillus* species on selenium dioxide
One hundred milliliters of DeMan–Rogosa–Sharpe (MRS) broth (Merck, Darmstadt, Germany) was used for inoculation of *L. plantarum* and *L. johnsonii* strains. The cultures were grown at 37°C in a shaker incubator for 24 h. After this time, selenium dioxide (Merck Schuchardt, Hohenbrunn, Germany) was dissolved in distilled water (289.5 mg/l) and sterilized by a Millipore filter apparatus (Millipore Corporation, Milford, MA, USA). This selenium dioxide solution was added aseptically to each of the *Lactobacillus* cultures to obtain a final concentration of 200 mg/l of Se. The cultures were further incubated at 37°C for 96 h. Two-milliliter samples were withdrawn at zero time and at intervals (24, 48, and 96 h) under aseptic conditions. The bacterial cells were removed from the cultures by centrifugation at $5,000 \times g$ for 10 min (Hettich Mikro 200, Tuttlingen, Germany). The supernatant at each time interval was used to measure the concentration of Se remaining in the medium by Somer and Kutay's spectrophotometric method [17]. The cell pellet from a culture of *L. plantarum* and isolated selenium nanoparticles (SeNPs) were examined at 100 kV by a Philips EM-208 transmission electron microscope (TEM) (FEI Ltd., Eindhoven, The Netherlands) to evaluate the presence and the size of Se NPs deposited inside the *L. plantarum* cells as previously described [18]. To determine the elemental composition of the nanoparticles (NPs), energy dispersive X-ray spectrum (EDX) microanalysis (Vega Tescan, Brno, Czech Republic) was also performed.

Preparation of *Lactobacillus* cultures for antifungal activity assays
Four flasks, each containing 100 ml MRS broth, were used for inoculation of two sets each of *L. plantarum* and *L. johnsonii* strains. The cultures were aerobically grown at 37°C in a shaker incubator for 24 h and one set of each bacterium was treated with selenium dioxide as previously described [16]. The cultures were incubated at 37°C for another 96 h. At zero time and every 24 h, 1 ml samples from all four sets of cultures were harvested under aseptic conditions. The samples were centrifuged at $5000 \times g$ for 15 min. All collected supernatants were

assayed for antifungal activity against *C. albicans*. Cultures incubated for additional time (96 h) were subjected to further centrifugations to isolate enough culture supernatants for the time-kill assay.

Assay for antifungal activity of *L. plantarum* and *L. johnsonii* grown with or without selenium dioxide
Both a conventional hole-plate diffusion method and a time-kill assay were used to detect antimicrobial activity in the samples. The supernatants of *L. plantarum* and *L. johnsonii*, grown with or without selenium dioxide, were sterilized by filtration through a 0.22 μm Millipore filter. Sabouraud dextrose agar (SDA) plates were inoculated with *C. albicans* and used to test anti-*Candida* effects of the collected supernatants from each culture. 14-mm diameter holes were punched aseptically in each plate and filled with 100 μl of the cell-free supernatants. As a negative control, sterile MRS liquid medium (100 μl) was used. The plates were incubated aerobically for 18 h at 37°C and the diameters of the inhibition zones (mm) were measured.

The effect of cell-free supernatants of 72-h cultures of *L. plantarum* and *L. johnsonii*, grown with or without selenium dioxide, on the survival of *C. albicans* was also evaluated by conventional time-kill assays. To the tubes containing each of the supernatants, *C. albicans* (3×10^6/ml) was added and incubated at 37°C. The viability of *C. albicans* was studied by plating samples taken at different intervals (0.5, 4, 8, 12, and 24 h) on SDA medium and counting the CFU of surviving *C. albicans*.

The antifungal activity of bacterial cells of *L. plantarum* and *L. johnsonii*, grown with or without selenium dioxide, was also assayed with *C. albicans*. Each of the bacterial pellets prepared as previously described was suspended in a normal saline solution containing 3×10^6 CFU/ml of *C. albicans*. The yeast: bacterial ratio in the suspension was approximately 1/1000 CFU/ml. Samples were withdrawn at different intervals (0.5, 4, 8, 12, and 24 h) for determining the number of surviving *C. albicans* in each challenge test. The samples were plated on SDA medium and incubated at 37°C overnight. The surviving *C. albicans* CFU were counted. These experiments were repeated three times.

Results
Selenium dioxide reduction
After 24 h incubation with both *L. plantarum* and *L. johnsonii*, the concentrations of selenium in the supernatants were considerably reduced. Figure 1 shows the concentration of selenium remaining in the culture medium taken every 24 h. The amount of Se remaining in the supernatants of *Lactobacillus* cultures after 72 h was approximately 3 mg/l, indicating that 98.5% of the selenium ions were reduced in each of the *Lactobacillus*

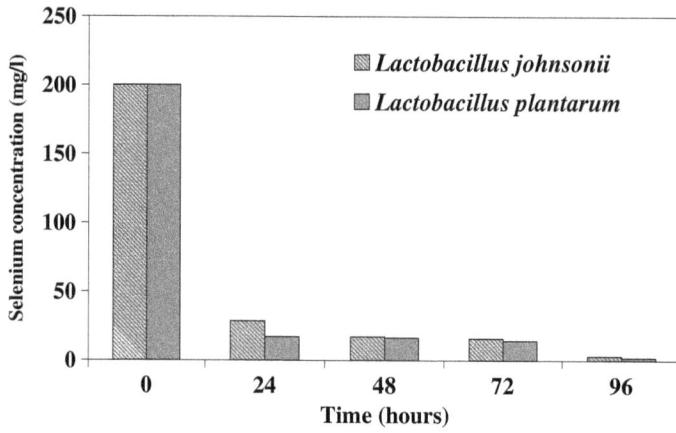

Figure 1 Reduction of selenium dioxide concentration in cultures of *L. johnsonii* or *L. plantarum*, as determined by a spectrophotometric method.

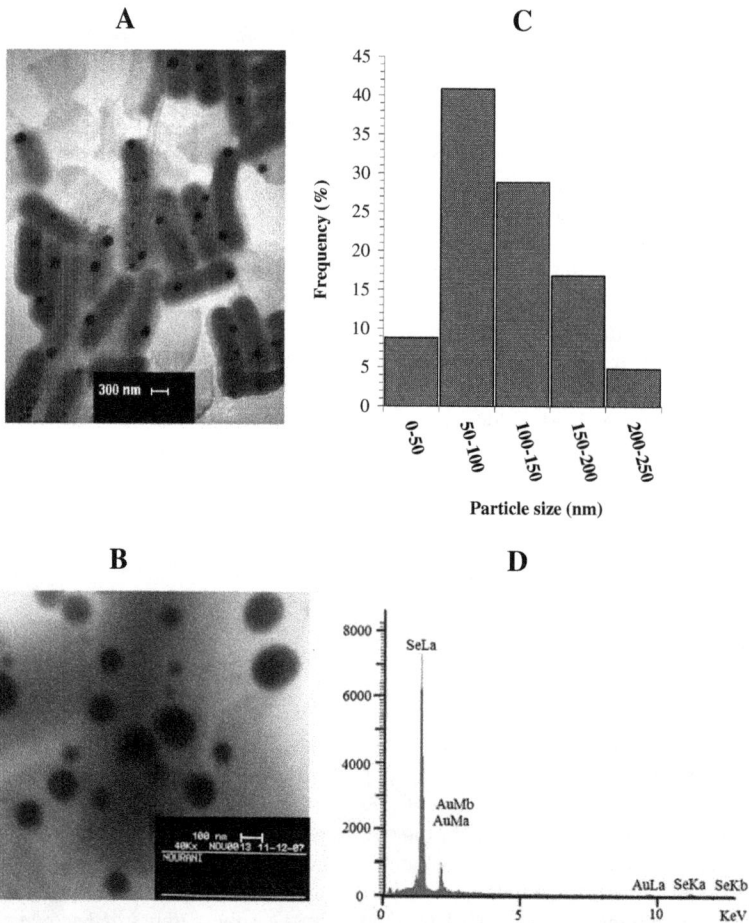

Figure 2 Characterization of SeNPs-enriched *L. plantarum* and purified SeNPs: TEM micrographs (images A and B), Particle size distribution histogram (C) and EDX spectrum of the particles (D).

cultures (Figure 1). No appreciable amount of Se was present in the culture supernatant of any of the strains after 96 h of incubation. The selenium-enriched *L. plantarum* cells were selected for a TEM experiment (Figure 2A). Spherical SeNPs of various sizes had formed inside the *L. plantarum* cells (Figure 2B). Figure 2C shows a size histogram of the SeNPs inside the cells; the particle sizes ranged from 25 to 250 nm. Furthermore, EDX microanalysis of the separated NPs exhibited Se absorption peaks consisting of SeLα, SeKα and SeKβ at 1.37, 11.22 and 12.49 keV, respectively (Figure 2D) and confirmed the presence of Se in the samples.

Anti-*Candida* effect of fermented broth of *L. plantarum* and *L. johnsonii*

The anti-*Candida* effects of the supernatants from *L. plantarum* and *L. johnsonii*, grown with and without selenium dioxide, were compared by measuring the zone of inhibition formed around each of the samples applied to the plates in the hole-plate diffusion method (Table 1). Negligible inhibition zones were observed on the plates containing culture supernatants of either of the species grown without selenium dioxide or sterile MRS broth supplemented with selenium dioxide (200 mg/l). Culture supernatants from *L. plantarum* and *L. johnsonii* grown with selenium dioxide for 48, 72, and 96 h showed potent anti-*Candida* activity and inhibited growth. The maximum antifungal activity was observed in 72 h cultures (Table 1). The time-kill assay, measuring the effect of culture supernatants of each strain, grown with or without selenium dioxide, on the viability of *C. albicans*, confirmed the increase in the antifungal activity of the strains grown with selenium dioxide (Figure 3). Whereas incubation of *C. albicans* with the supernatants of all cultures decreased viability, the number of surviving *C. albicans* cells substantially decreased when incubated with the supernatants of cultures grown for 72 h with selenium dioxide. The difference in the effect, which was observed even after

0.5 h incubation, increased with time. No viable *C. albicans* was present after 4 h incubation with culture supernatants of either species grown with selenium dioxide, but some viable *C. albicans* cells were present even after 24 h incubation with culture supernatants of species grown without selenium dioxide.

Antifungal effect of *L. plantarum* and *L. johnsonii* cells against *C. albicans*

The anti-*Candida* effects of the selenium-enriched and non-enriched cells of *L. plantarum* and *L. johnsonii* were also evaluated. The viability of *C. albicans* decreased following co-culture with both bacteria (Figure 4), but cells from selenium-enriched cultures were more effective at killing *C. albicans* (Figure 4). After 0.5 h incubation of *C. albicans* with the *Lactobacillus* strains grown without selenium dioxide, viability of *C. albicans* had decreased by approximately 10-fold, whereas a 1000-fold decrease was seen when incubated with the SeNPs-enriched species (Figure 4). However, the number of viable cells did not decrease with increased incubation time.

Discussion

Inhibition of *C. albicans* by some strains of *Lactobacillus* species is known and results of clinical trials have shown the effectiveness of some strains of *Lactobacillus* spp. in prevention of *C. albicans* infections [19]. In this study, we have evaluated the interaction of *L. plantarum* and *L. johnsonii* with selenium dioxide on the antifungal activity of these bacteria for *C. albicans*. Both strains converted selenium dioxide to SeNPs of various sizes, which accumulated inside the cells. Whereas both cells and culture supernatants had anti-*C. albicans* activity, substantially higher antifungal activity was observed in the culture supernatants of strains grown with selenium dioxide. It appears that selenium dioxide in the cultures enhanced production of soluble metabolites involved in killing *C. albicans* cells.

The antifungal activity of *L. plantarum* is related to the production of specific compounds, such as phenyllactic acid and 4-hydrophenyllactic acid [20]. When *C. albicans* was mixed with the SeNPs enriched *Lactobacillus* cells or the cell-free fermented broth, clear decreases in viability were observed. The addition of selenium dioxide to the culture medium of either *Lactobacillus* species led to potent increases in antifungal activity against *C. albicans*. Other studies indicate that the adverse effect of LAB can result from production of lactic acid, acetic acid, H_2O_2, CO_2, bacteriocins, and uncharacterized compounds [10-13]. Therefore, selenium dioxide may induce the production of these exometabolites or induce the synthesis of novel anti-*Candida* compounds. At this time, the nature of the exometabolites responsible for the observed antimicrobial activity is not known, and further bioassay-

Table 1 The antimicrobial activity of spent broth of L. johnsonii and L. plantarum cultures grown with or without selenium dioxide against C. albicans, as measured by the diameter of the zone of inhibition formed in the hole-plate diffusion assay

Supernatant samples	Inhibition zone diameter (mm)			
	24 h	48 h	72 h	96 h
L. plantarum	-ᵃ	-	-	-
Selenium-enriched *L. plantarum*	-	23 ± 0.5	28 ± 1	28 ± 0.5
L. johnsonii	-	-	-	-
Selenium-enriched *L. johnsonii*	-	22 ± 1	25 ± 0.5	26 ± 0.5
Sterile SeO₂ supplemented MRS broth	-	-	-	-

ᵃNegligible inhibition zone was observed (<9 mm).

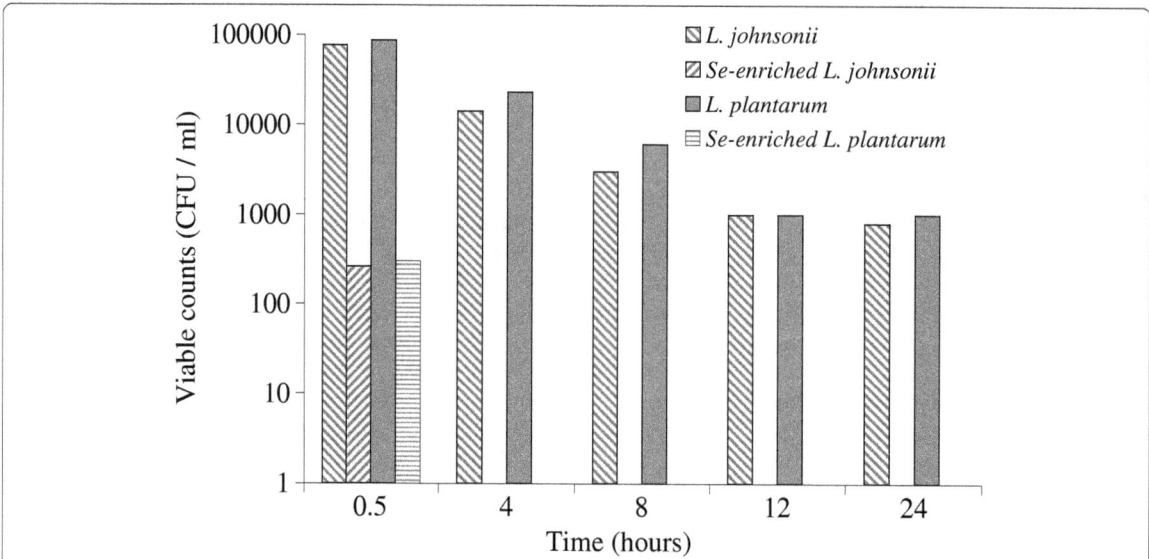

Figure 3 Viability of *C. albicans* after incubation in culture supernatants of *L. johnsonii* or *L. plantarum*, grown with or without selenium dioxide.

guided fractionation assays should be used to isolate and characterize the active constituent(s).

During the cultivation of *Lactobacillus* spp. in MRS broth containing selenium dioxide, this compound was reduced to elemental SeNPs, which accumulated in intracellular spaces of *Lactobacillus* spp. and may have contributed to the increased antifungal activity of the treated cells.

The modification of the microenvironment of LAB is being considered as a means of preventing infections of the urogenital and intestinal tracts [6-8]. The application of SeNPs enriched- *Lactobacillus* may be a good approach for the design of new strategies in enhancing the activities of probiotics for curing infections caused by urogenital pathogens, such as *C. albicans*.

Conclusions

The present work assessed the viability of *C. albicans* following exposure to selenium NPs-enriched *Lactobacillus*

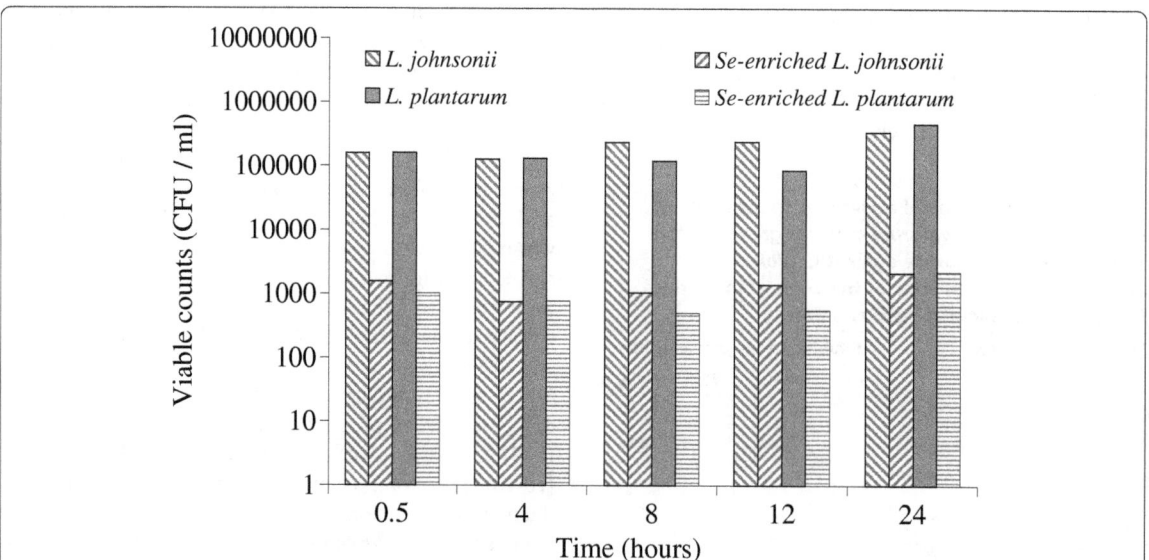

Figure 4 Viability of *C. albicans* after co-incubation with *L. johnsonii* and *L. plantarum* containing SeNPs.

species or their cell-free culture media. A greater decrease in viability of *C. albicans* was seen for bacteria grown with selenium dioxide than for non-Se-enriched bacteria. A direct antifungal effect was observed when SeNPs-enriched *Lactobacillus* spp. were co-cultured with *C. albicans*. In addition, evidence for release of potent exometabolites was indicated by the strong inhibition of growth of *C. albicans* treated with cell-free culture media from the SeNPs-enriched *Lactobacillus* species. This is the first time in which antifungal activity of the combination of *Lactobacillus* spp. and selenium has been studied. This phenomenon should be further evaluated for its practical application.

Competing interests

The authors declare that they have no competing interests.

Authors' contributions

EK: Conducted experiments. FR: Supervised antifungal experiments and revision of manuscript. MHY and AAS: Participated in microbiological experiments. ARS: Project design and manuscript preparation. MRO: Participated in discussion on experimental procedures. All authors read and approved the final manuscript.

Acknowledgment

This work was supported by the Deputy of Research, Tehran University of Medical Sciences, Tehran, Iran. There is no conflict of interest for authors in this work. The views presented in this article do not necessarily reflect those of the U. S. Food and Drug Administration.

Author details

[1]Department of Pharmaceutical Biotechnology and Biotechnology Research Center, Faculty of Pharmacy, Tehran University of Medical Sciences, Tehran, Iran. [2]Science and Research Branch, Azad University, Tehran, Iran. [3]Division of Microbiology, National Center for Toxicological Research, U.S. FDA, Jefferson, AR 72079, USA. [4]Department of Medical Biotechnology, School of Advanced Medical Technologies, Tehran University of Medical Sciences, Tehran, Iran. [5]Department of Food and Drug Control, Faculty of Pharmacy, Tehran University of Medical Sciences, Tehran, Iran.

References

1. Calderone RA, Fonzi WA: Virulence factors of *Candida albicans*. *Trends Microbiol* 2001, **9**:327–335.
2. Koga-Ito CY, Martins CAP, Jorge AOC: Estudo do gênero *Candida*. In *Jorge AOC*. 1st edition. Editora Santos, São Paulo, Brazil: Princípios de Microbiologia e Imunologia; 2006.
3. Vieira JDG, Ribeiro EL, Campos CC, Pimenta FC, Toledo OA, Nagato GM, Souza NA, Ferreira WM, Cardoso CG, Dias SMS, Araújo CA, Zatta DT, Santos JS: *Candida albicans* isoladas da cavidade bucal de crianças com síndrome de Down: ocorrência e inibição do crescimento por *Streptomyces* sp. *Rev Soc Bras Med Trop* 2005, **38**:383–386.
4. Savino F, Cordisco L, Tarasco V, Locatelli E, Di Gioia D, Oggero R, Matteuzzi D: Antagonistic effect of *Lactobacillus* strains against gas-producing coliforms isolated from colicky infants. *BMC Microbiol* 2011, **11**:157.
5. Jacobsen CN, Nielsen VR, Hayford AE, Moller PL, Michael Sen KF, Paerregaard A, Sandström B, Tvede M, Jacobsen M: Screening of probiotic activities of forty-seven strains of *Lactobacillus* spp. by *in vitro* techniques and evaluation of the colonization ability of five selected strains in humans. *Appl Environ Microbiol* 1999, **11**:4949–4956.
6. Eschenbach DA, Hillier SL, Critchlow C, Stevens C, De Rouen T, Holmes KK: Diagnosis and clinical manifestations of bacterial vaginosis. *Am J Obstet Gynecol* 1988, **158**:819–828.
7. Galask RP: Vaginal colonization by bacteria and yeast. *Am J Obstet Gynecol* 1989, **158**:993–995.
8. Klebanoff SJ, Hillier SL, Eschenbach DA, Waltersdorph AM: Control of the microbial flora of the vagina by H_2O_2-generating lactobacilli. *J Infect Dis* 1991, **164**:94–100.
9. McGoarty JA: Probiotic use of lactobacilli in the human female urogenital tract. *FEMS Immunol Med Microbiol* 1993, **6**:251–264.
10. Jay JM: Antimicrobial properties of diacetyl. *Appl Environ Microbiol* 1982, **44**:525–532.
11. Klaenhammer TR: Bacteriocins of lactic acid bacteria. *Biochimie* 1988, **70**:337–349.
12. Piard JC, Desmazeaud M: Inhibiting factors produced by lactic acid bacteria: 1. Oxygen metabolites and catabolism end products. *Lait* 1991, **71**:525–541.
13. Pikkemaat MG, Oostra-van Dijk S, Schouten J, Rapallini M, Egmond HJ: A new microbial screening method for the detection of antimicrobial residues in slaughter animals: The Nouws antibiotic test (NAT-screening). *Food Cont* 2008, **19**:781–789.
14. Reid G, Jass J, Sebulsky T, Sebulsky MT, McCormick JK: Potential uses of probiotics in clinical practice. *Clin Microbiol Rev* 2003, **16**:658–672.
15. Yang J, Huang K, Qin S, Wu X, Zhao Z, Chen F: Antibacterial action of selenium-enriched probiotics against pathogenic *Escherichia coli*. *Dig Dis Sci* 2009, **54**:246–254.
16. Yazdi MH, Mahdavi M, Setayesh N, Esfandyar M, Shahverdi AR: Selenium nanoparticle-enriched *Lactobacillus brevis* causes more efficient immune responses in vivo and reduces the liver metastasis in metastatic form of mouse breast cancer. *Daru* 2013, **21**:33. Doi: 10.1186/2008-2231-21-33.
17. Somer G, Kutay N: A new and simple spectrophotometric method for the determination of selenium in the presence of copper and tellurium. *Can J Chem* 1993, **71**:834–835.
18. Yazdi MH, Mahdavi M, Kheradmand E, Shahverdi AR: The preventive oral supplementation of a selenium nanoparticle-enriched probiotic increases the immune response and lifespan of 4T1 breast cancer bearing mice. *Arzneimittelforschung* 2012, **62**:525–531.
19. Falagas ME, Betsi GI, Athanasiou S: Probiotics for prevention of recurrent vulvovaginal candidiasis: a review. *J Antimicrob Chemother* 2006, **58**:266–272.
20. Lavermicocca P, Valerio F, Evidente A, Lazzaroni S, Corsetti A, Gobetti M: Purification and characterization of novel antifungal compounds from the sourdough *Lactobacillus plantarum* strain 21B. *Appl Environ Microbiol* 2000, **66**:4084–4090.

10

Proteomic screening of molecular targets of crocin

Hossein Hosseinzadeh[1], Soghra Mehri[1], Ali Heshmati[2], Mohammad Ramezani[3], Amirhossein Sahebkar[4] and Khalil Abnous[5*]

Abstract

Background: Traditional drug discovery approaches are mainly relied on the observed phenotypic changes following administration of a plant extract, drug candidate or natural product. Recently, target-based approaches are becoming more popular. The present study aimed to identify the cellular targets of crocin, the bioactive dietary carotenoid present in saffron, using an affinity-based method.

Methods: Heart, kidney and brain tissues of BALB/c mice were homogenized and extracted for the experiments. Target deconvolution was carried out by first passing cell lysate through an affinity column prepared by covalently attaching crocin to agarose beads. Isolated proteins were separated on a 2D gel, trypsinized *in situ* and identified by MALDI-TOF/TOF mass spectrometry. MASCOT search engine was used to analyze Mass Data.

Results: Part of proteome that physically interacts with crocin was found to consist of beta-actin-like protein 2, cytochrome b-c1 complex subunit 1, ATP synthase subunit beta, tubulin beta-3 chain, tubulin beta-6 chain, 14-3-3 protein beta/alpha, V-type proton ATPase catalytic subunitA, 60 kDa heat shock protein, creatine kinase b-type, peroxiredoxin-2, cytochrome b-c1 complex subunit 2, acetyl-coA acetyltransferase, cytochrome c1, proteasome subunit alpha type-6 and proteasome subunit alpha type-4.

Conclusion: The present findings revealed that crocin physically binds to a wide range of cellular proteins such as structural proteins, membrane transporters, and enzymes involved in ATP and redox homeostasis and signal transduction.

Keywords: *Crocus sativus* L, Crocin, Target Deconvolution, Affinity chromatography, Target deconvolution, Electrophoresis

Introduction

Dried stigma of *Crocus sativus* L. (Iridaceae), called saffron, is a widely used dietary spice and food colorant [1]. Aside from culinary purposes, saffron has been used in several traditional systems of medicine for the treatment of numerous diseases such as cough, colic, insomnia, chronic uterine hemorrhage, cardiovascular disorders and tumors [2].

Crocin (Figure 1) is a bioactive carotenoid present in *C. sativus*, and is responsible for the golden-yellow color of saffron [3]. Modern scientific investigations have unveiled several interesting pharmacological activities for

crocin including, but not limited to, antitumor [2], radical scavenging [4], antidepressant [5] and memory-enhancing effects [6]. In addition, crocin has been shown to possess high antioxidant and anti-proliferative capacities in both *in-vitro* and *in-vivo* conditions [7-11]. Yet, it must be taken into accurate account that the anti-tumor properties of crocin, like some other phytochemicals, are likely to be independent of the well-known antioxidant actions. The notion of antioxidants as potential anti-cancer agents has recently been questioned due to some observations on the lack of efficacy of antioxidant therapy in the treatment of cancer [12]. Besides, it is known that some chemotherapy agents exert their cytotoxic effects via induction of oxidative stress [13]. Finally, the fact that crocin induces apoptosis in cancerous cells – a phenomonen usually associated with increased generationof free radicals – is

* Correspondence: abnouskh@mums.ac.ir
[5]Pharmaceutical Research Center, Department of Medicinal Chemistry, School of Pharmacy, Mashhad University of Medical Sciences, 91775-1365 Mashhad, Iran
Full list of author information is available at the end of the article

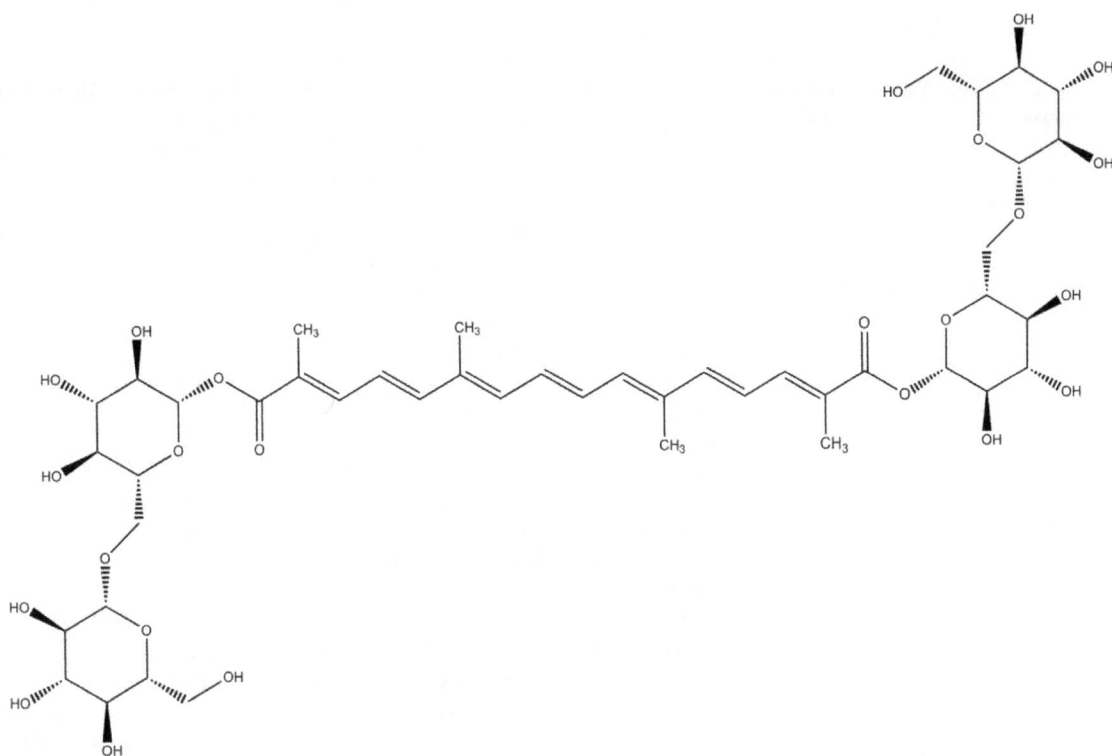

Figure 1 Chemical structure of crocin.

another proof for the lack of association between antioxidant and anti-cancer properties of this compound [14,15]. It has been hypothesized that phytochemicals with dual antioxidant/anti-cancer properties may exert the latter effect via epigenetic mechanisms including promotion of DNA demethylation, histone modification and RNA interference [16,17]. However, unraveling the mechanisms underlying the antioxidant and anti-cancer properties of crocin is warranted for further clarification in this context. Moreover, dose-effect studies need to be undertaken in order to identify optimal doses at which antioxidant and anti-cancer effects of crocin predominate.

In spite of proven benefits, molecular mechanisms that account for the pharmacological effects of crocin have remained largely unknown. However, several lines of evidence have demonstrated that phytochemicals promote their biological and health promoting effects through interaction with a variety of structural and functional proteins [18].

Traditional approach toward drug discovery has been mainly based on the observation of a phenotypic change following application of a plant extract, drug candidate or a natural product. Recently, target-based approaches are becoming more popular. The identification of target proteins for newly developed drugs or natural products

is regarded as "target deconvolution" [19,20]. Such an identification of the potential targets of a small pharmacologically active molecule helps elucidating the primary mechanism of action, prediction of side effects and unwanted off-target interactions, and finding new potential therapeutic effects.

The present study hypothesized that pharmacological activities of crocin depend, at least in part, on its physical interaction with cellular proteins. Hence, part of the cellular proteome that binds to crocin was isolated from tissue lysates using affinity chromatography and subjected to mass specterometry (MS)-based proteomic analysis to identify the potential molecular targets of this phytochemical.

Material and methods

Crocin extraction and purification

Stigmas of *C. sativus* L. were collected from Ghaen, Khorasan province, Northeast of Iran, and provided by Novin Saffron Co. (Mashhad, Iran). Analysis and quality control of samples was conducted in accordance to the ISO/TS 3632–2 standards. Extraction and purification of crocin from saffron was carried out as previously described by Hadizadeh and colleagues [21].

Animals

Twelve BALB/c mice (20–25 g) were killed by decapitation. Heart, kidney and brain tissues of mice were collected and washed using 0.9% normal saline solution. Tissues were immediately frozen in liquid nitrogen and transferred to –80°C until use. All animal experiments were carried out in accordance with the acts of the Mashhad University of Medical Sciences Ethics Committee (code 87772).

Preparation of tissue extracts

Each sample (200–400 mg) was homogenized 1:5 (w:v) in extraction buffer containing 50 mM Tris (pH 7.4), 2 mM EGTA, 2 mM EDTA, 2 mM Na_3VO_4, 1% Triton X-100 and 10 mM 2-mercaptoethanol with further addition of a few crystals of the protease inhibitor, phenylmethylsulfonyl fluoride (PMSF) immediately before homogenization of tissue. Samples were homogenized using a Polytron Homogenizer (Kinematica, Switzerland) for 10 sec followed by sonication (UP100H, Hielscher) for 40 sec and centrifugation (Hettich Universal 320R, Germany) at 25,000 g for 10 min at 4°C. The supernatant was then removed and stored on ice. Protein contents were measured using Bradford protein assay (BioRad). The protein contents of all samples were adjusted to 2 mg/mL.

Preparation of crocin-resin conjugate

Crocin affinity matrix was prepared using pharmaLink Kit (Pierce) according to the manufacturer's instructions. Briefly, agarose beads containing immobilized diaminodipropylamine (DADPA) were equilibrated in 4 mL coupling buffer (0.1 M MES, 0.15 M NaCl, pH 4.7). Crocin (100 mg) was dissolved in 2 mL of coupling buffer and transferred to the aforementioned resin slurry. Coupling reaction was started by adding 200 µL of coupling reagent (37% formaldehyde solution) to the resin/crocin mixture. Reaction mixture was incubated for 72 h in 50°C. To remove free crocin, resin slurry was transferred to a column and washed 12 times each time with 2 mL of wash buffer (0.1 M Tris, pH 8.0). Flowthrough fractions were collected and pooled. Quantity of free crocin was calculated by measuring absorbance of pooled flowthrough fractions at 441.6 nm using visible spectroscopy (CECIL 9000 Series). Efficiency of crocin conjugation to resin was calculated using the following equation:

$$\% \ Resin-conjugated \ crocin = \frac{mg \ (totatl \ crocin) - mg \ (free \ crocin)}{mg \ (total \ crocin)}$$

Affinity chromatography

Affinity chromatography was performed to isolate molecular targets of crocin. Briefly, both controlss (affinity column without crocin) and affinity column were equilibrated in binding buffer [50 mM Tris (pH 7.4), 2 mM EGTA, 2 mM EDTA, 2 mM Na_3VO_4, 1% Triton X-100, and 10 mM 2-ME]. Tissue extracts were incubated with control column resin for 30 min at 4°C. After a brief centrifugation at 1000 g, supernatants were transferred to the affinity column. Following incubation for 30 min at 4°C, affinity column was washed 4 times each time with 2 mL of binding buffer. Crocin target proteins were eluted using 2 mL of 2 M NaCl in binding buffer. The elution was repeated 3 more times and fractions were pooled. The presence of proteins in fractions was tested using Bradford protein assay kit (BioRad). The pooled fractions were dialyzed at a 2000 Da cut-off to remove electrolytes. To concentrate target proteins, samples were freeze-dried and stored at –20°C until use.

2D gel electrophoresis

Freeze-dried samples were dissolved to a final concentration of 125 µg/125 µL in rehydration buffer containing 6 M urea, 2 M thiourea, 2% (3-[(3-Cholamidopropyl)-dimethylammonio]-1-propane sulfonate) (CHAPS), 50 mM dithiothreitol (DTT) and 20% Bio-Lyte (BioRad). Non-linear immobilized pH gradients (IPGs) (pH 3–10; BioRad) were used to separate crocin target proteins based on their isoelectric point [1]. For passive rehydration, IPGs and protein solutions were incubated at room temperature for 12 h. Isoelectric focusing was performed using PROTEAN IEF cell (BioRad) at 4000 V for 11 h. After isoelectric focusing, IPGs were incubated in equilibration buffer [375 mM Tris (pH 8.8), 6 M Urea, 2.5% SDS and 30% glycerol] for 20 min. Then, IPGs were placed on top of 12% sodium dodecyl sulfate-polyacrylamide gel electrophoresis (SDS-PAGE) and sealed with heated agarose solution (25 mM Tris (pH 8.8), 84 mM glycine, 0.5% agarose, 0.1% SDS and small amount of tracking dye bromophenol blue). Electrophoresis was performed for 80 min at 120 V. Gels were silver stained and protein spots were excised and collected in microtubes.

In-gel digestion

Gel slices were incubated in destaining buffer (50% MeOH, 5% acetic acid) overnight at room temperature. Destaining was repeated with fresh buffer for 2 more h. Gel slices were dehydrated in acetonitrile for 30 min and dried in vacufuge. Afterwards, gels were covered with reducing buffer (1.5 mg/mL DTT in 100 mM ammonium bicarbonate) for 1 h. Protein alkylation was performed by incubation of gel slices in 100 µL of 10 mg/mL iodoacetamide in 100 mM ammonium bicarbonate for 30 min at room temperature. Gel slices were washed using 0.5 mL of 100 mM ammonium bicarbonate followed by dehydration using acetonitrile and drying in vacufuge. Then, 50 µL of 20 µg/mL trypsin was added to each gel slice and incubated overnight at 4°C. Peptides were

extracted in 3 steps by adding 100 μL of 100 mM ammonium bicarbonate, 100 μL extraction solution (50%
acetonitrile and 5% formic acid) and finally 150 μL extraction solution. Samples were dried down to a final
volume of 15 μL in vacufuge and desalted using ZipTip®
μC-18 (Millipore). Eluted samples were stored at −20°C
until use.

Mass analysis

Mass analysis was performed at Genome Research
Centre at the University of Hong Kong using a 4800
MALDI-TOF/TOF analyzer (ABI). In-house MASCOT
search engine was used to analyze Mass Data. Data were
BLASTed against both NCBInr and SwissProt databases.
MASCOT parameters were set as follow: Taxonomy:
mouse, fixed modification: carbamidomethyl (C), variable modification: oxidation (M), MS/MS fragment tolerance: 0.2 Da, precursor tolerance: 75 ppm, peptide
charge: +1, monoisotopic. MASCOT cut-off scores were
set to 30. Only the peptides ranked first with p-values
smaller than 0.05 were accepted.

Results

Affinity chromatography was performed to find cellular
targets of crocin in different organs. There are two types
of interactions between stationary phase and cellular
proteins in affinity chromatography: specific interaction
between crocin and its targets or unspecific binding of
proteins to other parts of stationary phase such as agarose beads. To reduce unspecific binding of non-target
proteins, tissue extracts were incubated with control
agarose beads. Unbound proteins were incubated with
crocin-resin beads. Target proteins were eluted using 2
M NaCl in binding buffer and subjected to 2D gel electrophoresis. After in-gel digestion of protein spots,
MALDI TOF/TOF was employed for their identification.
Mass data were analyzed using MASCOT (Figure 2;
Additional file 1).

Crocin-resin conjugation

Crocin was covalently attached to diaminodipropylamine side chain of agarose beads using Mannich reaction. Briefly, formaldehyde reacts with primary amino
group to produce highly reactive iminium group. This
group can react with active hydrogen on hydroxyl
groups of sugar residues on crocin. Yield of crocin conjugation to agarose beads was calculated to be 70%. In
FT-IR spectrum of crocin-resin conjugate, hydroxyl
groups (−OH) of crocin glycosides were observed at
3410.06 cm^{-1} which is identical with that of pure crocin
(Figure 3). Besides other peaks in the crocin-resin conjugate were overlapped with those of pure crocin, suggesting the presence of crocin with its functional groups
within the conjugate.

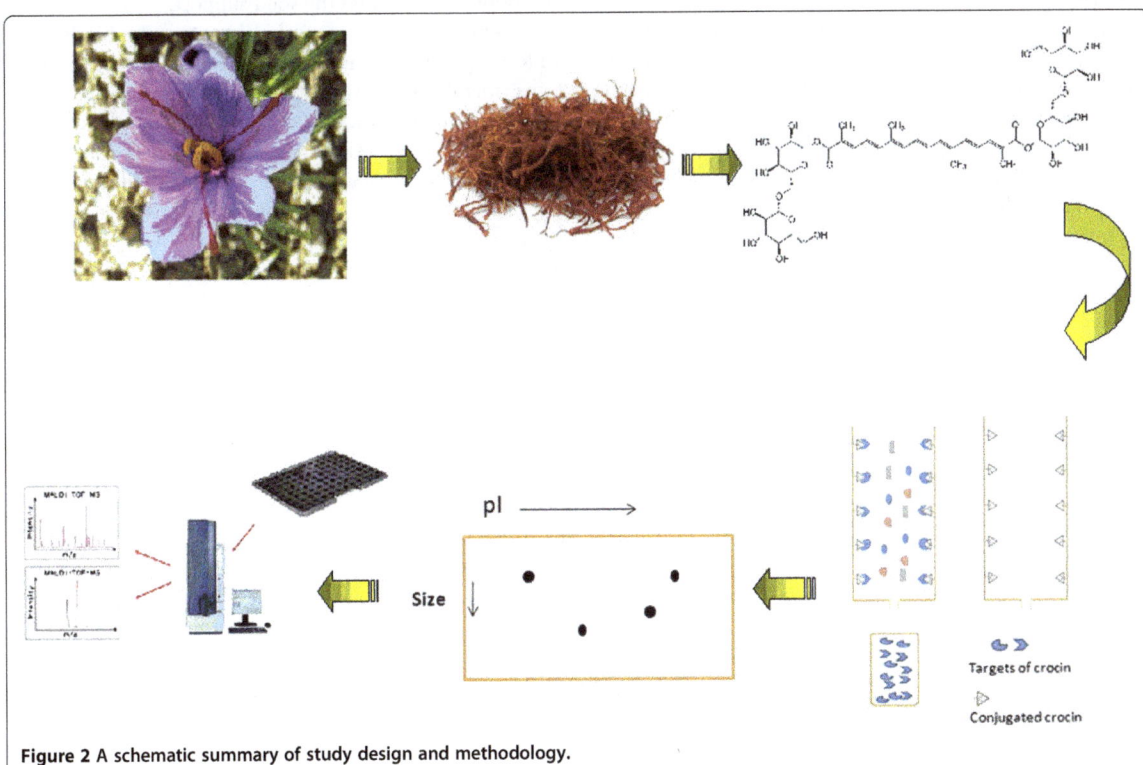

Figure 2 A schematic summary of study design and methodology.

Target proteins of crocin in kidney

Beta-actin-like protein 2, cytochrome c1, proteasome subunit alpha type-6 and proteasome subunit alpha type-4 were identified as cellular targets of crocin in kidney (Figure 4 and Table 1).

Target proteins of crocin in heart

Data indicated that crocin binds to mitochondrial ATP synthase subunit beta, beta-actin-like protein 2, cytochrome b-c1 complex subunit 1 and subunit 2, and acetyl-CoA acetyltransferase in heart (Figure 5 and Table 1).

Target proteins of crocin in Brain

Target proteins of crocin in brain were identified as tubulin beta-3 chain, tubulin beta-6 chain, mitochondrial ATP synthase, beta-actin-like protein 2, 14-3-3 protein beta/alpha, tyrosine 3-monooxygenase, V-type proton ATPase catalytic subunit A, 60 kDa heat shock protein, creatine kinase B-type and peroxiredoxin-2 (Figure 6 and Table 1).

Discussion

Saffron has been mentioned in the folk medicine to have a warm and dry temperament [22]. This plant is endowed with a variety of health benefits including exhilarant, liver tonic and deobstruent, aphrodisiac, labour-inducing, emmenagogue, digestive, hypnotic, cardioprotective, anti-inflammatory and bronchodilatory properties [22,23]. Interestingly, most of these traditional uses are consistent with the findings of modern pharmacological research [23].

In the present study, affinity purification was exploited to identify cellular proteins that could physically interact with crocin. This technique has a distinct superiority to other deconvolution methods such as biochemical fractionation, phage display and expression cloning as it is more relevant to be used with crude cellular samples in which the proteins are in their intact biological form [24].

Drugs are normally discovered based on their ability to show a certain desired biological outcome. For instance, crude natural product mixtures are tested for a specific pharmacological activity and then active ingredient is purified. The retrospective identification of the molecular targets that underlie the observed phenotypic responses is called target deconvolution. Unveiling the cellular targets of a given molecular entity is necessary for a better understanding of its mechanism of action, prediction of potential pharmacological activities as well as plausible side effects and off-target toxicities.

Affinity-based target deconvolution method is complicated by the risk of identifying interactions with proteins that have no pharmacological relevance (false positives), despite being targets of the compound. Therefore, activity- or phenotype-based assays are essential to discriminate between positive and false-positive interactions and to confirm true functional effects [19]. Another major challenge in affinity chromatography-coupled MS technology is the non-specific interaction of proteins with the immobilized support and/or linker [24]. In the current investigation, the referred problem was minimized by applying a control column and eliminating the cellular proteins that are more prone to bind the solid support.

Proteomic findings revealed that crocin binds to a wide range of cellular proteins such as structural proteins, membrane transporters, and enzymes involved in ATP and redox homeostasis and signal transduction. Beta-actin-like protein 2 was identified as one of the target proteins of crocin. Actin filaments help maintaining cell morphology and mediate functions such as

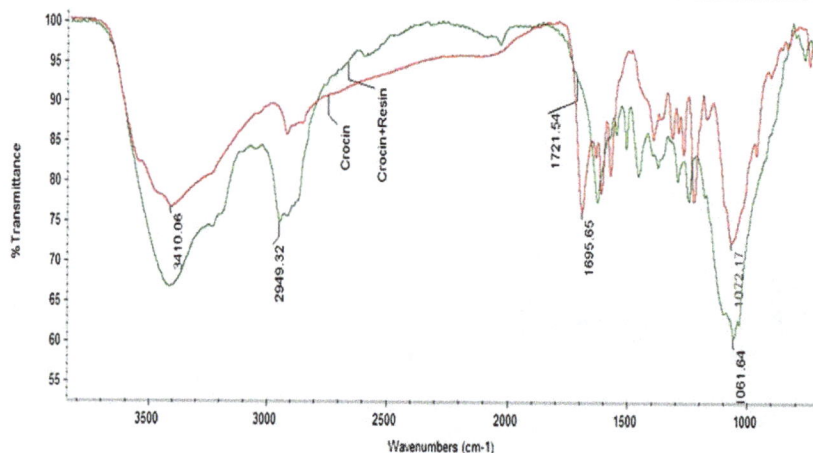

Figure 3 FT-IR spectrum of crocin (red) and crocin-resin conjugate (green).

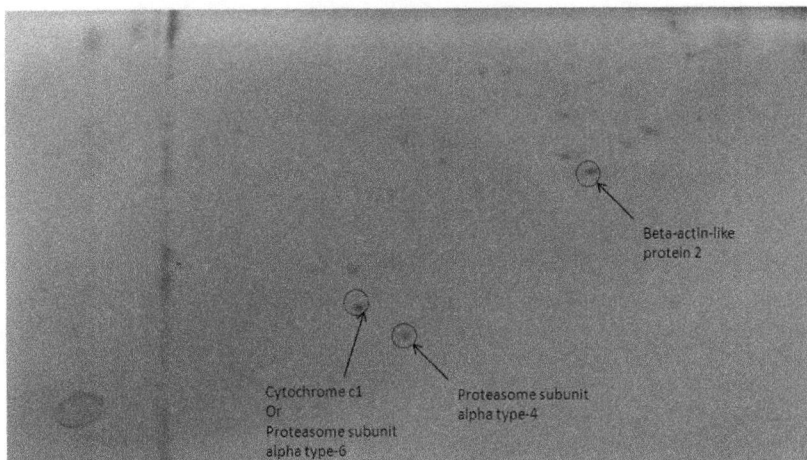

Figure 4 2D gel electrophoresis of crocin targets in kidney extract. Spots were identified as Beta-actin-like protein 2, cytochrome c1, proteasome subunit alpha type-6 and proteasome subunit alpha type-4.

adhesion, motility, exocytosis, endocytosis and cell division. Natural products like cytochalasin and jasklapinolide that interact with actin polymerization have cytotoxic effects [25].

Tubulin beta 3 and 6 are also cytoskeletal proteins that interact with crocin. Microtubules are long, hollow, cylindrical protein polymers composed of α/β-tubulin heterodimers. An important function of microtubules is to move cellular structures such as chromosomes, mitotic spindles and other organelles inside the cell [26]. Several microtubule-inhibiting agents such as vincristine, vinblastine, taxol and colchicine have shown potent activity against the proliferation of various cancer cells [27].

Crocin has been reported to significantly inhibit the growth of different types of cancerous cell lines such as colorectal cancer cells [11]. Effects of crocin on tubulin polymerization has been already studied [28]. Crocin may alter the tubulin polymerization through direct binding.

ATP synthase is a key enzyme of mitochondrial energy conversion [29]. Ahmad and Laughlin [30] discussed that dietary polyphenols and amphibian antimicrobial/antitumor peptides inhibit ATP synthase. Inhibition of ATP synthase may cause energy deprivation and increase ROS production. High ROS content induces cellular necrosis and/or apoptosis [29]. Our experiment showed

Table 1 Target proteins of crocin as identified by MALDI-TOF/TOF and MASCOT

	Protein name	Protein score	Protein score C.I.%	MW/pI	Accession number
1	Acetyl-CoA acetyltransferase	81	99	45KDa/8.7	Gi 21450129
2	V-type proton ATPase catalytic subunitA	113	100	68.6KDa/5.42	P50516.2
3	Proteasome subunit alpha type-4	159	100	30/KDa/7.59	Q9R1P0.1
4	14-3-3 protein beta/alpha	160	100	28KDa/4.77	Q9CQV8.3
5	Tubulin beta-6 chain	169	100	50.5KDa/4.8	Q922F4.1
6	Proteasome subunit alpha type-6	170	100	28KDa/6.34	Q9QUM9.1
7	Beta-actin-like protein 2	215	100	42KDa/5.3	Q8BFZ3
8	Tubulin beta-3 chain	258	100	51KDa/4.82	Q9ERD7.1
9	Cytochrome b-c1 complex subunit 1	265	100	53KDa/5.75	Q9CZ13.1
10	Cytochrome c1	277	100	35.5KDa/9.24	Q9DOM3.1
11	Peroxiredoxin-2	283	100	22KDa/5.2	Q61171.3
12	Cytochrome b-c1 complex subunit 2	323	100	48KDa/9.26	Q9DB77.1
13	60 kDa heat shock protein	348	100	61KDa/6.33	Gi 247242
14	Creatine kinase B-type	388	100	43KDa/5.4	Q04447.1
15	ATP synthase subunit beta	485	100	56KDa/5.19	P56480.2

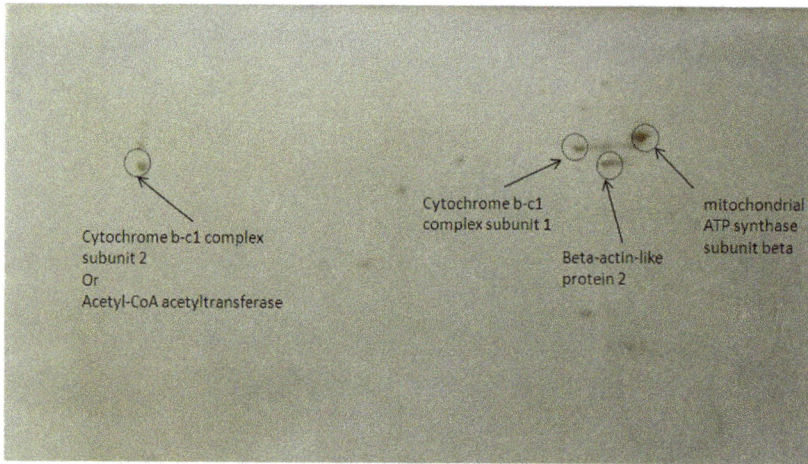

Figure 5 2D gel electrophoresis of crocin targets in heart extract. Spots were identified as mitochondrial ATP synthase subunit beta, beta-actin-like protein 2, cytochrome b-c1 complex subunit 1 and subunit 2 and *acetyl-CoA acetyltransferase*.

that crocin may physically interact with this enzyme, which is consistent with the findings of a previous study with safranal as another important constituent of saffron [31]. However, contrasting evidence has shown that crocin reduces ROS generation in cells exposed to acrylamide [32]. Overall, the majority of previous findings favor the antioxidant role of crocin and this may be due to the inhibitory effect of this phytochemical on other sources of ROS production, in particular lipid peroxidation, as well enhancement of free radical neutralization via stimulating the activity of superoxide dismutase and increasing intracellular glutathione content [33,34].

Creatine kinase (CK) catalyzes transfer of phosphate group from ATP to creatine to produce phosphocreatine and *vice versa*. CK works as an energy buffer and is found in tissues with high and/or fluctuating energy demand such as heart, muscle and brain [35]. Incubation of crocin-resin with brain homogenate showed that crocin has affinity for CK-B. Any change in CK activity may affect energy homeostasis in cell. Dahlstedt and Westerblad [36] showed that creatine kinase inhibition may reduce the rate of fatigue induced by decrease in tetanic Ca^{2+} in mouse skeletal muscle [37]. The oral administration of crocetin (another carotenoid of saffron) has been reported to improve physical capacity during fatigue-induced workload tests in men [38].

Crocin was also found to interact with cytochrome c1 and cytochrome b-c1. The most conserved role of these

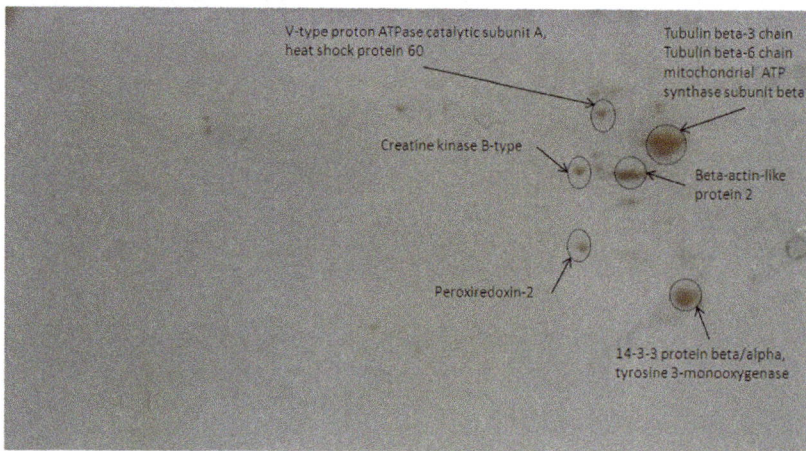

Figure 6 2D gel electrophoresis of crocin targets in brain extract. Spots were identified as tubulin beta-3 chain, tubulin beta-6 chain, mitochondrial ATP synthase, beta-actin-like protein 2, 14-3-3 protein beta/alpha, tyrosine 3-monooxygenase, V-type proton ATPase catalytic subunit A, 60 kDa heat shock protein, creatine kinase B-type and peroxiredoxin-2.

cytochromes is in the electron transport chain and oxidative phosphorylation. Moreover, cytochrome c release into the cytosol is particularly associated with activation of the intrinsic apoptotic pathway [39]. In previous studies, saffron carotenoids including crocin have been shown to modulate apoptosis through different mechanisms such as inhibition of ROS production [32,33] and direct interaction with caspase-3 and caspase-8 [14,15]. Crocin has been reported to promote apoptosis in tumor cells while exerting anti-apoptotic effects in non-tumor cells [40,41]. In view of the present finding, interaction of crocin with cytochrome c might play an important role in the stimulatory and inhibitory activities of this phytochemical on the apoptosis pathway and deserves further attention.

V-ATPase inhibitors such as bafilomycin A1 may induce apoptosis through intracellular acidosis. Effects of physical binding of crocin on V-ATPase activity should be studied in detail. It has been discussed that V-ATPase inhibitors can potentially be used in the treatment of solid tumors with overexpressed levels of this enzyme [42].

Crocin may also interact with biosynthetic pathways through direct interaction with acetyl-coenzyme A acetyl transferases (ACAT). ACAT converts two units of acetyl-CoA to acetoacetyl CoA in poly beta-hydroxybutyrate synthesis or steroid biogenesis [43].

Our study also showed that crocin binds to proteasome α type 4 and 6. Proteasome degrades misfolded and/or ubiquitin-tagged proteins. Proteasome inhibitors, like disulfiram, have been recently studied for cancer therapy [44,45]. Affinity of crocin for proteasome may explain its cytotoxic effect at higher concentrations.

Another crocin target was identified as 14-3-3 protein beta/alpha. 14-3-3 proteins are implicated in the regulation of key proteins such as Raf, bad, and Cbl, and are implicated in various biological processes such as signal transduction, transcriptional control, cell proliferation, apoptosis and ion channel physiology [46]. 14-3-3 protein zeta interacts with insulin resistance substrate-1 (IRS-1) protein and might therefore play a role in regulating insulin sensitivity. Crocin and safranal have been reported to reduce blood glucose and HbA1c levels but increase blood insulin levels significantly without any significant effect on liver and kidney functions in alloxan-induced diabetic rats [47].

Affinity of crocin for heat shock protein 60 may explain some the protective effects of saffron. Heat shock proteins are chaperones that assist proteins for proper folding, stability and transport across cellular membranes [48]. There is evidence indicating the cardioprotective effects of saffron and improvement of histopathologic and biochemical parameters in the cardiac tissue following stress [49,50]. Overexpression of heat shock protein 60 in myocardium is a defensive biological mechanism for the preservation of cardiac function upon exposure to cardiotoxic agents or other stressors [51]. Physical interaction of crocin with heat shock protein 60 might influence the function of this chaperone and improves its protective effects.

Peroxiredoxin-2 also shows some degrees of physical affinity to crocin. Peroxiredoxin-2 reduces the level of H_2O_2 in cells. Both crocin and peroxiredoxin may play an antioxidant protective role in cells. Physical interaction of these two enzymes may alter their antioxidant capacity.

In summary, the present data revealed that tubulin beta-3 chain, tubulin beta-6 chain, ATP synthase subunit beta, beta-actin-like protein 2, 14-3-3 protein beta/alpha, V-type proton ATPase, 60 kDa heat shock protein, creatine kinase B-type, peroxiredoxin-2, cytochrome b-c1 complex, cytochrome c1, heme protein, acetyl-CoA acetyltransferase, proteasome subunit alpha type-4 and type-6, protein disulfide-isomerase and delta-aminolevulinic acid dehydratase could serve as potential cellular targets for crocin. Although physical interaction of crocin with these proteins may explain some of its pharmacological effects, activity- or phenotype-based assays are essential to discriminate between positive and false-positive interactions.

Additional file

Additional file 1: Results of MASCOT search are available as supporting information.

Abbreviations

PMSF: Phenylmethylsulfonyl fluoride; DADPA: Diaminodipropylamine; CHAPS: (3-[(3-Cholamidopropyl)-dimethylammonio]-1-propane sulfonate); DTT: Dithiothreitol; IPGs: Immobilized pH gradient; SDS-PAGE: Sodium dodecyl sulfate-polyacrylamide gel electrophoresis; IEF: Isoelectric focusing; MALDI: Matrix-assisted laser desorption ionization; TOF: Time-of-flight; CoA: Coenzyme A; EDTA: Ethylenediaminetetraacetic acid; EGTA: Ethylene glycol tetraacetic acid; IRS-1: Insulin resistance substrate-1; ATP: Adenosine triphosphate; ACAT: Acetyl-coenzyme A acetyl transferases; CK: Creatine kinase; MS: Mass spectrometry.

Competing interests

The authors have no competing interest to declare.

Authors' contributions

KA, HH and MR conceived the study and designed the experiments. SM and AH did the experimental works. KA, SM, AH and AS performed literature review and were involved in the drafting and submission of the manuscript. All authors read and approved the final manuscript.

Acknowledgments

The authors are thankful the vice chancellor of research, Mashhad University of Medical Sciences for financial support. This study was part of Pharm.D thesis of A.H.

Author details

[1]Pharmaceutical Research Center, Department of Pharmacodynamics and Toxicology, School of Pharmacy, Mashhad University of Medical Sciences, Mashhad, Iran. [2]School of Pharmacy, Mashhad University of Medical Sciences, Mashhad, Iran. [3]Pharmaceutical and Biotechnology Research Centers, School of Pharmacy, Mashhad University of Medical Sciences, Mashhad, Iran. [4]Biotechnology Research Center, Mashhad University of Medical Sciences, Mashhad, Iran. [5]Pharmaceutical Research Center, Department of Medicinal

Chemistry, School of Pharmacy, Mashhad University of Medical Sciences, 91775-1365 Mashhad, Iran.

References

1. Abdullaev FI: Biological effects of saffron. *Biofactors* 1993, **4**:83–86.
2. Abdullaev FI, Espinosa-Aguirre JJ: Biomedical properties of saffron and its potential use in cancer therapy and chemoprevention trials. *Cancer Detect Prev* 2004, **28**:426–432.
3. Ríos JL, Recio MC, Giner RM, Meñez S: An update review of saffron and its active constituents. *Phytother Res* 1996, **10**:189–193.
4. Assimopoulou AN, Sinakos Z, Papageorgiou VP: Radical scavenging activity of *Crocus sativus* L. extract and its bioactive constituents. *Phytother Res* 2005, **19**:997–1000.
5. Hosseinzadeh H, Karimi G, Niapoor M: Antidepressant effects of *Crocus sativus* stigma extracts and its constituents, crocin and safranal, in mice. *J Med Plants* 2004, **3**(48):58.
6. Hosseinzadeh H, Ziaei T: Effects of *Crocus sativus* stigma extract and its constituents, crocin and safranal, on intact memory and scopolamine-induced learning deficits in rats performing the Morris water maze task. *J Med Plants* 2006, **5**:40–50.
7. Ochiai T, Shimeno H, Mishima K, Iwasaki K, Fujiwara M, Tanaka H, Shoyama Y, Toda A, Eyanagi R, Soeda S: Protective effects of carotenoids from saffron on neuronal injury *in vitro* and *in vivo*. *Biochim Biophys Acta* 2007, **1770**:578–584.
8. Ochiai T, Soeda S, Ohno S, Tanaka H, Shoyama Y, Shimeno H: Crocin prevents the death of PC-12 cells through sphingomyelinase-ceramide signaling by increasing glutathione synthesis. *Neurochem Int* 2004, **44**:321–330.
9. Hosseinzadeh H, Shamsaie F, Mehri S: Antioxidant activity of aqueous and ethanolic extracts of *Crocus sativus* L. stigma and its bioactive constituent, crocin and safranal. *Pharmacogn Mag* 2009, **5**:419–424.
10. Hosseinzadeh H, Modaghegh MH, Saffari Z: *Crocus sativus* L. (saffron) extract and its active constituents (crocin and safranal) on ischemia-reperfusion in rat skeletal muscle. *Evid Based Complement Alternat Med* 2009, **6**:343–350.
11. Aung HH, Wang CZ, Ni M, Fishbein A, Mehendale SR, Xie JT, Shoyama CY, Yuan CS: Crocin from Crocus sativus possesses significant anti-proliferation effects on human colorectal cancer cells. *Exp Oncol* 2007, **29**:175–180.
12. Bjelakovic G, Nikolova D, Gluud L, Simonetti R, Gluud C: Mortality in randomized trials of antioxidant supplements for primary and secondary prevention. *JAMA* 2007, **297**:842–857.
13. Ramanathan B, Jan KY, Chen CH, Hour TC, Yu HJ, Pu YS: Resistance to paclitaxel is proportional to cellular total antioxidant capacity. *Cancer Res* 2005, **65**:8455–8460.
14. Li X, Huang T, Jiang G, Gong W, Qian H, Zou C: Synergistic apoptotic effect of crocin and cisplatin on osteosarcoma cells via caspase induced apoptosis. *Toxicol Lett* 2013, **221**:197–204.
15. Razavi BM, Hosseinzadeh H, Movassaghi AR, Imenshahidi M, Abnous K: Protective effect of crocin on diazinon induced cardiotoxicity in rats in subchronic exposure. *Chem Biol Interact* 2013, **203**:547–555.
16. Schneider-Stock R, Ghantous A, Bajbouj K, Saikali M, Darwiche N: Epigenetic mechanisms of plant-derived anticancer drugs. *Front Biosci* 2012, **17**:129–173.
17. Saeidnia S, Abdollahi M: Antioxidants: Friends or foe in prevention or treatment of cancer: The debate of the century. *Toxicol Appl Pharmacol* 2013, **271**:49–63.
18. Murakami A, Ohnishi K: Target molecules of food phytochemicals: Food science bound for the next dimension. *Food Funct* 2012, **3**:462–476.
19. Guiffant D, Tribouillard D, Gug F, Galons H, Meijer L, Blondel M, Bach S: Identification of intracellular targets of small molecular weight chemical compounds using affinity chromatography. *Biotechnol J* 2007, **2**:68–75.
20. Terstappen GC, Schlupen C, Raggiaschi R, Gaviraghi G: Target deconvolution strategies in drug discovery. *Nat Rev Drug Discov* 2007, **6**:891–903.
21. Hadizadeh F, Mohajeri SA, Seifi M: Extraction and purification of crocin from saffron stigmas employing a simple and efficient crystallization method. *Pakistan J Biol Sci* 2010, **13**:691–698.
22. Javadi B, Sahebkar A, Emami A: A Survey on Saffron in Major Islamic Traditional Medicine Books. *Iran J Basic Med Sci* 2013, **16**:1–11.
23. Hosseinzadeh H, Nassiri-Asl M: Avicenna's (Ibn Sina) the Canon of Medicine and saffron (Crocus sativus): a review. *Phytother Res* 2013, **27**:475–483.
24. Saxena C, Higgs RE, Zhen E, Hale JE: Small-molecule affinity chromatography coupled mass spectrometry for drug target deconvolution. *Exp Opin Drug Discov* 2009, **4**:701–714.
25. Rao J, Li N: Microfilament actin remodeling as a potential target for cancer drug development. *Curr Cancer Drug Targets* 2004, **4**:345–354.
26. Howard J, Hyman AA: Dynamics and mechanics of the microtubule plus end. *Nature* 2003, **422**:753–758.
27. Zhou J, Giannakakou P: Targeting microtubules for cancer chemotherapy. *Curr Med Chem Anticancer Agents* 2005, **5**:65–71.
28. Alijanianzadeh M, Zarei HJ: Saffron carotenoid effects on the polymerization of microtubules and Hela cell growth. *Biol Sci* 2009, **4**:31–39.
29. Houstek J, Pícková A, Vojtísková A, Mrácek T, Pecina P, Jesina P: Mitochondrial diseases and genetic defects of ATP synthase. *Biochim Biophys Acta* 2006, **1757**:1400–1405.
30. Ahmad Z, Laughlin TF: Medicinal chemistry of ATP synthase: a potential drug target of dietary polyphenols and amphibian antimicrobial peptides. *Curr Med Chem* 2010, **17**:2822–2836.
31. Hosseinzadeh H, Mehri S, Abolhassani MM, Ramezani M, Sahebkar A, Abnous K: Affinity-based target deconvolution of safranal. *Daru* 2013, **21**:25.
32. Mehri S, Abnous K, Mousavi SH, Shariaty VM, Hosseinzadeh H: Neuroprotective effect of crocin on acrylamide-induced cytotoxicity in PC12 cells. *Cell Mol Neurobiol* 2012, **32**:227–235.
33. Ochiai T, Ohno S, Soeda S, Tanaka H, Shoyama Y, Shimeno H: Crocin prevents the death of rat pheochromocytoma (PC-12) cells by its antioxidant effects stronger than those of a-tocopherol. *Neurosci Lett* 2004, **362**:61–64.
34. Jnaneshwari S, Hemshekhar M, Santhosh MS, Sunitha K, Thushara R, Thirunavukkarasu C, Kemparaju K, Girish KS: Crocin, a dietary colorant mitigates cyclophosphamide-induced organ toxicity by modulating antioxidant status and inflammatory cytokines. *J Pharm Pharmacol* 2013, **65**:604–614.
35. Abnous K, Storey KB: Regulation of skeletal muscle creatine kinase from a hibernating mammal. *Arch Biochem Biophys* 2007, **467**:10–19.
36. Dahlstedt AJ, Westerblad H: Inhibition of creatine kinase reduces the rate of fatigue-induced decrease in tetanic [Ca(2+)](i) in mouse skeletal muscle. *J Physiol* 2001, **533**:639–649.
37. Abe K, Sugiura M, Shoyama Y, Saito H: Crocin antagonizes ethanol inhibition of NMDA receptor-mediated responses in rat hippocampal neurons. *Brain Res* 1998, **787**:132–138.
38. Mizuma H, Tanaka M, Nozaki S, Mizuno K, Tahara T, Ataka S, Sugino T, Shirai T, Kajimoto Y, Kuratsune H, Kajimoto O, Watanabe Y: Daily oral administration of crocetin attenuates physical fatigue in human subjects. *Nutr Res* 2009, **29**:145–150.
39. Mei Y, Yong J, Stonestrom A, Yang X: tRNA and cytochrome c in cell death and beyond. *Cell Cycle* 2010, **9**:2936–2939.
40. Gong Q, Shi DB, Cai WB, Yang ZH, Tan WG, Liao CY, Peng C, Liu C, Gao GQ, Yang X: Effect and mechanism of HeLa cell apoptosis induced by crocin. *Chinese J Cancer Prev Treat* 2009, **16**:1445–1447+1462.
41. Xu G, Gong Z, Yu W, Gao L, He S, Qian Z: Increased expression ratio of bcl-2/bax is associated with crocin-mediated apoptosis in bovine aortic endothelial cells. *Basic Clin Pharmacol Toxicol* 2007, **100**:31–35.
42. Izumi H, Torigoe T, Ishiguchi H, Uramoto H, Yoshida Y, Tanabe M, Ise T, Murakami T, Yoshida T, Nomoto M, Kohno K: Cellular pH regulators: potentially promising molecular targets for cancer chemotherapy. *Cancer Treat Rev* 2003, **29**:541–549.
43. Wood EJ: In *Harper's biochemistry*. 24th edition. Edited by Murray RK, Granner DK, Mayes PA, Rodwell VW. Stamford, CT: Appleton & Lange; 1996:237.
44. Lövborg H, Oberg F, Rickardson L, Gullbo J, Nygren P, Larsson R: Inhibition of proteasome activity, nuclear factor-KappaB translocation and cell survival by the antialcoholism drug disulfiram. *Int J Cancer* 2006, **118**:1577–1580.
45. Wickström M, Danielsson K, Rickardson L, Gullbo J, Nygren P, Isaksson A, Larsson R, Lövborg H: Pharmacological profiling of disulfiram using

human tumor cell lines and human tumor cells from patients. *Biochem Pharmacol* 2007, **73**:25–33.

46. Minamida S, Iwamura M, Kodera Y, Kawashima Y, Tabata K, Matsumoto K, Fujita T, Satoh T, Maeda T, Baba S: **14-3-3 protein beta/alpha as a urinary biomarker for renal cell carcinoma: proteomic analysis of cyst fluid.** *Anal Bioanal Chem* 2011, **401**:245–252.

47. Kianbakht S, Hajiaghaee R: **Anti-hyperglycemic effects of saffron and its active constituents, crocin and safranal, in alloxan-induced diabetic rats.** *J Med Plants* 2011, **10**:82–89.

48. Didelot C, Lanneau D, Brunet M, Joly AL, De Thonel A, Chiosis G, Garrido C: **Anti-cancer therapeutic approaches based on intracellular and extracellular heat shock proteins.** *Curr Med Chem* 2007, **14**:2839–2847.

49. Kamalipour M, Akhondzadeh S: **Cardiovascular effects of saffron: An evidence-based review.** *Journal of Tehran University Heart Center* 2011, **6**:59–61.

50. Joukar S, Najafipour H, Khaksari M, Sepehri G, Shahrokhi N, Dabiri S, Gholamhoseinian A, Hasanzadeh S: **The effect of saffron consumption on biochemical and histopathological heart indices of rats with myocardial infarction.** *Cardiovasc Toxicol* 2010, **10**:66–71.

51. Bonanad C, Núñez J, Sanchis J, Bodi V, Chaustre F, Chillet M, Miñana G, Forteza MJ, Palau P, Núñez E, Navarro D, Llàcer A, Chorro FJ: **Serum Heat Shock Protein 60 in acute heart failure: a new biomarker?** *Congest Heart Fail* 2013, **19**:6–10.

11

Synthesis of chemically cross-linked polyvinyl alcohol-co-poly (methacrylic acid) hydrogels by copolymerization; a potential graft-polymeric carrier for oral delivery of 5-fluorouracil

Muhammad Usman Minhas, Mahmood Ahmad[*], Liaqat Ali and Muhammad Sohail

Abstract

Background of the Study: The propose of the present work was to develop chemically cross-linked polyvinyl alcohol-co-poly(methacrylic acid) hydrogel (PVA-MAA hydrogel) for pH responsive delivery of 5-Fluorouracil (5-FU).

Methods: PVA based hydrogels were prepared by free radical copolymerization. PVA has been cross-linked chemically with monomer (methacrylic acid) in aqueous medium, cross-linking agent was ethylene glycol di-methacrylate (EGDMA) and benzoyl peroxide was added as reaction initiator. 5-FU was loaded as model drug. FTIR, XRD, TGA and DSC were performed for characterization of copolymer. Surface morphology was studied by SEM. pH sensitive properties were evaluated by swelling dynamics and equilibrium swelling ratio at low and higher pH.

Results: FTIR, XRD, TGA and DSC studies confirmed the formation of new copolymer. Formulations with higher MAA contents showed maximum swelling at 7.4 pH. High drug loading and higher drug release has been observed at pH 7.4.

Conclusions: The current study concludes that a stable copolymeric network of PVA was developed with MAA. The prepared hydrogels were highly pH responsive. This polymeric network could be a potential delivery system for colon targeting of 5-FU in colorectal cancers.

Keywords: Polyvinyl alcohol, Methacrylic acid, Hydrogel, 5-Fluorouracil, pH-responsive

Introduction

The term "hydrogel" is being considered for water insoluble polymeric network that has capacity to absorb large amount of water [1-5]. Synthetic or natural polymers, homopolymer or copolymer, are used to make three dimensional networks by molecular entanglements or by chemical crosslinking [6]. Physical or reversible hydrogels are synthesized by entanglements of polymer molecules or by hydrophobic interactions. Physical hydrogels can absorb the water but inhomogeneities or network defects may occur due to free chain ends or chain loops [7,8]. The network defects or loose aggregates in physical gels may cause the problem in drug loading and release formed by covalent crosslinking of polymers [9]. Chemical or permanent hydrogels are formed by covalent crosslinking of polymers [9]. Chemically cross-linked hydrogels do not change the shape under the ordinary pressure and erratic movements in GIT do not break the drug carrier systems. Therefore such stable system could be effective in site specific delivery of various agents.

First synthetic hydrogels of HEMA with EGDMA as cross-linker were prepared for biological use and later used for production of contact lenses [10]. Polyvinyl alcohol (PVA) based hydrogels have advantageous characteristics of good mechanical strength and high water retaining ability along with properties of biocompatibility, flexibility and can also be used as artificial soft tissue [11]. Mostly PVA hydrogels have been prepared by freezing and thawing cycles and by UV radiation crosslinking methods. PVA based hydrogels of different mechanical strengths can be produced by Freeze-thaw technique by controlling the freeze-thaw cycles but this would render the synthesis process time-consumption

* Correspondence: ma786_786@yahoo.com
Faculty of Pharmacy and Alternative Medicine, the Islamia University of Bahawalpur-63100, Punjab, Pakistan

[12]. Various methods have been reported for physical cross-linking or non-chemical cross-linking methods of PVA graft polymers involving many processing steps and prolonged processes [13-16]. Chemical cross-linkers have employed in synthesis of number of non-PVA hydrogels. Previously PVA cross-linked membranes were synthesized using glutaraldehyde as cross-linking agent [17]. In present work, chemical cross-linking method has been developed for suitable polymer monomer ratio. The actual challenge was to study the reaction parameters, suitable polymer-monomer ratio and their optimization for temperature, time and concentrations of reactants to synthesize pH sensitive PVA graft MAA hydrogels. The study method could be considered a rapid and simple method for synthesis of PVA-co-poly(methacrylic acid)

hydrogels by chemical cross-linking with EGDMA. A monomer MAA was used to impart pH sensitive characteristics. The study was undertaken to synthesize and characterize the pH sensitive chemically cross-linked PVA hydrogels and to introduce a promising delivery system for colonic delivery of 5-fluorouracil in colorectal cancer (5-FU is a first line anticancer drug in colorectal cancer therapy). Chemical structures of polymer, monomer and presumptive cross-linked hydrogel structure as well as their abbreviations have been listed in Table 1.

Materials and methods
Chemicals
5-Fluorouracil was obtained as a kind gift from Pharmedic Laboratories (Pvt.) Ltd. Lahore, Pakistan.

Table 1 Chemical structures of Polymer, monomer and possible cross-linked structure of hydrogels

Monomer/Polymer	Abbreviation	Chemical structure
Methacrylic acid	MAA	
Polyvinyl alcohol	PVA	
Ethylene glycol di-methacrylate	EGDMA	
Cross-linked polyvinyl-co-poly (Methacrylic acid) hydrogels	PVA-co-poly (MAA)	

Polyvinyl alcohol (PVA), methacrylic acid (MAA), ethylene glycol dimethacrylate (EGDMA), benzoyl peroxide were purchased from Sigma Aldrich, UK., Deionized distilled water was obtained from our laboratory.

Synthesis of PVA-co-polyMAA hydrogels

Free radical copolymerization method was adopted and various formulations were prepared that have been presented in Table 2. A specific quantity of PVA was weighed and dissolved in water by continuous stirring at 800 rpm and heating of the reaction mixture was maintained at 90°C, until a transparent solution was obtained. The reaction mixture was purged under the nitrogen stream for 30 min to exclude the dissolved oxygen. A separate solution was prepared in which benzoyl peroxide as initiator was dissolved in weighed amount of MAA. The benzoyl peroxide-MAA mixture was added slowly (drop wise) in PVA solution at 50°C. Finally ethylene glycol diamine methacrylate (EGDMA) was added (0.5 mol% of monomer) to the reaction mixture (Table 2). The resultant reaction mixture was carefully transferred to glass tubes of same dimensions and heated in water bath at 55°C for 4 hours, 60°C for 6 hours and 65°C for 12 hours. After this treatment, all tubes were cooled to room temperature and cylindrical hydrogels were cut into small discs (8 mm in length). These discs were washed with ethanol-water (70:30) to remove un-reacted monomers and catalyst, until no change in pH of solvents mixture before and after washing of discs. Initially the discs were dried in laminar flow air for 24 h and then in vacuum oven at 40°C for one week.

Characterization

FT-IR

The FT-IR spectra of pure PVA and MAA were recorded. Samples were thoroughly ground and analyzed

Table 2 Formulations of PVA-co-poly(MAA) hydrogels

Formulation code	Polyvinyl alcohol (g/100 g)	Methacrylic acid (g/100 g)	EGDMA mol% of monomer
PVH-1	0.500	20.0	0.10
PVH-2	1.00	20.0	0.10
PVH-3	2.00	20.0	0.10
PVH-4	2.00	20.0	0.10
PVH-5	2.00	30.0	0.10
PVH-6	2.00	40.0	0.10
PVH-7	1.00	20.0	0.20
PVH-8	1.00	20.0	0.25
PVH-9	1.00	20.0	0.30

by attenuated total reflectance ATR-FTIR (Shimadzu, Germany) in range of 4000–650 cm^{-1}. All the hydrogel formulations were examined by FT-IR.

TGA and DSC

Thermal analysis was performed by thermogravimetric analysis (TGA) of TA instruments Q5000 series Thermal Analysis System (TA instruments,WestSussex, UK) and differential scanning calorimetry (DSC) of TA instruments Q2000 Series Thermal Analysis system (TA Instrument WestSussex, UK). The hydrogel samples were ground and passed through mesh 40. For TGA, amount between 0.5-5 mg was placed in an open pan (platinum 100 µl) attached to a microbalance .The samples were heated at 20°C/min from 25-500°C under dry nitrogen at standard mode with ramp test type. All the measurements were made in triplicate. For DSC, samples of PVA, MAA and formulations (0.5-3 mg) were precisely weighed into an aluminum pan onto which aluminum lid with a central pierced hole was crimped. The samples were then scanned under a stream of nitrogen gas from 0-400°C using heating rate 20°C/min.

PXRD

Bruker D-8 powder diffractometer (Bruker Kahlsruhl, Germany) was used to record the XRD pattern, at room temperature. Powdered samples were filled on to plastic sample holder and smoothing the surface with a glass slide. Samples were scanned over range 5-50° 2θ at a rate of 1° 2θ/min using a copper Kα radiation source with a wavelength of 1.542 Å and 1 mm slits.

Morphology of networks

Surface morphology of hydrogels was investigated using scanning electron microscopy (SEM) by a Quanta 400 SEM (FEI Company, Cambridge, UK). Completely dried discs of hydrogels were cut to optimum sizes to fix on a double-adhesive tape stuck to an aluminum stub. The stubs were coated with gold to a thickness of ~300 Å under an argon atmosphere using a gold sputter module in a high-vacuum evaporator. The coated samples were randomly scanned and photomicrographs were recorded to reveal surface morphology.

Equilibrium swelling ratio

Swelling studies were performed to evaluate the pH sensitivity of the hydrogels. Dried discs of hydrogels were weighed and immersed in 0.1 M HCl pH 1.2 and in phosphate buffer solutions of 5.8, 7.4 at 37°C. The samples were removed at specific intervals and weighed after removing excess of water by blotting with filter paper. The degree of swelling and equilibrium water contents were calculated using Eq. 1 and 2 [18].

$$Q = \frac{M_s}{M_d} \qquad (1)$$

$$EWC\% = \frac{M_{eq}M_d}{M_d} \times 100 \qquad (2)$$

Where M_s indicates mass of swelling at predetermined time interval, M_{eq} is weight at equilibrium swelling and M_d represents the weight of dry gel before initiation of swelling experiments.

Drug loading and release studies

5-Fluorouracil (5-FU) was loaded in hydrogels by absorption method [17,19,20] as model drug by diffusion method. Dried circle PVA-co-MAA hydrogels discs (8 mm) were immersed into 100 ml 5-FU solution (1.0%) in phosphate buffer of pH 7.4 for 72 hours at room temperature. Higher pH and solvent was selected in which drug showed maximum solubility and higher swelling. The discs were immediately washed with distilled water and first dried at room temperature and then placed in oven at 40°C.

Percentage of drug loading was assessed by extracting the weighed amount of polymer with same solvent used for drug loading. Each time 25 ml of fresh buffer solution was used to extract the drug from discs. Extraction was repeated until no drug found in solution. Drug contents were determined by preparing calibration curve of 5-FU dilutions in phosphate buffer using UV–vis-spectrophotometer (UV-1601Shimadzu). The sample was scanned first to determine the λ_{max} that was found 266 nm.

Drug release was investigated at low and high pH values to confirm the pH dependant delivery of 5-FU from PVA/MAA hydrogel network. Drug loaded disks were evaluated for 5-FU release in 900 ml solutions of pH 1.2 and 7.4 in USP dissolution apparatus-II at 37 ± 0.5°C. These samples were analysed at 266 nm using UV–vis-spectrophotometer (UV-1601Shimadzu).

Results and discussion

Physical appearance of hydrogels

Polymerization of PVA with MAA after the crosslinking formed stable polymeric networks. Gels with higher MAA concentration revealed glass like transparent appearance while gels with low MAA contents showed milky white characteristics. An excellent mechanical strength was observed in gelled copolymer that retained the shape even after swelling. Hydrogels with high MAA ratio showed higher mechanical strength than hydrogels with higher polymer (PVA) contents. Discs in swelled form have been shown in Figure 1.

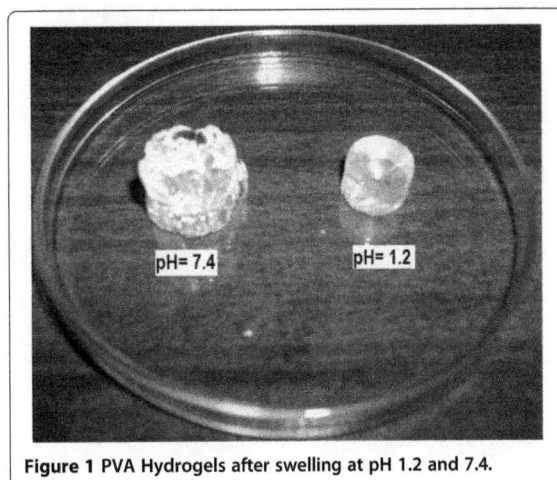

Figure 1 PVA Hydrogels after swelling at pH 1.2 and 7.4.

Structure analysis

FT-IR spectra of PVA, MAA and PVA-co-poly(MAA) hydrogel have been shown in Figure 2. PVA spectra showed broad absorption at region of 3400 cm^{-1} indicating the presence O-H stretching vibrations. Peak at 2940 cm^{-1} is related to presence of –CH$_2$ groups. A band at region of 1449 cm^{-1} showed –OH deformation. The FT-IR spectrum of methacrylic acid indicates peak at 2929 cm^{-1} that indicates the presence of methyl C–H asymmetric stretching. Band range in 1725–1700 cm^{-1} is assigned for carboxylic acid (1699 cm^{-1} indicate carboxylic acid groups) and the peak at 1633 cm^{-1} shows the C=C stretching vibrations.

The spectrum from cross-linked hydrogel formulations showed different peaks from the parent components (polyvinyl alcohol and methacrylic acid). Broad absorption at 3467 cm^{-1} showed –OH stretching and a absorption at region of 1700 cm^{-1} revealed the presence of carbonyl group that was not present in pure PVA spectrum which indicates the esterification between PVA and MAA.

TGA and DSC measurements were performed for the pure PVA, MAA and PVA-MAA hydrogels, shown in Figures 3 and 4. Thermogram analysis was performed to determine the thermal stability. Initial loss in mass was due the water loss. TGA curves showed that PVA was stable up to 250°C and decomposition occur above the 265°C. Complete loss of pure MAA occur above 100°C. However PVA-MAA hydrogel revealed first endothermic peak from 225°C to 325°C and decomposition curve from 400°C to 475°C. PVA-co-MAA showed higher thermal stability pattern, it indicates that cross-linking between the PVA and MAA increase the thermal stability of PVA. This showed that the formed hydrogels could be processed at reasonably higher temperature than its individual components (PVA, MAA and EGDMA).

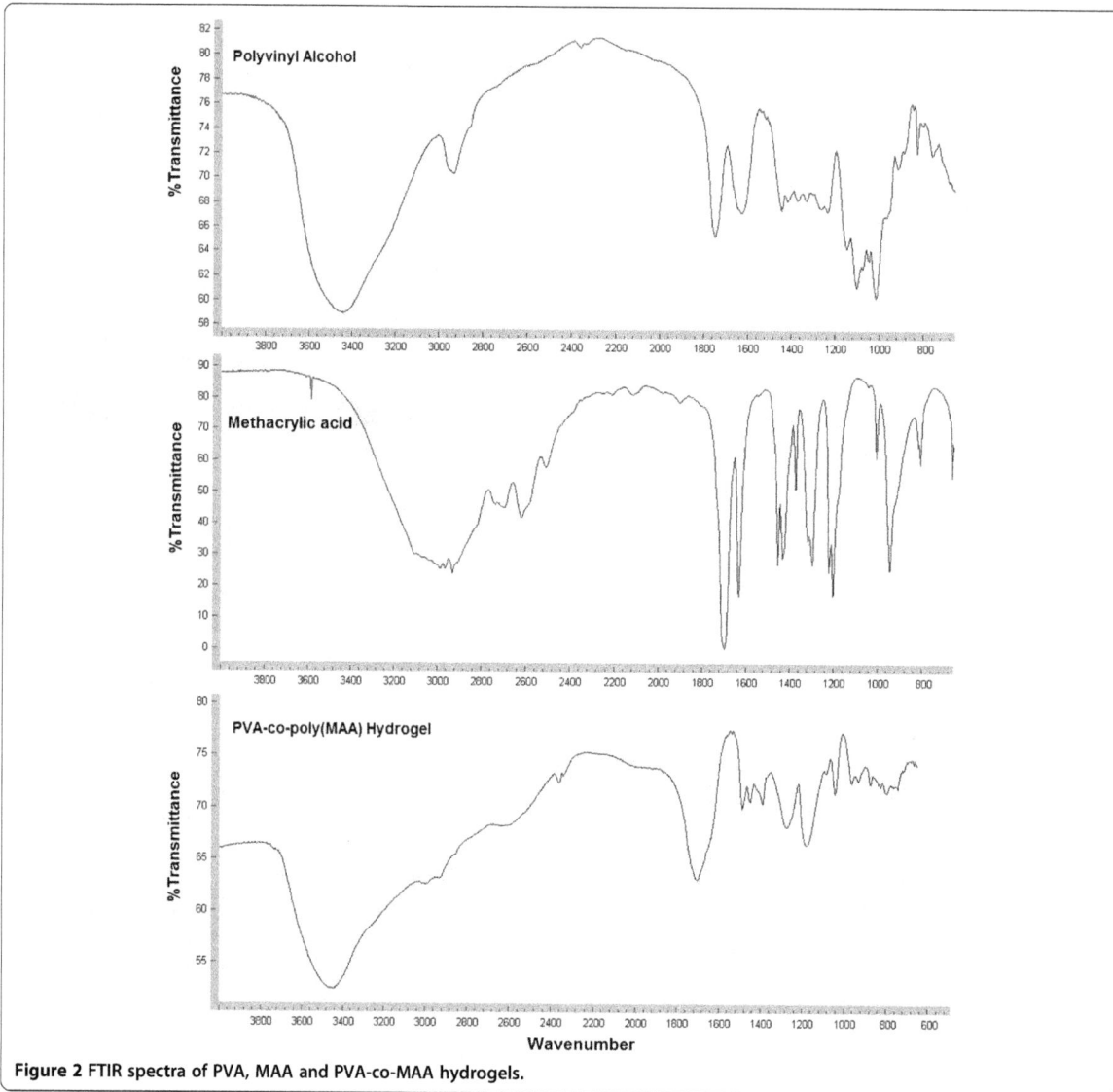

Figure 2 FTIR spectra of PVA, MAA and PVA-co-MAA hydrogels.

DSC endothermic peaks of pure PVA and MAA were different from the cross-linked PVA-MAA macromolecule. The DSC endothermic peak of PVA at 85°C can be attributed as Tg and decomposition start at 200°C that is melting temperature. Complete mass loss was observed for MAA at 25°C. DSC thermograms of PVA-MAA hydrogel formulations showed two major endothermic peaks, mass loss at 100°C could be attributed to water loss from preparation. However peak at 240°C showed the decomposition of cross-linked polymer-monomer networks, similar reponse by TGA thermogram has been recorded that indicates the decomposition range from 180 to 325°C. TGA and DSC thermograms indicate different thermal pattern of pure PVA and MAA from prepared hydrogels. Cross-linking between PVA and MAA increases the

thermal stability and these cross-linked matrices could provide a good delivering capacity for various types of drug molecules.

PXRD pattern of pure PVA and PVA-MAA hydrogels was recorded that has been shown in Figure 5. A sharp peak at $2\theta=20.1°$ is the characteristic of PVA. PVA-MAA hydrogel showed different XRD pattern from the pure PVA that confirmed the formation of a new polymer. The peak at $2\theta=20.1°$ is weekend significantly and another broad peak also appeared at $2\theta=50.0°$. The XRD pattern of PVA-MAA hydrogels showed decrease in the crystallinity. The cross-linking between the PVA and MAA decrease the crystalline behavior of PVA.

Morphological studies were performed for intact surface studies of hydrogels and cross-sectional part by

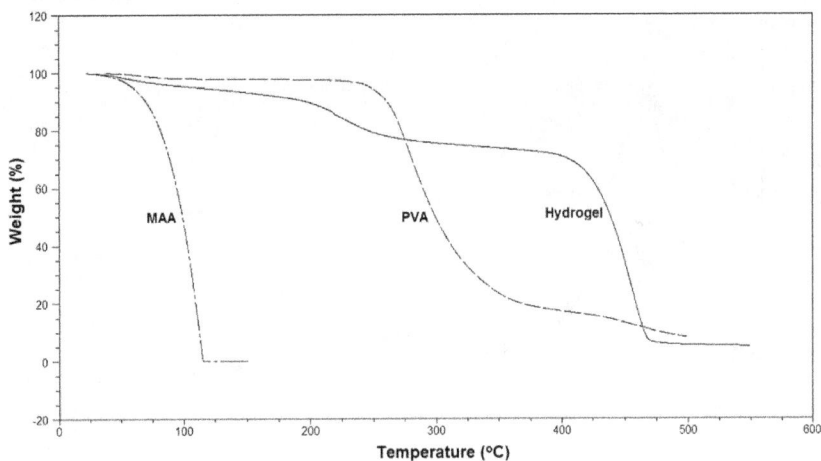

Figure 3 TGA of PVA, MAA and PVA-co-MAA hydrogels.

SEM. SEM micrographs revealed that hydrogel formulations with low polymer contents but high monomer contents indicates comparatively smooth outer surface while hydrogels with higher polymer concentration showed wavy surface. Surface morphology of intact discs and cross-sections are presented in Figure 6, hydrogels with higher monomer (MAA) contents revealed less wavy surface than Hydrogel discs with higher polymer ratio. Cross-sectional images of hydrogels with low polymer contents revealed large pores and dense areas (Figure 6). However smaller but number of pores were observed in cross-sectional images of hydrogels with high polymer. Generally a porous structure has been observed in morphological studies.

Effect of polymer, monomer and cross-linker on swelling
Various formulations were prepared with varying the polymer, monomer and cross-linker ratio. Three sets of sample series were prepared to evaluate the effect of polymer (PVA), monomer (MAA) and cross-linker (EGDMA) contents on dynamic swelling of hydrogels. Dynamic swelling was studied to evaluate the swelling with respect to time and representative swelling has been shown in Figure 7. Formulation series PVAH-1 to PVAH-3 with increasing concentration of polymer (PVA), PVAH-4 to PVAH-6 with increasing contents of monomer (Methacrylic acid) and PVAH-7 to PVAH-9 with increasing the cross-linker's concentration were prepared. In prepared hydrogels pH dependent swelling was observed that could be attributed

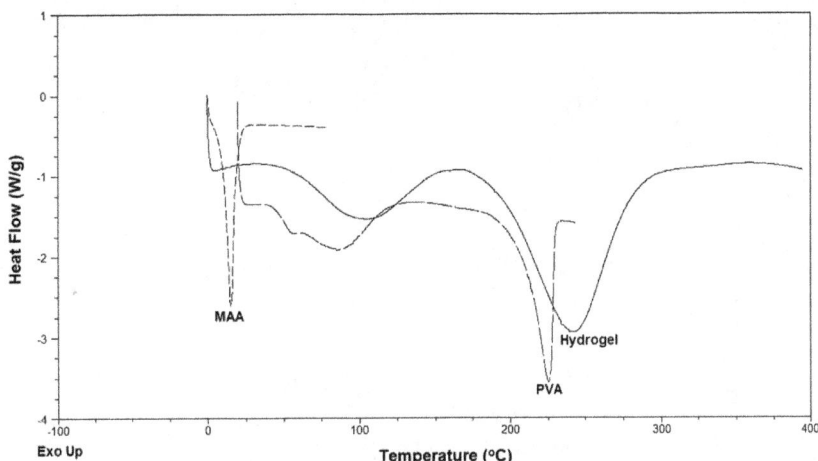

Figure 4 DSC of PVA, MAA and PVA-co-MAA hydrogels.

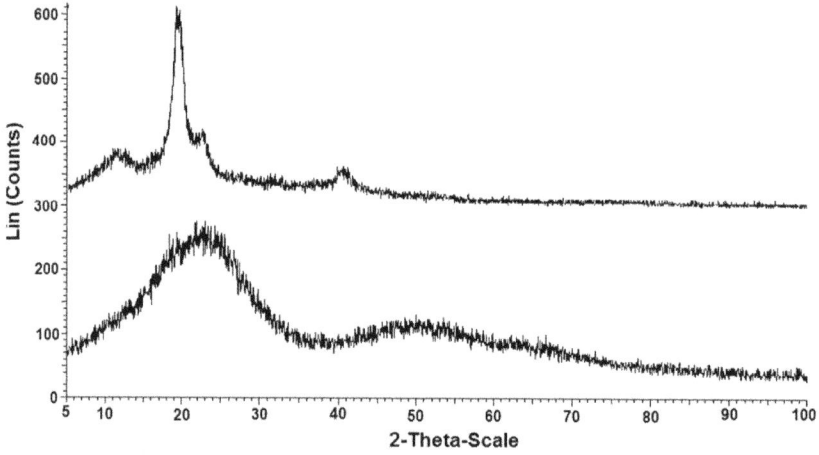

Figure 5 XRD patterns of pure PVA and PVA-co-MAA hydrogels.

to ionizable functional groups. PVA contain high hydroxyl groups that make this polymer highly interactive with water. Large pendent carboxylic groups associated with methacrylic acid made the coploymeric system a pH responsive that could be observed from swelling characteristics. At high pH these carboxylic groups ionized and repel each other. The repulsive forces impart the swelling properties to gels. Effect of polymer, monomer and cross-linker on swelling (equilibrium swelling index) at various pH has been presented in Figure 8. Dynamic swelling was studied to evaluate the swelling with respect to time and representative swelling has been shown in Figure 7. Hydrogels with increasing ratio of polymer (PVAH-1 to PVAH-3) did not show significant difference in dynamic swelling up to 12 hrs from each other.

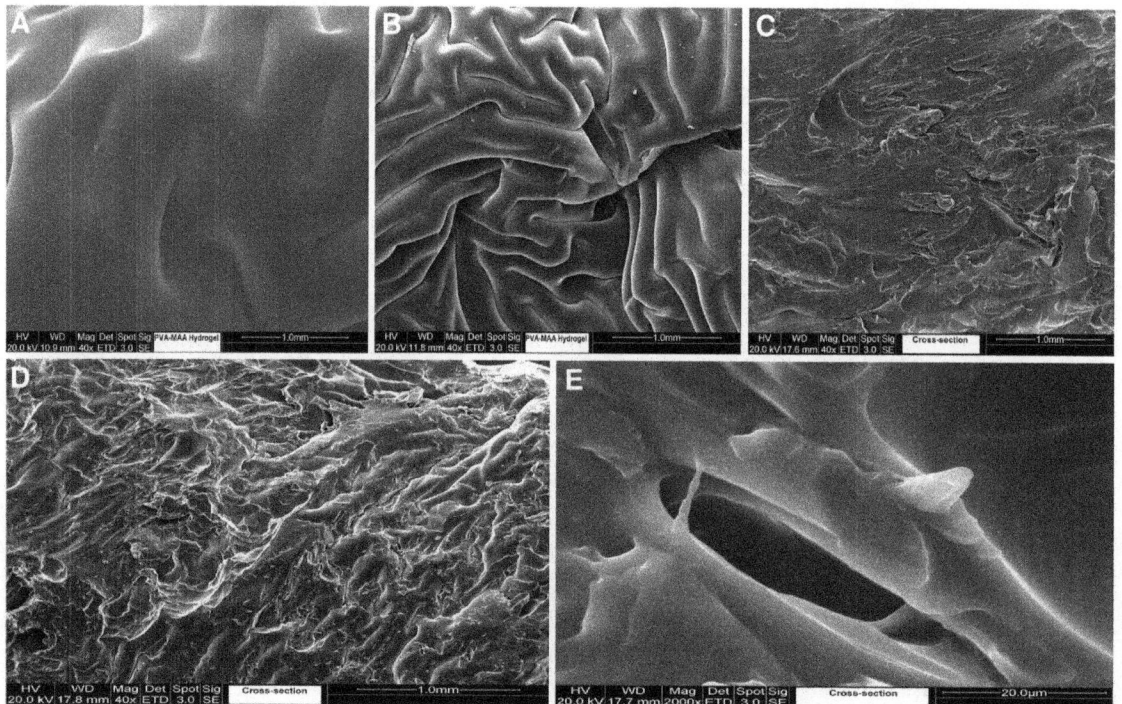

Figure 6 SEM micrographs of PVA-co-MAA hydrogels; (A) & (B) intact surface, (C) (D) & (E) cross-section.

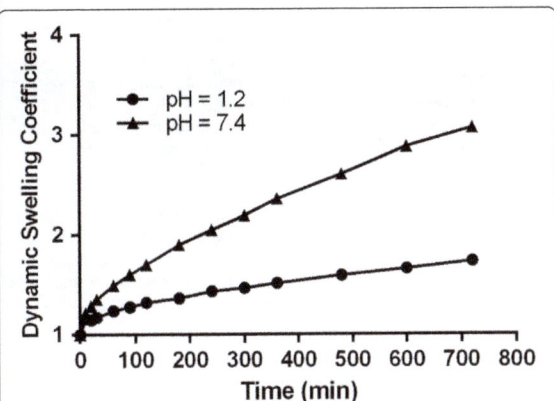

Figure 7 Effect of PVA, MAA and EGDMA on swelling index.

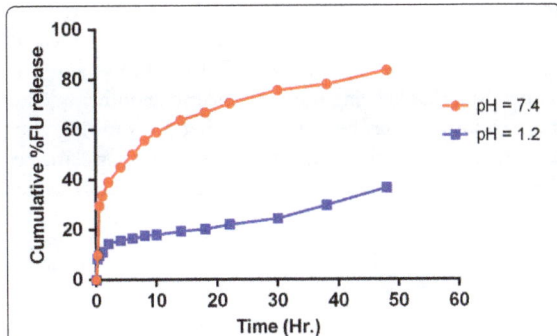

Figure 9 FU release studies from PVA-MAA hydrogels (PVH-3) at pH 1.2 and 7.4 up to 48 hrs.

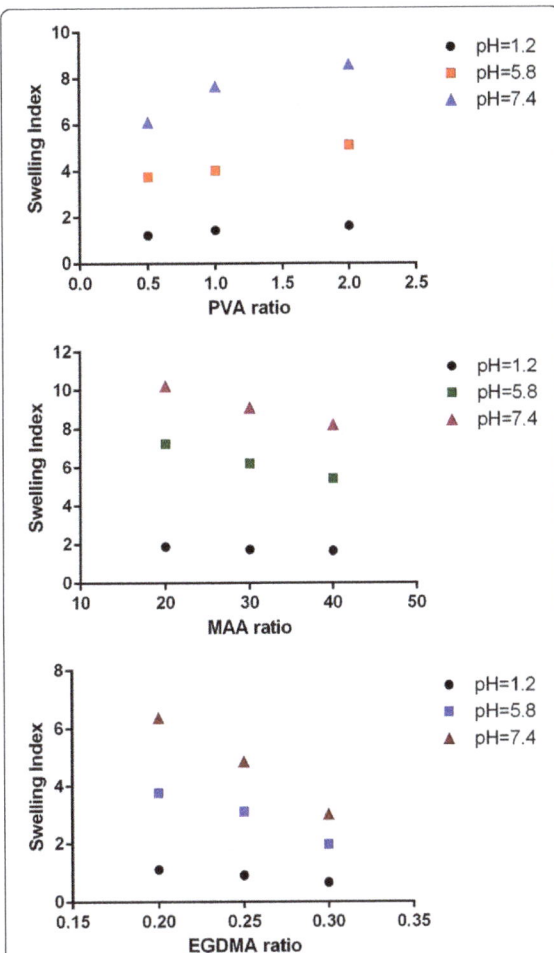

Figure 8 Dynamic swelling characteristics of PVA-MAA hydrogels (PVH-3).

Drug loading and release studies

5-Fluorouracil was loaded as model drug to evaluate its delivery against the pH stimuli. Drug loading was found 0.115 ± 0.02 mg of FU/mg of hydrogel. Higher drug loading was observed in discs that showed higher swelling. Percent release studies of 5FU at pH 1.2 and 7.4 have been presented in Figure 9. Low drug released at pH 1.2 but higher at pH 7.4. The prepared hydrogels showed drug release up to 48 hours in phosphate buffer of pH 7.4. The pH responsive delivery of this anticancer drug could be highly important because the prepared hydrogels showed higher 5-FU at high pH for longer period of time (approximately 80% during 48 hours. Percentage of drug release has also been presented in Table 3 to evaluate the effect of ratio (up to 24 hours).

Conclusions

Chemical cross-linking between polyvinyl alcohol and methacrylic acid modified the characteristics of individual components and formed a pH responsive co-polymeric matrix system. The chemical cross-linking of PVA by EGDMA impart a good strength, very low water

Table 3 Effect of reaction variables on drug loading and percent release

Formulation code	5FU loading mg/0.5 g of dry gel	% release of 5FU up to 24 hrs.		
		pH 1.2	pH 5.8	pH 7.4
PVH-1	72.62	4.66	32.2	63.67
PVH-2	79.22	5.19	39.3	68.23
PVH-3	88.81	6.01	44.1	73.29
PVH-4	89.65	7.21	51.1	78.55
PVH-5	84.44	6.22	47.3	74.19
PVH-6	75.23	5.98	41.2	70.37
PVH-7	81.71	6.63	34.4	70.32
PVH-8	72.91	5.32	28.8	63.35
PVH-9	67.26	3.81	22.2	56.44

absorption at low pH and high at high pH. The prepared hydrogels showed a pH responsive behavior as well as higher drug release at high pH. 5-FU has been loaded as model drug that is being used in cancer chemotherapy but intravenously. It can be concluded that a promising chemically cross-linked pH responsive co-polymeric matrix delivery would be highly effective in colorectal cancer therapies.

Abbreviations

PVA: Polyvinyl alcohol; MAA: Methacrylic acid; 5-FU: 5-Fluorouracil.

Competing interests

All authors declared that they have no competing interests.

Authors' contributions

All the authors have substantial contribution in completion of this study. MUM prepared the formulations, analyzed and wrote the manuscript. MA supervised the study and reviewed the manuscript. LA and MS participated in experimental work. All authors read and approved the final manuscript.

Acknowledgement

Authors are thankful to Higher Education Commission of Pakistan to finance the study.

References

1. Nguyen KT, West JL: **Photopolymerizable hydrogels for tissue engineering applications**. *Biomater* 2002, **23**:4307–4314.
2. Peppas NA, Bures P, Leobandung W, Ichikawa H: **Hydrogels in pharmaceutical formulations**. *Eur J Pharm Biopharm* 2000, **50**:27–46.
3. Sawhney AS, Pathak CP, van Rensburg JJ, Dunn RC, Hubbell JA: **Optimization of photopolymerized bioerodible hydrogel properties for adhesion prevention**. *J Biomed Mat Res* 1994, **28**:831–838.
4. Miyata T, Uragami T, Nakamae K: **Biomolecule-sensitive hydrogels**. *Adv Drug Deliv Rev* 2002, **54**:79–98.
5. Chang C, Duan B, Cai J, Zhang L: **Superabsorbent hydrogels based on cellulose for smart swelling and controllable delivery**. *Eur Polym J* 2010, **46**:92–100.
6. Langer R, Peppas NA: **Advances in biomaterials, drug delivery, and biotechnology**. *Bioeng Food & Nat Prod* 2003, **49**:2990–3006.
7. Campoccia D, Doherty P, Radice M, Brun P, Abatangelo G, Williams DF: **Semisynthetic resorbable materials from hyaluronan esterification**. *Biomater* 1998, **19**:2101–2127.
8. Prestwich GD, Marecak DM, Marecak JF, Vercruysse KP, Ziebell MR: **Controlled chemical modification of hyaluronic acid**. *J Cont Rel* 1998, **53**:93–103.
9. Hoffman AS: **Hydrogels for biomedical applications**. *Adv Drug Deliv Rev* 2002, **43**:3–12.
10. Wichterle O, Lim D: **Hydrophilic gels in biologic use**. *Nature* 1960, **185**:117–118.
11. Gibas I, Janik H: **Review: synthetic polymer hydrogels for biomedical applications**. *Chemistry Chemical technol* 2010, **4**:297–304.
12. Liu Y, Vrana NE, Cahill PA, McGuinness GB: **Physically crosslinked composite hydrogels of pva with natural macromolecules: structure, mechanical properties, and endothelial cell compatibility**. *J Biomed Mater Res B Appl Biomater* 2009, **90**:492–502.
13. Wu M, Bao B, Yoshii F, Makuuchi K: **Irradiation of crosslinked, Poly(Vinyl Alcohol) blended hydrogel for wound dressing**. *J Radioanal Nuclear Chem* 2001, **250**:391–395.
14. Yusong P, Dangsheng X, Xiaolin C: **Mechanical properties of nanohydroxyapatite reinforced poly(vinyl alcohol) gel composites as biomaterial**. *J Mater Sci* 2007, **42**:5129–5134.
15. Fenglan X, Yubao L, Jiang WX: **Preparation and characterization of nano-hydroxyl apatite polyvinyl alcohol hydrogel biocomposite**. *J Mater Sci* 2004, **39**:5669–5672.
16. Cascone MG, Lazzeri L, Sparvoli E, Scatena M, Serino LP, Danti S: **Morphological evaluation of bioartificial hydrogels as potential tissue engineering scaffolds**. *J Mater Sci: Mater In Medicine* 2004, **15**:1309–1313.
17. Alemzadeh I, Vossoughi M: **Controlled release of paraquat from poly vinyl alcohol hydrogel**. *Chem Eng Process* 2002, **41**:707–710.
18. Peppas NA, Barr-Howell BD: **Characterization of the crosslinked structures of hydrogels**. In *Hydrogels in medicine and pharmacy, Fundamentals.* Edited by Pappas NA. Boca Raton, Florida: CRC Press; 1986:27–57.
19. Bettini R, Colombo P, Peppas NA: **Solubility effects on drug transport through pH-sensitive, swelling-controlled release systems: transport of theophylline and metoclopramide monohydrochloride**. *J Cont Rel* 1995, **37**:105–111.
20. Chen J, Rong L, Lin H, Xiao R, Wu H: **Radiation synthesis of pH-sensitive hydrogels from β-cyclodextrin-grafted PEG and acrylic acid for drug delivery**. *Mater Chem Phys* 2009, **116**:148–152.

12

A stability indicating HPLC method for the determination of clobazam and its basic degradation product characterization

Effat Souri[1*], Amin Dastjani Farahani[1], Reza Ahmadkhaniha[2] and Mohsen Amini[1]

Abstract

Background: Clobazam is used for the treatment of different types of seizure and epilepsy. The present research is undertaken to study the systematic forced degradation of clobazam and to identify its main degradation product under basic conditions.

Methods: The degradation of clobazam was studied under different conditions. Clobazam and its degradation products were separated using a Nova-Pak C18 column and a mixture of KH_2PO_4 50 mM (pH 8.5) and acetonitrile (50:50, v/v) as the mobile phase with UV detection at 230 nm.

Results: The within-day and between-day precision values in the calibration range of 0.1-20 µg/ml were within 0.5-1.5%. Clobazam was relatively stable in solid from under exposure to visible and UV light and also heat. The clobazam aqueous solution of clobazam was more labile under exposure to visible and UV light. The bulk drug was significantly degraded under exposure to 2 M HCl, 0.1 M NaOH or 3% H_2O_2. Using the tablet powder, higher degradation rates were observed under different stress conditions. The main degradation product of clobazam under basic condition was subsequently characterized.

Conclusion: The developed method could be used for the determination of clobazam in the presence of its degradation products with acceptable precision and accuracy. The applicability of the proposed method was evaluated in commercial dosage forms analysis.

Keywords: Clobazam, HPLC, Stability indicating, Stress degradation

Introduction

Clobazam, 7-chloro-1-methyl-5-phenyl-1, 5-benzodiazepine-2, 4 (3H-dione) (Figure 1), is a benzodiazepine derivative which is used for the treatment of various seizure types and epilepsy [1]. Clobazam belongs to the 1, 5-benzodiazepine class with a pk_a value of 6.65. Clobazam bulk powder is a white crystal with molecular weight of 300.7. The drug is slightly soluble in water and soluble in alcoholic solvents. A number of HPLC methods have been reported before for the determination of clobazam and its metabolite in human plasma [2-6]. Also, HPLC method has been developed for the determination of clobazam in tablet dosage forms [7]. Clobazam is official in British Pharmacopeia (BP) and The United States Pharmacopeia (USP) and an HPLC method is reported for the assay determination of this drug in capsule dosage forms.

Literature survey showed that there is no stability indicating HPLC method for the determination of clobazam in the presence of its degradation products or its degradation behavior under stress conditions. Hence, it is important to develop an accurate, rapid and specific stability indicating analytical method, which is suitable for routine quality control analysis of clobazam in pharmaceutical dosage forms. Stress testing provides important information about the stability of the drug substance under different conditions. Moreover, the suitability of the proposed analysis technique could be verified. In this study, reversed-phase HPLC method is proposed for the determination of clobazam in bulk drug and pharmaceutical dosage forms. The stability tests were performed under

* Correspondence: souri@sina.tums.ac.ir
[1]Department of Medicinal Chemistry, Faculty of Pharmacy and Drug Design and Development Research Center, Tehran University of Medical Sciences, Tehran 14155-6451, Iran
Full list of author information is available at the end of the article

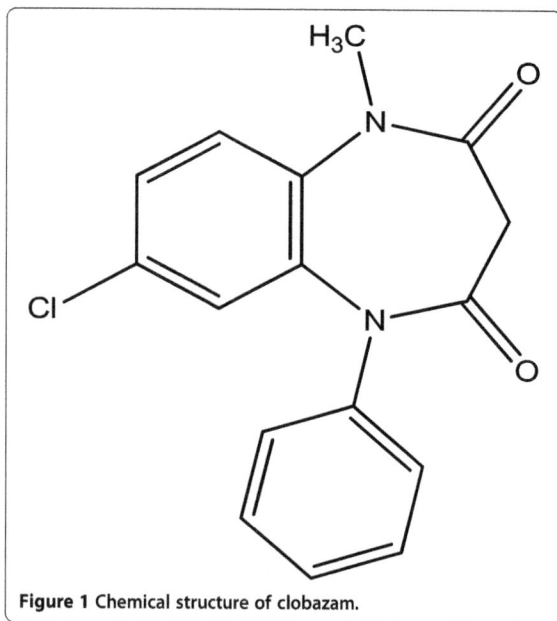

Figure 1 Chemical structure of clobazam.

different conditions according to the International Conference on Harmonization (ICH) guidelines to find out the suitability of the proposed analytical technique in the presence of degradation products.

Methods
Chemicals
The clobazam bulk powder was kindly provided by Hakim Pharmaceutical Company (Tehran, Iran). HPLC grade acetonitrile and analytical grade potassium dihydrogen phosphate were purchased from Merck (Darmstadt, Germany). Clobazam tablets (10 mg) were from Dr Abidi Pharmaceutical Laboratory, Tehran, Iran and obtained from a local pharmacy.

Instrumentation
The analysis was performed by using a chromatographic system from Waters (Milford, USA) consisting of a Model 515 isocratic pump, a Model 710 plus autosampler and a Model 480 UV–vis detector. The data processing system was the version 1.5x of a multi-channel Chrom&Spec software for chromatography. For heat studies, a dry air oven (Melag, Germany) was used. A 100 W Tungsten lamp and a low-pressure Mercury lamp 100 W were used as visible or UV light source, respectively.

The ^{1}H-NMR spectrum was obtained in $CDCl_3$ using a Bruker FT-500 Spectrometer (Bruker, Rheinstetten, Germany). The chemical shifts (δ) relative to tetramethylsilane as internal standard were reported in part per million (ppm). The mass spectrum was achieved on an Agilent 5975C Spectrometer. The IR spectrum was

obtained by using a Nicolet 550-FT Spectrophotometer (Nicolet, Maison, WI, USA).

Peak purity of the samples resulted from stress degradation was checked using an Agilent 1100 HPLC system (Agilent Technologies, USA), equipped with a quaternary pump, an on-line degasser, an auto-sampler, a column oven, and a Photodiode Array (PDA) detector coupled with a ChemStation Software version B.04.01 (Agilent Technologies, USA). For the peak purity analysis, the spectra were corrected for background absorption caused by the mobile phase or matrix compounds, by subtracting the appropriate reference spectra. The spectra were assessed in the range of 225–254 nm and the mode of "best possible match of the entire spectrum" was selected as the mode of normalization.

Chromatographic conditions
A Nova-pak C_{18} column (150 mm × 3.9 mm, 4 μm, Waters, Milford, USA) was used for the chromatographic separation. The mobile phase was composed of 50 mM KH_2PO_4 (pH 8.5) and acetonitrile in the ratio of 50:50 (v/v) and pumped at room temperature, at a flow rate of 1 ml/min. The wavelength of the UV detector was set at 230 nm. The mobile phase was degassed by filtration through a 0.45 μm filter and sonication for 5 min.

Stock standard solutions
A 50 μg/ml stock standard solution of clobazam was prepared in acetonitrile. Calibration solutions of clobazam at 0.1, 0.2, 0.5, 1, 2, 5, 10 and 20 μg/ml were prepared by transferring various aliquots of clobazam solution (50 μg/ml) into a series of 10 ml volumetric flasks and completing the volume to the mark with mobile phase.

Linearity
Six sets of calibration standard solutions of clobazam were prepared in mobile phase in the range of 0.1-20 μg/ml. The solutions were analyzed according to the optimized chromatographic conditions and the peak area was plotted over the clobazam concentration. The statistical data were calculated.

Precision and accuracy
Three different concentrations of clobazam (0.2, 2 and 20 μg/ml) within the calibration range were prepared and analyzed in triplicate during one day and three consecutive days. The coefficient of variation (CV) and error values were determined to find out the precision and accuracy of the analytical method.

Robustness
To find out the robustness of the proposed method, the chromatographic conditions were changed. The influence

of the pH value of the mobile phase and also the percent composition of the mobile phase were studied.

Analysis of tablets

The average weight of twenty finely powdered clobazam tablets (10 mg) was calculated. An amount of powdered tablet equivalent to one tablet was weighed and transferred into a 100 ml volumetric flask. After addition of about 70 ml of water and acetonitrile (50:50, v/v), the mixture was vortex-mixed for 15 min. The solution was diluted to mark with the same solvent and centrifuged at 4000 rpm for 10 min. The solution was subjected to the analysis method after four times dilution and filtration through a 0.45 μm polypropylene syringe filter (Teknokroma, Spain).

Recovery

The standard addition method was used to evaluate the relative recovery of clobazam from dosage forms. Standard concentrations of clobazam were added to a solution resulted from tablet sample and analyzed. The resulted peak area was compared with a standard solution at the same concentration level and the relative recovery was calculated.

Stress degradation

Acid and base induced degradation

Clobazam solutions containing 500 μg/ml in 1 M HCl, 2 M HCl and 0.1 M NaOH were allowed to stand at room temperature or 60°C. For the HPLC analysis, 0.5 ml of the solution was transferred into a 10 ml volumetric flask and the excess of acid or base were neutralized with NaOH or HCl, respectively. After diluting to the mark with the mobile phase, the solution was injected to the HPLC system. The peak area was compared with freshly prepared samples at the same initial concentration value. The same procedure was performed using tablet powder instead of clobazam bulk powder. All experiments were performed in triplicate.

Hydrogen peroxide induced degradation

Clobazam solutions in 3% H_2O_2 (500 μg/ml) prepared from bulk drug or tablet powder were kept at room temperature or 60°C. After twenty times dilution with the mobile phase, the resulted solution was injected to the HPLC system and the peak area compared with a standard solution at the same concentration.

Photolytic degradation

To study the effect of light on drug substance, 100 mg of the bulk powder and also tablet powder were spread in a watch glass and directly exposed to visible or UV-light. The distance between the light source and the samples was 20 cm. For HPLC analysis, 5 mg of the powder was weighed and dissolved in 10 ml mobile phase and injected to the HPLC system after 20 times dilution. Clobazam solutions in water (500 μg/ml) prepared from bulk powder or tablet powder was also exposed to visible or UV-light. The solution was diluted in mobile phase to give a claimed concentration of 25 μg/ml

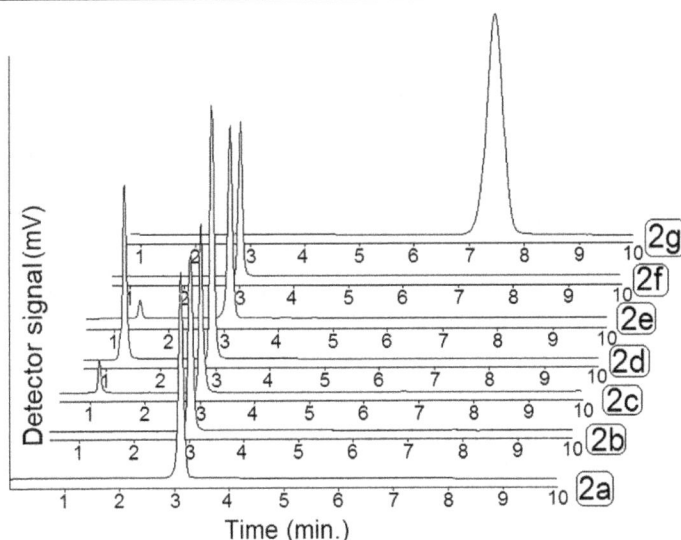

Figure 2 Typical chromatograms obtained from stability studies of clobazam. (a) clobazam standard solution (25 μg/ml); **(b)** clobazam solution in 2 M HCl after 1 h at 60°C; **(c)** clobazam solution in 0.1 M NaOH after 1 h at room temperature; **(d)** clobazam solution in 3% H_2O_2 after 1 h at 60°C; **(e)** clobazam solution in water after 5 days exposure to UV light; **(f)** clobazam dosage form solution in water after 5 days exposure to heat; **(g)** degradation product of clobazam in 0.1 M NaOH.

Table 1 System suitability parameters

Parameters	Found	Acceptable limits
USP theoretical plates (n = 6)	4100	N > 1500
USP tailing factor (n = 6)	1.2	T < 1.5
Repeatability (t$_R$) (n = 6)	0.48	RSD < 1%
Repeatability (peak area) (n = 6)	0.87	RSD < 1%

t_R: Retention time (min); N: Theoretical plate; T: Tailing factor; RSD: Relative Standard Deviation.

and 20 µl was injected for HPLC analysis. The percentage of the remained clobazam was calculated using a freshly prepared standard solution at the same concentration.

Heat degradation

To find out the thermal stability, clobazam bulk powder and tablet powder were incubated in a dry oven at 80°C for 5 days. Also, aqueous solutions of clobazam bulk powder and tablet powder were incubated in a dry oven at 80°C for 5 days. Solution prepared from these samples were injected to the HPLC system and compared with a standard solution to calculate the percent of degradation.

Isolation of the basic degradation product of clobazam

The degradation product formed in 0.1 M NaOH after 5 h at 60°C was a white crystal. The crystals were separated and dried in a vacuum desiccator. The purity of this product was proved by injecting a sample solution to the HPLC system. The retention time of the product was about 7.5 min. The structure of this product was elucidated by using its ^{1}H-NMR, mass and IR spectra.

Results and discussion

Chromatographic conditions

By using a Nova-Pak C18 column and a mobile phase consisting of 50 mM KH_2PO_4 (pH 8.5) and acetonitrile (50:50, v/v), the clobazam and its degradation products were well resolved. The representative chromatograms (Figure 2) showed no peak interfering from excipients or degradation products with analyte. Analysis of the samples after stress degradation studies showed that the HPLC method is stability indicating.

Table 2 Statistical data of calibration curves of clobazam (n = 6)

Parameters	Results
Linearity range	0.1-20 µg/ml
Regression equation	y = 183.39 x + 22.22
Standard deviation of slope	0.89
Relative standard deviation of slope (%)	0.49
Standard deviation of intercept	2.75
Correlation coefficient (r^2)	0.9997
Limit of quantification (LOQ)	0.15 µg/ml
Limit of detection (LOD)	0.05 µg/ml

Table 3 Precision and accuracy of the method for determination of clobazam (3 sets for 3 days)

Concentration added (µg/ml)	Concentration found (µg/ml)	CV (%)	Error (%)
Within day (n = 3)			
0.200	0.199 ± 0.003	1.52	−0.50
2.000	1.977 ± 0.020	1.01	−1.15
20.000	19.967 ± 0.153	0.77	−0.17
Between day (n = 9)			
0.200	0.200 ± 0.003	1.51	0.00
2.000	1.980 ± 0.021	1.04	−1.00
20.000	19.940 ± 0.092	0.46	−0.30

The system suitability parameters (peak symmetry and repeatability) were evaluated by six replicates injecting of a clobazam solution (25 µg/ml) in mobile phase. The results shown in Table 1 are within the acceptable range.

Linearity

Calibration plots over the clobazam concentration range of 0.1-20 µg/ml showed acceptable correlation coefficients. The statistical data of the repeated calibration curves are shown in Table 2. The limit of quantification (LOQ) and limit of determination (LOD) were calculated according to the following equations [8] and are presented in Table 2.

$$LOQ = 10\sigma/s \text{ and } LOD = 3.3\sigma/s$$

where σ is the standard deviation of intercept and s is the slope of the calibration graph.

Stability

The clobazam solutions showed acceptable stability (>99%) relative to freshly prepared standard solutions after 7 days in refrigerator.

Table 4 The influence of small changes in mobile phase composition (method robustness)

Mobile phase composition	Retention time (min)	Peak area
KH_2PO_4 50 mM (pH 8.8)-Acetonitrile (50:50)	3.12	8063
KH_2PO_4 50 mM (pH 8.8)-Acetonitrile (52:48)	3.82	8078
KH_2PO_4 50 mM (pH 8.8)-Acetonitrile (48:52)	3.06	8178
KH_2PO_4 50 mM (pH 8.5)-Acetonitrile (50:50)	3.40	8117
KH_2PO_4 50 mM (pH 8.5)-Acetonitrile (52:48)	3.92	8087
KH_2PO_4 50 mM (pH 8.5)-Acetonitrile (48:52)	3.13	8147
KH_2PO_4 50 mM (pH 8.2)-Acetonitrile (50:50)	3.14	8205
KH_2PO_4 50 mM (pH 8.2)-Acetonitrile (52:48)	3.59	8180
KH_2PO_4 50 mM (pH 8.2)-Acetonitrile (60:52)	3.12	8107

Table 5 The results of the stress degradation tests on clobazam bulk powder using different conditions

Stress test condition	Solvent	Temperature	Time	% of clobazam	Peak homogeneity
Acidic	1 M HCl	Room temperature	1 h	85.2	Pass
	2 M HCl	Room temperature	2 days	57.8	
	2 M HCl	60°C	1 h	71.4	
Basic	0.1 M NaOH	Room temperature	1 h	64.8	Pass
	0.1 M NaOH	Room temperature	48 h	1.2	
	0.1 M NaOH	60°C	1 h	13.8	
Oxidative	3% H₂O₂	Room temperature	48 h	75.3	Pass
	3% H₂O₂	60°C	1 h	91.4	
Photolytic					
UV light	Solid form	Room temperature	5 days	98.1	Pass
UV light	Water	Room temperature	5 days	65.0	
Visible light	Solid form	Room temperature	5 days	99.8	Pass
Visible light	Water	Room temperature	5 days	95.2	
Heat	Solid form	80°C	5 days	99.9	Pass
	Water	80°C	5 days	99.8	

Precision and accuracy

To find out the repeatability of the developed method, triplicate analysis of clobazam solutions at three different concentration levels were performed (in one day and three consecutive days). The calculated CV (%) and errors (%) values are presented in Table 3 which indicates high precision and accuracy of the method.

Small variations in the pH value of the phosphate buffer and also composition of the mobile phase did not show significant effect on the peak area or peak shape (Table 4) which showed the robustness of the proposed method.

Recovery

Recovery was evaluated by the determination of the analyte in solutions prepared by the standard addition technique. The mean percentage recovery of 98.3 ± 0.5% was achieved.

Degradation studies

Acid and base induced degradation

Under acidic conditions, degradation was dependent to the strength of hydrochloric acid and also exposure time (Table 5). No new peak was observed in the chromatogram after degradation (Figure 2b). The rate of degradation of clobazam tablet powder was comparatively higher than clobazam bulk powder under the same conditions (Table 6).

In the presence of 0.1 M NaOH solution, a very fast degradation was observed. The degradation was about 35% and 99% after 1 h or 48 h at room temperature (Table 5). The degradation of tablet powder was more under the same conditions (Table 6). Under basic conditions, the formation of a small peak at the retention time of 1.2 min was evident (Figure 2c). Also a white crystal was produced which was increased by increasing the

Table 6 The results of the stress degradation tests on clobazam tablet powder using different conditions

Stress test condition	Solvent	Temperature	Time	% of clobazam	Peak homogeneity
Acidic	2 M HCl	60°C	1 h	74.4	Pass
Basic	0.1 M NaOH	Room temperature	1 h	42.3	Pass
Oxidative	3% H₂O₂	60°C	1 h	87.3	Pass
Photolytic					
UV light	Solid form	Room temperature	5 days	87.1	Pass
UV light	Water	Room temperature	5 days	24.9	
Visible light	Solid form	Room temperature	5 days	99.5	Pass
Visible light	Water	Room temperature	5 days	70.0	
Heat	Solid form	80°C	5 days	51.2	Pass
	Water	80°C	5 days	55.1	

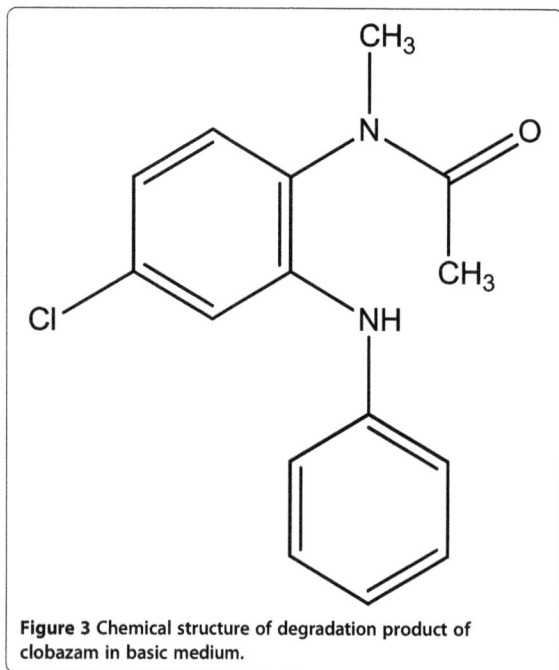

Figure 3 Chemical structure of degradation product of clobazam in basic medium.

exposure time. After 48 h exposure time at room temperature, the complete degradation of clobazam to this product was observed.

Hydrogen peroxide induced degradation
Significant degradation of clobazam bulk powder and also tablet powder was observed after exposure of clobazam to hydrogen peroxide at room temperature or 60°C (Tables 5 and 6). The hydrogen peroxide peak was observed at the retention time of about 1.2 without any other peak related to degradation products of clobazam (Figure 2d).

Photolytic degradation
Clobazam bulk powder was relatively stable in solid state after exposure to visible or UV-light. On the other hand,

the aqueous solution of clobazam bulk powder showed significant degradation of about 5% and 35% (Table 5). Clobazam tablet powder showed about 13% degradation after 5 days exposure to UV light (Table 6 and Figure 2e)). Higher degradation rates were observed for the aqueous solution of tablet powder under visible light (30%) or UV light (75%) after 5 Days (Table 6).

Heat degradation
Clobazam bulk powder was relatively stable under heat after 5 days (Table 5). On the other hand, the clobazam tablet powder and its aqueous solution were significantly labile under heat and about 49% and 45% of degradation was observed after 5 days exposure to 80°C (Table 6 and Figure 2f).

Peak purity studies
The peak purity of the samples resulted from stress degradation was checked by using a photo diode array detector. Peak purity results derived from the PDA detector confirmed that the clobazam peak was homogeneous and pure and there is no interfering peak from the diluents or degradation products. These results confirmed the stability indicating capability of the proposed method for determination of clobazam in the presence of its degradation products.

Characterization of the basic degradation product
According to the experimental method, the degradation product in basic conditions was isolated. The isolated compound was pure and showed a single peak at the retention time of 7.5 (Figure 2g). On the basis of the ^{1}H-NMR, mass and IR spectral data, the chemical structure of this product was assigned as N-[4-chloro-2-(phenyl amino) phenyl]-N-methylacetamide (Figure 3), impurity E, which has been reported in the European Pharmacopeia. The spectral data are as followed:
^{1}H-NMR (CDCl$_3$): δ (ppm); 1.93 (s, 3H, CH$_3$-CO), 3.23 (s, 3H, NCH$_3$), 6.84 (dd, J = 8.1 Hz and J = 2.0 Hz,

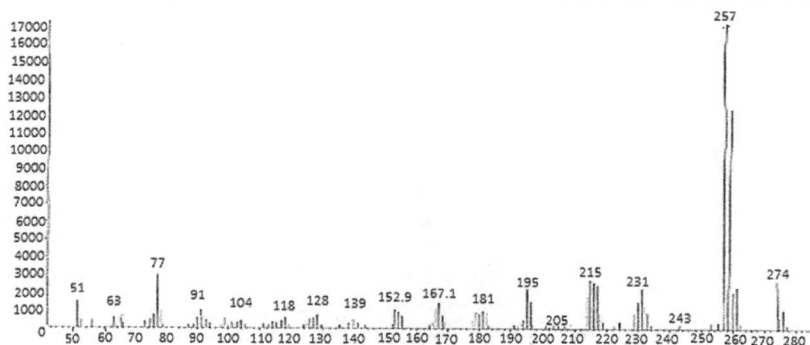

Figure 4 Mass spectrum of degradation product of clobazam in basic medium.

2H), 7.03 (d, J = 8.1 Hz, 1H), 7.10-7.17 (m, 3H), 7.25 (d, J = 2.0 Hz, 1H), 7.34-7.41 (m, 2H).

Mass: m/z (%) 276 (7), 274 (21), 259 (33), 257 (100), 231 (15), 215 (18), 195 (13), 181 (7), 167 (8), 153 (7), 91 (7) (Figure 4).

IR (KBr): v cm^{-1} 3267 (NH), 1644 (CO).

Analysis of tablet dosage form

The active ingredient in clobazam tablets (10 mg) was determined using the developed method. Good agreement with the label claimed amount (10.29 ± 0.11 mg per tablet) was observed with no interference from excipeients.

Conclusion

In this study clobazam was exposed to different stress conditions recommended in ICH guidelines. In the developed HPLC method, clobazam and its degradation products were resolved in a single isocratic run. Clobazam showed significant degradation under basic, acidic or oxidative conditions. The bulk drug remained unaffected under heat, UV light or visible light in the solid form, while significant degradation in these conditions was observed in aqueous solutions. The tablet powder was more labile under studied degradation conditions. The main degradation product under 0.1 M NaOH was separated and its chemical structure was elucidated. The proposed analytical method was relatively simple and accurate and could be used for the determination of clobazam in pharmaceutical dosage forms in the presence of its degradation products.

Competing interests
The authors declare that there is no competing interests.

Authors' contribution
ES has supervised the project and prepared the article. ADE has done the experimental part of the project. RA has performed the peak purity tests and obtained the mass spectrum. MA has performed the characterization of the degradation product. All authors read and approved the final manuscript.

Author details
[1]Department of Medicinal Chemistry, Faculty of Pharmacy and Drug Design and Development Research Center, Tehran University of Medical Sciences, Tehran 14155-6451, Iran. [2]Department of Human Ecology, School of Public Health, Tehran University of Medical Sciences, Tehran 1417614411, Iran.

References
1. Remy C: Clobazam in the treatment of epilepsy: a review of the literature. *Epilepsia* 1994, **35**:88–91.
2. Knapp J, Boknik P, Gumbinger HG, Linck B, Luss H, Muller FU, Schmitz W, Vahlensieck U, Neumann J: Quantitation of clobazam in human plasma using high-performance liquid chromatography. *J Chromatogr Sci* 1999, **37**:145–149.
3. Kunicki PK: Simple and sensitive high-performance liquid chromatographic method for the determination of 1, 5-benzodiazepine clobazam and its active metabolite N-desmethylclobazam in human serum and urine with application to 1, 4-benzodiazepine analysis. *J Chromatogr B* 2001, **750**:41–49.
4. Bolner A, Tagliaro F, Lomeo A: Optimized determination of clobazam in human plasma with extraction and high-performance liquid chromatography analysis. *J Chromatogr B* 2001, **750**:177–180.
5. Pistos C, Stewart JT: Direct injection HPLC method for the determination of selected benzodiazepines in plasma using a Hisep column. *J Pharm Biomed Anal* 2003, **33**:1135–1142.
6. Rouini M, Ardakani YH, Hakemi L, Mokhberi M, Badri G: Simultaneous determination of clobazam and its major metabolite in human plasma by a rapid HPLC method. *J Chromatogr B* 2005, **823**:167–171.
7. Gopalakrishnan S, Jeyashree B, Backialakshmi S, Chenthilnathan A: A new validated RP-HPLC method for the estimation of clobazam in tablet dosage form. *Asian J Res Chem* 2011, **4**(6):882–886.
8. Shabir GA: Validation of high-performance liquid chromatography methods for pharmaceutical analysis. Understanding the differences and similarities between validation requirements of the US food and drug administration, the US Pharmacopeia and the International Conference on Harmonization. *J Chromatogr A* 2003, **987**:57–66.

13

A system dynamics model for national drug policy

Akbar Abdollahiasl[1*], Abbas Kebriaeezadeh[1,2*], Rassoul Dinarvand[3], Mohammad Abdollahi[2], Abdol Majid Cheraghali[4,5], Mona Jaberidoost[1] and Shekoufeh Nikfar[1]

Abstract

Background: Data modeling techniques can create a virtual world to analyze decision systems. National drug authorities can use such techniques to take care of their deficiencies in decision making processes. This study was designed to build a system dynamics model to simulate the effects of market mix variables (5 P's) on the national drug policy (NDP) indicators including availability, affordability, quality, and rationality. This was aimed to investigate how to increase the rationality of decision making, evaluate different alternatives, reduce the costs and identify the system obstacles. System dynamics is a computer-based approach for analyzing and designing complex systems over time. In this study the cognitive casualty map was developed to make a concept about the system then the stock-flow model was set up based on the market demand and supply concept.

Results: The model demonstrates the interdependencies between the NDP variables through four cognitive maps. Some issues in availability, willingness to pay, rational use and quality of medicines are pointed in the model. The stock-flow diagram shows how the demand for a medicine is formed and how it is responded through NDP objectives. The effects of changing variables on the other NDP variables can be studied after running the stock-flow model.

Conclusion: The model can initiate a fundamental structure for analyzing NDP. The conceptual model made a cognitive map to show many causes' and effects' trees and reveals some relations between NDP variables that are usually forgotten in the medicines affairs. The model also provides an opportunity to be expanded with more details on a specific disease for better policy making about medication.

Keywords: National drug policy, System dynamics, Modeling

Background

Everyone has the inevitable right to achieve the high standard health services, thus this is the duty of health policy makers to promote national drug policies (NDP) in line with national health objectives [1,2]. The NDP objectives are defined as making essential quality medicines available in affordable price for rational use. The NDP as a framework of integrated activities is influenced by various factors especially those arisen from inside the government and the decision making systems. The market-mix variables including product, price, promotion, place and people are also added to other complexities and issues that should be taken into account by national drug authorities (NDAs) [3].

The NDP key indicators should be compatible with health system objectives in terms of effectiveness, financial fairness and responsiveness. Monitoring the processes and their results is so essential, however lack of the live key indicators make it difficult to have a clear picture of the consequences of decisions made by NDAs [4,5].

The NDA and different parties in the ministry of health (MOH) have problems in making unified decisions that would result in amelioration or deterioration of NDP indicators. Surely, the drug systems and decision makers have limited resources and technologies to predict and evaluate the consequences of their decisions. Exploring the previous studies shows a retrospective nature of appraising evidences and key performance indicators that influence the decision making processes in the health systems [6]. In fact the consequences of some NDAs' decisions are appeared when it cannot be compensated. To overcome such a deficit in decision making, the role of simulation systems for solving the problems is reasonable [7,8].

* Correspondence: abdollahiasl@gmail.com; kebriaee@sina.tums.ac.ir
[1]Department of Pharmacoeconomics and Pharmaceutical administration, Pharmaceutical policy research center and Faculty of Pharmacy, Tehran University of Medical Sciences (TUMS), Tehran, Iran
[2]Department of Toxicology and Pharmacology, Faculty of Pharmacy and Pharmaceutical Sciences Research Center, TUMS, Tehran, Iran
Full list of author information is available at the end of the article

The NDP is a complex system involving many variables; therefore, a system thinking approach is needed to analyze the roles of influencing factors [9]. To enhance the system efficiency and integrating activities, analysis of processes and evaluation the negative/positive effects of key variables must be addressed.

Qualitative and quantitative improvement in health system necessitates NDAs to provide higher quality services but considering government downsizing and budget constraints, there is no opportunity to increase human and capital resources. Therefore, simulation-based systems can facilitate and accelerate the decision process in order to help policy makers.

System dynamic (SD) is a modeling concept that supports decision systems by breaking them into simpler and smaller subsystems. It helps:

- Shortening the decision process
- Increasing the rationality of actions
- Evaluating the different alternatives
- Reducing the costs
- Decreasing the human-derived mistakes
- Increasing reliability and validity
- Providing potentials for sensitivity analysis and repeatability.

SD founded by Jay Forrester is used to analyze the performance of complex systems [10]. It is typically used for models that represent relationships between system variables, rates of change over time and unequivocal feedbacks [11].

A rational relationship between the functions of the NDP core components and market-mixed variables as the main variables of decision making would enhance the outcomes and effectiveness of decisions. To use SD method, it is essential to add some other constant variables and relations to the model.

Although modeling technique is not a new approach in policy making, it is new in pharmaceutical affairs [12,13]. Nowadays there is no such systematic decision module in Iran while NDAs need such a tool to take care of deficiencies in decision making process. There are some negative and positive variables which affect the NDP. Therefore, building a systemic model can identify, analyze and monitor the negative/positive effects of influential factors and at the end reduces the negative effects and improves positive effects which causes the NDP to promote.

Taking the case of Iran pharmaceutical sector into account, we designed this study to analyze the effects of market mix on the NDP indicators. This study was aimed to investigate the NDP components, helps to rationalize activities and decision making, evaluates different alternatives and increases the cost-effectiveness of interventions.

Method

In fact SD models are crucial and effective tools for focusing on stock variables and the flows between them. Therefore, it seems using SD as a well-adjusted modeling technique is authentic to respond to the requirements of this study [14,15].

The model should dynamically and quantitatively simulate the core components of NDP (availability, affordability, quality and rational use). Furthermore, it should reflect the interactions between the components and the market-mix variables (price, product, place, people, and promotion). The model should also address the key influencing factors for improvement of health policies.

The NDP is composed of four subsystems: availability, affordability, quality, and rationality. The related variables were listed (Table 1) and the model was developed in a deductive basis in three phases:

- Conceptualization: in this phase, the purpose of the model, the main structure, the boundaries of system and subsystems were developed and the results were demonstrated through a casual network or a cognitive map [16-19]. In addition to the articles and documents, an expert panel (including three decision maker in IR FDA, one expert of SD and two pharmacoeconomists) formed to justify the model.
- Stock-flow modeling: the variables are categorized to level, auxiliary and constant. Then the adjusted model and mathematical equations between the variable were developed. For running the model Vensim PLE software were used. This software makes an opportunity to develop and run system dynamics models in educational or proffessional level [10,20].
- Testing and sensitivity analysis; the model was verified and validated to increase the realty of the simulation. There are some testing methods in SD that would explain in result part [21-23].

Results

Study area

The NDA in Iran -under supervision of MOH- oversees and regulates the provision and utilization of medicines through pharmaceutical division of Food and Drug Administration (IR FDA). The demand of medicines is mainly responded through registered products that are supplied by the public and private manufacturers and importers. IR FDA follows the generic approach and tries to protect domestically produced generic medicines in the market. Two-third of the Iran's 3.5 billion USD market has been supplied by local manufacturers. A half of manufacturers are presented in the stock market and their main stocks holders are the Social Security Investment Company, Melli Bank Investing Company and Alborz

Table 1 The list of variables those used in the models' subsystems (A: Auxiliary, C: Constant variable)

	Variable	Description	Availability	Affordability	Quality	Rationality
1	Affordability	Affordability	C	A		
2	Availability of domestic products	Availability of domestic products	A	C		
3	Availability of imported products	Availability of imported products	A	C		C
4	Brand Strength Dom.	Brand Strength domestic products				A
5	Brand Strength Imp.	Brand Strength imported products				A
6	Community promotion	Community promotion				A
7	Competition Dom.	Competition domestic products	A		A	
8	Consumption Dom	Consumption domestic products	A	A		
9	Consumption Imp.	Consumption imported products	A	A		
10	Cost of production	Cost of production			A	
11	Demand Dom.	Demand domestic products	A		A	
12	Demand dom/imp	Share of domestic products' demand	A		A	
13	Demand Imp	Demand imported products	A		A	
14	Diagnosis accouracy	Diagnosis accouracy				A
15	Distributors stock dom.	Distributors stock domestic products	A			
16	Distributors stock Imp	Distributors stock imported products	A			
17	Drug costs Dom.	Average costs of domestic products	A	A		
18	Drug costs Imp.	Average costs of imported products	A	A		
19	Drug Price Dom.	Average price domestic products	C	C	A	A
20	Drug price Imp.	Average price imported products	C	C	A	A
21	Efficacy	Efficacy				A
22	GDP/Capita	GDP per Capita			C	
23	Global density of pharmacies	Average density of pharmacies in the country	A			
24	Good dispensing practice	Good dispensing practice				C
25	Good lableing	Good lableing				C
26	HouseHold costs	HouseHold costs			C	
27	Import	Volume of imported products	A			
28	Importers	Number of importers	A			
29	Income	Gross national income per capita			C	
30	Induced demand	Induced demand	A			A
31	Informed consumer	Informed consumer				A
32	Intractions	Medicinal intractions				A
33	Market saturation	Market saturation	C			
34	No. distributors	Number of distributors	A			
35	No. Known Patients	Number of known patients				A
36	No. pharmacies	Number of pharmacies	A			
37	No. pharmacists	Number of pharmacists	A			
38	No. physicians	Number of physicians				C
39	No. producers	Number of producers	A			
40	OoP/Household cost	OoP/Household cost			A	
41	OoP/Income	OoP/Income			A	
42	OoP/GDP	OoP/GDP			A	
43	Out of pocket	Out of pocket	A	A		
44	Packaging quality	Packaging quality			A	

Table 1 The list of variables those used in the models' subsystems (A: Auxiliary, C: Constant variable) *(Continued)*

#	Variable	Description				
45	Patients purchase domestic	Patients purchase domestic products	A	A		
46	Patients purchase Imp.	Patients purchase imported products	A	A		
47	Pharmacies purchase dom.	Pharmacies purchase domestic products	A			
48	Pharmacies purchase Imp	Pharmacies purchase imported products	A			
49	Pharmacies stock domestic	Pharmacies stock domestic products	A			
50	Pharmacies stock Imp	Pharmacies stock imported products	A			
51	Physicians' K.A.P.	Physicians' Knoledge/Attitude/practice about rationality				A
52	Polypharmacy	Polypharmacy				A
53	Population	Population	C			
54	Prescriber acceptance	Prescriber acceptance				A
55	Prescription	Prescription				A
56	Prescription with injectables	Prescription with injections				A
57	Prescriptions with Ab	Prescriptions with antibiotic				A
58	Producer profit	Producer profit			A	
59	Producers' stock	Producers' stock	A			
60	Production	Production	A	A		
61	Promotion Dom.	Promotion on domestic products	A	A		A
62	Promotion Imp.	Promotion on imported products	A	A		A
63	Quality budget Dom.	Budget for quality improvement of domestic products			A	
64	Quality budget Imp.	Budget for quality improvement of imported products			A	
65	Quality Dom.	Quality index of domestic products	C		A	C
66	Quality Imp.	Quality index of imported products	C		A	C
67	R&D budget	R&D budget			A	
68	Rational prescribing	Rational prescribing				A
69	Rational use	Rational use				A
70	Rationality	Rationality	A			A
71	Real demand	Real demand				A
72	Regional density of medical centers	Regional density of medical centers	A			
73	Regional density of pharmacies	Regional density of pharmacies	A			
74	Regulatory power	Regualatory power			C	
75	RX as OTC	dispensing RX products without prescription				A
76	Safety stock	Safety stock	C			
77	Sales costs	Sales costs			A	
78	Sales value Dom.	Sales value of domestic products	A		A	A
79	Sales value Imp.	Sales value Imported of products	A		A	A
80	Saving/OOP	Saving/OOP		A		
81	Self-treatment	Self-treatment				A
82	Side effects	Side effects				A
83	Social information	Social information				A
84	Stock imported	Stock of imported products	A			
85	Total demand	Total demand	A	A		A
86	Treatment	Treatment		A	A	A
87	User stock Dom.	Stock of domestic products in homes	A			
88	User stock Imp.	Stock of imported products in homes	A			
89	Waste & Exp. Dom.	Waste & expired domestic products	A			

Table 1 The list of variables those used in the models' subsystems (A: Auxiliary, C: Constant variable) *(Continued)*

90	Waste & Exp. Imp.	Waste & expired imported products	A		
91	Willing to use	Willing to use			A
92	WTP	Willingness to pay	A	A	

Investing Company; the other half of manufacturing companies and the most importers are owned by private sectors. There are tens of distributors that distribute medicines around the country but the top five covers about 80 percent of the market. The price of all medicines is set by the government through the commission of pricing in IR FDA. The official method of pricing is cost-plus for generic medicines and external reference pricing for branded products; although some country-specific factors such as market size, anti-inflation policies, national economics and some political issues are determinants. Clinical services are provided by both public and private sectors but patients pay the same price for medicines in both sectors. The majority of the people are covered for their treatment costs by three main basic health insurers; they cover about 45 percent of health costs. The medication costs for certain illness including AIDS, TB, Malaria, Hemophilia, Thalasemia, transplantation and vaccination are covered totally by the MOH [24]. The survey on access to medicines found that most general medicines are available and affordable for all - the lowest paid workers as indicator- in both public and private sectors [25,26].

Logical framework of the model

Our suggested SD conceptual model is composed of two subsystems: NDP objectives and market mix variables. NDP is aimed to improve quality of human life mainly by equitable providing affordable quality drugs for patients who rationally need them. Market mix (5 P's) are components of a market that are aimed by marketing strategies. The interaction between NDP objectives and market mix components shaped the framework of the model.

Health system is too wide and complicated to be modeled completely in a detailed study; the framework of the model determines how deep the model is supposed to study interactions between NDP and market mix. For exploring the interactions among the variables a SD model is proposed which mainly was structured on the demand of medicines.

Firstly, a summarized cognitive map of causal loops was described (Figure 1). As mentioned before, the NDP objectives play an important role in helping the policy makers to determine the demand of patients' medicines. Therefore, the twelve main variables -Affordability, Availability, Consumption, Demand, Distribution-Points, Price, Product Supply, Promotion, Quality, Rationality, Treatment, Willingness to pay (WTP)- formed an overview on the system through the sixteen causal loops. But it was

totally obvious that many other variables should be defined to justify the model. All relations in primary structure expanded to a network of variables; to justify the subsystems some other constant or auxiliary variables were added to the model (Figure 2). The expanded model is a casual network that shows the relationships between all variables in NDP. This vast model is for demonstrating the complexity of the system and is essential to break it to smaller parts for detailed analysis.

In Iran, there are two different governmental approaches against imported medicines and domestically produced ones, therefore it was tried to consider these two approaches in studying the main NDP variables. The nature of the model leads to study it in two parts; the conceptual cognitive map was explored in part 1 and quantifying the variables and running their relationships are explained in part 2 in a stock-flow model.

Part 1–1: Availability

According to the logical framework of NDP, the causal diagram of the availability was designed based on two approaches; domestically produced products and imported ones (Figure 3). Availability has been defined as having the essential stock of the product in determined distribution points [1]. Then the number of pharmacies who distribute the product, the distance between them and the level of

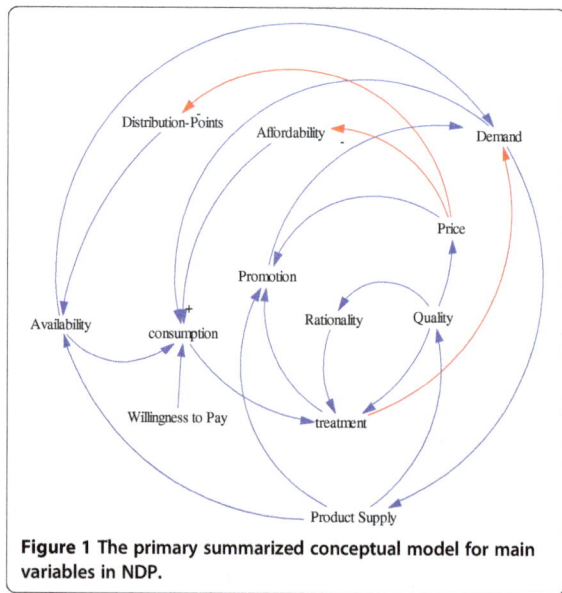

Figure 1 The primary summarized conceptual model for main variables in NDP.

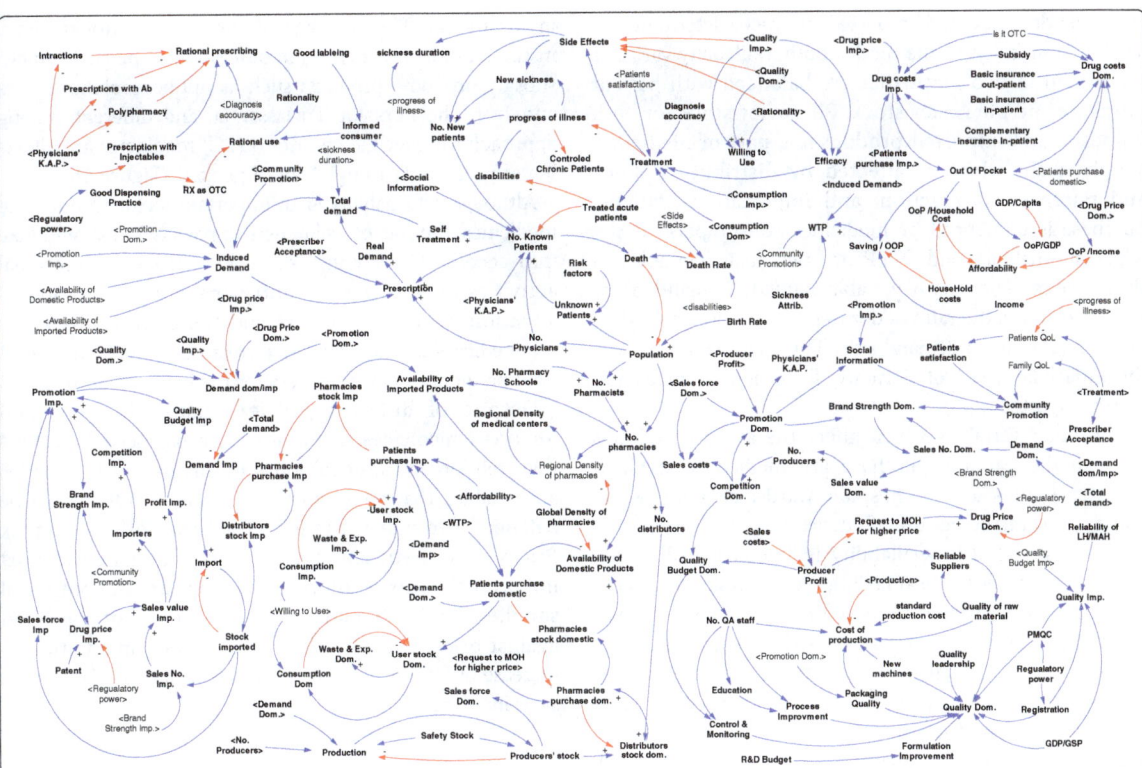

Figure 2 The expanded conceptual model for NDP.

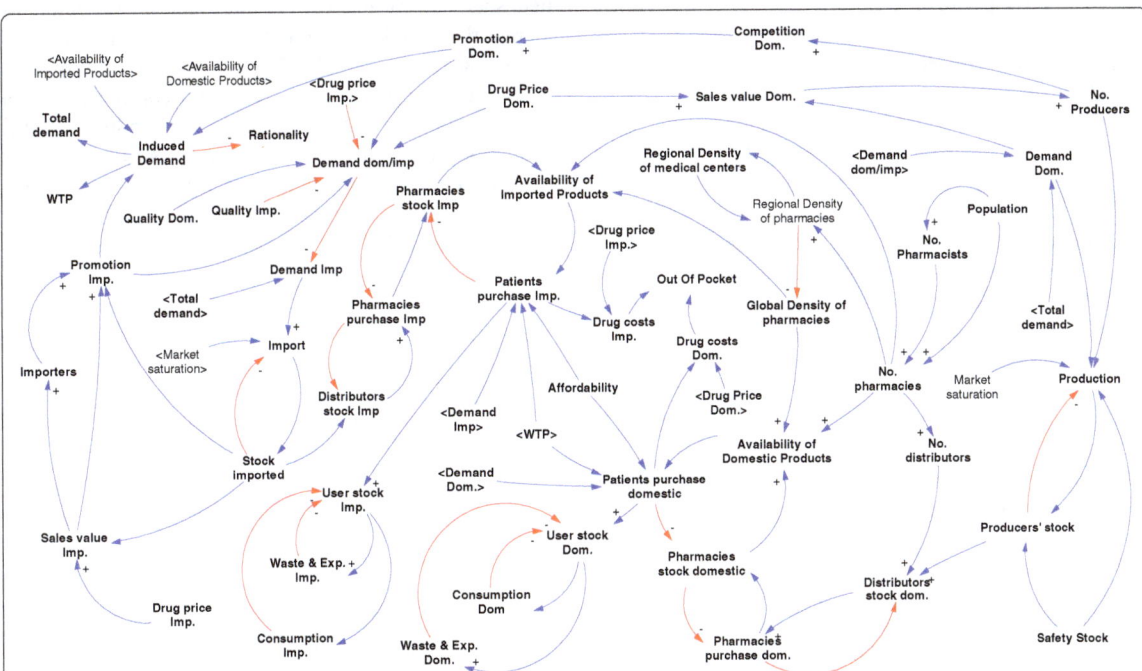

Figure 3 The conceptual model for availability.

stock for domestic and imported products determine the level of availability. In the model, both availability variables are placed in two loops that are balanced with patient purchase and pharmacy stock. Pharmacy stock for both domestic and imported product is a part of medicines supply chain which is affected by distributors' stock and purchase, production, and importation. Patients purchase is influenced by medicines consumption cycles while affordability and WTP are two main variables in these cycles. There is a variable named "demand dom/imp" that shows the ratio of domestically produced product in the market from demand side. This item would balance the availability level of domestically produced medicines versus imported ones.

The other variables which affect the availability loops through the patients purchase are medicines' stock in patient's homes and in hospital wards; also the waste and expired medicines are effective.

The other issue in availability is "medical malls" that are places that all medical facilities and physicians' offices have been concentrated in; based on the current regulations, the number of pharmacies as the dispensing places of medicines is a function of population, distance to other pharmacies and density of medical centers. Medical malls are ideal locations for founding pharmacies but they are against the physical availability of medicines. The IR FDA as the authorized organization for regulating pharmacies allows increasing the number of pharmacies in these regions regardless to the distance to promote the fair income of pharmacies. It makes a reinforced loop to gather more medical firms in such areas and decrease the uniform distribution of pharmacies around the cities; then the level of availability declines.

Availability is not only an essential factor for access to medicines but it can induce the demand in the market. High level of stock which is in favor of availability would increase the financial costs of suppliers then they increase their sales forces whenever they are overstocked; this is one of the causes of the induced demand. Although in the market the data of demand direct the supply, the role of potential market could not be ignored. Potential market that we showed it in the model as "market saturation ratio" is the extra stock of a medicine that should be supplied in addition to real demand for market confidence. "Market saturation" variable that directly related to the safety stock of a medicine in the country, is affecting significantly on other main variable in the model.

Part 1-2: affordability

Affordability as having enough money to pay for the medicines has involved many contributors in health system. Out of pocket (OOP) /household costs, OOP/income and OOP/gross domestic products (GDP) per capita are three indicators used to show the affordability of medicines

in the model. The coverage of basic and complementary insurances for in-patients and out-patients, the government subsidy on some products such as antihemophilic factors and Iron chelators for Thalassemia, and different pricing approach for over the counter (OTC) medicines are affecting affordability through "out of pocket" (Figure 4).

Although affordability is an important factor to purchase medicines, the role of willingness to pay (WTP) should take into account. Family and social knowledge, promotional activities by suppliers, country and family economical situation, severity of illness and the opportunity costs for medication (the alternative treatments that may exist) tend patients to pay more/less for medicines (Figure 5).

Despite of different policies against domestic and imported medicines, there are more balanced (negative) than reinforced (positive) loops in this part of the model; all variables that could increase patients' OOP, would be balanced through reduction of affordability (Figure 6). Prices of domestic and imported drugs that are the most important inputs of affordability loops are the output of suppliers' requests and negotiation power of the NDA against price increase. The price variables in addition to increase of OOP, can be input of the quality system through sales increase.

Part 1-3: quality

The quality of medicines not only initiates their safety, efficacy, WTP and patient acceptance but also affects on their share in the market. A wide range of variables influence the quality of domestically produced medicines but a few factors could affect the quality of imported ones (Figure 7). Because NDA has no complete control on the quality of imported medicines in production level in the country of origin, completing registration process and enforcing post marketing quality controls are two main tools for assuring the quality.

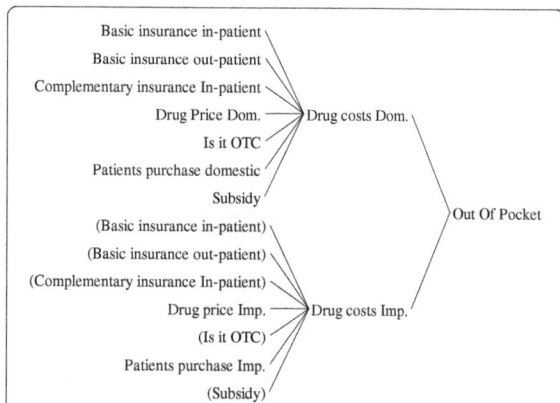

Figure 4 The causes tree for "out of pocket".

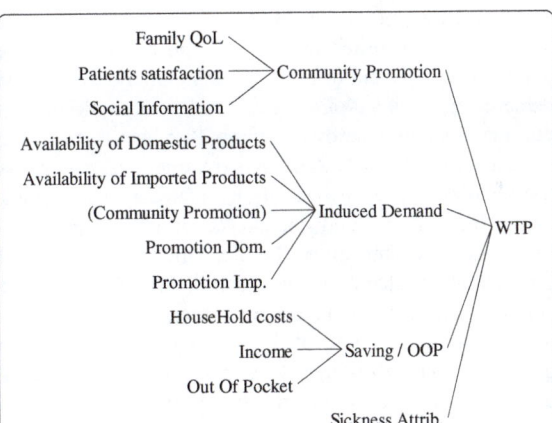

Figure 5 The causes tree for "willingness to pay".

The quality of domestic products placed in two feedback loops: the main balanced loop comes from the cost of quality which increases the cost of production and leads to decrease the quality budget due to the profit reduction. The second loop is a reinforced one coming from the

increase of demand, sales and market share due to the quality. For imported medicines, there is an only reinforced loop coming from investing on the post manufacturing quality controls and quality promotion (Figure 8).

The role of NDA is crucial in improving quality; NDA can promote the concept of quality management in local pharmaceutical companies, create the opportunity for investing on the quality with rationalizing the prices, regulating and auditing good manufacturing/distributing/storage/laboratory practices in drug supply chain, empowering registration process and post marketing quality control practices.

Part 1–4: rational use

Rational drug use as an important pillar of NDP could clinically, socially, and economically help the health system. In this model rational prescribing, good dispensing practice and giving information to patients are the main determinants of rationality. All promotional and advertising activities not only affect on the public health but also change the demand and subsequently modify activities of supply chains. Sales and promotion reinforce each other in two

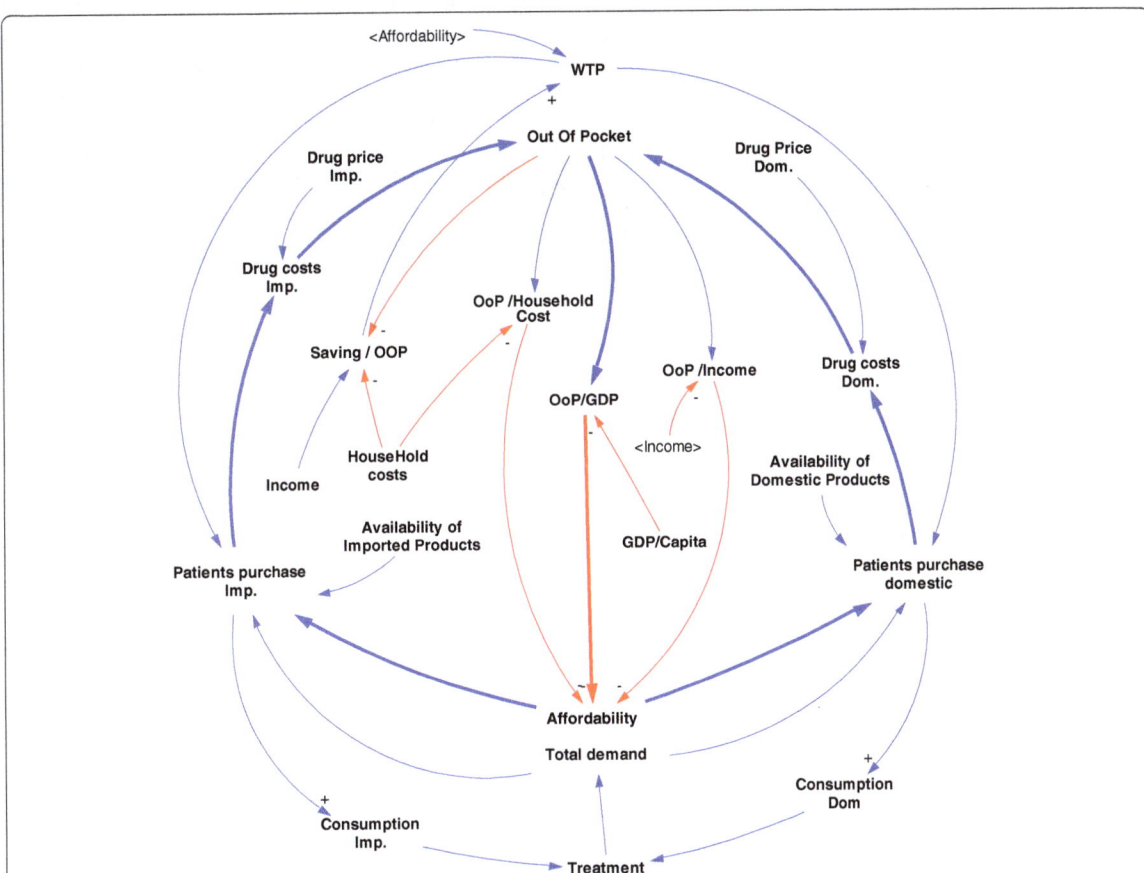

Figure 6 The conceptual model based on affordability.

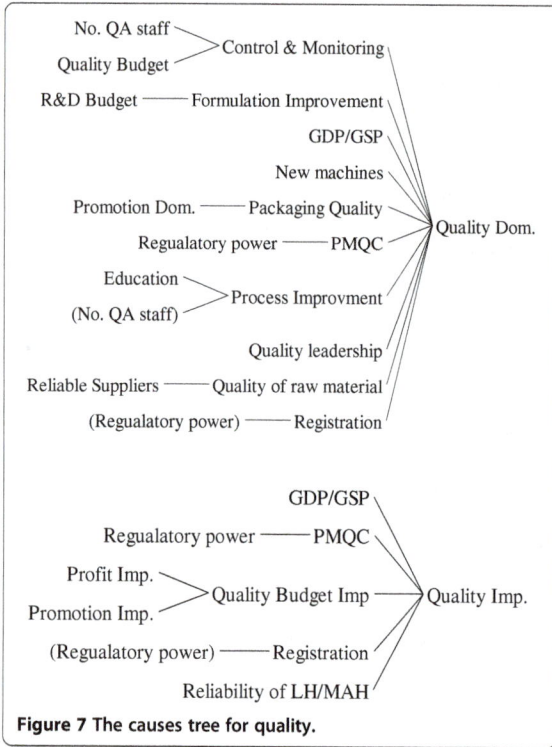

Figure 7 The causes tree for quality.

Part 1–5: Other important variables

There are some other variables in the model including population, birth and death rate, total demand, responded demand, epidemiological indices, number of physicians and pharmacists and diagnosis accuracy that help to complete system for simulation. Although treatment of patients is the main objective of medication, right diagnose, patient compliance, efficacy and side effects can change the treatment progress. Consuming the medicine is not the end of the treatment chain, many chronic diseases are never cured and patients should consume their medicine forever to control the progress of the disease or improve their quality of lives; thus they always stay on the medicine demand cycle. In spite of the demand for main illness treatment, treating the side effects and new sicknesses have some other negative forces on the treatment cycle and leads to new demands. The patients' death in chronic diseases and healing in acute ones removes the patients from the treatment cycle and reduce the demand.

Part 2–1: The stock-flow model

Figure 10 shows the stock flow diagram developed based on the mentioned conceptual casualty network. Population, demand and stock are three bunches of stock variables in the model. Population has divided into four stock variables due to age structure of the country. The incidence rates for each age group, the diagnosis rate and the standard dose of medicine would project the number of susceptible people for treatment that makes the demand. The unit used for demand variables was defined daily dose [27]. Every demand –"susceptible to

positive loops (Figure 9). Because there is an information asymmetry in health system, all activities that improve social information about the medicines and change knowledge, attitude and practice of practitioners can positively affect the rational use and prescribing behavior of the medicines.

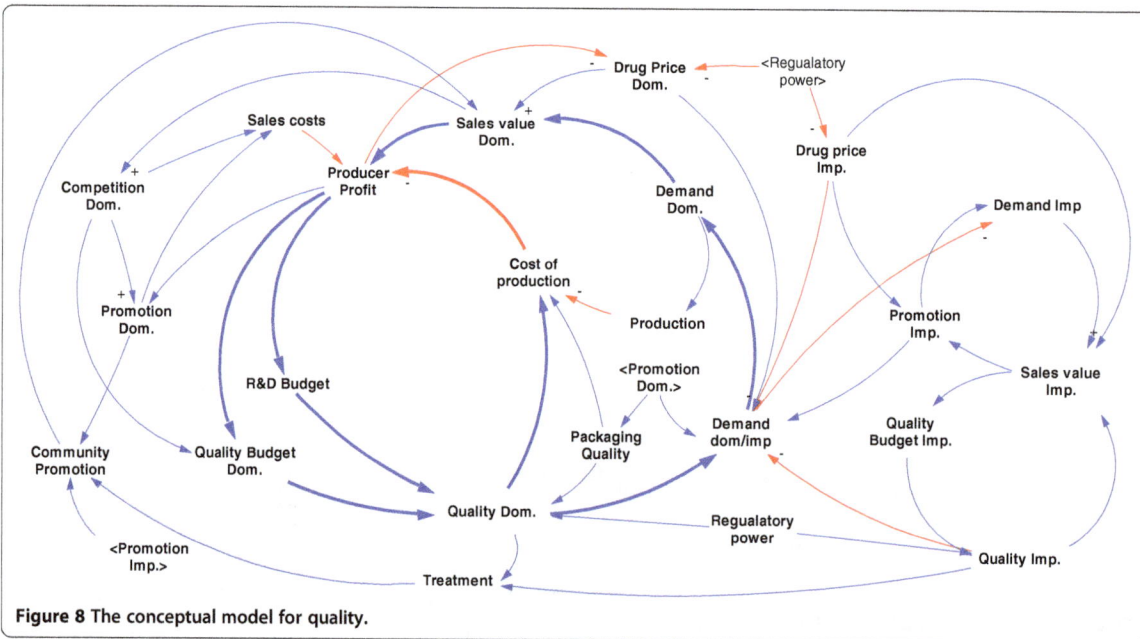

Figure 8 The conceptual model for quality.

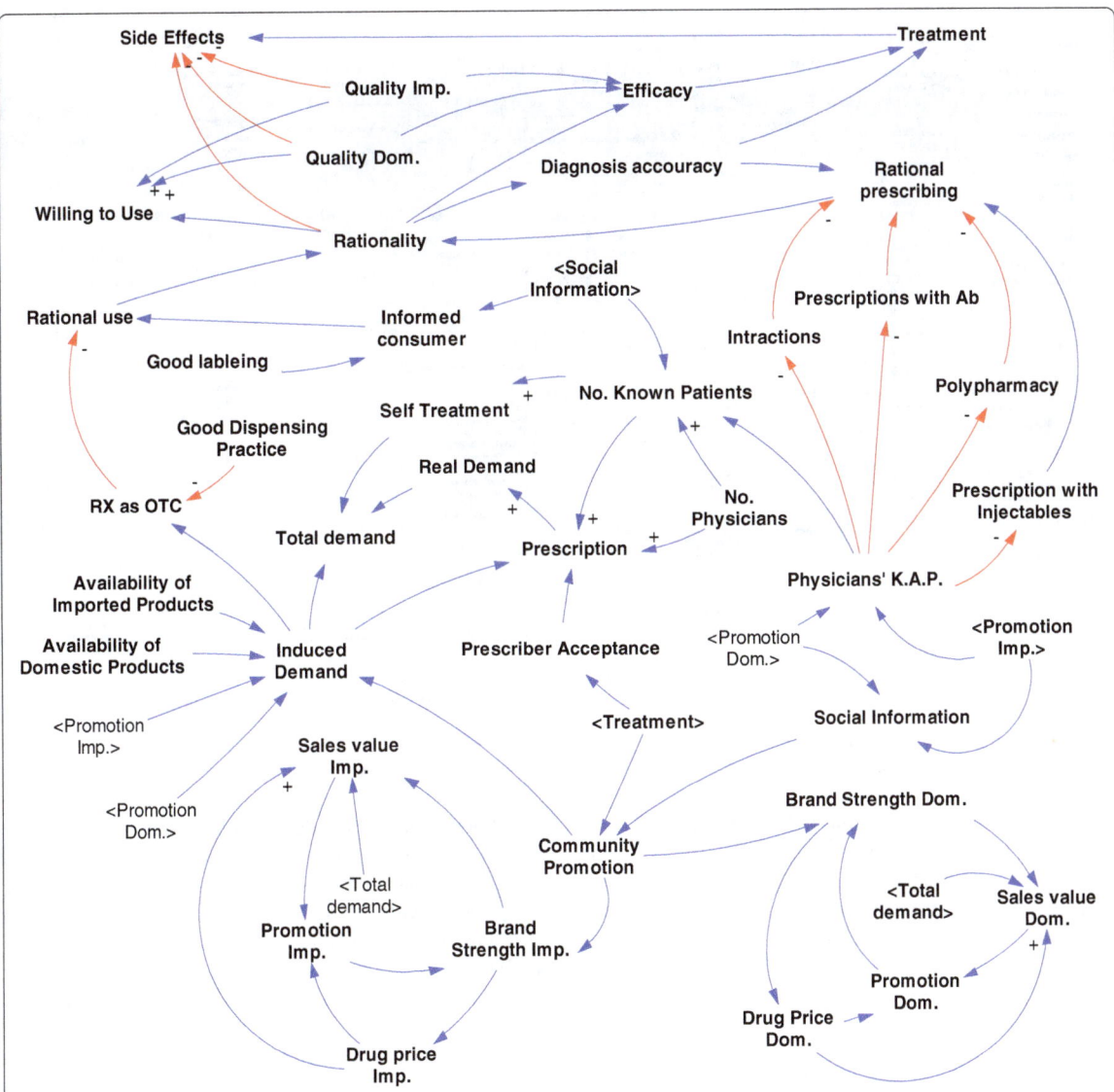

Figure 9 The conceptual model for rationality.

treat"- that is responded - diagnosed, afforded, provided, purchased and consumed -will move to the variable named "responded demand" (Figure 10). Death and stopping treatment are the exit ways of this stock variable for chronic patients; treating rate is the other exit way for acute ones.

All domestic producers and importers collect their supplied medicine in a stock variable called medicine stock. The level of medicine stock variable is higher than the demand based on market saturation rate. The variable "Medicine stock" has two existence way; all demands that can be responded including new demands and current chronic consumers would reduce the medicine

stock through these existence ways called "purchase rates" channels. The purchase rate has made by affordability, availability and WTP.

The quality and rationality related variables put their effects on auxiliary variables called "stop rate" that reduce the number of current consumers.

The variables, their units and the equations were defined on Vensim PLE (academic version) and the model was executed for a 120 months period.

The model was run without any mistakes and the influence of any changes on any variables could be explored on the time trend graphs on other variables that were made by the software.

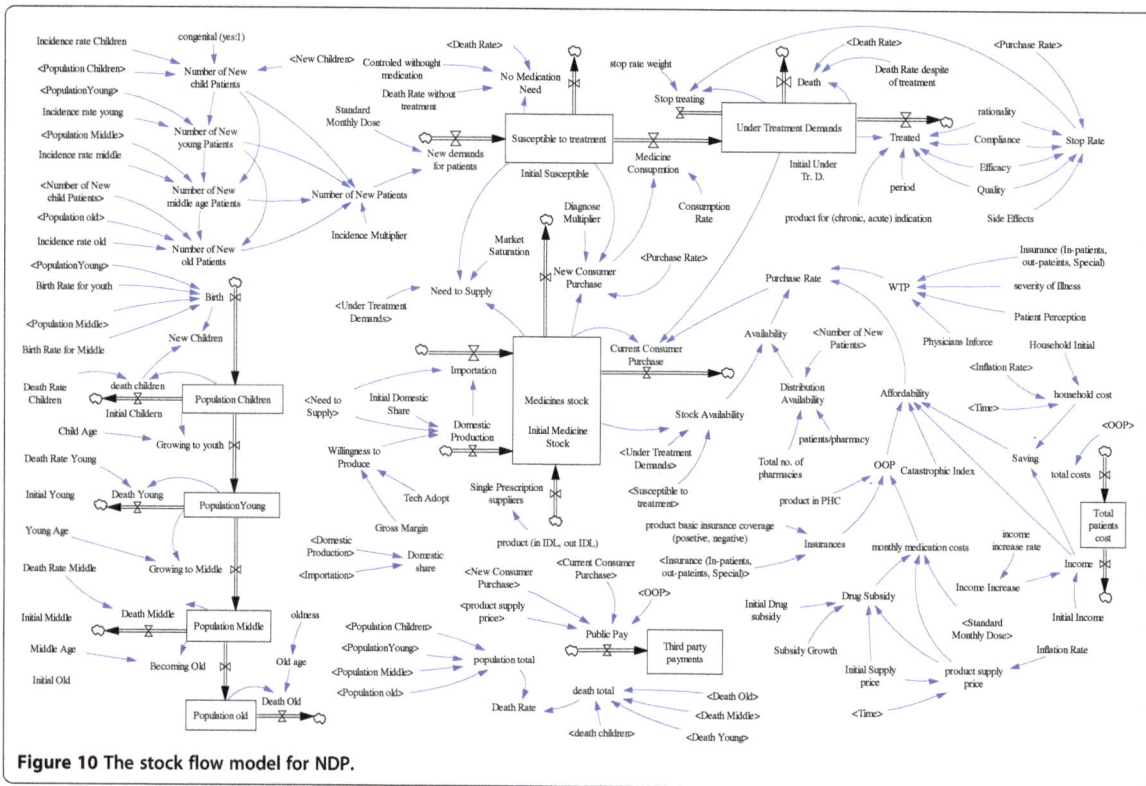

Figure 10 The stock flow model for NDP.

Part 3–1: Validity Tests and sensitivity analysis

There are a wide variety of tests for verification and validation of SD models. To assess the structure, dimensional consistency, extreme conditions and robustness of equations under stress situations are used. For testing behavior reproduction the pattern of outputs are compared with real data. Then the model was tested not only for outputs but also for internal structure [23]. Direct structure tests including extreme-conditions and dimensional consistency was done on all major variables by the software (Vensim). Also the expert panel of the study was revising the structure and casualty relations for many times to reach to the optimum situation.

For testing the structure behavior, some major variables including population groups were compared to real data but for some variables we had no real data for comparing and the expert panel tried to justify them.

Because the concept of modeling in NDP is new in Iran and there are a few written documents about it, reaching to a consensus in the expert panel on the result of the model was difficult; it is challengeable for other experts yet. Some extreme and different conditions that the model tested on them were acute versus chronic, high prevalence versus rare disease, cheap versus expensive treatment and rational high quality drugs versus irrational low quality.

Although for testing the validity, a kind of sensitivity analysis was done but for performing sensitivity analysis all rate variables and initial values are changed in a wide range (even wider than real situation) and the behavior of the model and the value of other major variables were studied. Because there are a lot of variables in the model that should be adjusted with a specific disease and its major treatments, the range of the variables' value significantly depend on the value of other variables. For example if we adjust the model with a rare congenital disease with a full subsidized medicines, availability, affordability and quality variables in the model is no sensitive to the ex-work price or death rate of adults; but it is hugely sensitive to the birth rate.

Discussion

The model is targeted to help policy makers as a decision support system (DSS) with analyzing interrelationships between availability, affordability, quality and rational use of medicines. The casual network was formed by about 140 selected variables made a crowded cognitive map in the conceptual phase that was too complex to interpret so it forced the model to break into four main subsystems. The challenges developed in defining the borders of the subsystems, caused some intersectional variables to be repeated in more than one subsystem.

The stock-flow model has been set based on the demand and supply concept. This demand was made by the population structure and incidence rates. We had to break the population to four stock variables due to the population structure of Iran. Because of the lack of disease epidemiology data in Iran we used any data from any country for covering incidence rates. It was thought this lack of data could be covered by the ability that is in SD to do a wide range of sensitivity analysis. The supply side was summarized to a few level and auxiliary variables that comes to the model as input variables, then it can be expanded to more detailed models in supplementary studies.

Availability subsystem consists of the supply side of the stock-flow model and number of pharmacies as the constant variable; although increasing the number of pharmacies can improve the availability, it cannot overwhelm the total stock situation; the total stock of the modeled medicine comes from the total demand through domestically production and imports. The number of pharmacies under the control of the government has a slow growth due to low population growth rate.

The insurance system and subsidization that play the main role in affordability subsystem present themselves as two constant variables in the stock-flow diagram. The role of insurance organizations can be explained based on the other variables in health financial system. There is a stock variable in the model that shows the cumulative medication costs of the illness and demonstrates the time when patients could fall in catastrophic expenses. The model shows only cancer and autoimmune patients can fall in the catastrophic expenses; medication for normal high burden diseases including cardiovascular, diabetes, central nervous disorders and gastro intestinal are too cheap to send patients to financial failure.

Quality and rationality in the stock-flow diagram are not in the core of the model; they can just affect the model as a foreign control knob.

It was attempted to use mathematical equations between variables than regression equations. Thus, we had to select some variables that can be adopted with it.

Conclusion

The model can initiate a fundamental structure for analyzing NDP. The conceptual model made a cognitive map for NDP that not only shows many causes and effects trees but also reveals some relations between NDP variables that are usually forgotten or ignored in the medicines affairs:

– The role of centralized medical centers in reducing the availability of medicines; although the model is silent on the effects of reducing profit of pharmacies on availability [28].

– It had already been demonstrated the increasing share of imported medicines in the market [29] but this study demonstrates the influence of importers' promotional activities on expanding the market and quality of domestically produced medicines.
– The effects of the patients' WTP on purchasing their medicines and the demand for the medicine.
– The bigger role of prescriber than consumer in rational use of medicines.
– The mutual effects of overstocking in domestic or imported products on supplying and promotion activities.
– The influence of quality and rational use on the patients' willingness to use.

There are also some special points in the model that play significant roles in the NDP that should be more notified:

– The amount of medicines that stocked in patients' homes. It can be the reason that the sales of pharmaceutical usually have no direct relation to health indices [30].
– The effects of medication on the population groups.
– The effect of brand names on the quality.
– The influence of regulatory power on the quality and the supply of medicines that was also explained in other studies [31,32].

Overall this model provides 52 control knobs for the modeler to adjust the model with a selected medicine in a specific disease. Then 121 level and auxiliary variable trends can clarify the consequences of any changes before making any decisions in the NDA.

Linking this model to some real live epidemiological and disease surveillance databases in the country could create a decision support system to help decision making.

The stock-flow model not only shows some relations between NDP variables but provide a framework for other more detailed studies.

Competing interests
The authors declare that they have no competing interests.

Authors' contributions
AA plan the project, set up the panels, developed the primary models, data analysis and drafted the paper, AK and RD conceived and revised the model and supervised the project, MA gave consultation on the study design and edited the draft, AC gave consultation on the conceptual model, SN revised the conceptual model and gave consultation on the medication procedures, MJ revised the stock-flow model and data analysis. All authors read and approved the final manuscript.

Acknowledgements
We thank Dr M. Fazeli, Dr H. Rasekh, Dr M. Cheraghali, the former managing directors of Pharmaceutical division in Iran FDA for their supports in developing the model especially in conceptualization and testing stages.

We would have a special thanks to Mr. M. Alaedini for his guidance in developing the system dynamics model.

Author details
[1]Department of Pharmacoeconomics and Pharmaceutical administration, Pharmaceutical policy research center and Faculty of Pharmacy, Tehran University of Medical Sciences (TUMS), Tehran, Iran. [2]Department of Toxicology and Pharmacology, Faculty of Pharmacy and Pharmaceutical Sciences Research Center, TUMS, Tehran, Iran. [3]Department of Pharmaceutics, Faculty of Pharmacy, TUMS, Tehran, Iran. [4]Food and Drug Organization, Ministry of Health and Medical Education, Tehran, Iran. [5]Department of Pharmacology, University of Baqiyatallah Medical Sciences, Tehran, Iran.

References
1. World Health Organization: *How to develop and implement a national drug policy.* Geneva: World Health Organization; 2002.
2. World Health Organization: *WHO medicines strategy: framework for action in essential drugs and medicines policy 2000–2003.* Geneva: WHO; 2000.
3. Kaplan A: Using the components of the marketing mix to market emergency services. *Health Mark Q* 1984, 2:53–62.
4. Nikfar S, Kebriaeezadeh A, Majdzadeh R, Abdollahi M: Monitoring of National Drug Policy (NDP) and its standardized indicators; conformity to decisions of the national drug selecting committee in Iran. *BMC Int Health Hum Rights* 2005, 5:5.
5. Kruk ME, Freedman LP: Assessing health system performance in developing countries: a review of the literature. *Health Policy* 2008, 85:263–276.
6. Paniz VM, Fassa AG, Maia MF, Domingues MR, Bertoldi AD: Measuring access to medicines: a review of quantitative methods used in household surveys. *BMC Health Serv Res* 2010, 10:146.
7. Abdollahiasl A, Nikfar S, Kebriaeezadeh A, Dinarvand R, Abdollahi M: A model for developing a decision support system to simulate national drug policy indicators. *Arch Med Sci* 2011, 7:744–746.
8. Lane DC, Husemann E: Steering without Circe: attending to reinforcing loops in social systems. *System dynamics review* 2008, 24:37–61.
9. Homer J, Milstein B: *Optimal decision making in a dynamic model of community health,* System Sciences, 2004 Proceedings of the 37th Annual Hawaii International Conference on. IEEE; 2004:11.
10. Sterman JD: System dynamics modeling. *California management review* 2001, 43:8–25.
11. Forrester JW: *System dynamics and the lessons of 35 years,* A systems-based approach to policymaking. Springer; 1993:199–240.
12. Homer JB, Hirsch GB: System dynamics modeling for public health: background and opportunities. *Am J Public Health* 2006, 96:452–458.
13. Koelling P, Schwandt MJ: Health systems: A dynamic system-benefits from system dynamics. *Proceedings of the 2005 Winter Simulation Conference* 2005, 1–4:1321–1327.
14. Pfaffenbichler P: Modelling with Systems Dynamics as a Method to Bridge the Gap between Politics, Planning and Science? Lessons Learnt from the Development of the Land Use and Transport Model MARS. *Transport Reviews* 2011, 31:267–289.
15. Forrester JW: *Learning through system dynamics as preparation for the 21st century.* Keynote Address for Systems Thinking and Dynamic Modelling Conference for K-12 Education; 1994.
16. Albin S, Forrester JW, Breierova L: *Building a System Dynamics Model: Part 1: Conceptualization.* MIT; 2001.
17. Eden C: Cognitive mapping and problem structuring for system dynamics model building. *System dynamics review* 1994, 10:257–276.
18. Größler A, Milling P: *Inductive and deductive system dynamics modeling.* The 2007 International Conference of the System Dynamics Society; 2007.
19. Grösser SN, Schaffernicht M: Mental models of dynamic systems: taking stock and looking ahead. *System dynamics review* 2012, 28:46–68.
20. Brailsford S, Hilton N: In *A comparison of discrete event simulation and system dynamics for modelling health care systems.* Edited by Riley J. Glasgow, Scotland: Proceedings from ORAHS 2000; 2001:18–39.
21. Forrester JW, Senge PM: *Tests for building confidence in system dynamics models.* Cambridge: System Dynamics Group, Sloan School of Management, Massachusetts Institute of Technology; 1978.
22. Merrill JA, Deegan M, Wilson RV, Kaushal R, Fredericks K: A system dynamics evaluation model: implementation of health information exchange for public health reporting. *J Am Med Inform Assoc* 2013, 20:e131–138.
23. Barlas Y: Formal aspects of model validity and validation in system dynamics. *System dynamics review* 1996, 12:183–210.
24. Iran FDA: *Iran Annual Pharmaceutical Statistics.* Iran Annual Pharmaceutical Statistics; 2012.
25. HAI/WHO: *IR. Iran, Medicine prices, availability, affordability and price components.* Geneva: Essential Medicines and Pharmaceutical Policies Unit, World Health Organization, Regional Office for the Eastern Mediterranean; 2010.
26. UNFPA: *State of World Population 2012.* Washington, D.C.: UNFPA; 2012.
27. WHO: *Guidelines for ATC classification and DDD assignment.* Oslo: Norsk Medisinal depot; 1996.
28. Keshavarz K, Kebriaeezadeh A, Meshkini AH, Nikfar S, Mirian I, Khoonsari H: Financial perspective of private pharmacies in Tehran (Iran); is it a lucrative business? *DARU J of Pharm Sci* 2012, 20:62.
29. Kebriaeezadeh A, Koopaei NN, Abdollahiasl A, Nikfar S, Mohamadi N: Trend analysis of the pharmaceutical market in Iran; 1997–2010; policy implications for developing countries. *DARU J Pharm Sci* 2013, 21:52.
30. Abdollahiasl A, Nikfar S, Abdollahi M: Pharmaceutical market and health system in the Middle Eastern and Central Asian countries: Time for innovations and changes in policies and actions. *Arch Med Sci* 2011, 7:365–367.
31. Jaberidoost M, Nikfar S, Abdollahiasl A, Dinarvand R: Pharmaceutical supply chain risks: a systematic review. *DARU J Pharm Sci* 2013, 12.
32. Nassiri-Koopaei N, Majdzadeh R, Kebriaeezadeh A, Rashidian A, Yazdi MT, Nedjat S, Nikfar S: Commercialization of biopharmaceutical knowledge in Iran; challenges and solutions. *DARU J Pharm Sci* 2014, 22:29.

14

Synthesis and psychobiological evaluation of modafinil analogs in mice

Arezou Lari[1], Isaac Karimi[2], Hadi Adibi[3], Alireza Aliabadi[3], Loghman Firoozpour[4] and Alireza Foroumadi[4,5*]

Abstract

Background and the purpose of the study: Modafinil, a novel wake-promoting agent with low potential for abuse and dependence, has a reliable structure to find some novel derivatives with better activity and lower potential for abuse and risk of dependency. This study was designed to evaluate psychobiological activity of some novel N-aryl modafinil derivatives.

Methods: Seven novel N-aryl modafinil derivatives were synthesized through three reactions: a) preparation of benzhydrylsulfanyl acetic acid through reaction of benzhydrol with thioglycolic acid, b) formation of desired amide by adding the substituted aniline to activated acid with EDC (1-ethyl-3-(3-dimethyl amino propyl) carbodiimide). This reaction was catalyzed by HOBt (N- hydroxylbenzotriazole), and c) oxidation of sulfur to sulfoxide group with H_2O_2. Then, their psychobiological effect on the performance of male albino mice were compared to that of modafinil as following: wakefulness by determining the effects of derivatives on phenobarbital-induced loss of the righting reflex (LOPR); exploratory activity by measuring activity in the open field test (OFT); depression by measuring immobility time (IT) during forced swimming test (FST) and the anxiogenic and anxiolytic like effects by using elevated plus-maze test (EPM). All tests were videotaped and analyzed for the frequency and duration of the behaviors during the procedures.

Conclusions: 2-(Benzhydrylsulfonyl)-N-(4-chlorophenyl)acetamide (**4c**) showed comparable result in LOPR test. However, all analogs were found to be stimulant except 2-(benzhydrylsulfinyl)-N-phenylacetamide (**4a**). Also **4c** led the most exploratory activity in mice among derivatives. FST results showed that 4a had the longest IT while modafinil, 2-(benzhydrylsulfinyl)-N-(3-chlorophenyl) acetamide (**4b**) and 2-(benzhydrylsulfinyl)-N-(4-ethylphenyl) acetamide (**4d**) had the shortest IT. In EPM, all derivatives showed anxiogenic-like behavior since they decreased open arms time and open arms entries and simultaneously increased close arms time.

Keywords: Modafinil, Wake-promoting agent, Narcolepsy

Introduction

Narcolepsy is a neurological sleep disorder that is estimated to affect as many as 200,000. It is as widespread as multiple sclerosis and more prevalent than cystic fibrosis, but it is less well known [1,2].

The main treatment of narcolepsy is using of central nervous system (CNS) stimulants such as amphetamine, methylphenidate and modafinil which is widely regarded as the first-line medication for narcolepsy (Figure 1) [1,3]. Amphetamine and methylphenidate are associated with a

significant abuse potential while modafinil which has lower abuse potential [4,5]. Surprisingly, modafinil is used sometimes to treat methamphetamine dependency; however this type of therapy has not been authoritized [6].

In one study, some modafinil analogs were evaluated for their CNS activity [7]. Most of the derivatives of nitrogen group like NHCH₃, NHCH (CH₃)₂, HCN (CH₃)₃ were stimulant, although some analogs with piperidine or morpholine groups were sedative. Here, synthesis and psychobiological evaluation of novel modafinil derivatives with different N-Aryl moieties were reported. These analogs with suitable Log P were chosen due to their easy transfer across the blood brain barrier. The tilted compounds were prepared according to Scheme 1. The key intermediate 2-(benzhydrylthio) acetic acid (**2**) was prepared from benzhydrol and thioglycolic acid. Amidation of appropriate

* Correspondence: aforoumadi@yahoo.com
[4]Drug Design and Development Research Center, Tehran University of Medical Sciences, Tehran, Iran
[5]Neuroscience Research Center, Institute of Neuropharmacology, Kerman University of Medical Sciences, Kerman, Iran
Full list of author information is available at the end of the article

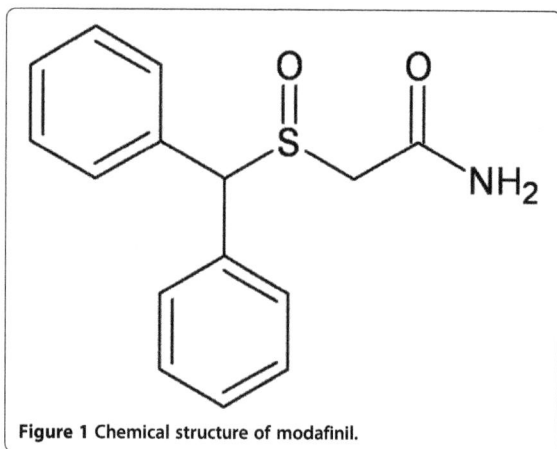

Figure 1 Chemical structure of modafinil.

Bruker 400 spectrometer (Bruker Bioscience, Billerica, MA, USA), and chemical shifts were expressed as δ (ppm) with tetramethylsilane as internal standard. The mass spectra were run on a Finigan TSQ-70 spectrometer (Finigan, USA) at 70 eV. Merck silica gel 60 F_{254} plates were used for analytical TLC.

Synthesis of 2-(benzhydrylthio)acetic acid (2)

A mixture of benzhydrol (50.0 g, 271.4 mmol) and thioglycolic acid (25.0 g, 271.4 mmol) in trifluoroacetic acid (300 mL) was stirred at room temperature for 3 h. The solvent was removed under reduced pressure to afford a crude solid. Water (300 ml) was added and the resulting precipitate collected by filtration. The solid was washed with *n*-hexane (400 ml) and dried to afford a white solid (69.2 g).

aniline with 2-(benzhydrylthio)acetic acid yielded the corresponding amide (**3a-3g**). The obtained amides (**3a-3g**) gently oxidized by H_2O_2 to form the corresponding sulfoxide derivatives (**4a-4g**).

Yield: 99%, mp: 126–129°C. IR (KBr, cm^{-1}); ū: 3071, 2570, 1941, 1860, 1809, 1689, 1596, 1491, 1301, 1203, 1137, 1209, 1021, 804. ^{1}H-NMR (CDCl$_3$, 400 MHz) δ (ppm): 3.1 + .3699 (s, 2H, -SCH$_2$CO-), 5.5 (s, 1H, Ph-CH-Ph), 7.13 (t, *J* = 7.6 Hz, aromatic), 7.22-7.25 (m, aromatic), 7.25 (m, aromatic), 7.33 (m, aromatic), 7.45 (m, aromatic) [8].

Material and methods

Chemistry

All chemical reagents and solvents used in this study were purchased from Merck AG (Darmstadt, Germany). Melting points were determined by Kofler hot stage apparatus and are not corrected. The IR spectra were obtained on a Shimadzu 470 spectrophotometer (potassium bromide disks). NMR spectra were appropriately recorded using a

General procedure for the synthesis of compounds 3a-3g

The mixture of 2-(benzhydrylthio) acetic acid (**2**), EDC (1-ethyl-3-(3-dimethylaminopropyl) carbodiimide) (1 mol) and HOBt (hydroxybenzotriazole) (1 mol) in acetonitrile solvent was kept under stirring for 30 min in order to activate acid group. Afterwards, appropriate aniline derivative was added and the mixture was stirred at room temperature for 24 h. The solvent was evaporated and

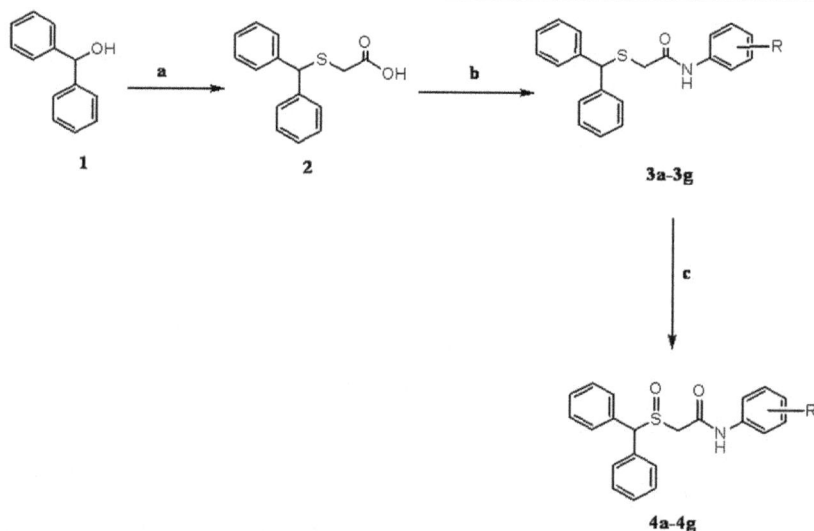

Scheme 1 Synthesis of target compounds 4a-4g (R: (a) = H, (b) = 3-Cl, (c) = 4-Cl, (d) = 4-Et, (e) = 3,4-Cl, (f) = 4-NO$_2$, (g) = 4-Br), Reagents and conditions: (a) Thioglycolic acid, TFA, 3 h; (b) appropriate amine, EDC, HOBt; (c) appropriate amide, H$_2$O$_2$, acetic acid.

ethyl acetate was added to the residue. The organic phase was washed with sulfuric acid 5%, sodium bicarbonate and brine. Then, the organic layer was dried over anhydrous sodium sulfate, filtered and evaporated to dryness. The residue was chromatographed on silica gel plate eluting with ethyl acetate/petroleum [9].

2-(benzhydrylthio)-N-phenylacetamide (3a)

Yield: 81%, mp: 90°C. IR (KBr, cm^{-1}); ū: 3431, 3243, 3060, 2959, 2854, 1655, 1597, 1547, 1491, 1443, 1325, 754, 696. ^{1}H-NMR (CDCl$_3$, 400 MHz) δ (ppm): 3.26 (s, 2H, -SCH$_2$CO-), 5.18 (s, 1H, Ph-CH-Ph), 7.13 (t, J = 7.6 Hz, aromatic), 7.22-7.25 (m, aromatic), 7.30-7.35 (m, aromatic), 7.41 (d, J = 8 Hz, aromatic), 7.48 (d, J = 8 Hz, aromatic), 8.41 (brs, 1H, NH).

2-(benzhydrylthio)-N-(3-chlorophenyl) acetamide (3b)

Yield: 73%, mp: 60°C. IR (KBr, cm^{-1}); ū: 3426, 3329, 3229, 3064, 2923, 1665, 1641, 1593, 1525, 1421, 1310, 1240, 1129, 1074, 878, 775, 698. ^{1}H-NMR (CDCl$_3$, 400 MHz) δ (ppm): 3.27 (s, 2H, -SCH$_2$CO-), 5.18 (s, 1H, PhCHPh), 7.15 (m, aromatic), 7.25-7.41 (m, aromatic), 8.42 (brs, 1H, NH).

2-(benzhydrylthio)-N-(4-chlorophenyl) acetamide (3c)

Yield: 78%, mp: 90°C. IR (KBr, cm^{-1}); ū: 3430, 3121, 3067, 2923, 2853, 1646, 1549, 1490, 1400, 1093, 1034, 823, 700. ^{1}H-NMR (CDCl$_3$, 400 MHz) δ (ppm): 3.27 (s, 2H, -SCH$_2$CO-), 5.15 (s, 1H, PhCHPh), 7.25-7.41 (m, 14H, aromatic), 8.41 (s, 1H, NH).

2-(benzhydrylthio)-N-(4-ethylphenyl) acetamide (3d)

Yield: 72%, mp: 87°C. IR (KBr, cm^{-1}); ū: 3258, 3060, 2962, 2925, 2873, 1638, 1599, 1535, 1449, 1410, 1321, 1124, 1073, 1025, 971, 825, 743, 697. ^{1}H-NMR (CDCl$_3$, 400 MHz) δ (ppm): 1.22 (t, 3H, CH$_3$), 2.62 (q, 2H, CH$_2$), 3.25 (s, 2H, -SCH$_2$CO-), 5.19 (s, 1H, PhCHPh), 7.15-7.42 (m, 14H, aromatic), 8.40 (s, 1H, NH).

2-(benzhydrylthio)-N-(3, 4-dichlorophenyl) acetamide (3e)

Yield: 75%, mp: 85°C. IR (KBr, cm^{-1}); ū: 3400, 3268, 3087, 2922, 1710, 1650, 1591, 1528, 1480, 1376, 1318, 1118, 1027, 870, 811, 748, 697. ^{1}H-NMR (CDCl$_3$, 400 MHz) δ (ppm): 3.28 (s, 2H, -SCH$_2$CO-), 5.14 (s, 1H, PhCHPh), 7.65 (s, 1H, H$_2$-Dichlorophenyl) and 7.24-7.40 (m, 12H, aromatic), 8.37 (brs, 1H, NH).

2-(benzhydrylthio)-N-(4-nitrophenyl) acetamide (3f)

Yield: 68%, mp: 80-84°C. IR (KBr, cm^{-1}); ū: 3313, 3087, 3017, 2923, 1675, 1616, 1596, 1552, 1500, 1334, 1307, 1255, 1117, 853, 748, 696. ^{1}H-NMR (CDCl$_3$, 400 MHz) δ (ppm): 3.34 (s, 2H, -SCH$_2$CO-), 5.16 (s, 1H, PhCHPh), 7.24 (d, J = 8Hz, aromatic), 7.31 (t, J = 4Hz, aromatic), 7.4 (d, J = 8Hz, aromatic), 7.61 (d, 2H, J = 8Hz, p-Nitrophenyl), 8.19 (d, 2H, J = 8.8Hz, p-Nitrophenyl), 8.64 (brs, 1H, NH).

2-(benzhydrylthio)-N-(4-bromophenyl) acetamide (3g)

Yield: 84%, mp: 92°C. IR (KBr, cm^{-1}); ū: 3237, 3027, 2927, 1714, 1641, 1593, 1533, 1490, 1396, 1314, 1125, 1072, 1008, 818, 746, 696. ^{1}H-NMR (CDCl$_3$, 400 MHz) δ (ppm): 3.28 (s, 2H, -SCH$_2$CO-), 5.17 (s, 1H, PhCHPh), 7.32-7.48 (m, 14H, aromatic), 8.42 (brs, 1H, NH).

General procedure for the synthesis of 2-(benzhydrylsulfinyl)-N-phenylacetamide (4a-4g)

2-(benzhydrylthio)-N-phenylacetamide (3.46 g, 0.013 mol) was taken in glacial acetic acid (14 ml) with stirring. 1.34 ml of 30% H$_2$O$_2$ was added with chilling in ice water. The mixture was left in the refrigerator for 4 h and thereafter worked up by treating with 70 ml of ice-cold water. The precipitated material was filtered under suction and washed with ice-cold water to give 1.5 g of white crystals (43%), mp: 159-160°C [10].

2-(benzhydrylsulfinyl)-N-phenyl acetamide (4a)

Yield: 70%, mp: 98°C. IR (KBr, cm^{-1}); ū: 3426, 3056, 2924, 2854, 1673, 1600, 1551, 1493, 1446, 1325, 1112, 1033, 755, 698.

^{1}H-NMR (d ppm, CDCl$_3$, 400 MHz): 3.23 (d, 1H, -SCH$_2$CO-, J = 12Hz), 3.66 (d, 1H, -SCH$_2$CO-, J = 12Hz), 5.25 (s, 1H, PhCHPh), 7.12 (t, J = 8Hz, aromatic), 7.26 (s, 1H, aromatic), 7.31 (t, J = 8Hz, aromatic), 7.36-7.52 (m, aromatic), 9.21 (brs, 1H, NH). ^{13}C-NMR (125 MHz, CDCl$_3$): δ 51.95 (S-CH$_2$), 71.54 (S-CH), 120.15 (C$_{2, 6}$ aniline), 124.64 (C$_4$ aniline), 128.77 (C$_{3, 5}$ aniline), 128.87 (C$_{3,5}$ phenyl), 128.97 (C$_4$ phenyl), 129.51 (C$_{2,6}$ phenyl), 133.78 (C$_1$ phenyl), 134.29 (C$_1$ aniline), 175.00 (C = O). MS (m/z): 349 (M$^+$), 309, 167, 119, 104, 93, 77, 65, 57, 43.

2-(benzhydrylsulfinyl)-N-(3-chlorophenyl) acetamide (4b)

Yield: 68%, mp: 160°C. IR (KBr, cm^{-1}); ū: 3441, 3250, 3184, 3066, 3026, 2923, 2856, 1682, 1596, 1546, 1480, 1430, 1372, 1320, 1035, 794, 700. ^{1}H-NMR (CDCl$_3$, 400 MHz) δ (ppm): 3.23 (d, 1H, -SCH$_2$CO-, J = 12Hz), 3.67 (d, 1H, -SCH$_2$CO-, J = 12Hz), 5.27 (s, 1H, PhCHPh), 7.08-7.50 (m, 13H, aromatic), 7.69 (s, 1H, H$_2$-m-Chlorophenyl), 9.35 (brs, 1H, NH). ^{13}C-NMR (125 MHz, CDCl$_3$): δ 52.34 (S-CH$_2$), 71.38 (S-CH), 117.88 (C$_3$ aniline), 120.04 (C$_2$ aniline), 124.55 (C$_4$ aniline), 128.84 (C$_{3, 5}$ phenyl), 128.90 (C$_4$ phenyl), 128.99 (C$_{2,6}$ phenyl), 129.51 (C$_6$ aniline), 131.94 (C$_5$ aniline), 133.67 (C$_1$ phenyl), 134.37 (C$_1$ aniline), 162.16 (C = O). MS (m/z): 385 (M$^+$+2), 383 (M$^+$), 293, 201, 167, 153, 127, 111, 91, 64, 47.

2-(benzhydrylsulfinyl)-N-(4-chlorophenyl) acetamide (4c)

Yield: 73%, mp: 170°C. IR (KBr, cm^{-1}); ū: 3444, 3248, 2920, 1684, 1597, 1541, 1489, 1398, 1320, 1246, 1037, 743, 701.

^{1}H-NMR (CDCl$_3$, 400 MHz) δ (ppm): 3.26 (d, 1H, -SCH$_2$CO-, $J=16$Hz), 3.66 (d, 1H, -SCH$_2$CO-, $J=16$Hz), 5.26 (s, 1H, PhCHPh), 7.24 (d, 2H, $J=8$Hz, p-Chlorophenyl), 725–7.50 (m, 12H, aromatic), 9.33 (brs, 1H, NH). ^{13}C-NMR (125 MHz, CDCl$_3$): δ 52.21 (S-CH$_2$), 71.52 (S-CH), 121.19 (C-Cl), 128.85 (C$_{2, 6}$ aniline), 128.91 (C$_{3,5}$ phenyl), 128.98 (C$_4$ phenyl), 129.52 (C$_{2,6}$ phenyl), 129.56 (C$_{3,5}$ aniline), 134.29 (C$_1$ phenyl), 136.18 (C$_1$ aniline), 162.08 (C = O). MS (m/z): 385 (M$^+$+2), 383 (M$^+$), 167, 153, 127, 111.

2-(benzhydrylsulfinyl)-N-(4-ethylphenyl) acetamide (4d)

Yield: 74%, mp: 158°C. IR (KBr, cm^{-1}) ū: 3253, 3185, 3058, 2957, 2923, 2858, 1679, 1540, 1412, 1322, 1043, 957, 832, 747, 701.

^{1}H NMR (CDCl$_3$, 400 MHz) δ (ppm): 1.23 (t, 3H, CH$_3$), 2.63 (q, 2H, CH$_2$), 3.23 (d, 1H, $J = 12$Hz, -SCH$_2$CO-), 3.66 (d, 1H, -SCH$_2$CO-, $J = 12$Hz), 5.21 (s, 1H, PhCHPh), 7.16-7.48 (m, 14H, aromatic), 9.21 (brs, 1H, NH). ^{13}C-NMR (125 MHz, CDCl$_3$): δ 15.66 (CH$_3$), 28.33 (CH$_2$), 36.97 (S-CH$_2$), 55.09 (S-CH), 120.22 (C$_4$ aniline), 127.53 (C$_{2, 6}$ aniline), 128.25 (C$_{3,5}$ phenyl), 128.34 (C$_4$ phenyl), 128.46 (C$_{2,6}$ phenyl), 128.84 (C$_{3,5}$ aniline), 135.02 (C$_1$ phenyl), 140.10 (C$_1$ aniline), 166.28 (C = O). MS (m/z): 377 (M$^+$), 284, 279, 191, 167, 149, 105, 85, 71, 57.

2-(benzhydrylsulfinyl)-N-(3, 4-dichlorophenyl) acetamide (4e)

Yield: 63%, mp: 140°C. IR (KBr, cm^{-1}); ū: 3293, 3258, 3101, 3052, 2912, 1711, 1686, 1587, 1383, 1312, 1224, 1146, 1036, 878, 820, 742, 698. ^{1}H NMR (CDCl$_3$, 400 MHz) δ (ppm): 3.24 (d, 1H, $J =16$Hz, -SCH$_2$CO-), 3.67 (d, 1H, $J=16$Hz, -SCH$_2$CO-), 5.32 (s, 1H, PhCHPh), 7.23-7.48 (m, 12H, aromatic), 7.77 (s, 1H, H$_2$-m-Chlorophenyl), 9.45 (brs, 1H, NH). ^{13}C-NMR (125 MHz, CDCl$_3$): δ 52.13 (S-CH$_2$), 71.41 (S-CH), 118.99 (C$_4$ aniline), 121.48 (C$_2$ aniline), 121.56 (C$_6$ aniline), 128.87 (C$_{3,5}$ phenyl), 129.04 (C$_4$ phenyl), 129.50 (C$_{2, 6}$ phenyl), 129.56 (C$_3$ aniline), 131.94 (C$_5$ aniline), 133.64 (C$_1$ phenyl), 134.19 (C$_1$ aniline), 162.14 (C = O). MS (m/z): 421 (M$^+$4), 419 (M$^+$+2), 417 (M$^+$), 199, 184, 167, 149, 105.

2-(benzhydrylsulfinyl)-N-(4-nitrophenyl) acetamide (4f)

Yield: 76%, mp: 198°C. IR (KBr, cm^{-1}); ū: 3448, 3202, 3078, 2922, 2852, 1702, 1618, 1598, 1566, 1497, 1335, 1251, 1159, 1039, 859, 748, 698. ^{1}H NMR (CDCl$_3$, 400 MHz) δ (ppm): 3.47 (d, 1H, -SCH$_2$CO-, $J=12$Hz), 3.76 (d, 1H, -SCH$_2$CO-, $J=12$Hz), 5.42 (s, 1H, PhCHPh), 7.35-7.41 (m, 8H, aromatic), 7.53 (d, 2H, $J=8.4$Hz, aromatic), 7.78(d, 2H, $J=8$Hz, p-Nitrophenyl), 8.16 (d, 2H, $J=8$Hz, p-Nitrophenyl), 10.40 (brs, 1H, NH). MS (m/z): 394 (M$^+$), 279, 257, 236, 167, 149, 69, 57, 43.

2-(benzhydrylsulfinyl)-N-(4-bromophenyl) acetamide (4g)

Yield: 66%, mp: 155°C. IR (KBr, cm^{-1}); ū: 3430, 2923, 2853, 1741, 1663, 1630, 1454, 1379, 1240, 1155, 1034,

837, 743, 700. ^{1}H NMR (CDCl$_3$, 400 MHz) δ (ppm): 3.24 (d, 1H, -SCH$_2$CO-, $J=16$Hz), 3.65 (d, 1H, -SCH$_2$CO-, $J=16$Hz), 5.33 (s, 1H, PhCHPh), 7.26-7.49 (m, 14H, aromatic), 9.44 (s, 1H, NH). ^{13}C-NMR (125 MHz, CDCl$_3$): δ 51.68 (S-CH$_2$), 71.76 (S-CH), 117.24 (C-Br), 121.82 (C$_{2, 6}$ aniline), 128.82 (C$_{3,5}$ phenyl), 129.00 (C$_4$ phenyl), 129.43 (C$_{2, 6}$ phenyl), 129.55 (C$_{3, 5}$ aniline), 131.94 (C$_1$ phenyl), 136.61 (C$_1$ aniline), 162.19 (C = O). MS (m/z): 429 (M$^+$+2), 428 (M$^+$+1), 368, 362, 167, 152, 69, 57, 43.

Psychobiological activity

Animals

This study approved by the Laboratory Animal Care Committee of School of Veterinary Medicine, Razi University, Kermanshah, Iran. The experiments were carried out on male albino mice weighing 20–25 g at the beginning of the experiments. The animals were maintained under standard laboratory conditions (12-h light/dark cycle, room temperature 21 ± 1°C) with free access to tap water and laboratory chow (Dan-e-pars Co., Kermanshah, Iran) except during brief periods of experiments, and were adapted to the laboratory conditions for at least 1 week. Each experimental group consisted of 5–6 animals.

Drugs

The compounds tested were: modafinil (Modiodal®, Cephalon, France), Phenobarbital (Chemi darou product, Iran) and our made modafinil derivatives. All agents were diluted to an adequate concentration using dimethyl sulfoxide (DMSO). They were administered intraperitoneally (i.p.) 30 min prior to each behavioral test. Control groups received DMSO injection at the same volume and by the same route. The doses of modafinil and its derivatives (100 mg/kg) employed in the present study was adopted from previous study [11]. The dose of phenobarbital (50 mg/kg) was chosen according to that commonly used dose reported in the literature [12]. In all tests, each mouse was tested once.

Phenobarbital-induced loss of righting reflex

Phenobarbital (50 mg/kg i.p.) was administered to each mouse. The loss of righting reflex (LORR) was measured as the time interval between losing and recovery of the righting reflex after phenobarbital administration. Recovery of the righting reflex was defined as the ability of the animal to return to its feet 3 times within 60 sec when placed on its back [13]. Mice received modafinil or its derivatives (100 mg/kg, i.p.) 30 min before i.p. injection of phenobarbital. The ethological room was illuminated with a soft light and external noise was attenuated.

Open field test (OFT)

The open field consisted of a square arena (60 × 60 cm^2), with a white floor divided into 36 squares (10 × 10 cm^2), enclosed by continuous, 25-cm-high walls made of glass. The test was initiated by placing a single mouse in the middle of the arena and letting him move freely for 5 min. The mice had not been pre-exposed to the arena. Mouse behavior was continuously videotaped by a video camera placed over the apparatus and the arena was carefully cleaned with alcohol and rinsed with water after every test to eliminate olfactory cues. Decrease of the latency to enter the central part was considered as an indicator of anxiolysis and locomotor activity was evaluated by counting the number of segments crossed with a 4-paw as described previously [14].

Forced swimming test (FST)

Mice were individually forced to swim in a plastic cylinder ($25 \times 25 \times 40$ cm^3) containing 18 cm of water at 22°C. This volume of water precluded mice touching the bottom with their feet or tails. Mice were submitted to the procedure for 15 min on the first day (pretest) and for 5 min on the second day test, 24 h later. Each mouse i.p. received the tested derivatives 30 min before forced swimming paradigm. At the end of the swimming exposition, the animals were removed from the water and gently dried. The initial 5 min of both swimming sessions were videotaped for behavioral analysis. The immobility time (IT) was recorded only during the last 4 min of these periods, and was defined as the sum of time that the animal was floating, with the face above the water surface and making only slight movements with the front paws to keep from submerging as described previously [15]. The frequency of alternation between mobility and immobility behaviors gradually decreased as time lapsed, the animals tending to remain much more immobile. The decrease and increase of immobility time were interpreted as antidepressive or depressive actions, respectively [16].

Elevated plus maze (EPM)

Behavioral effect of modafinil and its derivatives were elevated in the mouse EPM paradigm. The experimental apparatus is shaped like a "plus" sign and consists of a central platform (5×5 cm), two open arms ($30 \times 15 \times 5$ cm) and two equal-sized closed arms opposite to each other. The maze is made of wood, elevated to a height of 50 cm above the floor. A video camera was mounted vertically about 1meter above the plus-maze for recording behavioral responses. The test consisted of placing a mouse in the central platform facing an enclosed arm and allowed it to freely explore the maze for 5 min. Entry into one arm was defined as the animal placing all four paws into that arm. The test arena was wiped with a damp cloth after each trial. The number of entries into the open and closed arms and the time spent in open arms were measured in the offline condition. Anxiolytic activity was indicated with increase of time spent in open arms or with

number of open arms entries while anxiogenic effects are characterized with decrease of these measures.

For the purpose of analysis, open-arm activity was quantified as the amount of time that the rat spent in the open arms relative to the total amount of time spent in open arm (open/total $\times$ 100), and the number of entries into the open arms was quantified relative to the total number of entries into open arm (open/total $\times$ 100) [17].

Statistics

The data are expressed as mean ± S.E.M. The statistical analyses were performed using one-way analyses of variance (ANOVA). Post-hoc comparison of means was carried out with the Tukey's test for multiple comparisons, when appropriate. All data were analyzed using the General Linear Models Procedure of SPSS ver.16 (SPSS Inc., Chicago, IL, USA). The confidence limit of P <0.05 was considered as statistically significant.

Results and discussion
Chemistry

Our synthetic route to target compounds **4a-4g** (Table 1) is shown in Scheme 1. The key intermediate 2-(benzhydrylthio) acetic acid **2** was prepared from benzhydrol and thioglycolic acid in trifluoroacetic acid (TFA). 1-Ethyl-3-(3-dimethylaminopropyl) carbodiimide (EDC) was treated with 2-(benzhydrylthio) acetic acid **2** in the presence of hydroxybenzotriazole (HOBt) and stirred for 30 min in acetonitrile. Then, appropriate amine derivative was added and stirring was continued overnight. Thereafter the mixture was washed sequentially with %5 NaHCO$_3$ and saturated NaCl solutions, and then dried over Na$_2$SO$_4$. Removal of the solvent under reduced pressure afforded the amide derivatives **3a-3g**. The obtained amide derivatives **3a-3g** were gently oxidized by H$_2$O$_2$ to form the corresponding sulfoxide derivatives **4a-4g** (Table 1) and analyzed by ^{1}H NMR, infrared, mass spectroscopy and melting point.

^{1}H NMR spectrum of intermediate **2** showed the benzylic hydrogen was more deshielded (5.50 ppm) than benzylic hydrogen of benzhydrol. Based on ^{1}H NMR analysis of intermediates **3a-3g**, the corresponding signals of protons CH benzylic, methylene group adjacent to carbonyl substituent, and NH were appeared within 5.0-5.2 ppm as a singlet, 3.2-3.5 ppm as a singlet, 8.40-8.65 ppm as a broad singlet respectively. Broad singlet peak of the NH proton is a good sign for formation of the amidic bond in this series. The aromatic hydrogens of the phenyl rings are generally appeared in the range between 7.0-8.0 ppm. The ^{1}H NMR spectra of compounds **4a-4g** corresponding to the methylene group between carbonyl and sulfoxide substituents showed a doublet of doublet splitting pattern. This behavior is due to existence of two diastereotopic hydrogens of the

Table 1 Effects of *N*-aryl derivatives of modafinil on behavior of albino mice in the elevated plus-maze

Compound	Open arms entries (O.E)	Open arms time spend (O.T)	Close arms entries (C.E)	Close arms time spend (C.T)
Modafinil	8.25(2.17)	71.7(10.5)	11.75(3.88)	228.2(10.5)
4a	1.00(1.00)[a]	1.5(1.5)[aab]	8.00(3.82)	221.2(23.8)[aa]
4b	7.25(1.25)	84.5(19.3)	6.25(0.47)	215.5(19.3)
4c	0.00(0.00)[aab]	0.0(0.0)[aab]	2.00(0.00)	285.0(6.4)[aa]
4d	3.50(1.50)	57.5(17.5)	4.50(1.50)	242.5(17.5)
4e	0.00(0.00)[a]	0.0(0.0)[aa]	1.50(0.50)	300.0(0.0)[aa]
4f	6.00(1.00)	120.0(10.0)	6.50(1.50)	180.0(10.0)
4g	2.50(1.190)[a]	16.75(10.0)[aa]	8.25(2.59)	216.2(26.7)[aa]
Control	12.25(2.86)	123.5(19.5)	10.50(3.92)	175.5(19.1)

Data are presented as mean ± S.E.M.
[a]$P < 0.05$ *vs.* control group, [aa]$P < 0.001$ *vs.* control group, [b]$P < 0.05$ *vs.* modafinil group.

methylene group. In addition, mass spectrometry analysis of the synthesized compounds **4a-4g** showed expectable fragmentation and hence established the structure of modafinil derivatives. Potassium bromide (KBr) disk was used to obtain the infra red (IR) spectrum related to each compound. The peak related to the carbonyl group appeared in <1700 cm^{-1} is a sign of the amidic carbonyl group in IR spectrum and it is a confirmation for the formation of the amidic moiety in these compounds.

Psychobiological activity
LORR
For comparability of data, we had to use same doses of derivatives. Based on previous study [10], 100 mg/kg of modafinil could be a suitable dose. In this dose, some analogs like **4c** made mice subconscious after i.p. administration of phenobarbital. On the other hand, some mice which received compound **4a**, died. This may be due to more sedative activity of this analog.

In comparison with control animals, compound **4a** significantly increased phenobarbital-induced LORR while other compounds demonstrated a decrease in the duration of LORR.

The experiment showed that compound **4c** was the best CNS stimulant among our synthetic derivatives however it was a slightly weaker than modafinil. Stimulant activity of used compounds is ranged in the following order:

Modafinil > **4c** > **4g** > **4d** > **4f** > **4b** > **4e** > DMSO (control) > **4a**

OFT
The results of the duration of active exploration in the OFT are presented in Figure 2. Mean square crossing of compound **4c**, **4d** and **4f** did not show significant differences when compared to the respective control and modafinil groups. Compound **4a**, **4b** and **4g** were recognized to significantly reduce square crossing compared

to control (**4a**, **4g**: p < 0.05, **4b**: p < 0.001). Furthermore, the square crossing of compounds **4a**, **4b**, **4e** and **4g** were significantly decreased compared to modafinil (**4a**, **4b** and **4g**: P < 0.001, #5: P < 0.05, respectively).

The results in Figure 3 showed that all compounds except compound **4f** failed to reach the statistically significant level in measuring the latency to enter the central part compared to control and modafinil groups. Compound **4f** showed had a reliable decrease in the latency to enter the central part compared to the both groups (P < 0.05).

FST
The effects of derivatives and modafinil on IT during trials were depicted in Figure 4. The control animals showed 45 ± 3 sec immobility duration during FST. Compounds **4a** and **4e** increased IT and showed considerable differences when compared to the respective control groups (P < 0.001). Compound **4g** also lengthened IT in comparison to control (P < 0.05). In addition,

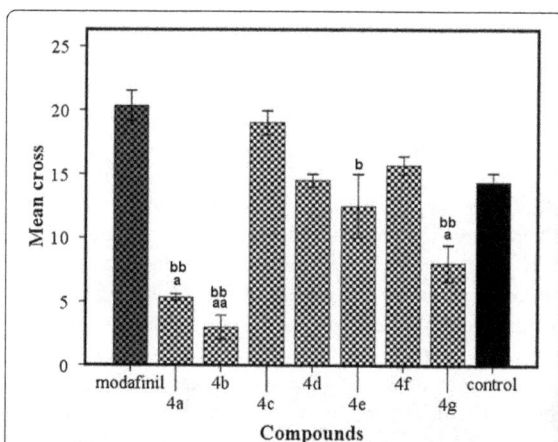

Figure 2 Exploratory activity (mean ± S.E.M.) in albino mice in the open field test. [a]$P < 0.05$, [aa]$P < .001$ *vs.* control and [b]$P < 0.05$, [bb]$P < 0.001$ *vs.* modafinil groups.

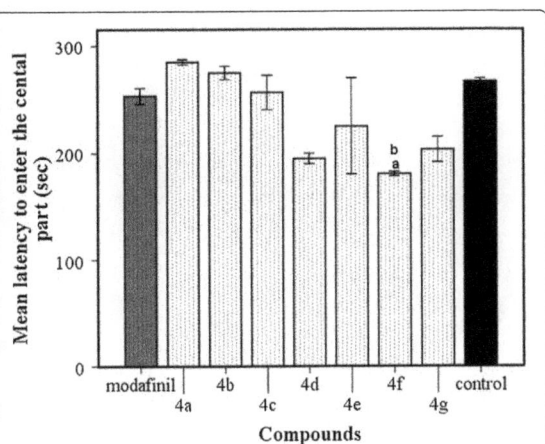

Figure 3 Effects of different derivatives in open field test in mice. Data are expressed as mean ± SEM of the latency to enter the central part. [a]P < 0.05 vs. control, [b]P < 0.05 vs. modafinil.

compounds **4a**, **4e**, **4g** and control showed a significant increase in IT compared to modafinil group (P < 0.001).

The rest of the compounds significantly decreased IT in comparison to control (P < 0.001).

EPM

Mice exposed to compounds **4a**, **4c**, **4e** and **4g** showed decline in open arms entries and open arms spent time in comparison to control mice (P < 0.05). However, modafinil, compounds **4b**, **4d** and control (DMSO) showed similar results (P > 0.05). (See Table 1.)

The percent of close arms entries revealed that all derivatives showed a non-significantly decrease in this parameter compared to those of control and modafinil groups.

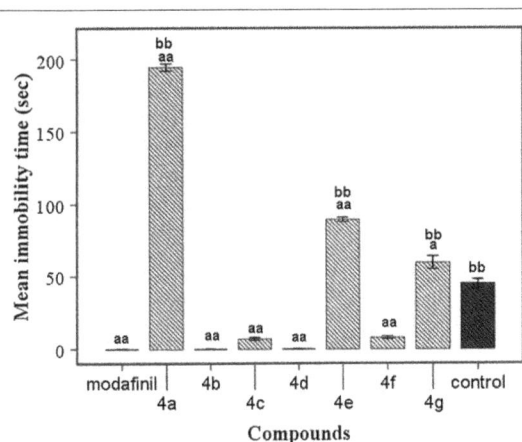

Figure 4 Effect of different derivatives of modafinil on the immobility response in forced swimming test ([a]P < .05, [aa]P < .001 vs. control and [bb]P < 0.001 vs. modafinil groups).

Compound **4a**, **4c**, **4e** and **4g** produced a reliable increase of close time spend (P < 0.05) than control group.

Conclusions

We have described a novel series of modafinil analogs (**4a-4g**) that displayed some kind of CNS activities. From our psychobiological results, compounds **4a**, **4c**, **4e** and **4g** decreased frequencies of open arms entries and duration of open arms spent times, suggesting an anxiogenic-like effect and as well as these derivatives increased close arms time significantly. Compounds **4a**, **4e** and **4g** also lengthened IT in FST, indicating that the derivatives exerted a depressive action, while other derivatives shortened IT and would be considered to have antidepressant effects. The square crossing numbers of compounds **4a**, **4b** and **4g** showed a significant reduction compared to modafinil and control groups which suggest this compound may be putative sedative. Compound **4f** induced an anxiolytic-like effect because it decreased the latency to enter the central part compared to other derivatives. The results of EPM also roughly confirmed the anxiolytic-like effect of compound **4f**. Based on LORR test, it is evident that most of the analogs exhibited stimulant activity in LORR test and compound **4c** is the most potent ones. Only compound **4a** (aniline substitution) was recognized as sedative analog. Finally, little discrepancies among results obtained from different psychobiological tests in this study may be related to the different mechanisms of actions of these derivatives and future studies are highly requested to exploit the structure-function relationships of these derivatives in more details.

Competing interests
The authors declare that they have no competing interests.

Authors' contributions
AL: Synthesis of target compounds and performing the biological tests. IK: supervision of the psychobiological part. HA: collaboration in identifying of the structures of target compounds and manuscript preparation. AA: collaboration in identification of synthesized compounds. LF: collaboration in synthesis of target compound and manuscript preparation. AF: Design of target compounds and supervision of the synthetic part. All authors read and approved the final manuscript.

Author details
[1]Students Research Committee, Faculty of Pharmacy, Kermanshah University of Medical Sciences, Kermanshah, Iran. [2]Laboratory of Molecular and Cellular Biology, School of Veterinary Medicine, Razi University, Kermanshah, Iran. [3]Novel Drug Delivery Research Center, Faculty of Pharmacy, Kermanshah University of Medical Sciences, Kermanshah, Iran. [4]Drug Design and Development Research Center, Tehran University of Medical Sciences, Tehran, Iran. [5]Neuroscience Research Center, Institute of Neuropharmacology, Kerman University of Medical Sciences, Kerman, Iran.

References
1.   Hublin C: Narcolepsy: current drug treatment options. *CNS Drugs* 1996, 5:426–436.

2. U.S. Modafinil in Narcolepsy Multicenter Study Group: **Randomized trial of modafinil as a treatment for excessive daytime somnolence of narcolepsy.** *Neurology* 2000, **54**:1166–1175.
3. Thorpy M: **Therapeutic advances in narcolepsy.** *Sleep Med* 2007, **8**:427–440.
4. Mitler MM, Harsh J, Hirshkowitz M, Guilleminaultd C: **Long-term efficacy and safety of modafinil (PROVIGIL) for the treatment of excessive daytime sleepiness associated with narcolepsy.** *Sleep Med* 2000, **1**:231–243.
5. Willie JT, Renthal W, Chemelli RM, Miller MS, Scammell TE, Yanagisawa M, *et al*: **Modafinil more effectively induces wakefulness in orexin-null mice than in wild-type littermates.** *Neuroscience* 2005, **130**:983–995.
6. Mehrjerdi ZA: **Crystal in Iran: methamphetamine or heroin kerack.** *Daru* 2013, **15**:21–22.
7. De Risi C, Ferraro L, Pollini GP, Tanganelli S, Valente F, Veronese AC: **Efficient synthesis and biological evaluation of two modafinil analogs.** *Bioorg Med Chem* 2008, **16**:9904–9910.
8. Prisinzano T, Podobinski J, Tidgewell K, Luo M, Swenson D: **Synthesis and determination of the absolute configuration of the enantiomers of modafinil.** *Tetrahedron* 2004, **15**:1053–1058.
9. Aliabadi A, Shamsa F, Ostad SN, Emami S, Shafiee A, Davoodi J, *et al*: **Synthesis and biological evaluation of 2-Phenylthiazole-4-carboxamide derivatives as anticancer agents.** *Eur J Med Chem* 2010, **11**:5384–5389.
10. Chatterjie N, Stables JP, Wang H, Alexander GJ: **Anti-narcoleptic agent modafinil and its sulfone: a novel facile synthesis and potential anti-epileptic activity.** *Neurochem Res* 2004, **29**:1481–1486.
11. Cao J, Prisinzano TE, Okunola OM, Kopajtic T, Shook M, *et al*: **SARs at the monoamine transporters for a novel series of modafinil analogues.** *ACS Med Chem Lett* 2011, **2**:48–52.
12. Yadav AV, Nade VS: **Anti-dopaminergic effect of the methanolic extract of Morus alba L. leaves.** *Indian J Pharmacol* 2008, **40**:221–226.
13. Wu CF, Zhang HL, Liu W: **Potentiation of ethanol-induced loss of the righting reflex by ascorbic acid in mice: interaction with dopamine antagonists.** *Pharmacol Biochem Behav* 2000, **66**:413–418.
14. Lalonde R, Strazielle C: **The relation between open-field and emergence tests in a hyperactive mouse model.** *Neuropharmacology* 2009, **57**:722–724.
15. Ferigolo M, Barros H, Marquadt A, Tannhauser M: **Comparison of behavioral effects of moclobemide and deprenyl during forced swimming.** *Pharmacol Biochem Behav* 1998, **60**:431–437.
16. Enríquez-Castillo A, Alamilla J, Barral J, Gourbière S, Flores-Serrano AG, *et al*: **Differential effects of caffeine on the antidepressant-like effect of ami-triptyline in female rat subpopulations with low and high immobility in the forced swimming test.** *Physiol Behav* 2008, **94**:501–509.
17. Miraghaee S, Karimi I, Becker LA: **Psychobiological assessment of smoke of agarwood (Aquilaria spp.) in male rats.** *J Appl Biol Sci* 2011, **5**:45–53.

15

Preparation, characterization and *in vitro* efficacy of magnetic nanoliposomes containing the artemisinin and transferrin

Amir Gharib[1*], Zohreh Faezizadeh[1], Seyed Ali Reza Mesbah-Namin[2] and Ramin Saravani[3]

Abstract

Background: Artemisinin is the major sesquiterpene lactones in sweet wormwood (*Artemisia annua* L.), and its combination with transferrin exhibits versatile anti-cancer activities. Their non-selective targeting for cancer cells, however, limits their application. The aim of this study was to prepare the artemisinin and transferrin-loaded magnetic nanoliposomes in thermosensitive and non-thermosensitive forms and evaluate their antiproliferative activity against MCF-7 and MDA-MB-231 cells for better tumor-targeted therapy.

Methods: Artemisinin and transferrin-loaded magnetic nanoliposomes was prepared by extrusion method using various concentrations of lipids. These formulations were characterized for particle size, zeta potential, polydispersity index and shape morphology. The artemisinin and transferrin-loading efficiencies were determined using HPLC. The content of magnetic iron oxide in the nanoliposomes was analysed by spectrophotometry. The in vitro release of artemisinin, transferrin and magnetic iron oxide from vesicles was assessed by keeping of the nanoliposomes at 37°C for 12 h. The in vitro cytotoxicity of prepared nanoliposomes was investigated against MCF-7 and MDA-MB-231 cells using MTT assay.

Results: The entrapment efficiencies of artemisinin, transferrin and magnetic iron oxide in the non-thermosensitive nanoliposomes were 89.11% ± 0.23, 85.09% ± 0.31 and 78.10% ± 0.24, respectively. Moreover, the thermosensitive formulation showed a suitable condition for thermal drug release at 42°C and exhibited high antiproliferative activity against MCF-7 and MDA-MB-231 cells in the presence of a magnetic field.

Conclusions: Our results showed that the thermosensitive artemisinin and transferrin-loaded magnetic nanoliposomes would be an effective choice for tumor-targeted therapy, due to its suitable stability and high effectiveness.

Keywords: Artemisinin, Transferrin, Liposome, MCF-7 cells, *In vitro*

Background

Artemisinin is the major sesquiterpene lactones in sweet wormwood (*Artemisia annua* L.), and it possesses a range of medicinal properties including anti-malaria and anti-cancer activities [1]. This compound has an endoperoxide bridge in its structure. When in contact with high iron concentrations, the molecule releases reactive oxygen species [2]. It has been documented that cancer cells need high iron levels to proliferate; hence cancer cells typically absorb a significantly larger amount of transferrin than normal cells and were more susceptible to artemisinin cytotoxicity [3]. However, the insolubility of artemisinin in the water and its non-selective targeting towards cancer cells could limit its use [4]. Later studies demonstrated that the encapsulation of artemisinin in drug delivery systems and covalently tagging artemisinin to transferrin could partly resolve the aforementioned problems, but it could not resolve the specific targeting of tumors [2,5]. In this case, other options such as preparing of magnetic nanoliposomes containing artemisinin and transferrin can be considered.

Magnetic liposomes are spherical and colloidal vesicles entrapping magnetic iron oxide (Fe_3O_4) and may range from tens of nanometers to several micrometers in

* Correspondence: amirgharib@gmail.com
[1]Department of Laboratory Sciences, Borujerd Branch, Islamic Azad University, Borujerd, Iran
Full list of author information is available at the end of the article

diameter [6]. Magnetic liposomes loaded with magnetic iron oxide were used as an important drug delivery system, because they can transport drugs to the therapeutic site for cancer treatment [7]. These carriers could congregate around the magnetic site and act as "intelligent" drug delivery systems [8]. Moreover, magnetic liposomes have multi-functionality applications such as image contrasting in magnetic resonance imaging (MRI) and hyperthermia cancer therapy [9].

We speculate that encapsulation of artemisinin and transferrin in magnetic nanoliposomes could increase the artemisinin and transferrin stability, whilst improving selective targeting towards cancerous tumors trough magnetic attraction and thermosensivity. The ability of co-encapsulation of artemisinin and transferrin in magnetic nanoliposomes has not yet been studied. The primary objective of this study was to prepare the thermosensitive and non-thermosensitive magnetic nanoliposomes containing artemisinin and transferrin and evaluate their physicochemical properties. A secondary objective was to investigate cytotoxicity of prepared nanoliposomes against MCF-7 and MDA-MB-231 cells using MTT assay.

Methods
Chemicals
Artemisinin (purity $\geq$ 98%), soy phosphatidylcholine (SPC), distearoyl phosphatidylcholine (DSPC), dipalmitoyl phosphatidylcholine (DPPC), cholesterol (CHOL), magnetic iron oxide, tamoxifen (an anti-cancer drug, as the positive control, purity $\geq$ 99%) and human transferrin (partially iron saturated, purity $\geq$ 98%) were obtained from Sigma (USA). Acetonitrile and ammonium sulphate were purchased from Merck (Germany). Alpha-modified Eagle's medium (aMEM) and fetal bovine serum (FBS) were obtained from Gibco (USA).

Cell culture
MCF-7 (NCBI C135) and MDA-MB-231 (ATCC HTB-26) breast cancer cell lines were purchased from National Cell Bank of Iran (Pasteur Institute, Tehran, Iran) and cultured as described previously [10]. In brief, cells were maintained in α-modified Eagle's medium supplemented with 10% FBS, 1% penicillin/streptomycin, 1 mM sodium pyruvate and 100 mM non-essential amino acids at 37°C and a 5% CO_2 environment.

Preparation of nanoliposomes
To preparation of artemisinin and transferrin-loaded magnetic nanoliposomes with thermosensitive and non-thermosensitive properties, the SPC, DSPC, DPPC and CHOL with different molar ratios (Table 1) were dissolved in chloroform and thoroughly dried on a rotary evaporator (Brinkman, Toronto, Canada) under vacuum and N_2 flow at 30°C. The dried lipids were dispersed by

Table 1 Lipid composition of magnetic nanoliposomes

Type of magnetic nanoliposomes	Lipids	Molar ratio of lipids* (µmols/mL)
Non-thermosensetive	SPC:CHOL	30:6
Thermosensetive	DPPC:DSPC:CHOL	26:4:6

agitation in 6 mL of PBS-ethanol solution (v:v/5:1, pH = 7.4) containing artemisinin (12 mg), transferrin (12 mg) and magnetic iron oxide (12 mg) and then sonicated at 4°C in ultrasonic bath (Braun-sonic 2000, Burlingame, USA). Finally, artemisinin and transferrin-loaded magnetic nanoliposomes were obtained by extruding the respective suspension through a polycarbonate membrane with 100 nm-sized pores 12 times, and separating the excess artemisinin, transferrin and larger lipid aggregation by ultracentrifugation (100000 g, 30 min). Moreover, the non-trapped magnetic iron oxide was separated by a previously described method [11]. The control magnetic nanoliposomes were prepared similarly, but PBS (pH, 7.4) was used instead of the artemisinin and transferrin solutions. Before the preparation of nanoliposomes, the phase transition temperatures of used phospholipids were tested by a differential scanning calorimetric (DSC) method, as reported previously [12].

Physiochemical characterization of nanoliposomes
Determination of encapsulation efficacy
The content of the artemisinin and transferrin in the nanoliposomes were determined by HPLC method following dissolution in 0.1% Triton X-100.

To determination of artemisinin, the 20 µL of nanoliposomal lysate was injected into the HPLC column. In the HPLC analysis, a C18 column (3.9 mm × 150 mm, 5 µm, Waters Co., Milford, USA) and diode array UV detector was used. The mobile phase was 2:1 (v:v) acetonitrile: water at a flow rate of 1 mL/min. The calibration curve was produced by diluting artemisinin stock solution in the mobile phase. To determination of transferrin, the 25 µL of nanoliposomal lysate was injected into a Polypropyl A HPLC column (PolyLC Inc., MD, USA). The column was eluted with a linear salt gradient from 2 M ammonium sulfate (pH 6.5) to 0.1 M potassium phosphate (pH 6.5) at a flow rate of 1 mL/min. The HPLC system was equipped with UV–vis detector (280 nm). The transferrin calibration curve was created by diluting its stock solution with mobile phase.

The content of magnetic iron oxide was determined using previously reported methods [13], with some modification. In brief, the magnetic iron oxide nanoparticles were separated using centrifugation after lyses of nanoliposomes. The precipitate was then dissolved in 0.1 N HCl solution under stirring and a 5 mL of the supernatant was dissolved in the 750 µL of sulfosalicylic acid dihydrate solution 10% (w/v). Subsequently, 750 μL of ammonia solution 25% (w/v) was added to the solution and was analysed by using spectra for the total iron complex at 425 nm. The absorbance of the diluted sample obtained from the magnetic iron oxide stock solution was used for standard curve preparation. Finally, the percentage of artemisinin, transferrin and magnetic iron oxide loading were then calculated as:

The amount of artemisinin or transferrin or magnetic iron oxide in nanoliposome × total volume tested × 100 / Total sample volume × Initial amount of artemisinin or transferrin or magnetic iron oxide.

Particle size, zeta-potential and polydispersity index determination

The mean particle size, zeta-potential and polydispersity index of the magnetic nanoliposomes were determined using Malvern zetasizer (Malvern instrument, Worcestershire, UK) apparatus, as reported previously [14]. Each experiment was done in triplicate.

Shape, surface morphology and magnetic properties

The size and structure of the thermosensitive and non-thermosensitive magnetic nanoliposomes that contained artemisinin and transferrin were analysed by cryo-transmission electron microscopy (cryo-TEM), as described previously [15]. Briefly, a grid was immersed in the nanoliposomal sample reservoirs at room temperature, blotted with blotting paper, drew the sample into the grid and vitrified in liquid ethane. Subsequently, the sample was transferred to liquid nitrogen for storage. Digital imaging was performed at 200 kV in a stage cooled by liquid nitrogen. Finally, size analysis was performed using ImageJ software (NIH, Bethesda, MD, USA). The magnetic properties of prepared nanoliposomes were measured using a vibrating sample magnetometer (Meghnatis Daghigh Kavir Co., Iran), as described previously [16].

In vitro release study, thermosensitive behaviors and size stability

To determination of artemisinin, transferrin and magnetic iron oxide released from the nanoliposomes, a cellulose membrane (molecular weight cut-off of 8000 kDa, Membrane Filtration Products, USA) was mounted between the donor and receptor compartments. The donor medium consisted of 1 mL of each magnetic nanoliposomal formulation. The receptor medium consisted of 10 mL of citrate-phosphate buffer (0.1 M, pH 7.4). During the dialysis, the temperature was kept at 37°C. At pre-determined time intervals, between 2 to 12 hours, the amount of the released artemisinin, transferrin and magnetic iron oxide were then determined by the above described methods. To confirm whether the prepared nanoliposomes exhibit a thermal sensitivity, their stability in 42°C for 4 h was

investigated. The size stability of artemisinin and transferrin-loaded magnetic nanoliposomes was assessed by measuring the particle sizes after 1 month storage at 4°C.

In vitro efficacy

In vitro selective targeting of MCF-7 and MDA-MB-231 cell lines by prepared magnetic nanoliposomes was performed using previously reported methods [17], with some modification. Briefly, 100 μL of the MCF-7 and MDA-MB-231 cells (3×10^4 cells/mL) was added into each well of a 96-well plate and allowed the cells to attach. In the absence or presence of a magnet, the proliferation of cells in the presence of different concentration of free and encapsulated artemisinin, transferrin and magnetic iron oxide for 12, 24, and 48 h was evaluated. Tamoxifen (7.43 μg/mL) was used as a positive control.

In order to evaluate the antiproliferative effects of free and encapsulated artemisinin, transferrin and magnetic iron oxide on MCF-7 and MDA-MB-231 cell lines in the presence of a magnetic field, a magnet (127.8 × 85.6 × 7 mm) was added to below the 96-well plate (with 24-well plate in between), and then the incubation was done.

At the end of the treatment, cells proliferation was analysed by 3-(4, 5-dimethylthiazol-2-yl)-2,5-diphenyl tetrazolium bromide (MTT) assay. In brief, 20 μL of MTT (5 mg/mL in PBS) was added to each well and samples were incubated for 4 h at 37°C. The MTT solution was removed, and 200 μL DMSO was added into each well to dissolve the precipitate. Then, optical density of the wells was measured at 570 nm.

Data analysis

All data were expressed as means ± standard deviation (SD). The analysis of variance was performed to determine the significance level among the tested groups. The P values less than 0.05 were considered statistically significant.

Results

The encapsulation efficacies of artemisinin, transferrin and magnetic iron oxide in the thermosensitive magnetic nanoliposomes were 83.06% ± 0.53, 80.12% ± 0.12 and 66.14% ± 0.42, respectively. Moreover, the encapsulation efficacies of artemisinin, transferrin and magnetic iron oxide in the non-thermosensitive nanoliposomes were 89.11% ± 0.23, 85.09% ± 0.31 and 78.10% ± 0.24, respectively.

Our results showed that the phase transition temperature of DPPC (as the main phospholipid of thermosensitive nanoliposomes) was lower than SPC (Figure 1).

The particle size, zeta-potential and polydispersity index of the non-thermosensetive nanoliposomes were 99.12 ± 0.11, −1.25 ± 0.23 and 0.21 ± 0.05, respectively. Likewise, the particle size, zeta-potential and polydispersity index

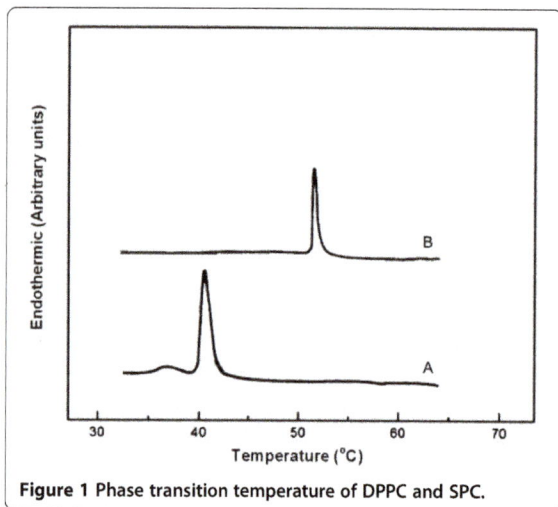

Figure 1 Phase transition temperature of DPPC and SPC.

of the thermosensetive nanoliposomes were 95.06 ± 0.15, −1.40 ± 0.22 and 0.19 ± 0.09, respectively.

Cryo-TEM analysis showed that the nanovesicles have a fine spherical shape and rough surface with a relatively monodispersed size distribution confirming the size distribution measurement studies (Figure 2).

The saturation magnetizations for thermosensitive and non-thermosensitive nanoliposomes were 30.5 and 35.7 electromagnetic unit per gram (emu/g), respectively. In addition, there was no hysteresis in the magnetization with both remanence and coercivity, indicating that these magnetic nanoliposomes were superparamagnetic.

The released amount of artemisinin, transferrin and magnetic iron oxide at 37°C from each nanoliposomal formulation were plotted as a function of time (Figure 3). The percentages of the artemisinin, transferrin and magnetic iron oxide recoveries for the thermosensitivity nanoliposomes after 12 h were 75.3% ± 2.1, 81.5% ± 2.3 and 91.1% ± 1.4, respectively (Figure 3A).

The incubation was conducted at 42°C for 4 h to determine the extent of spontaneous and nanoliposomal-mediated artemisinin, transferrin and magnetic iron oxide released from the prepared nanoliposomes (Figure 4). The

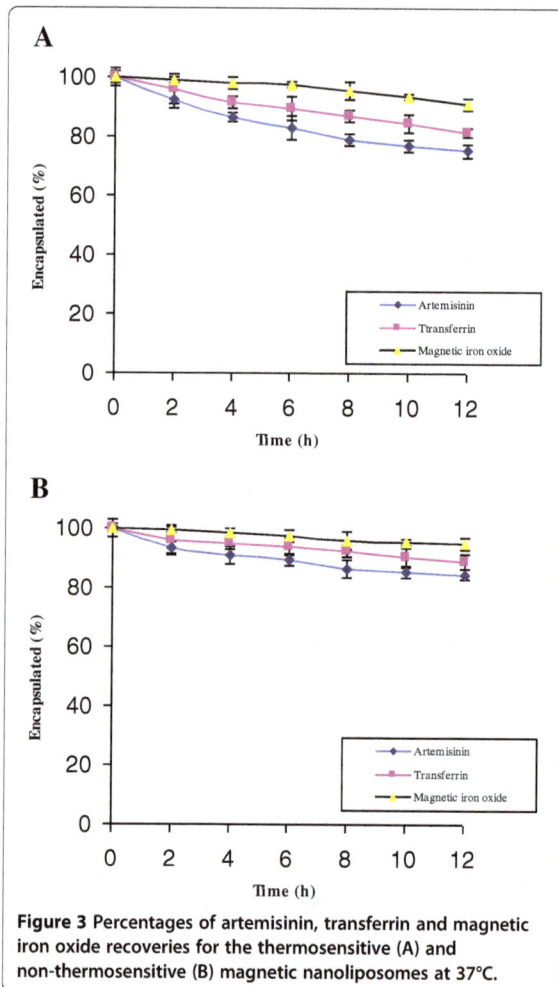

Figure 3 Percentages of artemisinin, transferrin and magnetic iron oxide recoveries for the thermosensitive (A) and non-thermosensitive (B) magnetic nanoliposomes at 37°C.

results showed an approximately 2-fold increase in artemisinin release from thermosensitivity nanoliposomes after 4 h at 42°C (Figure 4A).

The physical stability of prepared nanoliposomes was evaluated by comparing different changes in mean diameters during their storage. Two formulations have minor size changes within 60 days storage at 4°C in PBS, so that the mean diameter of thermosensitive and non-thermosensitive nanoliposomes was 98.25 ± 0.14 and 106.20 ± 0.12 nm, respectively.

In the presence or absence of an external magnetic field, the effect of the combination of artemisinin, transferrin and magnetic iron oxide in the free and encapsulated forms on MCF-7 and MDA-MB-231 cellular growth were examined by MTT assay. The results showed that the cell proliferation was inhibited in the MCF-7 and MDA-MB-231 cells in a dose- and time-dependent manner (Figure 5). Under identical conditions, the viability ratios of treated MCF-7 cells were lower than MDA-MB-231 cells. In all

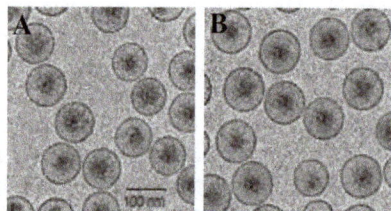

Figure 2 Cryo-transmission electron micrographs of the thermosensitive (A), and non-thermosensitive (B) magnetic nanoliposomes loaded with artemisinin and transferrin.

A

B

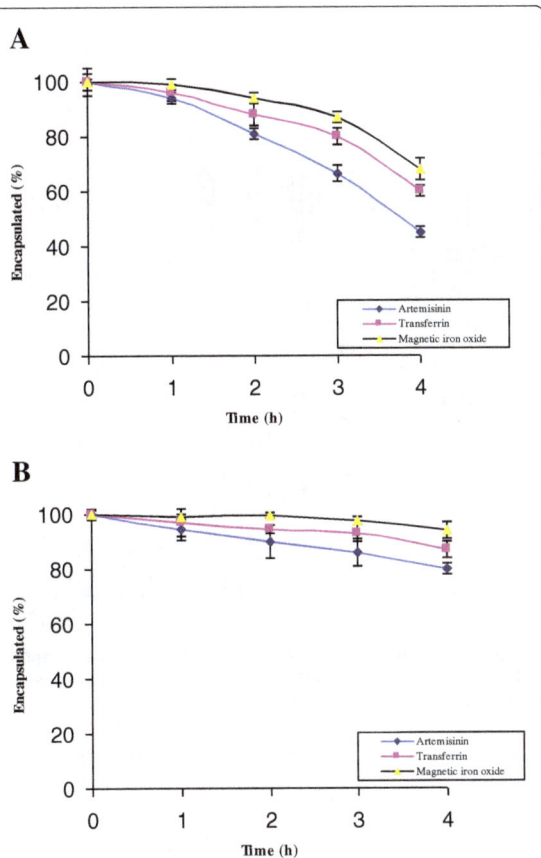

Figure 4 Percentages of artemisinin, transferrin and magnetic iron oxide recoveries for the thermosensitive (A) and non-thermosensitive (B) magnetic nanoliposomes at 42°C.

that the magnetic nanoliposomes that contained doxorubicin or adriamycin were tailored to target cancer cells, and the application of a magnetic field could increase drug concentration in the tumors [22,23].

Artemisinin is a sesquiterpene lactone and phytochemical found naturally in *Artemisia annua* L. [1]. Evidence for artemisinin's benefit was strongest for anti-malaria, anti-oxidative, anti-inflammatory, and anti-cancer effects [2,5]. It is reported that the anti-cancer effect of artemisinin in the presence of iron sources such as transferrin was increased several fold [3].

In this study, we evaluated the potential of incorporating artemisinin and transferrin into magnetic nanoliposomes. We found that the encapsulation efficiencies of artemisinin and transferrin in the thermosensitivity nanoliposomes were suitable. According to the literature, this result was related to some condition, such as liposomal lipid content [24].

The liposomal particle size is highly dependent on the molar ratio of membrane lipids [25]. Our results showed that the increasing of the DPPC molar ratio could reduce the size of prepared nanoliposomes. Previous researches showed that the DPPC have excellent biocompatibility to form small nanoliposomes due to the ratio of head group size compared to hydrocarbon tail [26].

In this research, we found that the thermosensitive artemisinin and transferrin-loaded magnetic nanoliposomes produced a greater reduction in the proliferation of MCF-7 and MDA-MB-231 cells. This finding is in accordance with previous studies showing that the size of magnetic nanoliposomes is an important factor for their *in vitro* and *in vivo* distributions, pharmacodynamics and effectiveness [27].

The polydispersity index is an important indicator of the physical stability of nanoliposomes. The polydispersity index values between 0.1 and 0.25 indicate acceptable uniformity, while values >0.5 are indicative of poor uniformity [28].

Our results showed that the thermosensitive magnetic nanoliposomes have an acceptable polydispersity index, size homogeneity as well as the stability in pH 7.4 citrate-phosphate buffers within 12 h at 37°C. Therefore, in accordance with previous reports the best prepared thermosensitive magnetic nanoliposomes not only have an appropriate particle size and stability for cancer therapy but also have an appropriate size for use as a targeted therapeutic agent [29].

According to the literature, the change in the physicochemical properties of nanoparticles could alter their biokinetics parameters such as their toxicity and bioavailability [30].

Our study showed that the thermosensitive magnetic nanoliposomes have a more negative charge than another formulation. It has been reported that the interactions

conditions, the artemisinin and transferrin-loaded magnetic nanoliposomes were more effective than those of free artemisinin, transferrin and magnetic iron oxide on MCF-7 and MDA-MB-231 cellular growth. As shown in Figure 5 C1 and C2, in the presence of magnetic field, the extent of inhibition increased significantly at 12 h with the lowest concentration of artemisinin, transferrin and magnetic iron oxide in the free and encapsulated forms which was continued to rise up, with 24 and 48 h durations at their maximum concentration.

Discussion

The use of plant derived-loaded nanoliposomes for cancer therapy has been widely investigated [18,19]. The main problem associated with the application of such liposomal formulations is insufficient delivery to the target site [20]. As an interesting approach to drug delivery research, magnetic iron oxides were incorporated into nanoliposomes under the action of a magnetic field could overcome this limitation [21]. It is documented

---

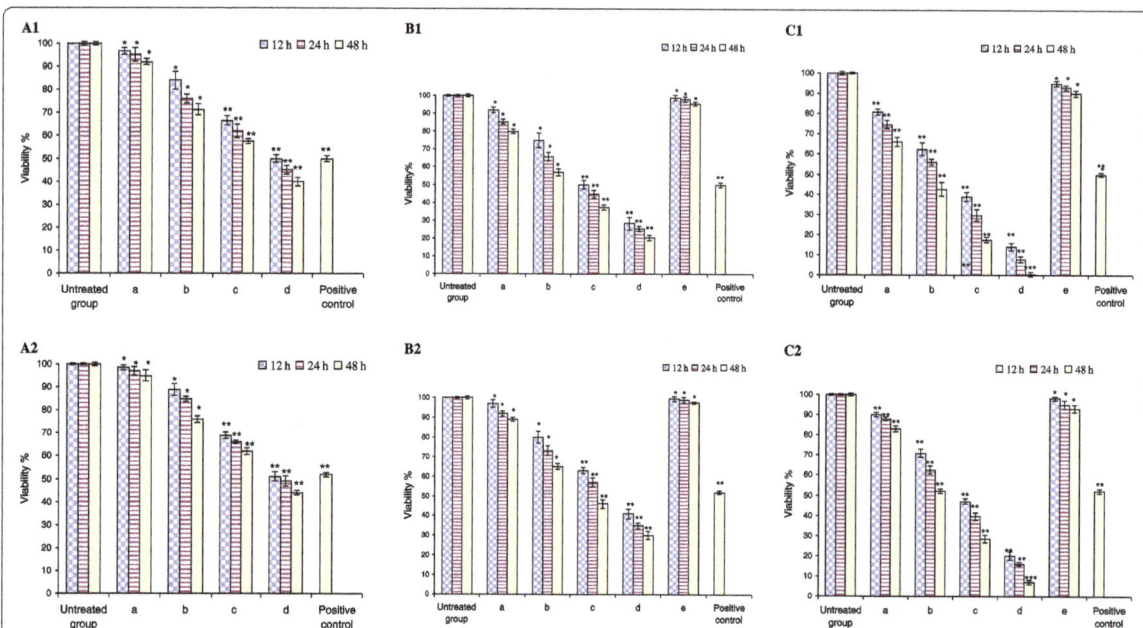

Figure 5 Dose- and time-dependent inhibition of MCF-7 and MDA-MB-231 cellular growth by the combined free artemisinin, transferrin and magnetic iron oxide in the presence of an external magnetic force (A1 and A2), and by the thermosensitive artemisinin and transferrin-loaded magnetic nanoliposomes without (B1 and B2), and with (C1 and C2) an external magnetic force. (a: Contained 12.50 µg/mL (44.27 µM) artemisinin, 12.80 µg/mL (0.16 µM) transferrin and 9.93 µg/mL (42.88 µM) magnetic iron oxide; **b**: 2 × **a**; **c**: 4 × **a**; **d**: 8 × **a**; **e**: control magnetic nanoliposones contained 9.93 µg/mL magnetic iron oxide). As a positive control, the tamoxifen (7.43 µg/mL, 20 µM) was used. Data were expressed as mean ± standard deviation from three independent experiments (*$p < 0.05$, **$p < 0.01$ and ***$p < 0.001$).

between the magnetic nanoliposomes and the some human cells such as capillary endothelium are zeta potential dependent [31]. Therefore, it revealed that the thermosensitive magnetic nanoliposomes would have a better potency for targeted therapy.

We found that the application of an external magnetic force could increase MCF-7 and MDA-MB-231 cellular death by artemisinin and transferrin. An approximately 12 h application of magnetic force elicits the maximum antiproliferation from thermosensitive magnetic nanoliposomes, as presently prepared. It was shown that the *in vitro* stability of magnetic nanoliposomes could also affect their performance [32], and our finding could explain this phenomenon. Magnetic artemisinin and transferrin-loaded nanoliposomes alone (without magnetic force) elicited higher antiproliferative activity on MCF-7 and MDA-MB-231 cells than free artemisinin, transferrin and magnetic iron oxide alone or in their combination. When nanoliposomes containing compounds were used *in vitro*, they can interact with the membranes of exposed cancer cells, and therefore decrease their viability and proliferation [33]. It is documented that the effect of the same nanoparticles on various cells is significantly different and could not be assumed for other cells [34]. Therefore, in accordance with "cell vision" effect, we noted that the prepared

nanoliposomes have antiproliferative effects on the examined cells, and their efficacy for the other cell types may be varied.

Conclusion

We have successfully prepared artemisinin and transferrin-loaded magnetic nanoliposomes in the thermosensitive and non-thermosensitive forms with acceptable uniformity, sustained release profile at 37°C and superparamagnetism. Current work demonstrated that artemisinin and transferrin-loaded magnetic nanoliposomes, in particular in the thermosensetive form have potent anti-growth effect on MCF-7 and MDA-MB-231 cells, and time-dependently inhibit cell growth in these cell lines. To the best of our knowledge, artemisinin and transferrin-loaded magnetic nanoliposomes treatment in combination with an external magnetic force resulted in an excellent decrease in proliferation of MCF-7 and MDA-MB-231 cells. Therefore, these novel formulations could be a promising approach for artemisinin and transferrin targeted cancer therapy.

Competing interests
The authors declare that they have no competing interests.

Authors' contributions
All authors have read and approved the final manuscript.

Acknowledgements
The author gratefully acknowledges financial support from the Iran National Science Foundation (INSF) under grant agreement no: 91001200.

Author details
[1]Department of Laboratory Sciences, Borujerd Branch, Islamic Azad University, Borujerd, Iran. [2]Department of Clinical Biochemistry, Faculty of Medical Sciences, Tarbiat Modares University, Tehran, Iran. [3]Department of Biochemistry, School of Medicine, Zahedan University of Medical Sciences, Zahedan, Iran.

References

1. Efferth T, Kaina B: **Toxicity of the antimalarial artemisinin and its derivatives.** *Crit Rev Toxicol* 2010, **40**:405–421.
2. Lai HC, Singh NP, Sasaki T: **Development of artemisinin compounds for cancer treatment.** *Invest New Drugs* 2012, **31**:230–246.
3. Efferth T, Benakis A, Romero MR, Tomicic M, Rauh R, Steinbach D, Häfer R, Stamminger T, Oesch F, Kaina B, Marschall M: **Enhancement of cytotoxicity of artemisinins toward cancer cells by ferrous iron.** *Free Radic Biol Med* 2004, **37**:998–1009.
4. Singh NP, Lai HC: **Artemisinin induces apoptosis in human cancer cells.** *Anticancer Res* 2004, **24**:2277–2280.
5. Nakase I, Gallis B, Takatani-Nakase T, Oh S, Lacoste E, Singh NP, Goodlett DR, Tanaka S, Futaki S, Lai H, Sasaki T: **Transferrin receptor-dependent cytotoxicity of artemisinin-transferrin conjugates on prostate cancer cells and induction of apoptosis.** *Cancer Lett* 2009, **274**:290–298.
6. Fattahi H, Laurent S, Liu F, Arsalani N, Vander Elst L, Muller RN: **Magnetoliposomes as multimodal contrast agents for molecular imaging and cancer nanotheragnostics.** *Nanomedicine (Lond)* 2011, **6**:529–544.
7. Hanuš J, Ullrich M, Dohnal J, Singh M, Stěpánek F: **Remotely controlled diffusion from magnetic liposome microgels.** *Langmuir* 2013, **29**:4381–4387.
8. Bakandritsos A, Fatourou AG, Fatouros DG: **Magnetoliposomes and their potential in the intelligent drug-delivery field.** *Ther Deliv* 2012, **3**:1469–1482.
9. Qiu D, An X: **Controllable release from magnetoliposomes by magnetic stimulation and thermal stimulation.** *Colloids Surf B Biointerfaces* 2013, **104**:326–329.
10. Tang Q, Cao B, Wu H, Cheng G: **Cholesterol-peptide hybrids to form liposome-like vesicles for gene delivery.** *PLoS One* 2013, **8**:e54460.
11. Frascione D, Diwoky C, Almer G, Opriessnig P, Vonach C, Gradauer K, Leitinger G, Mangge H, Stollberger R, Prassl R: **Ultrasmall superparamagnetic iron oxide (USPIO)-based liposomes as magnetic resonance imaging probes.** *Int J Nanomedicine* 2012, **7**:2349–2359.
12. Liu XM, Zhang Y, Chen F, Khutsishvili I, Fehringer EV, Marky LA, Bayles KW, Wang D: **Prevention of orthopedic device-associated osteomyelitis using oxacillin-containing biomineral-binding liposomes.** *Pharm Res* 2012, **29**:3169–3179.
13. Silva-Freitas EL, Carvalho JF, Pontes TR, Araújo-Neto RP, Carriço AS, Egito ES: **Magnetite content evaluation on magnetic drug delivery systems by spectrophotometry: a technical note.** *AAPS Pharm Sci Tech* 2011, **12**:521–524.
14. Rudra A, Deepa RM, Ghosh MK, Ghosh S, Mukherjee B: **Doxorubicin-loaded phosphatidylethanolamine-conjugated nanoliposomes: *in vitro* characterization and their accumulation in liver, kidneys, and lungs in rats.** *Int J Nanomedicine* 2010, **5**:811–823.
15. Bothun GD, Lelis A, Chen Y, Scully K, Anderson LE, Stoner MA: **Multicomponent folate-targeted magnetoliposomes: design, characterization, and cellular uptake.** *Nanomedicine* 2011, **7**:797–805.
16. Akbarzadeh A, Samiei M, Joo SW, Anzaby M, Hanifehpour Y, Tayefi Nasrabadi H, Davaran S: **Synthesis, characterization and *in vitro* studies of doxorubicin-loaded magnetic nanoparticles grafted to smart copolymers on A549 lung cancer cell line.** *J Nanobiotechnology* 2012, **10**:46.
17. Foy SP, Stine A, Jain KT, Labhasetwar V: **Magnetic Nanoparticles for Drug Delivery.** In *Methods in Bioengineering: Nanoscale Bioengineering and Nanomedicine*. Edited by Rege K, Medintz IL. Norwood: Artech House Publishers; 2009:123–135.
18. Thangapazham RL, Puri A, Tele S, Blumenthal R, Maheshwari RK: **Evaluation of a nanotechnology based carrier for delivery of curcumin in prostate cancer cells.** *Int J Oncol* 2008, **32**:1119–1123.
19. Podhajcer OL, Friedlander M, Graziani Y: **Effect of liposome-encapsulated quercetin on DNA synthesis, lactate production, and cyclic adenosine 3':5'-monophosphate level in Ehrlich ascites tumor cells.** *Cancer Res* 1980, **40**:1344–1350.
20. Coimbra M, Isacchi B, van Bloois L, Torano JS, Ket A, Wu X, Broere F, Metselaar JM, Rijcken CJ, Storm G, Bilia R, Schiffelers RM: **Improving solubility and chemical stability of natural compounds for medicinal use by incorporation into liposomes.** *Int J Pharm* 2011, **416**:433–442.
21. Wang ZY, Wang L, Zhang J, Li YT, Zhang DS: **A study on the preparation and characterization of plasmid DNA and drug-containing magnetic nanoliposomes for the treatment of tumors.** *Int J Nanomedicine* 2011, **6**:871–875.
22. Nobuto H, Sugita T, Kubo T, Shimose S, Yasunaga Y, Murakami T, Ochi M: **Evaluation of systemic chemotherapy with magnetic liposomal doxorubicin and a dipole external electromagnet.** *Int J Cancer* 2004, **109**:627–635.
23. Kubo T, Sugita T, Shimose S, Nitta Y, Ikuta Y, Murakami T: **Targeted systemic chemotherapy using magnetic liposomes with incorporated adriamycin for osteosarcoma in hamsters.** *Int J Oncol* 2001, **18**:121–125.
24. Gharib A, Faezizadeh Z, Mesbah-Namin SA: **In vitro and in vivo antibacterial activities of cyanidinum chloride-loaded liposomes against a resistant strain of *Pseudomonas aeruginosa*.** *Planta Med* 2013, **79**:15–19.
25. Qian S, Li C, Zuo Z: **Pharmacokinetics and disposition of various drug loaded liposomes.** *Curr Drug Metab* 2012, **13**:372–395.
26. Malmsten M, Lassen B: **Competitive protein adsorption at phospholipid surfaces.** *Colloids surfaces B: Biointerface* 1995, **4**:173–184.
27. Meledandri CJ, Ninjbadgar T, Brougham DF: **Size-controlled magnetoliposomes with tunable magnetic resonance relaxation enhancements.** *J Mater Chem* 2011, **21**:214–222.
28. Cheng M, Gao X, Wang Y, Chen H, He B, Hongzhi X, Li Y: **Synthesis of glycyrrhetinic acid-modified chitosan 5-fluorouracil nanoparticles and its inhibition of liver cancer characteristics in vitro and in vivo.** *Mar Drugs* 2013, **11**:3517–3536.
29. Mikhaylov G, Mikac U, Magaeva AA, Itin VI, Naiden EP, Psakhye I, Babes L, Reinheckel T, Peters C, Zeiser R, Bogyo M, Turk V, Psakhye SG, Turk B, Vasiljeva O: **Ferri-liposomes as an MRI-visible drug-delivery system for targeting tumours and their microenvironment.** *Nat Nanotechnol* 2011, **6**:594–602.
30. Mostafalou S, Mohammadi H, Ramazani A, Abdollahi M: **Different biokinetics of nanomedicines linking to their toxicity; an overview.** *Daru* 2013, **21**:14.
31. Paulis LE, Jacobs I, van den Akker NM, Geelen T, Molin DG, Starmans LW, Nicolay K, Strijkers GJ: **Targeting of ICAM-1 on vascular endothelium under static and shear stress conditions using a liposomal Gd-based MRI contrast agent.** *J Nanobiotechnology* 2012, **10**:25.
32. Long Q, Xiel Y, Huang Y, Wu Q, Zhang H, Xiong S, Liu Y, Chen L, Wei Y, Zhao X, Gong C: **Induction of apoptosis and inhibition of angiogenesis by PEGylated liposomal quercetin in both cisplatin-sensitive and cisplatin-resistant ovarian cancers.** *J Biomed Nanotechnol* 2013, **9**:965–975.
33. Isacchi B, Arrigucci S, Ia Marca G, Bergonzi MC, Vannucchi MG, Novelli A, Bilia AR: **Conventional and long-circulating liposomes of artemisinin: preparation, characterization, and pharmacokinetic profile in mice.** *J Liposome Res* 2011, **21**:237–244.
34. Laurent S, Burtea C, Thirifays C, Häfeli UO, Mahmoudi M: **Crucial ignored parameters on nanotoxicology: the importance of toxicity assay modifications and "cell vision".** *PLoS One* 2012, **7**:e29997.

16

Synthesis and molecular modeling of six novel monastrol analogues: evaluation of cytotoxicity and kinesin inhibitory activity against HeLa cell line

Khalil Abnous[1], Batoul Barati[2], Soghra Mehri[3], Mohammad Reza Masboghi Farimani[2], Mona Alibolandi[4], Fatemeh Mohammadpour[2], Morteza Ghandadi[2] and Farzin Hadizadeh[4*]

Abstract

Background and the purpose of the study: A common approach in cancer chemotherapy is development of drugs that interrupt the mitosis phase of cell division. Dimethylenastron is a known kinesin inhibitor. In this study, six novel dimethylenastron analogues (**4a-f**), in which 3-hydroxyphenyl substituent has been replaced with substituted benzylimidazolyl, were synthesized through Biginelli reaction.

Methods: Six novel Biginelli compounds (**4a-f**) were synthesized through one step Biginelli reaction of imidazole aldehydes (**3a-c**), dimedone and urea or thioura. In vitro cytotoxicities of prepared compounds were investigated using MTT assay. Furthermore the ELIPA kit was implemented to study inhibitory effects of synthesized compounds on ATPase activity of kinesin by measuring of organic phosphate.

Results: Our results indicated that analogue **4c** is the most toxic and analogues **4f**, **4b** and dimethylenasteron were less cytotoxic in compare with other analogues. On the other hand, analogue **4a**, **4b**, **4c** and **4e** showed stronger Kinesin inhibition as compared with analogue **4f** and dimethylenasteron. None of synthesized compounds were as potent kinesin inhibitor as Taxol. Docking analysis revealed that hydrogen bond formation and hydrophobic interactions were the key factors affecting inhibitory effects of these compounds.

Conclusion: Newly synthesized compounds were found to have moderate to good cytotoxicity against HeLa cancer cell. Our results may be helpful in further design of dihydropyrimidine as potential anticancer agents.

Keywords: Biginelli reaction, Dihydropyrimidine, Mitotic kinesin Eg5, Dimethylenastron

Background

A common approach in cancer chemotherapy is development of drugs that interrupt the mitosis phase of cell division. The mitotic spindle is an important target in cancer chemotherapy [1]. Compounds that perturb the spindle assembly checkpoint by interfering microtubule polymerization or depolymerization, arrest the cell cycle in mitosis due to prevention of the microtubule dynamics.

Nowadays, Taxol, the undisputed star, which inhibit the depolymerisation of microtubules to disassemble the mitotic spindle during cell division, is frequently used in cancer chemotherapy [2].

For the first time in 1999, Mayer *et al.*, [3] identified a novel cell-permeable small molecule, named monastrol. Unlike taxol, monastrol as an antimitotic agent has not exhibited neuronal cytotoxicity.

Monastrol induces a mono-astral conformation of microtubules by inhibiting the mitotic kinesin Eg5 [4,5].

Exploration of monastrol, commenced a new stage in Biginelli 3,4-dihydropyrimidine-2(1H)-one chemistry. Although many researches have been devoted to reveal the anti-mitotic mechanism of monastrol in the cell cycle [6-8], there are few examples concerning the anticancer activity [9-11]. Leizerman *et al.* [12] described the antiproliferative

* Correspondence: hadizadehf@mums.ac.ir
[4]Biotechnology Research Center, School of Pharmacy, Mashhad University of Medical Sciences, P. O. Box 91775–1365, Mashhad, Iran
Full list of author information is available at the end of the article

effect of monastrol on AGS and HT-29 cell lines as compared with taxol. Since the antimitotic activity of monastrol is not very high, structural variants could be verified to have better activity. Russowsky *et al.* [13], investigated the differential antiproliferative activity of monastrol, oxo-monastrol and oxygenated analogs on seven human cancer cell lines. In another study, more potent analogs of monastrol such as dimethylenastron [14] and quinazoline-2(1H)-thione [15] (Figure 1) were provided by skeleton modifications of monastrol in the parent ring by annelation across the C-5–C-6 bond. Notable work has also been dedicated to delineate the structure-activity relationship in the monastrol derivatives [16]. In this work six novel compounds (**4a-f**) were synthesized through Biginelli reaction in which hydroxyphenyl at C-4 position in dimethylenastron has been replaced with substituted benzylimidazolyl (Figure 2).

Methods
Chemistry
Melting points were determined using an Electrothermal Capillary apparatus and are uncorrected. ^{1}H-NMR spectra were recorded using Bruker AC-80 NMR spectrometer. The chemical shift values are on δ scale and the coupling constant values (J) are in ppm relative to tetramethylsilane as internal standard. Errors of elemental analyses were within ±0.4% of theoretical values.

The desired compounds were synthesized by the reactions outlined in Figure 2. Imidazole aldehydes [**3a-c**] was synthesized as described previously [17].

General procedure for synthesis of 4a-f
The suspension of **3a-c** (2 mmoles), dimedone (2 mmoles) and urea or thiourea (2.4 mmoles) in TMSCl (0.25 ml), DMF (0.8 ml) and acetonitrile (1.6 ml) was stirred for 4 h. The solid was separated by centrifugation and washed with distilled water followed by methanol. The residue was completely dried to give compound **4**.

4-[1-benzyl-2-(methylthio)-1H-imidazol-5-yl]- 3,4,7,8-tetrahydro- 7,7 dimethyl- quinazoline-2,5-(1H,6H)-diones (4a)
This compound was obtained in 44% yield; mp 169°C; ^{1}H-NMR (DMSO-d_6): 9.5(s, 1H, NH), 8 (s, 1H, NH), 7.82–6.94 (m, 6H, arom, H-imidazole), 6.21–5.44 (3H, CH$_2$N, C-H quinazoline), 2.91 -2.52 (m, 7H, SCH$_3$, 6,8, CH$_2$ quinazoline), 1.111-0.93 (m, 6H,CH$_3$ quinazoline). Anal. Calcd for C$_{21}$H$_{24}$N$_4$O$_2$S: C, 63.61; H, 6.10; N, 14.13. Found: C, 63.48; H, 6.07; N, 14.07.

4-[1-benzyl-2-(methylthio)-1H-imidazol-5-yl]-1,2,3,4,7,8-hexahydro- 7,7 dimethyl-2-thio oxoquinazoline-5-(6H)-one (4b)
This compound was obtained in 36% yield; mp 157°C; ^{1}H-NMR (DMSO-d_6): 9.5 (s, 1H, NH), 8.00 (S, 1H, NH), 7.62 –6.95 (m, 6H, arom, H-imidazole), 5.54 (3H, CH$_2$N, C-H quinazoline), 2.93 - 2.54 (m, 7H, SCH$_3$, 6,8,CH$_2$ quinazoline) 1.11-0.83 (m, 6H, CH$_3$ quinazoline). Anal. Calcd for C$_{21}$H$_{24}$N$_4$OS$_2$: C, 63.13; H, 5.86; N, 13.58. Found: C, 61.27; H, 5.88; N, 13.63.

4-[1-(2-chlorobenzyl)-2-(methylthio)-1H-imidazol-5-yl]-3,4,7,8- tetrahydro- 7,7 dimethyl quinazoline-2,5-(1H,6H)-diones (4c)
This compound was obtained in 61% yield; mp 149°C; ^{1}H-NMR (DMSO-d_6): 9.5(s, 1H, NH), 8.1(s, 1H, NH), 7.43-6.02 (m, 5H, arom, H-imdazole), 5.53 (3H, CH$_2$N, C-H quinazoline), 2.82 -2.53 (m, 7H, SCH$_3$, 6,8- CH$_2$ quinazoline), 1.11-0.74 (m, 6H, CH$_3$ quinazoline). Anal. Calcd for C$_{21}$H$_{23}$ClN$_4$O$_2$S: C, 58.53; H, 5.38; N, 13.00. Found: C, 58.68; H, 5.40; N, 12.94.

4-[1-(2-chlorobenyl)-2-methylthio-1H-imidazol-5-yl]-1,2,3,4,7,8- hexahydro-7,7 dimethyl-2-thio oxoquinazoline-5-(6H)-one (4d)
This compound was obtained in 58.1% yield; mp 142°C; ^{1}H-NMR (DMSO-d_6): 9.5 (s, 1H,NH), 8.13 (s, 1H, NH) 7.63-6.41 (m, 5H, arom, H-imdazole) 5.52 (3H, CH$_2$N,

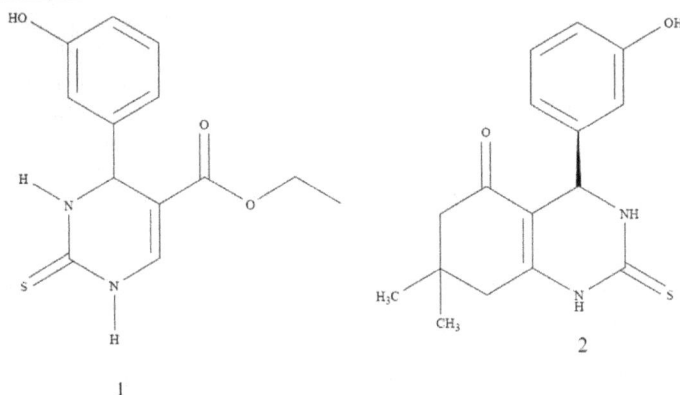

Figure 1 Monastrol (1) and dimethylenastron (2) structures.

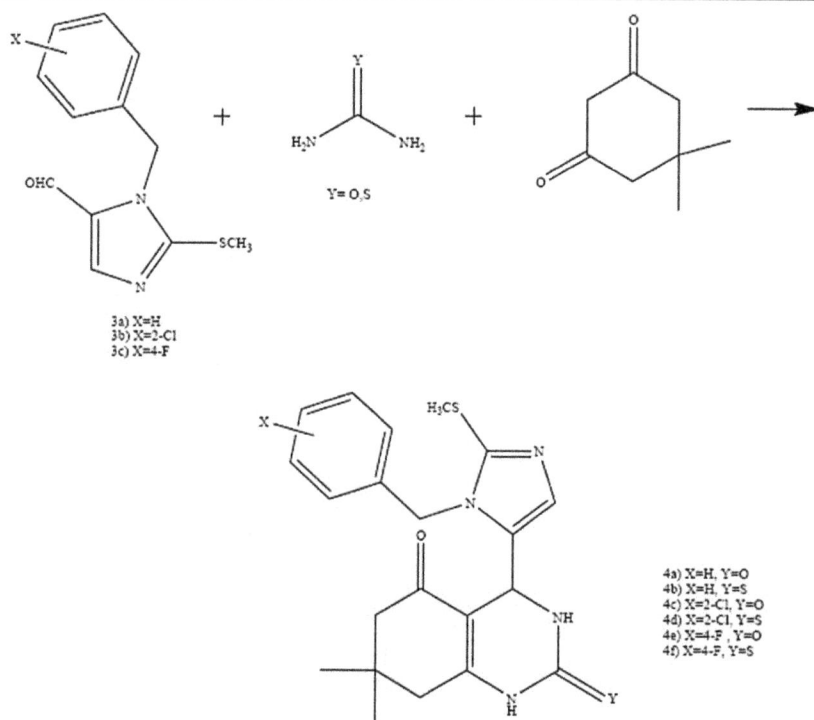

Figure 2 Synthesis of 4-imidazolyl tetrahydroquinazolines (4a-f) under Biginelli condition.

C-H quinazoline), 2.83 -2.45 (m, 7H, SCH$_3$, 6,8- CH$_2$ quinazoline), 1.23-1.02 (m, 6H, CH$_3$ quinazoline). Anal. Calcd for C$_{21}$H$_{23}$ClN$_4$OS$_2$: C, 56.42; H, 5.19; N, 12.53. Found: C, 56.31; H, 5.21; N, 12.45.

4-[1-(4-fluorobenzyl)-2-(methylthio)-1H-imidazol-5-yl]-3,4,7,8 – tetrahydro-7,7 dimethyl quinazoline-2,5-(1H,6H)-diones (4e)

This compound was obtained in 68.7% yield; mp 82°C; ^{1}H-NMR (DMSO-d$_6$): 9.52 (s, 1H, NH), 7.91 (s, 1H, NH), 7.14- 7.11 (m, 5H, arom, H-imdazole), 5.41-5.23 (3H, CH$_2$N, C-H quinazoline), 2.81- 2.05 (m, 7H, SCH$_3$, 6,8- CH$_2$ quinazoline), 1.22 -0.92 (m, 6H, CH$_3$ quinazoline). Anal. Calcd for C$_{21}$H$_{23}$FN$_4$O$_2$S: C, 60.85; H, 5.59; N, 13.52. Found: C, 60.80; H, 5.61; N, 13.46.

4-[1-(4-fluorobenzyl)-2-methylthio-1H-imidazol-5-yl]-1,2,3,4,7,8 -hexahydro-7,7-dimethyl-2-thiooxoquinazoline-5-(6H)-one (4f)

This compound was obtained in 58% yield; mp 149°C; ^{1}H-NMR (DMSO-d$_6$): 9.5 (s, 1H, NH), 8.1 (s, 1H, NH), 7.33-7.10 (m, 5H, arom, H-imdazole), 5.43 (3H, CH$_2$N, C-H quinazoline), 2.85- 2.12 (m, 7H, SCH$_3$, 6,8-CH$_2$ quinazoline), 2.81 -2.43 (m, 3H, SCH$_3$), 1.22-0.94 (m, 6H, CH$_3$ quinazoline). Anal. Calcd for C$_{21}$H$_{23}$FN$_4$OS$_2$: C,

58.58; H, 5.38; N, 13.01. Found: C, 58.61; H, 5.39; N, 13.06.

Docking

The X-ray crystal structure of Eg5-enastron complex (Protein Data Bank ID: 2X7C) was obtained from the Protein Data Bank. The three-dimensional structures of the derivatives were constructed using molecular mechanic force field (MM+), pre-optimization and AM1 semiemperical calculation in Hyperchem 7 software. The final corrected PDB file of the protein and synthesized analogs were submitted to AutoDock tools in order to run docking process. Docking studies were performed by AutoDock software Version 4. Searching was conducted within a specified 3D docking box (40 angstrom in all aspects) around enastron and the number of GA runs adjusted to 20 using Lamarckian genetic algorithm and all other parameters set as default. At the final stage through the docked structures of all analogs, best conformation was selected and saved as PDB file.

PDB files of best docked analogs along with Eg5 protein were submitted to MOE 2007.11 (License purchased from Chemical Computing Group by Mashhad University Medical Sciences, http://www.chemcomp.com/ for preparing figures and running protein ligand interaction fingerprint (PLIF).

The virtual physicochemical parameters of the synthesized compounds were also determined using MOE 2007.11 software.

Cell culture

HeLa cell line was obtained from National Cell Bank of Iran, Pasteur Institute of Iran. Cells were cultured in DMEM medium (Gibco, USA) supplemented with 10% (v/v) heat-inactivated fetal bovine serum (Gibco, USA), 100 U/ml penicillin (Biosera, UK), and 100 mg/ml streptomycin (Biosera, UK) at 37°C in a humidified atmosphere (95%) containing 5% CO_2.

Cell viability

Cytotoxic effects of synthesized compounds were determined using the MTT [3-(4,5-dimethylthiazol-2-yl)-2,5-diphenyltetrazolium bromide] assay [18-20]. Briefly, 5000 HeLa cells/well were seeded in a 96-well plate and cultured overnight. Different concentrations of synthesized compounds were added to each well. After incubation for 24 h, cells were treated with MTT solution (final concentration 0.5 mg/ml; Sigma, USA) for 4 h at 37°C. Then, the medium was removed, and the purple formazan crystals were dissolved in 150 µl dimethylsulfoxide (Merck, Germany). Absorbance was measured at 545 nm (630 nm as a reference) in Synergy H4 Hybrid Multi-Mode Microplate Reader (Biotek, Model: H4MLFPTAD). IC_{50} was calculated using CalcuSyn (BioSoft).

Kinesins activity assay

Briefly MT ELIPA master mix was prepared using 2 ml of reaction buffer containing 15 mM PIPES pH 7, 5 mM $MgCl_2$, 160 µl of 1 µg/µl tubuline solution in reaction buffer, 480 µl of ELIPA reagent 1 containing 1 mM 2-amino-6-mercapto-7-methylpurine riboside (MESG) and 24 µl of ELIPA reagent 2 containing 0.1 units/µl of purine nucleoside phosphorylase (PNP). Final reaction mixture was prepared by adding 75 µl of ELIPA master mix, 1 µl of 2.5 mg/ml kinesin heavy chain Motor (Cytoskeleton, Cat # KR01-A) and 20 µl of different concentrations of synthesized inhibitors and Taxol. Reaction was started by adding 8 µl of 100 mM ATP stock solution (Sigma, Cat # A3377). Absorbance of each well was recorded on a kinetic mode at λ_{360} nm wavelength using Synergy H4 Hybrid Multi-Mode Microplate Reader (Biotek, Model: H4MLFPTAD). Phosphate standard curve was constructed by adding 0–25 µl of 0.5 mM phosphate stock, to ELIPA master mix (Without tubulin). Activity of kinesin was reported as nmole Pi/min/2.5 µg kinesin.

Statistical analysis

Data are expressed as mean ± SD. Statistical analyses were performed with ANOVA followed by Tukey–Kramer test to compare the differences between means.

Differences were considered statistically significant when $P < 0.05$.

Results and discussion

Chemistry

In this study the new dimethylenastron derivatives (4a-f) were produced by substitution of 3-hydroxyphenyl in dimethylenastron with substituted benzyl imidazolyl under Biginelli condition.

The purity of the compounds was checked by TLC and melting points. The structure of the compounds was confirmed on the basis of its ^{1}H NMR spectral data and elemental analyses. All spectral data are in accordance with assigned structures. In IR spectra, N-H and C-O stretching bands were observed at spectra expected values. In the ^{1}H NMR spectra, methyl protons were seen at 0.90-1.00 ppm as separated singlets. Aromatic, methylene, methine and NH protons were found at expected values.

Docking analysis

Accuracy of docking protocol was examined by docking enastron in active site of Eg5 enzyme. Figure 3 shows docked enastron and co-crystallized one in almost same position among the receptor (RMSD = 1.24Å) that confirmed validation of docking protocol. All dimethylenastron derivatives were docked into active site of Eg5.

Table 1 shows estimated free energy of binding and calculated ki of synthesized compounds extracted from docking studies, these data in addition to Figure 4 which indicates synthetic ligands were in suitable position between active site of enzyme approve suitable interaction between ligands and protein.

According to PLIF, the most consistence interaction is H-bound between side chain of Glu116 and nitrogen atom on quinazoline ring. Compounds 4a, 4b, 4c and 4d have shown mentioned interaction and a backbone H-bound donor interaction was also detected between Glu118 and nitrogen atom in imidazolic ring of compound 4a. On the other hand by calculating ligand-protein interactions using LigX module in MOE software, except these H-bound interactions, surface contact interactions (arene-cation) between imidazolic ring of ligands and Arg 221 were identified. (Figure 5) Figure 5 represents 2D graph of interactions between synthesized compound 4b and Eg5 protein calculated by LigX module.

Docking analysis revealed that the all compounds interacted with Eg5 in good manner and confirms the importance of H-bound donor group in quinazoline ring and the role of imidazole ring as well as benzene ring in surface contact interaction on antiproliferative effects of synthesized compounds.

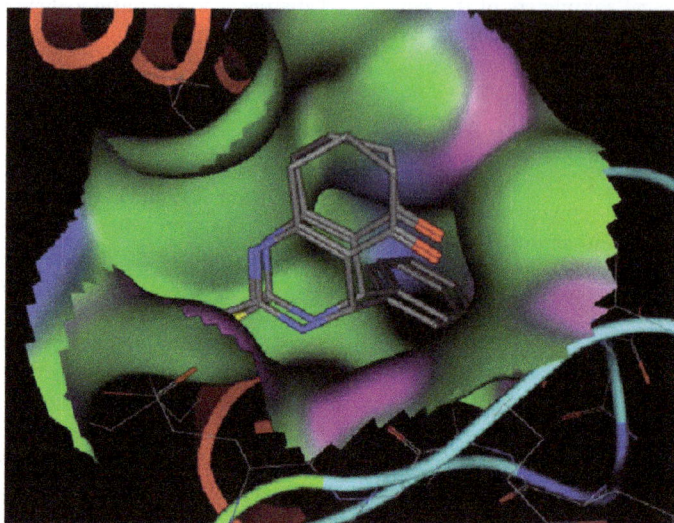

Figure 3 Docked and co-crystalized enasteron in Eg5 enzyme.

Effects of synthesized compounds on cell viability

Cytotoxicity of synthesized compounds was evaluated using MTT assay (Table 1). HeLa cells were incubated with different concentrations of newly synthesized compounds for 24 h and cytotoxicities were evaluated using MTT assay. Our data showed that analogue **4c** (X = 2-Cl Y = O, IC_{50}: 98 ± 19 µg/ml) was the most toxic compound among the newly synthesized compounds. Analogue **4f** (X = 4-F Y = S, IC_{50}: 339 ± 23 µg/ml), **4b** (X = H Y = S, IC_{50}: 301 ± 22 µg/ml) and dimethylenasteron (IC_{50}: 338 ± 26 µg/ml) showed less cytotoxicities.

The significant difference between cytotoxicity of analogues **4f** (X = 4-F Y = S, IC_{50}: 339 ± 23 µg/ml) and **4e** (X = 4-F Y = O, IC_{50}: 110 ± 28 µg/ml) or analogue **4b** (X = H Y = S, IC_{50}: 301 ± 22 µg/ml) and **4a** (X = H Y = O, IC_{50}: 210 ± 21 µg/ml)demonstrated the essential role of carbonyl group at position C2 of tetrahydro-quinazoline on antiproliferative effect of synthesized compounds.

Meanwhile there was no big difference between cytotoxicity of compound **4c** (X = 2-Cl Y = O, IC_{50}: 98 ± 19 µg/ml) and **4e** (X = 4-F Y = O, IC_{50}: 110 ± 28 µg/ml); they had so much better cytotoxic effect in comparison with compounds **4b** (X = H Y = S, IC_{50}: 301 ± 22 µg/ml) and **4a** (X = H Y = O, IC_{50}: 210 ± 21 µg/ml). The obtained results illustrated the presence of an electron withdrawing groups (F or Cl) on the benzylimidazolyl substituent at position C4 of tetrahydro-quinazoline structure could increase the cytotoxicity of prepared compounds.

Table 1 Cytotoxicity on HeLa cell line (n = 5), inhibition of Kinesin activity (n = 2) and docking results of synthesized analogues 4a-f

Compound	X*	Y*	IC_{50} (µg/ml) ± SD on HeLa cell line	IC_{50} (µg/ml) for Kinesin inhibition	Estimated** free energy of binding	Calculated*** Ki (nM) for Kinesin inhibition
4a	H	O	210 ± 21	72	−8.94	281.5 nM
4b	H	S	301 ± 22	77	−8.67	438.63 nM
4c	2-Cl	O	98 ± 19	79	−9.39	130.76 nM
4d	2-Cl	S	ND**	ND**	−8.83	334.27 nM
4e	4-F	O	110 ± 28	96	−8.55	536.29 nM
4f	4-F	S	339 ± 23	198	−8.52	573.33 nM
dimethylenastrone	-	-	338 ± 26	210	−8.72	409.07 nM
Taxol	-	-	ND**	7	ND	ND

*X and Y were represented in Figure 2.
**Not determined.
***Docking results.

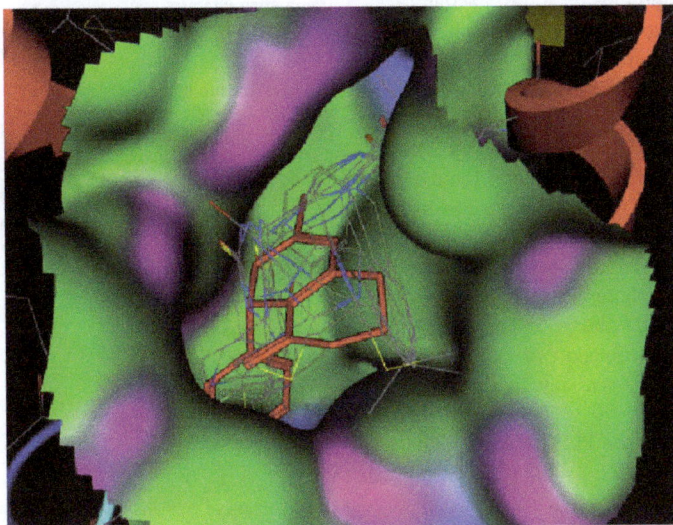

Figure 4 Map surface of docked analogs in active site of enzyme (Green: hydrophobic; Violet: H bonding; Blue: mild polar). Crystallized enasteron is indicated by red and stick lines.

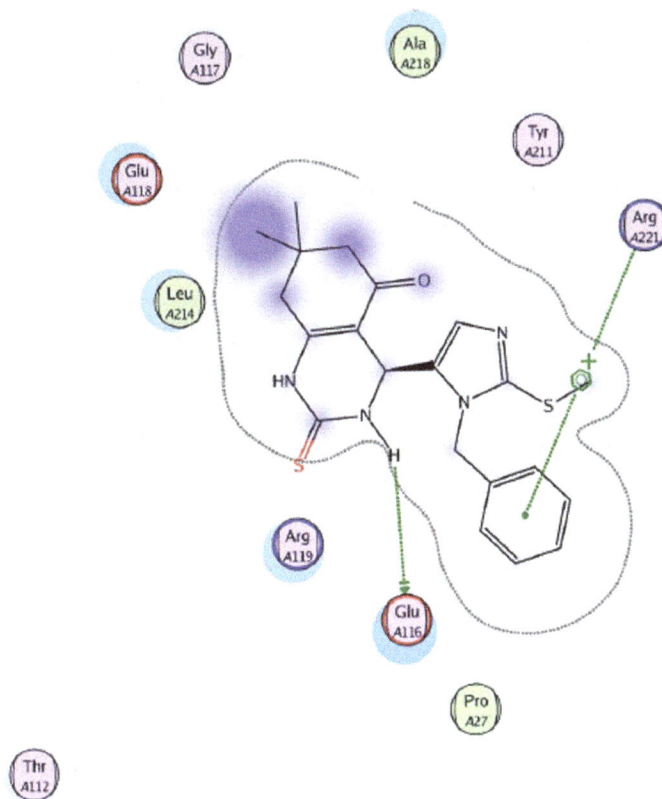

Figure 5 2D graph of interactions between synthesized compound 4b and protein made by LigX module of MOE software. In the 2D graphs hydrophobic/aromatic residues are colored in green, whereas polar amino acids are shown in magenta. H-bonds and all π-stacking interactions are represented as green dotted lines. The active site contour is also shown.

Effects of synthesized compounds on Kinesin activity

Kinesins operate by utilizing the energy of ATP hydrolysis, generating Pi, to move along microtubule (MT) substrates. To determine activity of kinesins, rate of Pi production was measured using ELIPA (Enzyme Linked Inorganic Phosphate Assay) Biochem kit (Cytoskeleton, cat # BK060). The assay was based on an absorbance shift (330–360 nm) that occurred when 2-amino-6-mercapto-7-methylpurine ribonucleoside (MESG) was catalytically converted to 2-amino-6-mercapto-7-methylpurine in the presence of inorganic phosphate (Pi). The reaction was catalyzed by purine nucleoside phosphorylase (PNP). One molecule of Pi produces one molecule of 2-amino-6-mercapto-7-methylpurine in an essentially irreversible reaction. Thus, the absorbance at 360 nm is directly proportional to the amount of Pi. Our data (Table 1) showed that analogue **4a** (X = H Y = O, IC_{50}: 72 µg/ml), **4b** (X = H Y = S, IC_{50}: 77 µg/ml), **4c** (X = 2-Cl Y = O, IC_{50}: 79 µg/ml) and **4e** (X = 4-F Y = O, IC_{50}: 96 µg/ml) were stronger Kinesin inhibitor as compared with analogue **4f** (X = 4-F Y = S, IC_{50}: 198 µg/ml) and dimethylenasteron (IC_{50}: 210 µg/ml. None of our compounds were able to inhibit kinesin as much as Taxol (IC_{50}: 7 µg/ml).

According to kinesin inhibitory effect of analogues **4f** and **4e**, the carbonyl group at C2 position of tetrahydroquinozoline was crucial in kinesin inhibitory activities of synthesized compounds. On the other hand, our results suggested that the presence of an electron withdrawing group in benzene ring of benzylimidazolyl at position C4 of tetrahydro-quinazoline structure had no significant effect either positive or negative on kinesin inhibitory activity of synthesized compounds.

Conclusion

In this study a series of six novel dimethylenastron analogs based on Biginelli reaction were synthesized with IC_{50} in the range of 98 to 210 µg/mL against HeLa cell line. Compared with dimethylenastron, these new series were found to have stronger antiproliferative activity against HeLa cell line. Structural-activity relationship study highlighted the important role of carbonyl substitution at C2 position of tetrahydro-quinazoline structure in antiproliferative and kinesin inhibitory effect of newly synthesized compounds. The reported results could be helpful in developing potential formulation of new anti-cancer drugs.

Abbreviations

DMF: Dimethylformamide; ELIPA: Enzyme linked inorganic phosphate assay; IR: Infrared; MESG: 2-amino-6-mercapto-7-methylpurine ribonucleoside; MTT: 3-(4,5-Dimethylthiazol-2-yl)-2,5-diphenyltetrazolium bromide; MT: Microtubule; NMR: Nuclear magnetic resonance; PLIF: Protein ligand interaction fingerprint; PNP: Purine nucleoside phosphorylase; RMSD: Root-mean-square deviation; TLC: Thin layer chromatography; TMSCL: Trimethylsilyl chloride.

Competing interests
The authors declare that they have no competing interests.

Authors' contributions
KA: Supervision of biological studies including cytotoxicity (MTT) and Kinesin inhibition assay. BB: performed synthesis of the target compounds. SM: Collaboration in biological studies, MRMF: Performed the cytotoxic tests and Kinesin Assay. MA: manuscript draft preparation and Collaboration in biological studies. FM: performed synthesis and identifying of the target compounds. MG: performed molecular modeling studies. FH: supervision of design and synthesis of target compounds and manuscript preparation. All authors read and approved the final manuscript.

Acknowledgements
The authors are thankful for financial support from the Research Council of Mashhad University of Medical Sciences. This work was part of Pharm.D thesis.

Author details
[1]Pharmaceutical Research Center, School of Pharmacy, Mashhad University of Medical Sciences, Mashhad, Iran. [2]School of Pharmacy, Mashhad University of Medical Sciences, Mashhad, Iran. [3]Department of Pharmacodynamics and Toxicology, School of Pharmacy, Mashhad University of Medical Sciences, Mashhad, Iran. [4]Biotechnology Research Center, School of Pharmacy, Mashhad University of Medical Sciences, P. O. Box 91775–1365, Mashhad, Iran.

References
1. Jun Z, Paraskevi G: Targeting microtubules for cancer chemotherapy. Curr Med Chem Anti Canc Agents 2005, 5:65–71.
2. Verweij J, Clavel M, Chevalier B: Paclitaxel (Taxol) and docetaxel (Taxotere): not simply two of a kind. Ann Oncol 1994, 5:495–505.
3. Mayer TU, Kapoor TM, Haggarty SJ, King RW, Schreiber SL, Mitchison TJ: Small molecule inhibitor of mitotic spindle bipolarity identified in a phenotype-based screen. Science 1999, 286:971–974.
4. Crews CM, Mohan R: Small-molecule inhibitors of the cell cycle. Curr Opin Chem Biol 2000, 4:47–53.
5. Liu X, Gong H, Huang K: Oncogenic role of kinesin proteins and targeting kinesin therapy. Cancer Sci 2013, 104:651–656.
6. Kapoor TM, Mayer TU, Coughlin ML, Mitchison TJ: Probing spindle assembly mechanisms with monastrol, a small molecule inhibitor of the mitotic kinesin, Eg5. J Cell Biol 2000, 150:975–988.
7. DeBonis S, Simorre J-P, Crevel I, Lebeau L, Skoufias DA, Blangy A, Ebel C, Gans P, Cross R, Hackney DD, et al: Interaction of the mitotic inhibitor monastrol with human kinesin Eg5. Biochemistry 2002, 42:338–349.
8. Cochran JC, Gilbert SP: ATPase mechanism of Eg5 in the absence of microtubules: insight into microtubule activation and allosteric inhibition by monastrol. Biochemistry 2005, 44:16633–16648.
9. Haque SA, Hasaka TP, Brooks AD, Lobanov PV, Baas PW: Monastrol, a prototype anti-cancer drug that inhibits a mitotic kinesin, induces rapid bursts of axonal outgrowth from cultured postmitotic neurons. Cell Motil Cytoskeleton 2004, 58:10–16.
10. Maliga Z, Kapoor TM, Mitchison TJ: Evidence that monastrol is an allosteric inhibitor of the mitotic kinesin Eg5. Chem Biol 2002, 9:989–996.
11. Muller C, Gross D, Sarli V, Gartner M, Giannis A, Bernhardt G, Buschauer A: Inhibitors of kinesin Eg5: antiproliferative activity of monastrol analogues against human glioblastoma cells. Cancer Chemother Pharmacol 2007, 59:157–164.
12. Leizerman I, Avunie-Masala R, Elkabets M, Fich A, Gheber L: Differential effects of monastrol in two human cell lines. Cell Molecular Life Sci 2004, 61:2060–2070.
13. Russowsky D, Canto RFS, Sanches SAA, DOca MGM, de Fatima A, Pilli RA, Kohn LK, Antonio MA, de Carvalho JE: Synthesis and differential antiproliferative activity of biginelli compounds against cancer cell lines: monastrol, oxo-monastrol and oxygenated analogues. Bioorg Chem 2006, 34:173–182.

14. Gartner M, Sunder-Plassmann N, Seiler J, Utz M, Vernos I, Surrey T, Giannis A: **Development and biological evaluation of potent and specific inhibitors of mitotic kinesin Eg5.** *Chem Bio Chem* 2005, **6:**1173–1177.

15. Sunder-Plassmann N, Sarli V, Gartner M, Utz M, Seiler J, Huemmer S, Mayer TU, Surrey T, Giannis A: **Synthesis and biological evaluation of new tetrahydro-β-carbolines as inhibitors of the mitotic kinesin Eg5.** *Bioor Med Chem* 2005, **13:**6094–6111.

16. Klein E, DeBonis S, Thiede B, Skoufias DA, Kozielski F, Lebeau L: **New chemical tools for investigating human mitotic kinesin Eg5.** *Bioor Med Chem* 2007, **15:**6474–6488.

17. Hadizadeh F, Mohajeri S, Hosseinzadeh H, Salami S, Motamedshariat F: **Synthesis of novel 4-[1-(4-fluorobenzyl)-5-imidazolyl] dihydropyridines and study of their effects on rat blood pressure.** *Iranian J. Basic Medical Sci* 2011, **14**(5):213–218.

18. Hadizadeh F, Moallem SA, Jaafari MR, Shahab M, Alahyari M, Rameshrad M, Samiei A: **Synthesis and immunomodulation of human lymphocyte proliferation and cytokine (interferon-gamma) production of four novel malonitrilamides.** *Chem Biol Drug Des* 2009, **73**(6):668–673.

19. Vosooghi M, Yahyavi H, Divsalar K, Shamsa H, Kheirollahi A, Safavi M, Ardestani SK, Sadeghi-Neshat S, Mohammadhosseini N, Edraki N, Khoshneviszadeh M, Shafiee A, Foroumadi A: **Synthesis and in vitro cytotoxic activity evaluation of (E)-16-(substituted benzylidene) derivatives of dehydroepiandrosterone.** *Daru J Pharmaceut Sci* 2013, **21:**34.

20. Noushini S, Alipour E, Emami S, Safavi M, Ardestani SK, Gohari AR, Shafiee A, Foroumadi A: **Synthesis and cytotoxic properties of novel (E)-3-benzylidene-7-methoxychroman-4-one derivatives.** *Daru J Pharmaceut Sci* 2013, **21:**31.

17

N-Substituted indole carbohydrazide derivatives: synthesis and evaluation of their antiplatelet aggregation activity

Seyedeh Sara Mirfazli[1], Farzad Kobarfard[2,3], Loghman Firoozpour[4], Ali Asadipour[5], Marjan Esfahanizadeh[2], Kimia Tabib[2], Abbas Shafiee[1] and Alireza Foroumadi[1,5*]

Abstract

Background: Platelet aggregation is one of the most important factors in the development of thrombotic disorders which plays a central role in thrombosis (clot formation). Prophylaxis and treatment of arterial thrombosis are achieved using anti-platelet drugs. In this study, a series of novel substituted indole carbohydrazide was synthesized and evaluated for anti-platelet aggregation activity induced by adenosine diphosphate (ADP), arachidonic acid (AA) and collagen.

Methods: Our synthetic route started from methyl 1H-indole-3-carboxylate (1) and ethyl 1H-indole-2-carboxylate (4) which were reacted with hydrazine monohydrate 99%. The aldol condensation of the later compound with aromatic aldehydes led to the formation of the title compounds. Sixteen indole acylhydrazone derivatives, **3d-m** and **6d-i** were tested for anti-platelet aggregation activity induced by adenosine diphosphate (ADP), arachidonic acid (AA) and collagen.

Results: Among the synthesized compounds, **6g** and **6h** with 100% inhibition, proved to be the most potent derivatives of the 2-substituted indole on platelet aggregation induced by AA and collagen, respectively. In 3-substituted indole **3m** with 100% inhibition and **3f** and **3i** caused 97% inhibition on platelet aggregation induced by collagen and AA, respectively.

Conclusion: In this study, compounds **6g, 6h, 3m, 3f** and **3i** showed better inhibition on platelet aggregation induced by AA and collagen among the title compounds. Quantitative structure–activity relationship (QSAR) analysis between the structural parameters of the investigated derivatives and their antiplatelet aggregation activity was performed with various molecular descriptors but, analysis of the physicochemical parameters doesn't show a significant correlation between the observed activities and general molecular parameters of the synthesized derivatives. Although, due to the existence of several receptors on the platelets surface which are responsible for controlling the platelet aggregation, the investigated compounds in the present study may exert their activities through binding to more than one of these receptors and therefore no straight forward SAR could be obtained for them.

Keyword: Anti-platelet aggregation, Indole, N-acylhydrazone

* Correspondence: aforoumadi@yahoo.com
[1]Department of Medicinal Chemistry, Faculty of Pharmacy and Pharmaceutical Sciences Research Center, Tehran University of Medical Sciences, Tehran, Iran
[5]Neuroscience Research Center, Institute of Neuropharmacology, Kerman University of Medical Sciences, Kerman, Iran
Full list of author information is available at the end of the article

Background

Cardiovascular diseases are responsible for the largest number of death and disability worldwide. Platelet adhesion and aggregation are key events in hemostasis and thrombosis which cause disrupted atherosclerotic plaques that is the initiator of most thrombotic disorders including heart attacks and strokes [1-3]. Platelets play the major role in the pathogenesis of thromboembolic disorders and activation of the platelets by complex biochemical pathways and mediators is the primary step in this process [4,5]. Endogenous agonists such as arachidonic acid (AA), adenosine 5′-diphosphate (ADP) that acts on purinergic receptors on the platelet-known as P_2Y receptors, thromboxane A_2 (TxA_2), thrombin, platelet activating factor (PAF), epinephrine (EPN) and collagen are among potent agonists that initiate the formation of stable platelet aggregates [6-8].

Clinical evidence has clearly proven that antiplatelet aggregation agents are useful for preventing thrombotic disorders. On the other hand, there are still some serious limitations to currently use agents which include weak inhibition of platelet function (aspirin), slow onset of action (clopidogrel), variable response to treatment among patients and high incidence of bleeding events which is dose dependent in both aspirin and clopidogrel drug therapy [9]. Considering the current situation, pursuit of finding novel scaffolds as new antiplatelet aggregation drugs which are more effective and safer with fewer side effects is very important [10].

A novel group of heterocyclic acylhydrazone derivatives with antiplatelet aggregation activity on rabbit platelet-rich plasma have been reported [11,12]. Furthermore, the N-acylhydrazone (NAH) moiety, have shown a series of biological activities such as analgesic, anti-inflammatory [13-20], protozoa proteases inhibition [21], HIV-1 reverse transcriptase dimmer destabilization [22], antibiotic and antifungal activities [23], and cardiovascular actions [24-28].

Indole ring is another structural moiety which has been reported to have antiplatelet aggregation activity [29]. Considering this background, a diverse group of derivatives have been synthesized in this study by molecular hybridization between indole and hydrazone moieties, to find the structure–antiplatelet activity relationship of the derivatives. The schematic structural backbone for these compounds which contain both indole and N-acylhydrazone is depicted in Figure 1.

Chemistry

The synthetic procedure planned to obtain the desired indole N-acylhydrazone derivatives, is shown in Scheme 1. The key intermediates were obtained by hydrazinolysis of **1** and **4** in 96% and 91% yield, respectively, using hydrazine monohydrate 99% in ethanol. The final indole

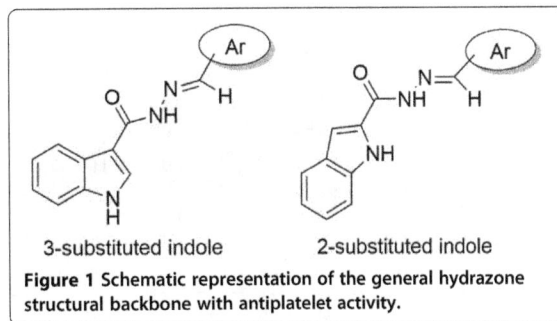

3-substituted indole   2-substituted indole

Figure 1 Schematic representation of the general hydrazone structural backbone with antiplatelet activity.

N-acylhydrazone derivatives were obtained by condensing the hydrazide intermediates with the proper aromatic aldehydes (ArCHO) in water and glacial acetic acid as the solvent, in good yields.

Material and methods
General
All commercial solvents, chemicals and reagents were purchased from either Merck or Sigma-Aldrich with the highest purity and used without further purification. Proton nuclear magnetic resonance (^{1}H NMR) spectra were recorded on a Bruker 500 MHz spectrometers (Bruker, Rheinstetten, Germany) and pick positions are illustrated in parts per million (δ) in DMSO-d_6 solution and tetramethylsilane (0.05% v/v) as internal standard and coupling constant values (J) are given in Hertz. Signal multiplicities are reported by: s (singlet), d (doublet), t (triplet), q (quadruplet), m (multiplet) and br (broad signal). For NMR spectral data assignments, the atom numbering of compounds is depicted in Table 1. Analytical thin layer chromatography (TLC) was performed with Merck silica gel plates and visualized with UV irradiation (254 nm) or iodine. Electrospray ionization mass spectra (ESI-MS) were obtained using Agilent 6410 Triple Quad. LC/MS. Melting points were obtained by an Electrothermal 9100 apparatus and are uncorrected. The IR spectra were taken by a Perkin-Elmer 843 spectrometer with KBr as diluent. The elemental analysis for C, H and N was performed by a Costech model 4010 and the percentage values agreed with the proposed structures within ±0.4% of the theoretical values. All described products showed ^{1}H NMR spectra according to the assigned structures. The physicochemical parameters including Clog P value, surface area, molecular volume, refractivity and polarizability were calculated by Hyperchem 8.0 software.

General procedure for the preparation of carbohydrazides (2, 5)
Compounds (**1** or **4**) (2.86 mmol) was added to a solution of hydrazine monohydrate 99% (2.14 mL; 2.18 g; 43.6 mmol) in ethanol (0.5 mL) and the reaction mixture

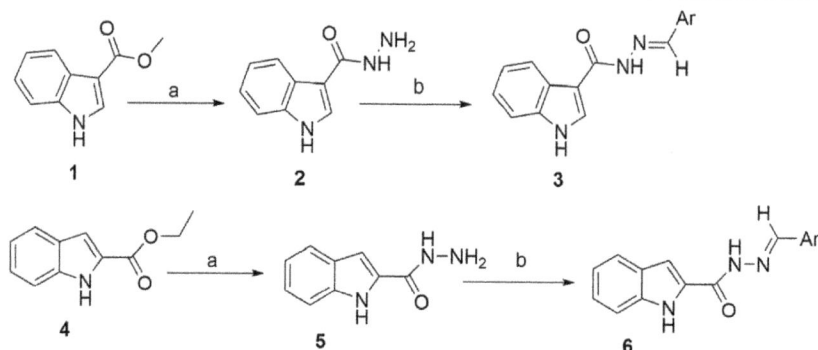

Scheme 1 The synthesis pathway for indole*N*-acylhydrazones. Reagents and reaction condition: **a)** Hydrazine monohydrate 99% (NH$_2$NH$_2$), Ethanol (a few drop), reflux at 80°C, 3 h **b)** ArCHO, H$_2$O, Glacial acetic acid (a few drop), reflux at 100°C, 3 h.

was stirred at about 80°C temperature, for 2 h. TLC indicated the end of reaction. The mixture was cooled by addition of a water/ice mixture. The solid was filtered in excellent yield (Scheme 1) [30-32].

1*H*- indole-3-carbohydrazide (**2**) and 1*H*- indole-2-carbohydrazide (**5**) were prepared according to a literature method [30-32].

General procedure for the preparation of N-acylhydrazone derivatives

Equimolar amount of appropriate aromatic aldehyde was added to a solution of hydrazide compound (**2** or **5**) in 10 mL of water, in presence of catalytic amount of glacial acetic acid (0.4 mL). Reaction mixture was heated under reflux with stirring for about 2 h and poured into ice/water mixture. The precipitate was filtered and washed with cold water (Scheme 1).

N'-(4-hydroxybenzylidene)-1*H*-indole-3-carbohydrazide (**3i**), *N'*-(3-hydroxybenzylidene)-1*H*-indole-3-carbohydrazide (**3j**), *N'*-benzylidene-1*H*-indole-3-carbohydrazide (**3 m**), *N'*-(2-hydroxybenzylidene)-1*H*-indole-2-carbohydrazide (**6e**), *N'*-(2-methoxybenzylidene)-1*H*-indole-2-carbohydrazide (**6f**) and *N'*-benzylidene-1*H*-indole-2-carbohydrazide (**6i**) were prepared according to a literature method [30-32].

N'-(2-hydroxybenzylidene)-1H-indole-3-carbohydrazide (3d)

Yield: 92%, mp 256- 259°C. IR (KBr) cm^{-1}: 3365 (v OH), 3283, 3041, 2927, 1660, 1614, 1596, 1577, 1564. ^{1}H NMR (500 MHz, DMSO): δ 11.79 (s, 1H, CONH), 11.71 (bs, 1H, Indole NH), 11.51 (bs, 1H, OH), 8.52 (s, 1H, —N=C*H*—) 8.21 (bs, 1H, —N=CH—C$_6$H$_5$, H$_2$), 8.20 (d, 1H, J = 7.85 Hz, —N=CH—C$_6$H$_5$,H$_4$), 7.52 (d, 1H, J = 7.5 Hz, —N=CH—C$_6$H$_5$, H$_6$), 7.50 (d, 1H, J = 7.8 Hz, —N=CH—C$_6$H$_5$, H$_4$), 7.29 (td, 1H, J = 7.0, 1.40 Hz, Indole H$_7$), 7.21 (td, 1H, J = 7.4, 1.45 Hz, Indole H$_5$), 7.17 (td, 1H, J = 7.0, 1.45 Hz, Indole H$_6$), 6.95- 6.91 (m, 2H, —N=CH—C$_6$H$_5$, H$_3$, H$_5$), ESI-Mass m/z: 280 [M + H]$^+$, 302 [M + Na]$^+$; Anal. Calcd. for C$_{16}$H$_{13}$N$_3$O$_2$: C,

68.81; H, 4.69; N, 15.05. Found: C, 68.64; H, 4.83; N, 14.92.

N'-(2-nitrobenzylidene)-1H-indole-3-carbohydrazide (3e)

Yield: 96%, mp 272- 274°C. IR (KBr) cm^{-1}: 3282, 3218, 3143, 3089, 1635, 1595, 1564, 1540 and 1353 (NO$_2$). ^{1}H NMR (500 MHz, DMSO): δ 11.83 (s, 1H, CONH), 11.81 (s, 1H, Indole NH), 8.72 (s, 1H, —N=CH—C$_6$H$_5$, H$_2$), 8.28 (bs, 1H, —N=C*H*—), 8.21 (d, 1H, J = 7.8 Hz, Indole H$_4$), 8.16 (d, 1H, J = 7.4 Hz, —N=CH—C$_6$H$_5$, H$_6$), 8.08 (dd, 1H, J = 7.20, 1.0 Hz, —N=CH—C$_6$H$_5$, H$_3$), 7.83 (t, 1H, J = 7.5 Hz, —N=CH—C$_6$H$_5$, H$_5$), 7.66 (td, 1H, J = 7.6, 1.35 Hz, —N=CH—C$_6$H$_5$, H$_4$), 7.49 (d, 1H, J = 7.9 Hz, Indole H$_7$), 7.23-7.16 (m, 2H, Indole H$_5$, H$_6$), ESI-Mass m/z: 309 [M + H]$^+$, 331 [M + Na]$^+$, 347 [M + K]$^+$; Anal. Calcd. for C$_{16}$H$_{12}$N$_4$O$_3$: C, 62.33; H, 3.92; N, 18.17. Found: C, 62.58; H, 4.08; N, 18.32.

N'-(2-methoxybenzylidene)-1H-indole-3-carbohydrazide (3f)

Yield: 69%, mp 229- 231°C. IR (KBr) cm^{-1}: 3300- 3200 (v NH), 3112, 3076, 1622, 1601, 1578, 1540; ^{1}H NMR (500 MHz, DMSO): δ 11.73 (s, 1H, CONH), 11.41 (s, 1H, Indole-NH), 8.65 (bs, 1H, Indole H$_2$), 8.22 (bs, 2H, Indole H$_4$, —N=C*H*—), 7.87 (d, 1H, J = 6.70 Hz, —N=CH—C$_6$H$_5$, H$_6$), 7.48 (d, 1H, J = 7. 85 Hz, Indole H$_7$), 7.41 (td, 1H, J = 7.3, 1.35 Hz, —N=CH—C$_6$H$_5$, H$_4$), 7.20 (t, 1H, J = 7.0 Hz, —N=CH—C$_6$H$_5$, H$_5$), 7.15 (t, 1H, J = 7.4 Hz, Indole H$_5$), 7.12 (d, 1H, J = 8.3 Hz, —N=CH—C$_6$H$_5$, H$_3$), 7.04 (t, 1H, J = 7.4 Hz, Indole H$_6$), 3.89 (s, 3H, —OCH$_3$); ESI-Mass m/z: 294 [M + H]$^+$, 316 [M + Na]$^+$; Anal. Calcd. for C$_{17}$H$_{15}$N$_3$O$_2$: C, 69.61; H, 5.15; N, 14.33. Found: C, 69.46; H, 5.33; N, 14.12.

N'-(3-chlorobenzylidene)-1H-indole-3-carbohydrazide (3 g)

Yield: 78%, mp 288- 291°C. IR (KBr) cm^{-1}: 3545, 3390, 3320, 3263, 3068, 1635, 1580, 1558,1548; ^{1}H NMR (500 MHz, DMSO): δ 11.78 (s, 1H, CONH), 11.50 (s, 1H,

Table 1 Effect of 3-substituted indole (3d-m) and 2-substituted indole (6d-i) derivatives at 1 mM concentration on *in-vitro* platelet aggregation induced by AA, ADP and collagen

Derivative	Structure	AA Inhibition (%)[b]	ADP	Collagen
3d		30.1 ± 3	31 ± 1.5	24.5 ± 2.1
3e		94 ± 5	20 ± 1.3	80 ± 4.3
3f		97 ± 4.9	41.5 ± 2.1	73.6 ± 2.9
3 g		94 ± 2.5	46 ± 2.5	65.6 ± 3.1
3h		95 ± 3.9	21.3 ± 1	44.6 ± 2.1
3i		97 ± 5.1	47.5 ± 1.2	74 ± 3.9
3j		96 ± 4.6	42.8 ± 0.9	81 ± 1.9
3 k		93 ± 1.9	55 ± 1.3	91 ± 2.7

Table 1 Effect of 3-substituted indole (3d-m) and 2-substituted indole (6d-i) derivatives at 1 mM concentration on *in-vitro* platelet aggregation induced by AA, ADP and collagen *(Continued)*

3 l		94 ± 3	53 ± 2.1	91 ± 0.9
3 m		94 ± 2.8	35 ± 1.2	100 ± 2.0
6d		96 ± 4.1	31.4 ± 1.4	61.6 ± 3.2
6e		35 ± 2.5	66.8 ± 1.1	8 ± 0.9
6f		94.5 ± 3.1	25.9 ± 0.6	61 ± 3
6 g		100 ± 3.8	26.8 ± 1	27.3 ± 1.2
6 h		96 ± 2.9	24 ± 0.8	100 ± 3.4
6i		98 ± 1.4	51 ± 1.3	80 ± 2.5
Indomethacin[a]		100 ± 4.3	42 ± 1.1	100 ± 2.8
Aspirin[a]		100 ± 2.8	21 ± 0.6	100 ± 3.1

[a]Aspirin and Indomethacin were used as a positive control.
[b]Values are presented as mean ± S.E. of three separate determination.

Indole-NH), 8.27 (bs, 1H, —N=C*H*—), 8.21 (s, 1H, Indole H$_2$), 8.20 (s, 1H, Indole H$_4$), 7.78 (s, 1H, —N=CH—C$_6$H$_5$, H$_2$), 7.68 (d, 1H, *J* = 7.0 Hz, —N=CH—C$_6$H$_5$, H$_6$), 7.51- 7.47 (m, 3H, Indole H$_7$, —N=CH—C$_6$H$_5$, H$_4$, H$_5$), 7.22- 7.15 (m, 2H, Indole H$_5$, H$_6$); ESI-Mass *m/z*: 298 [M + H]$^+$, 320 [M + Na]$^+$; Anal. Calcd. for C$_{16}$H$_{12}$ClN$_3$O: C, 64.54; H, 4.06; N, 11.91. Found: C, 64.19; H, 4.24; N, 11.76.

N'-(4-chlorobenzylidene)-1H-indole-3-carbohydrazide (3 h)
Yield: 74%, mp 265- 267°C. IR (KBr) cm^{-1}: 3394, 3240, 3060, 1637, 1603, 1555, 1536; ^{1}H NMR (500 MHz, DMSO): δ 11.76 (s, 1H, CONH), 11.45 (s, 1H, Indole-NH), 8.35- 8.21 (m, 3H, —N=C*H*—, Indole H$_2$, H$_4$), 7.75 (d, 2H, *J* = 8.5 Hz, —N=CH—C$_6$H$_5$, H$_2$, H$_6$), 7.53 (d, 2H, *J* = 8.5 Hz, —N=CH—C$_6$H$_5$, H$_3$, H$_5$), 7.49 (d, 1H, *J* = 8.0 Hz, Indole H$_7$), 7.22- 7.15 (m, 2H, Indole H$_5$, H$_6$); ESI-Mass *m/z*: 298 [M + H]$^+$, 320 [M + Na]$^+$; Anal. Calcd. for C$_{16}$H$_{12}$ClN$_3$O: C, 64.54; H, 4.06; N, 11.91. Found: C, 64.43; H, 3.91; N, 12.16.

N'-(2-fluorobenzylidene)-1H-indole-3-carbohydrazide (3 k)
Yield: 90%, mp 239- 240°C. IR (KBr) cm^{-1}: 3299- 3073 (v NH), 3032, 2956, 1636, 1614, 1586, 1555. ^{1}H NMR (500 MHz, DMSO): δ 11.77 (s, 1H, CONH), 11.50 (bs, 1H, Indole NH), 8.55 (bs, 1H, —N=C*H*—), 8.22 (d, 1H, *J* = 7.5 Hz, Indole H$_4$), 7.94 (t, 1H, *J* = 6.8 Hz, —N=CH—C$_6$H$_5$, H$_4$), 7.50- 7.45 (m, 3H, —N=CH—C$_6$H$_5$, H$_6$, Indole H$_2$, H$_7$), 7.33- 7.29 (m, 2H, —N=CH—C$_6$H$_5$, H$_3$, H$_5$), 7.21 (td, 1H, *J* = 6.5, 1.3 Hz, Indole H$_5$), 7.16 (td, 1H, *J* = 6.5, 1.3 Hz, Indole H$_6$); ESI-Mass *m/z*: 282 [M + H]$^+$, 304 [M + Na]$^+$; Anal. Calcd. for C$_{16}$H$_{12}$FN$_3$O: C, 68.32; H, 4.30; N, 14.94. Found: C, 68.64; H, 4.13; N, 14.62.

N'-(3-fluorobenzylidene)-1H-indole-3-carbohydrazide (3 l)
Yield: 87%, mp 278- 281°C. IR (KBr) cm^{-1}: 3319- 3200 (v NH), 3139, 3089, 1647, 1591, 1558, 1500. ^{1}H NMR (500 MHz, DMSO): δ 11.76 (s, 1H, CONH), 11.50 (bs, 1H, Indole NH), 8.34- 8.27 (m, 3H, —N=C*H*—, Indole H$_4$, H$_2$), 7.57- 7.48 (m, 4H, —N=CH—C$_6$H$_5$,H$_2$, H$_5$, H6, Indole, H$_7$), 7.28- 7.24 (m, 1H, —N=CH—C$_6$H$_5$, H$_4$), 7.21 (td, 1H, *J* = 6.8, 1.2 Hz, Indole H$_5$), 7.16 (td, 1H, *J* = 6.8, 1.2 Hz, Indole H$_6$); ESI-Mass *m/z*: 282 [M + H]$^+$, 304 [M + Na]$^+$; Anal. Calcd. for C$_{16}$H$_{12}$FN$_3$O: C, 68.32; H, 4.30; N, 14.94. Found: C, 68.14; H, 4.03; N, 15.02.

N'-(2-fluorobenzylidene)-1H-indole-2-carbohydrazide (6d)
Yield: 98%, mp 186- 188°C. IR (KBr) cm^{-1}: 3450, 3227, 3038, 2922, 1643, 1621, 1612, 1593, and 1564. ^{1}H NMR (500 MHz, DMSO): δ 12.03 (s, 1H, CONH), 11.85 (s, 1H, Indole NH), 8.71 (s, 1H, —N=C*H*—), 7.98 (t, 1H, *J* = 7.3 Hz, —N=CH—C$_6$H$_5$,H$_4$), 7.70 (d, 1H, *J* = 7.8 Hz, —N=CH—C$_6$H$_5$,H$_6$), 7.52- 7.47 (m, 2H, Indole

H$_4$, H$_7$), 7.35- 7.32 (m, 2H, Indole H$_5$, H$_6$), 7.24 (t, 1H, *J* = 7.4 Hz, —N=CH—C$_6$H$_5$, H$_3$), 7.08 (t, 1H, *J* = 7.4 Hz, —N=CH—C$_6$H$_5$, H$_5$); ESI-Mass *m/z*: 282 [M + H]$^+$; Anal. Calcd. for C$_{16}$H$_{12}$FN$_3$O: C, 68.32; H, 4.30; N, 14.94. Found: C, 68.14; H, 4.63; N, 15.12.

N'-(3-fluorobenzylidene)-1H-indole-2-carbohydrazide (6 g)
Yield: 88%, mp 171- 173°C. IR (KBr) cm^{-1}: 3448, 3313, 3264, 3126, 3071, 1629, 1597, 1577, 1529; ^{1}H NMR (500 MHz, DMSO): δ 12.02 (s, 1H, CONH), 11.84 (s, 1H, Indole NH), 8.47 (s, 1H, —N=C*H*—), 7.70 (d, 1H, *J* = 8.0 Hz, —N=CH—C$_6$H$_5$,H$_2$),7.61 (d, 1H, *J* = 7.3 Hz, Indole H$_7$), 7.58- 7.52 (m, 2H, —N=CH—C$_6$H$_5$ H$_5$, Indole, H$_4$), 7.48 (d, 1H, *J* = 8.0 Hz, —N=CH—C$_6$H$_5$, H$_6$), 7.34 (s, 1H, Indole H$_3$), 7.30 (t, 1H, *J* = 8.5 Hz, —N=CH—C$_6$H$_5$, H$_6$), 7.24 (t, 1H, *J* = 7.5 Hz, Indole H$_6$), 7.08 (t, 1H, *J* = 7.5 Hz, Indole H$_5$); ESI-Mass *m/z*: 282 [M + H]$^+$, 304 [M + Na]$^+$; Anal. Calcd. for C$_{16}$H$_{12}$FN$_3$O: C, 68.32; H, 4.30; N, 14.94. Found: C, 68.01; H, 4.33; N, 14.62.

N'-(3-hydroxybenzylidene)-1H-indole-2-carbohydrazide (6 h)
Yield: 89%, mp 278- 281°C. IR (KBr) cm^{-1}: 3412 (v OH), 3227, 3185, 3048, 2924, 1624, 1599, 1583, 1564, 1507; ^{1}H NMR (500 MHz, DMSO): δ 12.05 (s, 1H, CONH), 11.84 (bs, 2H, Indole NH, OH), 8.44 (s, 1H, —N=C*H*—), 7.82 (s, 1H, —N=CH—C$_6$H$_5$, H$_2$), 7.74- 7.68 (m, 2H, Indole H$_4$, H$_7$), 7.53- 7.51 (m, 2H, —N=CH—C$_6$H$_5$, H$_5$, H$_6$), 7.47 (d, 1H, *J* = 8.3 Hz, —N=CH—C$_6$H$_5$, H$_4$), 7.34 (s, 1H, Indole H$_3$), 7.24 (t, 1H, *J* = 7.1 Hz, Indole H$_6$), 7.08 (t, 1H, *J* = 7.1 Hz, Indole H$_5$); ESI-Mass *m/z*: 280 [M + H]$^+$, 302 [M + Na]$^+$; Anal. Calcd. for C$_{16}$H$_{13}$N$_3$O$_2$: C, 68.81; H, 4.69; N, 15.05. Found: C, 69.04; H, 4.41; N, 14.92.

Biological assay
In vitro evaluation of anti-platelet aggregation activity
Human plasma used to measure the derivatives anti-platelet aggregation activity. Fresh blood was obtained from healthy volunteer with negative history of drug consumption from 15 days prior to the test. Platelet-rich plasma (PRP) was obtained from citrated whole blood (9:1 by volume) which centrifuged at 1,000 rpm for 8 min. The remained layer was centrifuged at 3,000 rpm for 15 min and the upper layer; PPP (Platelet poor plasma) was collected as the blank. The platelet count was adjusted to 250,000 plts/mL by diluting PRP with appropriate amount of PPP. To the PRP samples, test compounds previously dissolved in DMSO (at 0.05% final concentration) were added and samples were incubated for 5 min at 37°C. Then ADP (5 μM), collagen (1.25 mg/mL) or AA (1.25 mg/mL) was added and platelet shape change and aggregation were monitored for 5 min. DMSO (0.5% v/v) was used as negative control and aspirin and indomethacin

were applied as standard drugs. The extent of platelet aggregation was calculated by the following formula:

$$Inhibition\% = [1-(D/S)] * 100$$

D = platelet aggregation in the presence of test compoundsS = platelet aggregation in the presence of solvent.

The platelet aggregation inhibitory activity was expressed as percent inhibition by comparison with that measured for the vehicle (DMSO) alone and IC_{50} values were obtained from log (concentration) – inhibition (%) diagram and was defined as the concentration of the test compound that inhibits the platelet aggregation by 50%. Data were presented as mean ± S.E.M. of three independent experiments performed in triplicate. IC_{50}values and inhibition data were analyzed with prism software.

Consent

The study was approved in the Institute Review Board with code number 93-6-10:1–1. Written informed consent was obtained from the patient for the publication of this report and any accompanying images.

Results

The synthetic pathway is disclosed in Scheme 1. Final desired derivatives were prepared by a two-step procedure. The structures were confirmed by spectroscopic techniques including IR, Mass and ^{1}H NMR. Molecular mass of all the derivatives was determined by Electronspray ionization mass spectrometry (ESI–MS) as M + 1 and/or M + 23 relating to hydrogen and sodium adducts of the intact molecules, respectively. All the synthesized compounds were evaluated for their ability to inhibit platelet aggregation of human platelet-rich plasma (PRP) induced by AA, ADP and collagen as potent aggregation inducers, and using indomethacin and aspirin were applied as standard drugs. The results of *in-vitro* antiplatelet aggregation activity for the title compounds were summarized in Table 1. All the derivatives were initially tested at 1 mM.

The physicochemical parameters of the derivatives were calculated and are listed in Table 2.

Discussion

Chemistry

All derivatives of 3-substituted indole and 2-substituted indole were obtained by the reaction of **2** and **5** with the proper aldehydes. *Synthesis of Schiff bases were* performed in ethanol with a few drops of glacial acetic acid. This reaction in the majority of the cases was straight forward; however, the products were soluble in ethanol and their separation was difficult. Therefore in another effort, the solvent was changed to water, a few drops of glacial acetic acid was added to the reaction mixture and

Table 2 General molecular parameters of the synthesized compounds

Compound	Clog P	R[a]	P[b]	V[c]	SA[d]	
					Approx.	Grid
3d	2.92	86.69	30.1	771.23	374.67	469.41
3e	-0.15	92.78	32.03	809.38	404.94	487.59
3f	3.35	88.16	30.83	781.07	373.02	472.72
3g	2.72	90.56	31.99	854.73	356.93	517.77
3h	3.85	91.28	32.12	807.06	402.79	488.39
3i	3.28	86.69	30.1	772.67	378.22	470.61
3j	2.72	88.16	30.83	784.59	381.64	474.45
3k	2.72	88.16	30.83	783.92	379.99	474.45
3l	3.85	91.28	32.12	807.9	403.8	488.87
3m	3.14	86.56	30.19	764.21	367.69	464.55
6d	3.26	87.96	30.1	775.75	381.25	476.6
6e	3.69	89.44	30.83	787.22	379.72	479.81
6f	3.06	94.21	32.66	844.8	422.2	515.34
6g	3.62	87.96	30.1	778.08	384.8	477.59
6h	3.06	89.44	30.83	791.05	387	482.43
6i	3.48	87.83	30.19	772.17	374	474.2

[a]Refractivity.
[b]Polarizability.
[c]Molecular volume.
[d]Surface area.

heated for 10 min. After completion of reaction, the products were obtained in excellent yields.

In the ^{1}H NMR spectra of these compounds the existence of two singlet at 11.00 to 12.00 ppm was assigned to hydrazide NH and indole NH. Also, singlet signal at 8.20-8.80 ppm was assigned to H—C = N. The ^{1}H NMR and ESI-mass data of compounds approved the exact structures.

Antiplatelet aggregation activity

Platelet activation and thrombus formation are major causes of cardiovascular diseases and thrombosis. Thus, antiplatelet therapy is a useful way to prevent or treat these diseases; these diseases; thus, antiplatelet agents such as aspirin, ticlopidine and dipyridamole have been clinically used for thrombus-related diseases [9]. However, the side effects of mentioned agents frequently have been reported and a new group of compounds with greater efficacy and safety are desired. Therefore, in the present study, the inhibitory effects of synthesized compounds on platelet aggregation were evaluated by turbidimetric method reported by Born and Cross [33] using APACT 4004 aggregometer. The baseline value was set using PRP and maximal transmission using PPP. Compounds **3d-m** and **6d-i** were tested for anti-platelet aggregation activity induced by adenosine diphosphate (ADP), arachidonic acid (AA) and collagen using indomethacin and aspirin as standards.

Interestingly, most of the tested derivatives selectively inhibited platelet aggregation induced by AA and collagen with satisfactory percent inhibition values. According to the literature [15]; herein, antiplatelet aggregation activity of N-acylhydrazones is probably related to modulation of AA cascade enzymes.

Among the synthesized indole-2-carbaldehyde derivatives compound 6g exhibited 100% inhibition of platelet aggregation at 1 mM when AA was used as agonist while this compound has no significant inhibitory activity against ADP and collagen induced platelet aggregation. Comparing the results obtained for indole derivatives, compounds 3m and 6h showed the best antiplatelet aggregation effect which induced by collagen. On the other hand, effects of the synthesized compounds on the platelet aggregation induced by ADP shows another pattern: all the compounds caused no significant inhibition on platelet aggregation except 6e which showed 66.7% inhibition.

The IC_{50} values were calculated for more potent compounds (3f, 3i, 3k, 3l, 3m, 6d, 6g, 6h and 6i) for the inhibition of AA and collagen-induced aggregation which are shown in Table 3.

However, the obtained results were compared with those reported by Kobarfard et al. on antiplatelet aggregation effect of some indole derivatives [4]. It was found that the insertion of acyl group to indole hydrazone moiety cannot improve platelet aggregation inhibitory activity.

In order to investigate the possible relationship between the structural parameters of the investigated derivatives and their antiplatelet aggregation activity, quantitative structure–activity relationship (QSAR) analysis was performed with various molecular descriptors. The calculated

octanol–water partition coefficient (Clog P) has been considered as descriptor for the hydrophobic effect. The steric effect has been described by means of the surface area (SA: approx and grid) and molecular volume (V) refractivity (R) and polarizability (P) have been used as descriptors for both volume and electronic state (London dispersive forces) properties of the molecules. For each descriptor, the best multilinear regression equation was obtained. The calculated physicochemical parameters of the derivatives are listed in Table 2. Analysis of the physicochemical parameters doesn't show a significant correlation between the observed activities and general molecular parameters of the synthesized derivatives.

Conclusion

In summary, we have synthesized sixteen N-acylhydrazone derivatives (3d-m and 6d-i) and evaluated their antiplatelet aggregation activity against collagen, ADP and AA as the aggregation inducers. Compounds 3e, 3g, 3h, 3i, 3j, 3k, 3l, 3m, 6d, 6f, 6g, 6h and 6i showed significant antiplatelet aggregation (>90%) when arachidonic acid was used as the inducer. While, 3l, 3k, 3m and 6h exhibited best (>90%) platelet aggregation inhibition induced by collagen among other compounds.

Failure to extract a clear correlation between activities and general molecular parameters of the synthesized compounds could be related to the existence of several receptors on the platelets surface which are responsible for controlling platelet aggregation. Platelets are activated by variety of metabolic pathways. The mechanism of platelet aggregation pathway is very complex and involves multiple components and it can be controlled by heterogeneous group of endogenous compounds such as ADP, ATP, collagen, tryptophan, epinephrine, thromboxane A_2 and calcium. Each can independently and together begin the process leading to platelet aggregation. These compounds on platelets have specific receptors and the investigated compounds in the present study may exert their activities through binding to more than one of these receptors and therefore no straight forward SAR could be obtained. The findings of this study will be helpful for the development of new antiplatelet compounds providing some directions in the area of antiplatelet drug discovery.

Table 3 IC$_{50}$values for the antiplatelet aggregation activity induced by collagen and AA[a]

Compound	Aryl	IC_{50} (µM)[b]	
		AA	Collagen
3f	2-methoxyphenyl	310±8.1	121.5±3.1
3i	4-hydroxyphenyl	290±5.3	188±2.8
3k	2-fluorophenyl	179±2.4	122±1.6
3l	3-fluorophenyl	321±3.9	120±4.0
3m	phenyl	182±5.2	21±0.9
6d	2-fluorophenyl	286±1.5	720±9.1
6g	3-fuorophenyl	140±4.3	>1000
6h	3-hydroxyphenyl	200±2.0	190±3.2
6i	phenyl	94±1.9	134±4.1
Indomethacin		3±0.2	1.2±0.1
Aspirin		30.3±2.6	9.7±0.6

[a]Data related to compounds 3 and 6 as shown in Scheme 1.
[b]IC$_{50}$ values represent mean ± S.E. of triplicate measurements from one of three independent experiments.

Competing interests
The authors declare that they have no competing interests.

Authors' contributions
SSM: Synthesis of the title compounds and collaboration in the antiplatelet aggregation test. FK: Design of target compounds and supervision of the synthetic and pharmacological parts. LF: Collaboration in computational study. AA: collaboration in the synthetic part. ME: Performed the antiplatelet aggregation test. KT: collaborated in the antiplatelet aggregation test and identifying the structures of target compounds. AS: Design of target compounds and supervision of the synthetic part. AF: Design of target compounds and supervision of the synthetic part. All authors read and approved the final manuscript.

Acknowledgements
The authors are thankful for financial support from the Research Council of Tehran University of Medical Sciences and Iran National Science Foundation (INSF).

Author details
[1]Department of Medicinal Chemistry, Faculty of Pharmacy and Pharmaceutical Sciences Research Center, Tehran University of Medical Sciences, Tehran, Iran. [2]Department of Medicinal Chemistry, School of Pharmacy, Shahid Beheshti University of Medical Sciences, Tehran, Iran. [3]Phytochemistry Research Center, Shahid Beheshti University of Medical Sciences, Tehran, Iran. [4]Drug Design and Development Research Center, Tehran University of Medical Sciences, Tehran, Iran. [5]Neuroscience Research Center, Institute of Neuropharmacology, Kerman University of Medical Sciences, Kerman, Iran.

References
1. Mendis S, Puska P, Norrving B: Global atlas on cardiovascular disease prevention and control. 2011, [http://www.world-heart-federation.org/publications/books/global-atlas-on-cvd-prevention-and-control/]
2. Reddy MV, Tsai WJ, Qian K, Lee KH, Wu TS: Structure–activity relationships of chalcone analogs as potential inhibitors of ADP- and collagen-induced platelet aggregation. Bioorg Med Chem 2011, 19:7711–7719.
3. Brito FCF, Kummerle AE, Lugnier C, Fraga CAM, Barreiro EJ, Miranda ALP: Novel thienylacylhydrazone derivatives inhibit platelet aggregation through cyclic nucleotides modulation and thromboxane A₂synthesis inhibition. Eur J Pharmacol 2010, 638:5–12.
4. Mashayekhi V, Hajmohammad Ebrahim Tehrani K, Amidi S, Kobarfard F: Synthesis of novel indole hydrazone derivatives and evaluation of their antiplatelet aggregation activity. Chem Pharm Bull 2013, 61:144–150.
5. DeCandia M, Liantonio F, Carotti A, De Cristofaro R, Altomare C: Fluorinated benzyloxyphenyl piperidine-4-carboxamides with dual function against thrombosis: inhibitors of factor Xa and platelet aggregation. J Med Chem 2009, 52:1018–1028.
6. Maree AO, Fitzgerald DJ: Variable platelet response to aspirin and clopidogrel in atherothrombotic disease. Circulation 2007, 115:2196–2207.
7. Meadows TA, Bhatt DL: Clinical aspects of platelet inhibitors and thrombus formation. Circ Res 2007, 100:1261–1275.
8. Fathiazad F, Matlobi A, Khorrami A, Hamedeyazdan S, Soraya H, Hammami M, Maleki-Dizaji N, Garjani A: Phytochemical screening and evaluation of cardioprotective activity of ethanolic extract of Ocimum basilicum L. (basil) against isoproterenol induced myocardial infarction in rats. DARU J Pharm Sci 2012, 20:87.
9. Eskandariyan Z, Esfahanizadeh M, Haj Mohammad Ebrahim Tehrani K, Mashayekhi V, Kobarfard F: Synthesis of thioether derivatives of quinazoline-4-one-2-thione and evaluation of their antiplatelet aggregation activity. Arch Pharm Res 2013, 37:332–339.
10. Siwek A, Stączek P, Stefańska J: Synthesis and structure activity relationship studies of 4-arylthiosemicarbazides as topoisomerase IV inhibitors with Gram-positive antibacterial activity. search for molecular basis of antibacterial activity of thiosemicarbazides. Eur J Med Chem 2011, 46:5717–5726.
11. Fraga AGM, Rodrigues CR, de Miranda ALP, Barreiro EJ, Fraga CAM: Synthesis and evaluation of novel heterotricyclic acylhydrazones derivatives, designed as PAF antagonist candidates. Eur J Pharm Sci 2000, 11:285–290.
12. Cunha AC, Figueiredo JM, Tributino JLM, Miranda ALP, Castro HC, Zingali RB, Fraga CAM, de Souza MCBV, Ferreira VF, Barreiro EJ: Antiplatelet properties of novelN-substituted-phenyl-1,2,3-triazole-4-acylhydrazone derivatives. Bioorg Med Chem 2003, 11:2051–2059.
13. Cunha AC, Tributino JLM, Miranda ALP, Fraga CAM, Barreiro EJ: Synthesis and pharmacological evaluation of novel antinociceptive N-substituted-phenylimidazolyl- 4-acylhydrazone derivatives. Il Farmaco 2002, 57:999–1007.
14. Lima PC, Lima LM, da Silva KC, Le'da PH, de Miranda AL, Fraga CAM, Barreiro EJ: Synthesis and analgesic activity of novelN-acylarylhydrazones and isosters, derived from natural safrole. Eur J Med Chem 2000, 35:187–203.
15. Silva GA, Costa LMM, Brito FCF, Miranda ALP, Barreiro EJ, Fraga CAM: New class of potent antinociceptive and antiplatelet 10H-phenothiazine-1-acylhydrazone derivatives. Bioorg Med Chem 2004, 12:3149–3158.
16. Bezerra-Neto HJC, Lacerda DI, Miranda ALP, Alves HM, Barreiro EJ, Fraga CAM: Design and synthesis of 3,4-methylenedioxy-6-nitrophenoxyacetylhydrazone derivatives obtained from natural safrole: new lead-agents with analgesic and antipyretic properties. Bioorg Med Chem 2006, 14:7924–7935.
17. Duarte CD, Tributino JLM, Lacerda DI, Martins MV, Alexandre-Moreira MS, Dutra F, Bechara EJH, De-Paula FS, Goulart MOF, Ferreira J, Calixto JB, Nunes MP, Bertho AL, Miranda ALP, Barreiro EJ, Fraga CAM: Synthesis, pharmacological evaluation and electrochemical studies of novel 6-nitro-3,4-methylenedioxyphenyl-N-acylhydrazone derivatives: discovery of LASSBio-881, a new ligand of cannabinoid receptors. Bioorg Med Chem 2007, 15:2421–2433.
18. Lima LM, Frattani FS, dos Santos JL, Castro HC, Fraga CAM, Zingali RB, Barreiro EJ: Synthesis and anti-platelet activity of novel arylsulfonateacylhydrazone derivatives, designed as antithrombotic candidates. Eur J Med Chem 2008, 43:348–356.
19. Tributino JLM, Duarte CD, Corrêa RS, Dorigetto AC, Ellena J, Romeiro NC, Castro NG, Miranda ALP, Barreiro EJ, Fraga CAM: Novel 6-methanesulfonamide- 3,4-methylenedioxy-phenyl- N-acylhydrazones: orally effective anti-inflammatory drug candidates. Biorg Med Chem 2009, 17:1125–1131.
20. Maia RC, Silva LL, Mazzeu EF, Fumian MM, de Rezende CM, Doriguetto AC, Corrêa RS, Miranda ALP, Barreiro EJ, Fraga MCA: Synthesis and analgesic profile of conformationally constrained N-acylhydrazone analogues: Discovery of novel N-arylideneamino quinazolin-4(3H)-one compounds derived from natural safrole. Bioorg Med Chem 2009, 17:6517–6525.
21. Chen R, Li X, Gong B, Selzer PM, Li Z, Davidson E, Kurzban G, Miller RE, Nuzum EO, McKerrow JH, Fletterick RJ, Gillmor SA, Craik CS, Kuntz ID, Cohen FE, Kenyon GL: Structure-based design of parasitic protease inhibitors. Bioorg Med Chem 1996, 4:1421–1427.
22. Sluis-Cremer N, Arion D, Parniak MA: Destabilization of the HIV-1 reverse transcriptase dimer upon interaction with N-acyl hydrazone inhibitors. Mol Pharmacol 2002, 62:398–405.
23. Dimmock JR, Baker GB, Taylor WG: Arylhydrazones. Part II. The ultraviolet spectroscopy and antimicrobial evaluation of some substituted aroylhydrazones. Can J Pharm Sci 1972, 7:100–103.
24. Sudo RT, Zapata-Sudo G, Barreiro EJ: The new compound, LASSBio 294, increases the contractility of intact and saponin-skinned cardiac muscle from Wistar rats. Br J Pharmacol 2001, 134:603–613.
25. Gonzalez-Serratos H, Chang R, Pereira EF, Castro NG, Aracava Y, Melo PA, Lima PC, Fraga CAM, Barreiro EJ, Albuquerque EX: A novel thienylhydrazone, (2- thienylidene) 3,4-methylenedioxybenzoylhydrazine, increases inotropism and decreases fatigue of skeletal muscle. J Pharmacol Exp Ther 2001, 229:558–566.
26. Silva CLM, Noe LF, Barreiro EJ: Cyclic GMP-dependent vasodilatory properties of LASSBio 294 in rat aorta. Br J Pharmacol 2002, 135:293–298.
27. Zapata-Sudo G, Sudo RT, Maronas PA, Silva GL, Moreira OR, Aguiar MI, Barreiro EJ: Thienylhydrazone derivative increases sarcoplasmic reticulum Ca²⁺release in mammalian skeletal muscle. Eur J Pharmacol 2003, 470:79–85.
28. Silva AG, Zapata-Sudo G, Kummerle AE, Fraga CAM, Barreiro EJ, Sudo RT: Synthesis and vasodilatory activity of newN-acylhydrazone derivatives, designed as LASSBio-294 analogues. Bioorg Med Chem 2005, 13:3431–3437.
29. Park MK, Rhee YH, Lee HJ, Lee EO, Kim KH, Park MJ, Jeon BH, Shim BS, Jung CH, Choi SH, Ahn KS, Kim SH: Antiplatelet and antithrombotic activity of indole-3-carbinol in vitro and in vivo. Phytother Res 2008, 22:58–64.
30. Alemany A, Bernabé M, Elorriaga C, Fernández AE, Lora-Tamayo M, Nieto O: Patent; Patron, Invest. Cie. Tech. Bull Soc Chim Fr 1966, 8:2486–2497.

31. Bao XP, Zheng PC, Liu Y, Tan Z, Zhou YH, Song BA: **Salicylaldehyde-indole-2-acylhydrazone: a simple, colorimetric and absorption ratiometric chemosensor for acetate ion.** *Supramol Chem* 2013, **25**:246–253.
32. Wareth A, Sarhan AO: **On the synthesis and reactions of indole-2-carboxylic acid hydrazide.** *Monatsh Chem* 2001, **132**:753–763.
33. Born GVR: **Aggregation of blood platelets by adenosine diphosphate and its reversal.** *Nature* 1962, **194**:927–929.

18

Curcumin as a double-edged sword for stem cells: dose, time and cell type-specific responses to curcumin

Fatemeh Attari[1,3], Maryam Zahmatkesh[1], Hadi Aligholi[1,3], Shahram Ejtemaei Mehr[4], Mohammad Sharifzadeh[5], Ali Gorji[3,7], Tahmineh Mokhtari[2], Mojtaba Khaksarian[6] and Gholamreza Hassanzadeh[1,2*]

Abstract

Background: The beneficial effects of curcumin which includes its antioxidant, anti-inflammatory and cancer chemo-preventive properties have been identified. Little information is available regarding the optimal dose and treatment periods of curcumin on the proliferation rate of different sources of stem cells.

Methods: In this study, the effect of various concentrations of curcumin on the survival and proliferation of two types of outstanding stem cells which includes bone marrow stem cells (BMSCs) and adult rat neural stem/progenitor cells (NS/PCs) at different time points was investigated. BMSCs were isolated from bilateral femora and tibias of adult Wistar rats. NS/PCs were obtained from subventricular zone of adult Wistar rat brain. The curcumin (0.1, 0.5, 1, 5 and 10 μM/L) was added into a culture medium for 48 or 72 h. Fluorescent density of 5-bromo-2′-deoxyuridine (Brdu)-positive cells was considered as proliferation index. In addition, cell viability was assessed by MTT assay.

Results: Treatment of BMSCs with curcumin after 48 h, increased cell survival and proliferation in a dose-dependent manner. However, it had no effect on NSCs proliferation except a toxic effect in the concentration of 10 μM of curcumin. After a 72 h treatment period, BMSCs and NS/PCs survived and proliferated with low doses of curcumin. However, high doses of curcumin administered for 72 h showed toxic effects on both stem cells.

Conclusions: These findings suggest that curcumin survival and proliferative effects depend on its concentration, treatment period and the type of stem cells. Appropriate application of these results may be helpful in the outcome of combination therapy of stem cells and curcumin.

Keywords: Curcumin, Bone marrow mesenchymal stem cells, Neural stem cells, Cell proliferation, Cell survival

Background

Curcumin (diferuloylmethane) is one of the active components of dietary spice turmeric (Curcuma longa Linn) which was first chemically characterized in 1910 [1, 2]. To date, a great number of studies have focused on the multifarious biological effects of curcumin including its antioxidant, anti-inflammatory and cancer chemo-preventive properties [3, 4]. In addition, some papers have reported that curcumin can decrease oxidative damage and improve cognitive deficiencies related to aging. Moreover, curcumin can also be useful for the treatment of neurodegenerative diseases such as Alzheimer's disease and brain ischemia [5, 6]. Furthermore, there are some reports on the synergistic effect of curcumin in conjunction with stem cell therapy vis-à-vis recovery from spinal cord injury [7]. In this regard, curcumin may enhance proliferation of stem cells for swift regeneration [7, 8]. Previous investigations have reported that curcumin has biphasic effects on the proliferation of some stem cells including spinal cord neural progenitor cells [9], embryonic neural progenitor cells [8] and 3 T3-L1 preadipocytes [10]. To find the optimal curcumin concentration as well as the administration time for treatment of different types of stem cells with curcumin, more studies are needed.

Among different sources of stem cells, bone marrow mesenchymal stem cells (BMSCs) are known to have

* Correspondence: hassanzadeh@tums.ac.ir
[1]Department of Neuroscience, School of Advanced Technologies in medicine, Tehran University of Medical Sciences, Tehran, Iran
[2]Department of Anatomy, School of Medicine, Tehran University of Medical Sciences, Tehran, Iran
Full list of author information is available at the end of the article

capacity for proliferation and differentiation into mesen-chymal and non-mesenchymal lineages. In many previ-ous study, these types of stem cells were used for cell and gene therapy due to their capacity for self-renewal in a number of non-hematopoietic tissues as well as their multi-potentiality for differentiation [11].

On the other hand, adult neural stem/progenitor cells (NS/PCs) are self-renewal and multi-potent cells located specially in the subventricular zone of the lateral wall of the lateral ventricle of an adult mammalian brain. These cells can be isolated and cultured in-vitro to produce true neural and glial cells and finally transplanted for the treat-ment of neurodegenerative diseases [12, 13]. Little is known about the effective dose and treatment periods of curcumin when it is utilized as a supportive element for BMSCs and NS/PCs. Hence, in this study, the effects of various concentrations of curcumin on survival and prolif-eration of BMSCs and NS/PCs at different time points were investigated.

Methods

BMSCs culture

BMSCs were extracted from the bone marrow of bilateral femora and tibias of 4 weeks old male Wistar rats. The cell suspension was centrifuged and plated on T-25 plastic flasks in Dulbecco's Modified Eagle Medium (DMEM/F12) (Invitrogen, USA), supplemented with 10 % fetal bovine serum (FBS, Invitrogen, USA), 100U/ml penicillin and 100 mg/ml streptomycin (Invitrogen, USA) and incubated at 37 °C with 5 % CO_2. When primary cultures became al-most confluent, the cells were passaged by trypsinization and cultured in the above compound. All of the experi-ments were performed using cells at passages 10-18 [14].

NS/PCs culture

SVZ specimens were harvested from the brain of young adult male Wistar rats (150-200 g) and transported in 10 % penicillin-streptomycin solution (prepared with 0.1 M cold PBS, PH 7.2-7.4). Next, 500 µl of 0.05 % trypsin/ EDTA so-lution (Invitrogen, USA, 5 min at 37 °C) was used for tissue dissection. The reaction was brought to a halt by the addition of 500 µl of Soybean trypsin inhibitor (Sigma, USA) to the dissociated tissue. After centrifugation, the cells were placed on T-25 plastic flasks in 5 mL of DMEM/F12 containing 1 % N2 supplement (Invitrogen, USA), 3 % B27 supplement (Invitrogen, USA), 2 µg/mL heparin (Sigma, USA), 1 % glutamax (Invitrogen, USA), 1 % penicil-lin/streptomycin (Invitrogen, USA), 10 ng/ml basic fibro-blast growth factor (bFGF; Millipore, Germany), 20 ng/ml epidermal growth factor (EGF; Miltenybiotech, Germany), at 37 °C in a humidified atmosphere with 5 % CO_2. Neuro-spheres were passaged by trypsinization and mechanically separated after 15 days [12, 15]. The NS/PCs obtained from the third passage were used for all experiments.

Cell viability assay

Cell viability was assessed by MTT (3-(4,5-dimethylthiazo-lyl-2) -2,5-diphenyltetrazolium bromide) assay. NS/PCs and BMSCs were seeded at a density of 1×10^4 cells in 96-well plates. Curcumin (Sigma, USA) was dissolved in Di-methyl Sulphoxide (DMSO) (Sigma, USA) and added in different concentrations of 0.1, 0.5, 1, 5 and 10 µM/L into the culture medium. In the control group, cells were treated with the DMSO. Forty-eight and seventy two hours after the treatment, the medium containing curcu-min was replaced with fresh medium containing 1 mg/ml MTT solution in 0.01 M PBS. The plates were incubated at a temperature of 37 °C for 4 h. The mitochondrial de-hydrogenase of viable cells broke down MTT and pro-duced purple formazan. The cells were disrupted in DMSO. The purple formazan dye was then measured with ELISA reader at 595 nm absorbance [16]. Each experi-ment was repeated three times.

Immunofluorescent assay

The cells were fixed with 4 % paraformaldehyde in PBS for 1 h then rinsed with PBS three times for 5 min and in-cubated with blocker solution (5 % normal goat serum and 1 % bovine serum albumin in PBS) for 60 min. Mouse anti-Nestin (1:100; Abcam, USA) [12], rabbit anti-CD73 (1:200; Abcam, USA) or rabbit anti-CD105 (1:100; Abcam, USA) [17] were used at 4 °C over night. After washing with PBS, goat anti-Mouse IgG (alexa flour 647, 1:600; invitrogen, USA) or goat anti-Rabbit IgG (FITC; 1:700; Abcam, USA) were added to the cells for 60 min at room temperature and the nuclei were stained with 4,6-diami-dino-2-phenylindole (DAPI, 1 g/ml, Santa Cruz, Germany) or Propidium Iodide (PI; invitrogen, USA). Immuno-labeled cells were assessed by a fluorescent microscope (Olympus, japan). In control samples, the primary anti-bodies were eliminated in a reaction in which no immuno-reactivity was detected.

Bromodeoxyuridine (BrdU) Immunocytochemistry

Cells were plated onto polyornithine (50 µg/ml) coated 96-well plates at a density of 1×10^4 cells. Cells were treated with either DMSO or curcumin at two time points (48 and 72 h). Adherent cells and neurospheres were then fixed in 4 % paraformaldehyde for 30 min. The cells were washed with 0.2 % Triton-X 100 in 0.1 M PBS (pH 7.4) three times for 5 min. DNA was denatured by exposing the cells to acid (2 M HCl, 30 min at 37 °C). After that, borate buffer (0.1 M) was added to the cells for 12 min at room temperature. Then, 5 % normal goat serum in 0.1 M PBS (pH 7.4) was added to block en-dogenous peroxidases. Next, the cells were incubated overnight with mouse anti-BrdU antibody (1:1000, Sigma, Germany) and thereafter exposed to FITC conju-gate anti-mouse IgG (1:1000, Sigma, Germany) for BMSCs or Alexa-Fluor 647-conjugated anti-mouse IgG (1:500, Abcam USA) for NS/PCs for 2 h at room temperature. Each experiment was repeated three times.

Proliferating cells and neurospheres were incubated by 10 μM/l BrdU for 48 h and analyzed by immuno-staining [18]. Fluorescent density of Brdu positive cells were measured using image J software [19, 20]. The study had the endorsement of the ethical committee of Tehran University of Medical Sciences.

Statistical analysis

The statistical significance was determined using the t-test and One-Way Analysis of Variance (ANOVA) and a Tukey post-hoc test. The results are expressed as mean ± SEM. The null hypothesis was rejected at the 0.05 level of significance.

Results

Isolation of BMSCs and NS/PCs

After primary culture, BMSCs were obtained as monolayer cells which expressed mesenchymal stem cell markers CD105 and CD73. Cultivation of SVZ specimen resulted in the production of neurospheres which expressed nestin as a marker of NS/PCs (Fig. 1).

Effect of curcumin on proliferation of BMSCs

As indicated in Fig. 2, in the aftermath of 48 h administration, curcumin enhanced the BrdU positive BMSCs in a dose dependent manner, suchthat the doses of 5 and 10 μM of curcumin enhancement was statistically significant compared to the DMSO group ($P < 0.01$).

After 72 h treatment with different doses of curcumin, the above pattern was not seen, only the concentration of 0.5 μM of curcumin could considerably increase the BrdU positive BMSCs compared to the DMSO group ($P < 0.001$).

Effect of curcumin on proliferation of NS/PCs

There were no significant differences among the groups after 48 h treatment of NS/PCs with various doses of curcumin except for the 10 μM curcumin group in which the fluorescent density of BrdU was significantly decreased compared to the DMSO group ($P < 0.05$, Fig. 3).

After 72 h administration of curcumin, there was an increase in BrdU positive NS/PCs in doses of 0.1, 0.5 ($P < 0.01$) and 1 μM ($P < 0.001$) of curcumin compared to the DMSO group. The proliferation rate of NS/PCs significantly decreased following the administration of 5 or 10 μM of curcumin when compared with that of the DMSO group ($P < 0.05$, Fig. 3).

Effect of curcumin on survival of BMSCs

The results of MTT assay showed that all concentrations of curcumin including 0.1, 0.5, 1 ($P < 0.05$), 5 and 10 μM ($P < 0.01$) could enhance the viability of BMSCs after 48 h compared to the DMSO group (Fig. 4). Following 72 h treatment, the survival of BMSCs significantly increased with 0.5 μM of curcumin (P < 0.001), but this index considerably decreased with 5 and 10 μM of curcumin ($P < 0.05$) compared to the DMSO group.

Effect of curcumin on survival of NS/PCs

According to the results of MTT assay, curcumin with concentrations of 5 and 10 μM significantly reduced viability of NS/PCs compared to the DMSO group after 48 h (Fig. 5, $P < 0.05$). Moreover, following 72 h of NS/PCs encounter with curcumin, the highest cell viability was seen by using 1 μM of curcumin ($P < 0.001$ compared to the DMSO group). However, high doses of curcumin (5 and 10 μM) considerably decreased the viability of NS/PCs in comparison with the DMSO group ($P < 0.05$).

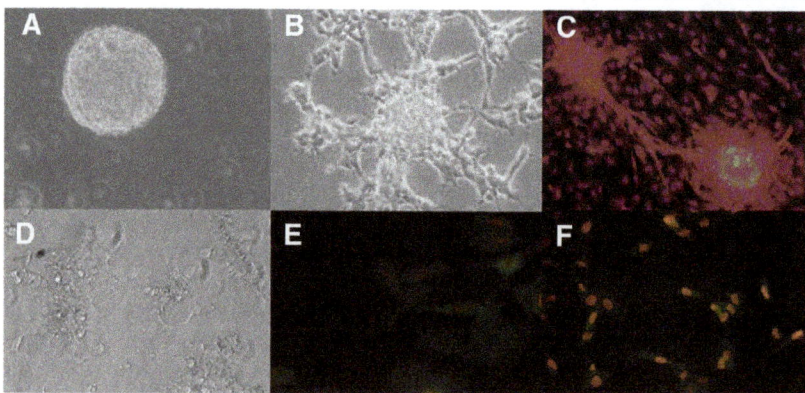

Fig. 1 Primary culture of NS/PCs and BMSCs. NS/PCs were cultured as flouting neurospheres (**a**) or slightly adherent cells (**b**) which expressed neural stem cell marker nestin (**c**). BMSCs were cultured as adherent cells (**d**) which expressed mesenchymal stem cell markers CD105 (**e**) and CD73 (**f**)

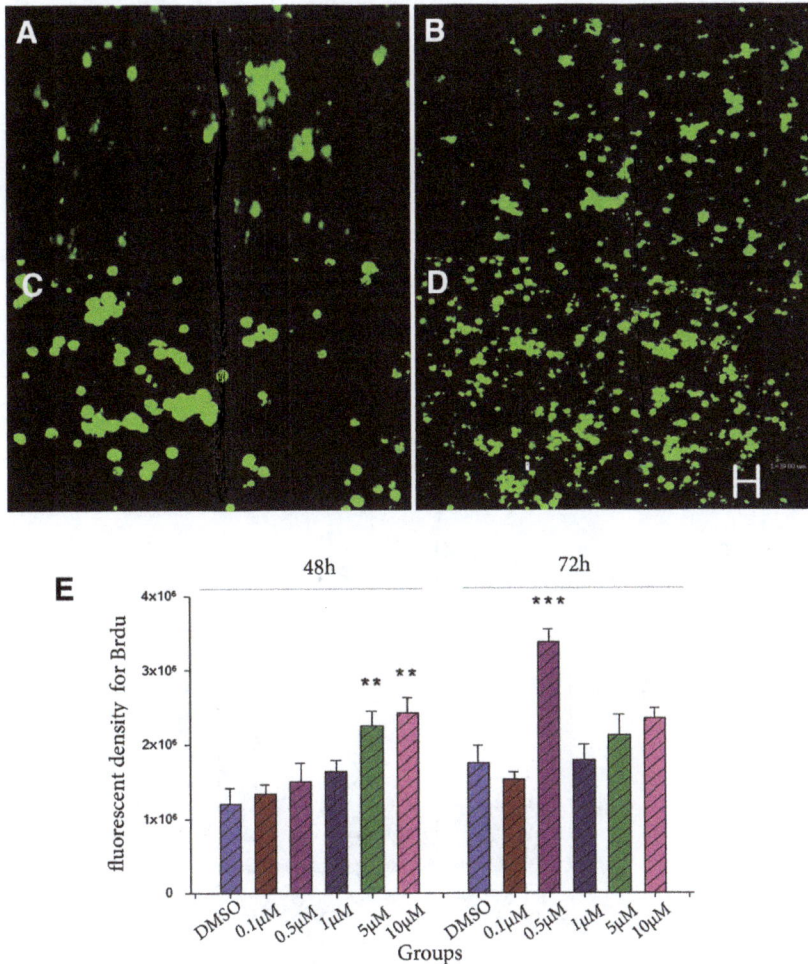

Fig. 2 The effect of various concentrations of curcumin on proliferation of BMSCs after 48 and 72 h. Different doses of curcumin (0.1, 0.5, 1, 5 and 10 µM) added 48 or 72 h into culture medium have various proliferative effects on BMSCs . The above pictures indicate the BrdU positive cells (green) in the DMSO 48 h group (**a**), 10 µM curcumin 48 h group (**b**), DMSO 72 h group (**c**) and 0.5 µM curcumin 72 h group (**d**). Scale bare:40 µm. **e**, fluorcent density for BrdU positive cells in different doses of curcumin after 48 or 72h, **: $P < 0.01$ or ***: $P < 0.001$ vs the DMSO group

Discussion

In the present study we observed multifarious effects of curcumin in terms of cell viability and stem cell proliferation. After administration of different doses of curcumin (0.1, 0.5, 1, 5 and 10 µM/L) to BMSCs, the high doses of curcumin enhanced the proliferation of BMSCs after 48 h However, when these cells were exposed to curcumin for 72 h, the increase in cell proliferation was seen only in doses of 0.5 µM of curcumin. On the other hand, the high doses of curcumin had adverse effects on the proliferation of NS/PCs while the doses of 0.1, 0.5 and 1 µM/L of curcumin administered for 72 h had beneficial effects on proliferation. The effect of curcumin on viability of BMSCs and NS/PCs was almost similar to its effect on proliferation of the cells.

Previous studies evaluated some of the effects of curcumin on the proliferation and viability of the cells. Kim et al. [8] revealed that after a 24 h treatment period, low concentration (0.5 µM) of curcumin was the most effective dose for increasing Brdu positive cells and cell viability of NS/PCs in cell culture. They opined that the stimulatory mechanism of low doses of curcumin on neural stem cells was facilitated by ERK and p38 MAP kinases [8]. In addition, Kim et al.[10] reported an increase in cell proliferation of preadipocytes with low concentrations of curcumin during a 24 h treatment period [10]. Moreover, Ormand et al. [7] reported that after 24 h, low doses of (0.5 µM) curcumin was the most effective concentration for increasing the neurosphere diameter of NS/PCs isolated from the adult rat SVZ, as

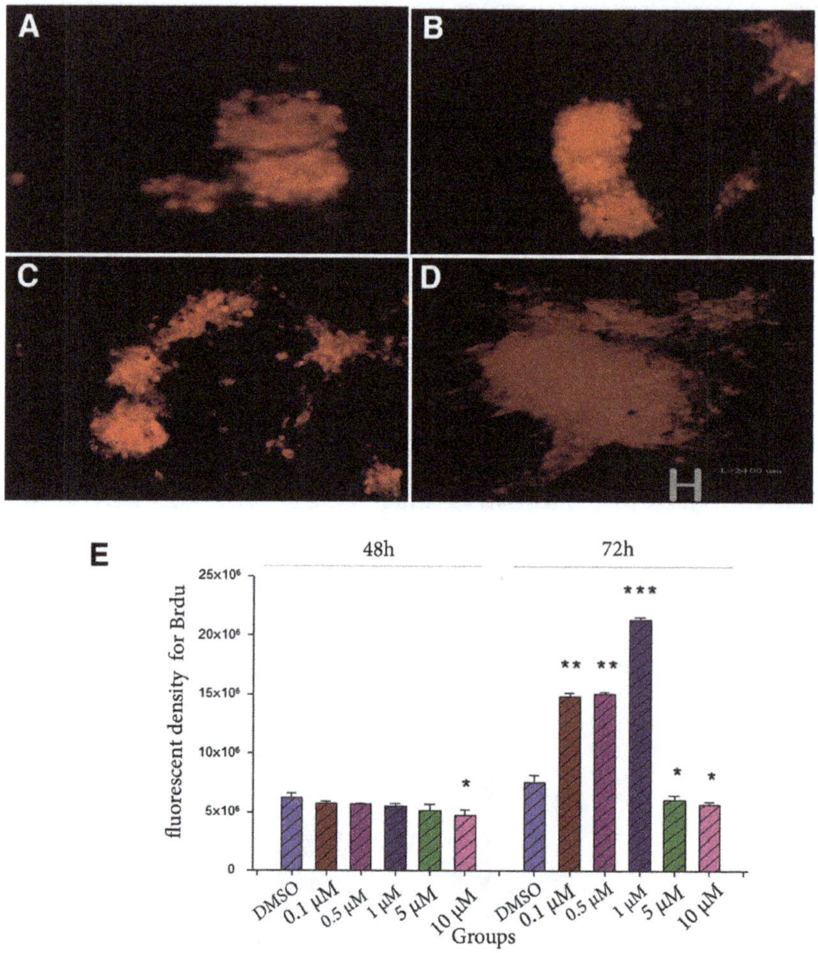

Fig. 3 The effect of various concentrations of curcumin on proliferation of NS/PCs after 48 and 72 h. Proliferation of NSCs was evaluated using fluorescent density for Brdu-positive cells. This index was different in the groups following 48 or 72 h treatment of NS/PCs with curcumin. The above photographs show the BrdU positive cells (red) in the DMSO 48 h group (**a**), 10 μM curcumin 48 h group (**b**), DMSO 72 h group (**c**) and 1 μM curcumin 72 h group (**d**). Scale bare:24 μm. **e**, fluorcent density for BrdU positive cells in different doses of curcumin after 48 or 72h, *: $P < 0.05$, **: $P < 0.01$ or ***: $P < 0.001$ vs the DMSO group

a proliferation index [7]. Previous studies have shown that curcumin can be utilized at low doses to induce heme oxygenase 1 at pharmacological levels, and its induction is accompanied by generation of non-lethal levels of reactive oxygen species [3]. On the other hand, Kim et al. [8] reported a cytotoxic effect with concentrations more than 10 μM of curcumin [8]. Ormand et al. [7] also demonstrated that curcumin at higher doses caused apoptosis [7]. Another report showed that the concentrations of 1-50 μM of curcumin increased cell viability while doses higher than 80 μM decreased it [16]. The discrepancies observed among the studies may be attributed in part to the different species, duration of curcumin exposure and the dose of curcumin. In the present study, the different doses of curcumin and

treatment duration were chosen based on a pilot study as well as previous reports [10, 8]. It is important to point out that according to the results of the present study; it seems that the toxic effects of curcumin on NS/PCs were more sensitive than that on BMSCs.

Indeed, in the light of latest investigations and results, curcumin acts as a double-edged sword. In other words, it can be toxic to cells and can also be helpful. It depends on the dose and type of cells. Based on this fact, curcumin should be used cautiously in future treatment strategies. Recent studies have shown that curcumin could reduce oxidative damage related to aging and was beneficial in the treatment of neurodegenerative diseases such as Alzheimer diseases, Parkinson disease, and stroke in animal models [21–25]. Xu et al. [26] showed that curcumin could reverse

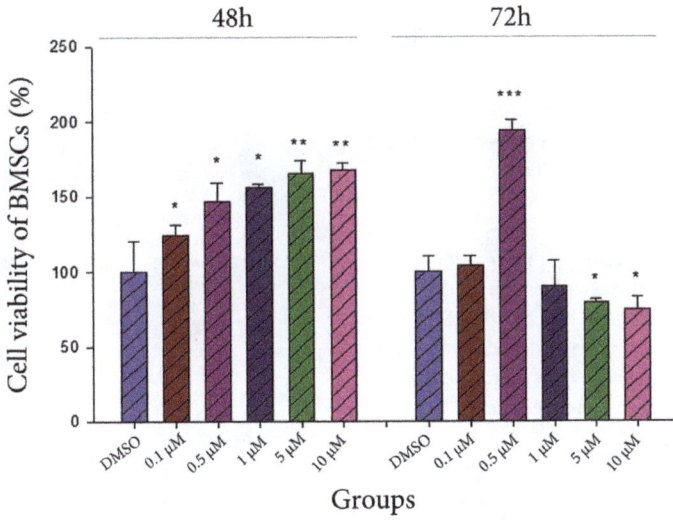

Fig. 4 The effect of various concentrations of curcumin on viability of BMSCs after 48 and 72 h. Cell viability of BMSCs was assessed using MTT assay method. The results indicated that dose and exposure time of curcumin were the factors infuence the cell viability. *: $P < 0.05$, **: $P < 0.01$ or ***: $P < 0.001$ vs the DMSO group

impaired hippocampal neurogenesis in rat model affected by chronic stress. Their results suggested that curcumin could increase the cell proliferation and neuronal populations in stress-induced behavioral abnormalities and hippocampal neuronal damage. Moreover, curcumin effects were induced by up-regulation of 5-HT$_{1A}$ receptors and BDNF [26]. Fadhel et al. [24] indicated that administration of 200 mg/kg of curcumin by intraperitoneal method immediately, 3 h and 24 h after transient forebrain, ischemia model significantly reduced neuronal damage. This protective effect did not differ among these three different times. Fusheng et al. [21] reported that five months administration of 500 ppm curcumin in aged APP transgenic mice suppressed amyloid accumulation. Kim et al. showed that when curcumin was administered intraperitoneally at a dose of 500 nmol/kg body weight of adult mice once daily for 4 days, the Numbers of Newly Generated Cells in the Hippocampus increased [8]. However, the translation

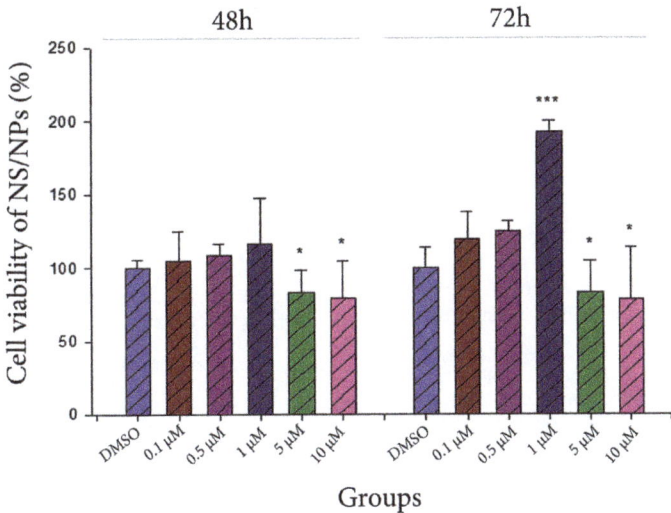

Fig. 5 The effect of various concentrations of curcumin on viability of NS/PCs after 48 and 72 h. Curcumin in different doses had various effects on survival of NS/PCs. In addition, the cell viabilty was affected by period of treatment. *: $P < 0.05$ or ***: $P < 0.001$ vs the DMSO group

of the results of animal studies to the clinic is not an easy job. The results of phase I clinical trials indicated that curcumin is safe even at high doses (12 g/day). Humans however exhibit poor bioavailability [27]. Considering the fact that curcumin in the face of stem cells exhibits a biphasic effect, further investigation is needed to determine specific effects of curcumin on different types of stem cells.

Conclusion

These findings suggest that curcumin proliferation effects depend on treatment period, its concentration, and the type of stem cells. These factors should be considered in stem cell therapy of degenerative and neurological disorders. Further studies are required to evaluate the synergistic effect of combination therapy of curcumin and stem cells.

Abbreviations
BMSCs: Bone marrow mesenchymal stem cells; NS/PCs: Neural stem/progenitor cells; DMEM/F12: Dulbecco's Modified Eagle Medium; DMSO: 3-(4, 5-dimethylthiazolyl-2)-2, Dimethyl Sulphoxide; MTT: 5-diphenyltetrazolium bromide; BrdU: Bromodeoxyuridine; ANOVA: One-Way Analysis of Variance.

Competing interests
The authors declare that they have no competing interests.

Authors' contributions
GH and FA carried out study concept and design, GH and AG carried out providing laboratory equipment, FA and GH carried out analysis and interpretation of data, FA carried out drafting of the manuscript, GH, MZ, HA, SE and MS carried out critical revision of the manuscript for important intellectual content, FA, TM and MK carried out statistical analysis. All authors read and approved the final manuscript.

Acknowledgments
This study was supported by a grant (90-3-87-14565) from Tehran University of Medical Sciences.

Author details
[1]Department of Neuroscience, School of Advanced Technologies in medicine, Tehran University of Medical Sciences, Tehran, Iran. [2]Department of Anatomy, School of Medicine, Tehran University of Medical Sciences, Tehran, Iran. [3]Shefa Neuroscience Research Center, Khatamolanbia Hospital, Tehran, Iran. [4]Department of Pharmacology, School of Medicine, Tehran University of Medical Sciences, Tehran, Iran. [5]Faculty of Pharmacy, and Pharmaceutical Sciences Research Center, Tehran University of Medical Sciences, Tehran, Iran. [6]Department of Physiology, Medical College, Lorestan University of Medical Sciences, Khorramabad, Iran. [7]Epilepsy Research Center, WestfälischeWilhelms-UniversitätMünster, Münster, Germany.

References
1. Milobedzka J, Kostanecki V, Lampe V. Structure. Chem Ber. 1910;43:2163.
2. Sharma R, Gescher A, Steward W. Curcumin: the story so far. Eur J Cancer. 2005;41(13):1955–68.
3. McNally SJ, Harrison EM, Ross JA, Garden OJ, Wigmore SJ. Curcumin induces heme oxygenase 1 through generation of reactive oxygen species, p38 activation and phosphatase inhibition. Int J Mol Med. 2007;19(1):165–72.
4. Goel A, Kunnumakkara AB, Aggarwal BB. Curcumin as "Curecumin": from kitchen to clinic. Biochem Pharmacol. 2008;75(4):787–809.
5. Ray B, Bisht S, Maitra A, Maitra A, Lahiri DK. Neuroprotective and neurorescue effects of a novel polymeric nanoparticle formulation of curcumin (NanoCurc™) in the neuronal cell culture and animal model: implications for Alzheimer's disease. J Alzheimers Dis. 2011;23(1):61–77.
6. Hatcher H, Planalp R, Cho J, Torti F, Torti S. Curcumin: from ancient medicine to current clinical trials. Cell Mol Life Sci. 2008;65(11):1631–52.
7. Ormond DR, Shannon C, Oppenheim J, Zeman R, Das K, Murali R, et al. Stem cell therapy and curcumin synergistically enhance recovery from spinal cord injury. PLoS One. 2014;9(2):e88916.
8. Kim SJ, Son TG, Park HR, Park M, Kim M-S, Kim HS, et al. Curcumin stimulates proliferation of embryonic neural progenitor cells and neurogenesis in the adult hippocampus. J Biol Chem. 2008;283(21):14497–505.
9. Son S, Kim K-T, Cho D-C, Kim H-J, Sung J-K, Bae J-S. Curcumin Stimulates Proliferation of Spinal Cord Neural Progenitor Cells via a Mitogen-Activated Protein Kinase Signaling Pathway. J Korean Neurosurg Soc. 2014;56(1):1–4.
10. Kim J-H, Park S-H, Nam S-W, Kwon H-J, Kim B-W, Kim W-J, et al. Curcumin stimulates proliferation, stemness acting signals and migration of 3T3-L1 preadipocytes. Int J Mol Med. 2011;28(3):429–35.
11. Chen J, Li Y, Wang L, Zhang Z, Lu D, Lu M, et al. Therapeutic benefit of intravenous administration of bone marrow stromal cells after cerebral ischemia in rats. Stroke. 2001;32(4):1005–11.
12. Aligholi H, Hassanzadeh G, Azari H, Rezayat SM, Mehr SE, Akbari M, et al. A new and safe method for stereotactically harvesting neural stem/progenitor cells from the adult rat subventricular zone. J Neurosci Methods. 2014;225:81–9.
13. Azari H, Rahman M, Sharififar S, Reynolds BA. Isolation and expansion of the adult mouse neural stem cells using the neurosphere assay. J Vis Exp. 2010;45:1–4.
14. Dahl J-A, Duggal S, Coulston N, Millar D, Melki J, Shandadfar A, et al. Genetic and epigenetic instability of human bone marrow mesenchymal stem cells expanded in autologous serum or fetal bovine serum. Int J Dev Biol. 2008;52(8):1033.
15. Azari H, Sharififar S, Rahman M, Ansari S, Reynolds BA. Establishing embryonic mouse neural stem cell culture using the neurosphere assay. J Vis Exp. 2011;47:1–4.
16. Ye J, Zhang Y. Curcumin protects against intracellular amyloid toxicity in rat primary neurons. Int J Clin Exp Med. 2012;5(1):44.
17. Dominici M, Le Blanc K, Mueller I, Slaper-Cortenbach I, Marini F, Krause D, et al. Minimal criteria for defining multipotent mesenchymal stromal cells. The International Society for Cellular Therapy position statement. Cytotherapy. 2006;8(4):315–7.
18. Zhang M, Jia G, Cheng J, Yang P, Lu Y, Wu X. In vitro analysis and in vivo tracing of BrdU-labeled rat bone marrow mesenchymal stem cells. Sichuan Da Xue Xue Bao Yi Xue Ban. 2012;43(2):266–70.
19. Jensen EC. Quantitative analysis of histological staining and fluorescence using image. J Anat R. 2013;296(3):378–81.
20. Wei W-L, Sun H-S, Olah ME, Sun X, Czerwinska E, Czerwinski W, et al. TRPM7 channels in hippocampal neurons detect levels of extracellular divalent cations. Proc Natl Acad Sci Proc Natl Acad Sci U S A. 2007;104(41):16323–8.
21. Yang F, Lim GP, Begum AN, Ubeda OJ, Simmons MR, Ambegaokar SS, et al. Curcumin inhibits formation of amyloid β oligomers and fibrils, binds plaques, and reduces amyloid in vivo. J Biol Chem. 2005;280(7):5892–901.
22. Calabrese V, Butterfield D, Stella A. Nutritional antioxidants and the heme oxygenase pathway of stress tolerance: novel targets for neuroprotection in Alzheimer's disease. Ital J Biochem. 2003;52(4):177–81.
23. Chen H, Zhang Z, Zhang Y, Zhou D. Curcumin inhibits cell proliferation by interfering with the cell cycle and inducing apoptosis in colon carcinoma cells. Anticancer Res. 1998;19(5A):3675–80.
24. Al-Omar FA, Nagi MN, Abdulgadir MM, Al Joni KS, Al-Majed AA. Immediate and delayed treatments with curcumin prevents forebrain ischemia-induced neuronal damage and oxidative insult in the rat hippocampus. Neurochem Res. 2006;31(5):611–8.
25. Zbarsky V, Datla KP, Parkar S, Rai DK, Aruoma OI, Dexter DT. Neuroprotective properties of the natural phenolic antioxidants curcumin and naringenin but not quercetin and fisetin in a 6-OHDA model of Parkinson's disease. Free Radic Res. 2005;39(10):1119–25.
26. Xu Y, Ku B, Cui L, Li X, Barish PA, Foster TC, et al. Curcumin reverses impaired hippocampal neurogenesis and increases serotonin receptor 1A mRNA and brain-derived neurotrophic factor expression in chronically stressed rats. Brain Res. 2007;1162:9–18.
27. Anand P, Kunnumakkara AB, Newman RA, Aggarwal BB. Bioavailability of curcumin: problems and promises. Mol Pharm. 2007;4(6):807–18.

The fruit extract of *Berberis crataegina* DC: exerts potent antioxidant activity and protects DNA integrity

Mohammad Charehsaz[1], Hande Sipahi[1], Engin Celep[2], Aylin Üstündağ[3], Özge Cemiloğlu Ülker[3], Yalçın Duydu[3], Ahmet Aydın[1] and Erdem Yesilada[2*]

Abstract

Background: Dried fruits of *Berberis crataegina* (Berberidaceae) have been frequently consumed as food garniture in Turkish cuisine, while its fruit paste has been used to increase stamina and in particular to prevent from cardiovascular dysfunctions in Northeastern Black Sea region of Turkey. This study investigated this folkloric information in order to explain the claimed healing effects as well as to evaluate possible risks.

Methods: Total phenolic, flavonoid and proanthocyanidin contents and antioxidant capacity of the methanolic fruit extract were evaluated through several *in vitro* assays. The cytotoxic and genotoxic effects of *B. crataegina* fruit extract were also assessed in both cervical cancer cell line (HeLa) and human peripheral blood lymphocytes.

Results: The extract showed protective effects against ferric-induced oxidative stress and had a relatively good antioxidant activity. It also ameliorated the H_2O_2 mediated DNA damage in lymphocytes, suggesting the protective effect against oxidative DNA damage.

Conclusion: The methanolic extract of *B. crataegina* fruits may be a potential antioxidant nutrient and also may exert a protective role against lipid peroxidation as well as oxidative DNA damage.

Keyword: *Berberis crataegina* DC, Folk medicine, Genotoxicity, Lipid peroxidation, Antioxidant

Background

Berberis species (Berberidaceae) are known to exert spasmolytic, cholagogue, analgesic, anti-inflammatory, anxiolytic, antipsychotic, antidepressant, and potent scolicidal effects [1-3]. There are four naturally occurring species of *Berberis* in Turkey. Among these species, *B. crataegina* DC. and its hybrids are widely distributed and its black fruits are often consumed as food, and used as diuretic and expectorant. Moreover, the roots and root barks of this plant have been used in Turkish folk medicine against various ailments including jaundice, hemorrhoids, dysuria and as febrifuges in feverish conditions as well as tonic and appetizer [4,5]. On the other hand, the red fruits of another species, *B. vulgaris* L., have been used as a garniture in Persian food culture owing to its color and mellow taste [2,6], while the aqueous extract of barks is reported to be used to treat rheumatism and fever in Azerbaijan folk medicine [5] and Bulgaria [7].

Similar utilizations for the roots of several other *Berberis* species have also been reported elsewhere. In Uzbekistan, condensed aqueous extract of *B. oblonga* root is reported to be prescribed for the effective treatment of lumbago [8], while in Nepal, the condensed aqueous extract of *B. asiatica* Roxb. root barks is reported to be used orally against fever and in Pakistan powdered roots of *B. lycium* Royle are used orally with milk to treat rheumatic and muscular pains [5].

As summarized above, the underground parts of *Berberis* species have been used particularly against inflammatory disorders in worldwide traditional medicines, while the fruits of *Berberis* species have frequently been used as food, rather than for healing purposes. According to a recent report, the fruit paste of *B. crataegina* has been used to

* Correspondence: yesilada@yeditepe.edu.tr
[2]Faculty of Pharmacy, Department of Pharmacognosy, Yeditepe University, 34755 Atasehir, Istanbul, Turkey
Full list of author information is available at the end of the article

increase stamina and in particular to prevent from cardio-vascular dysfunctions in Northeastern Black Sea region of Turkey [9].

Reactive oxygen species (ROS) and reactive nitrogen species (RNS), either generated exogenously or produced endogenously, are involved in a variety of biological phenomena such as pathogenesis of many diseases, mutation, carcinogenesis and aging [10,11]. Fortunately, there are several defense mechanisms for protection against these reactive molecules under physiological steady state conditions. Among these various defense mechanisms, the antioxidant system is extremely important due to its direct removal of pro-oxidants and maximum protection for biological sites [10]. Furthermore, it is important to protect the balance between oxidative stress and antioxidant defense mechanisms in order to prevent the adverse effects generated by oxidative stress [12]. Scientific investigations have demonstrated that phytochemicals are a great source for antioxidants, particularly the phenolic components, which have the structural requirements for free radical scavenging activity [1,12,13]. Ethanolic extracts of roots, twigs and leaves of B. vulgaris L. and also B. croatica Horvat showed some radical scavenging activity in correlation with the content of phenolic compounds [1]. In another study, Hanachi et al. [14] showed that B. vulgaris fruits exhibit antioxidant activity and have the ability to reduce the cell viability in human liver cancer cell line.

The present survey was aimed to evaluate the antioxidant effects of the fruit paste of B. crataegina in order to explain the claimed healing effects as well as to define the possible risks. For this purpose, the in vitro antioxidant potential of B. crataegina fruits extract was evaluated through several chemical and biochemical assays, including 2,2′-diphenyl-1-picrylhydrazyl (DPPH) radical-scavenging activity, superoxide anion radical scavenging activity, ferric reducing antioxidant power (FRAP), cupric reducing antioxidant capacity (CUPRAC), β-carotene bleaching, total antioxidant capacity (TOAC) and Trolox equivalent antioxidant capacity (TEAC). Also, the cytotoxic and genotoxic effects of B. crataegina fruits extract were investigated in both human cervical cancer cell line (HeLa) and human peripheral blood lymphocytes. In addition to these tests, the total contents of phenolic, flavonoid and proanthocyanidin of the fruits were also determined.

Material and methods
Preparation of fruit extract
The dried B. crataegina fruits (2 kg) were provided from Bayburt province (Turkey) and authenticated by one of the authors (E.Y.). A voucher specimen was deposited in the Herbarium of Faculty of Pharmacy, Yeditepe University (YEF 10018). The fruits were washed, mashed in a blender with 500 mL of warm distilled water and freeze-dried (Christ Alpha 2-4 LD). Then 200 g of dried fruit sample were extracted twice with 50 mL of 80% methanol (Sigma) at 45°C for 4 hours with continuous stirring. The combined extract was filtered through a filter paper and then was evaporated to dryness under reduced pressure. Finally, the sticky residue was dissolved in distilled water and freeze-dried [BCFE] (yield, 9.2%).

Phytochemical screening of the extract
The method previously described was used for determination of total phenolic content [15]. Accordingly, 20 μL of properly diluted BCFE sample were mixed with Folin–Ciocalteu reagent (Sigma) and Na_2CO_3 (20%) (Riedel de Hean). Then, samples were incubated at 45°C for 30 minutes. At the end of this period, the absorbance was measured at 765 nm by UV-Vis spectrophotometer (Thermo, Evolution 300). Results were expressed as mg gallic acid equivalents (GAE) per gram of dried extract.

For the determination of total flavonoid content, 500 μL of properly diluted BCFE sample were mixed with 10% $AlCl_3$ (Merck) and 1 M sodium acetate (Riedel de Hean). Following the incubation period (30 minutes at room temperature), the absorbance was recorded at 415 nm. Results were expressed as mg quercetin equivalents (QE) per g of dried extract [13].

The total proanthocyanidin content of the BCFE sample was measured by adding of 2.5 mL of vanillin (1%) (Fluka) and 2.5 mL of 9 M HCl (Sigma) in methanol to properly diluted extracts. After incubating at 30°C for 20 min, the absorbance was measured at 500 nm. Total proanthocyanidin content of samples was expressed as mg epigallocatechingallate equivalents (EGCG-E) per g of dry extract [13].

Measurement of in vitro antioxidant activity
DPPH radical-scavenging activity, superoxide anion radical scavenging activity, FRAP, CUPRAC, β-carotene bleaching, TOAC and TEAC were measured spectrophotometrically by the methods previously described by Celep et al. [13].

In vitro cytotoxicity and genotoxicity studies
Treatment of human peripheral lymphocytes
The donor was a 30 years old woman (non-smoker) and her health status was completely compatible with the WHO guideline on the blood donor selection criteria.

Treatment procedure I Lymphocytes were isolated from the whole blood by using LeucoSep® (greiner bio-one) centrifuge tubes according to the instruction manual provided by the manufacturer. Briefly, the anticoagulated blood sample was poured into the Leucosep tube and centrifuged for 10 min (1000xg). The lymphocytes appeared at the interface between the plasma (top layer) and separation medium (Ficoll, 1.077 g/ml). This enriched cell fraction was harvested by means of a Pasteur pipette, washed with 10 ml of phosphate-buffered saline (PBS), and centrifuged for 10 min at 250 x g. Afterwards, 50 µL aliquots of the cell (lymphocyte) suspension were dispensed into micro centrifuge tubes ($1x10^4$-$2x10^4$ cells/50 µL). 1 mL aliquots of BCFE (0.001, 0.005, 0.01, 0.05, 0.1, 0.2, 0.5, 1, 2, and 4 mg/mL) were added into related micro-centrifuge tubes and incubated for 2 hours. Two micro-centrifuge tubes were allocated as positive control and treated with 50 µM and 100 µM H_2O_2 at the last 5 minutes of the incubation period. The micro-centrifuge tubes were centrifuged at 250 g and the supernatants were discarded. The DNA damage in lymphocytes was identified by using the alkaline comet assay.

Treatment procedure II The same procedure described above was applied with the following exception; the micro-centrifuge tubes containing BCFE were treated with 50 µM H_2O_2 at the last 5 minutes of the 2 hours incubation period. Afterwards, the procedure proceeded with centrifugation as was described above. The DNA repair in lymphocytes was identified by using the alkaline comet assay.

Comet assay
Preparation of the cells
The same comet assay procedure was used for both HeLa cells and lymphocytes. The details of the procedure were formerly described [16,17]. Briefly; 50 µL aliquots of the cell suspension ($1x10^4$ - $2x10^4$ HeLa cells or lymphocytes/50 µL) were mixed with 100 µL of low melting point agarose (0.5% LMA) (Sigma) and dispensed onto the microscope slides previously coated with normal melting point agarose (1% NMA) (Sigma). The suspension spread by using a coverslip and left on an ice-cold flat tray for 5 minutes. After removal of the cover slip, the slides were immersed in lysing solution.

Lysing
The slides were immersed into formerly prepared cold (4°C) lysing solution containing 2.5 M NaCl (Sigma), 100 mM Na_2EDTA (Sigma), 10 mM Tris (Sigma), 1% sodium sarcosinate (Sigma), (pH 10) with 1% Triton-X 100 (Sigma) and 10% DMSO (Sigma) and left there for 1 hour, afterwards the slides were removed from the lysing solution and drained.

Electrophoresis
The slides were placed in horizontal gel electrophoresis tank containing the electrophoresis solution (1 mM Na_2EDTA and 300 mM NaOH, pH 13). Electrophoresis was then conducted for 20 min by applying an electric current of 25 V/300 mA to allow damaged DNA to migrate from the nucleus toward the anode.

Neutralization: The slides were then drained, placed on tray and washed with three changes of neutralization buffer (0.4 M Tris, pH 7.5) for 5 minutes each. The slides were left to drain before staining.

Staining
The slides were stained with 50 µL (20 µg/mL) ethidium bromide (Sigma) and covered with a coverslip. Then the slides were viewed using a fluorescence microscope (Leica DM1000) equipped with an excitation filter of 515-560 nm. A single scorer randomly selected and captured 100 cells using the Perceptive Instruments COMET Assay IV analysis system. Tail % intensity was selected as the image analysis parameter. Two slides were prepared for each single sample. The results are given as the mean of both slides.

Trypan blue viability test
The cell suspension (lymphocytes) was diluted (1:1) with 0.4% trypan blue solution (Sigma) and carefully filled the hemocytometer (Improved Neubauer) chamber. The viable (unstained) and non-viable cells (blue) were counted under a microscope.

Treatment of HeLa cells
The HeLa cell line was cultured as a monolayer in an appropriate tissue culture flask at 37°C with 5% CO_2 in F12 HAM containing 10% heat inactivated fetal bovine serum (Sigma), 50 µg/mL penicillin (Biological Industries) and 50 µg/mL streptomycin (Biological Industries). When cells approach confluence, they were removed from the flask by trypsinization. After counting the cells, the culture is seeded into two 24-well plates ($5x10^4$ cells/well) and incubated at 37°C with 5% CO_2 for 24 hours. Afterwards, 1 mL aliquots of BCFE (0.001, 0.005, 0.01, 0.05, 0.1, 0.2, 0.5, 1, 2, and 4 mg/mL) were added into related wells and incubated for 2 hours. Two wells were allocated as positive control and treated with 50 µM and 100 µM H_2O_2 (Merck) at the last 5 minutes of the incubation period. The cells were removed from the wells by trypsinization and the supernatant was discarded after centrifugation at 2500 rpm for 5 minutes. The DNA damage in HeLa cells was identified by using the alkaline comet assay.

In another set of 24-well plates, the HeLa cells were exposed 24 hours to the equal concentrations of BCFE by using the same procedure described above.

Neutral Red Uptake (NRU) cytotoxicity test
The HeLa cells were cultured as described above then seeded into a 96-well microtiter plate ($1x10^4$ cells/well) and incubated at 37°C with 5% CO_2 for 24 hours. Afterwards, the culture medium was removed and the cells were treated with 100 µl treatment medium containing

either 8 concentrations of BCFE or the positive control (sodium dodecyl sulfate, SDS) (Merck). After 24 hours of treatment period, medium were removed and the cells were washed with 150 µl PBS (Thermo). Thereafter, PBS was aspirated and the cells were incubated in 100 µl of neutral red medium (Sigma) for additional 3 hours. After this final incubation period, neutral red medium were discarded and washed with 150 µl PBS. Finally 150 µl ethanol (Sigma)/acetic acid (Sigma) (1% glacial acetic acid, 50% ethanol, %49 H_2O) solution were added to all wells and the 96-well plate was shaken for 10 minutes in a micro plate shaker. The absorption of the colored solution was measured at 540 nm by a micro plate reader (SpectraMax 190) and the related IC_{50} values were computed [18].

Statistical evaluation

All of the results are expressed as the mean ± SD. For in vivo data, the differences between the groups were evaluated with Kruskal-Wallis analysis of variance and comparisons between two independent groups were made with the Mann-Whitney U-test. For the data of the comet assay, the analysis of variance (ANOVA) was used to determine whether there are any significant differences between the means of the groups. The Dunnett test was used as part of the ANOVA test to determine whether means were different from mean of the control. All statistical tests were performed with SPSS for Windows Release 11. $p < 0.05$ was considered statistically significant.

Results and discussion

Phytochemical screening of the extract

Phenolic compounds are the major class of bioactive components. Previous reports have shown that the fruits of various Berberis species are rich in polyphenolic constituents and eventually fruit extracts have shown to possess potent free radical-scavenging activity [19-21] due to the polyphenolic compound's ability to act as hydrogen donors, reducing agents and radical scavengers [1].

Flavonoids and proanthocyanidins are one of the major polyphenolic constituents of plants because of the radical scavenging ability conferred by their hydroxyl groups at various positions; particularly of an ortho-dihydroxy structure in their B ring [15]. A previous study revealed that polyphenols can also prevent oxidative stress-mediated DNA damage [22].

Limited numbers of studies have previously been reported the phenolic contents of the fruits of Berberis species, i.e. B. vulgaris, [23] while no report have been found on the polyphenolics of B. crataegina fruits in a reference survey. In present study, total phenolics, flavonoids and proanthocyanidins contents of 80% methanolic extracts of BCFE were evaluated and results were expressed as mg gallic acid, quercetin and epigallocatechingallate equivalents, respectively (Table 1).

In vitro antioxidant activity

Since free radicals are one of the main causes of oxidative stress, the ability of BCFE on free radical scavenging was assessed by DPPH, superoxide radical scavenging and TEAC tests in this study [15]. As given in Table 2, DPPH radical scavenging activity of BCFE was about 30% of reference substance BHT and superoxide radical scavenging activity was about 2% of reference substance gallic acid. These results indicate that BCFE does not have a good activity against superoxide radicals but have a relatively good activity against other stable radicals like DPPH. On the other hand, Fe^{3+} and Cu^{2+} involve in the formation of free radicals and the reduction of ferric as well as cupric ions indicate another mechanism of antioxidant potential [13]. As shown in Table 2, ferric reducing power of BCFE was higher than that of reference substance BHT and copper reducing activity was about the 5.6% of ascorbic acid. These results indicate that BCFE can prevent ferric induced oxidative stress efficiently but not for copper. As an indicator of the prevention of lipid peroxidation, β-carotene bleaching assay demonstrated that BCFE to possess about 80% of activity of reference substance BHT, suggesting a good activity against lipid peroxidation (Table 2). Furthermore, total antioxidant capacity of BCFE was about 8.6% of ascorbic acid and 20% of Trolox, indicating a relatively good antioxidant activity (Table 2).

In vitro evaluation of genotoxicity and cytotoxicity

The genotoxic potential of the BCFE in HeLa cells was tested at concentrations lower than its IC_{50} value. Since the DNA damaging potential of H_2O_2 is well known and has been reported previously in several published studies [16,17], H_2O_2 (50 and 100 µM) was used as a positive control. The HeLa cells were treated with increasing concentrations of BCFE in order to assess its effect on

Table 1 The total phenolic, flavonoid and proanthocyanidin content of 80% MeOH extract of B. crataegina fruit (BCFE)[A]

	Total phenolic content (mg GAE/g extract)[B]	Total flavonoid content (mg QE/g extract)[C]	Total proanthocyanidin content (mg EGCG-E/g extract)[D]
BCFE	53.51 ± 3.62	27.42 ± 1.34	548 ± 19.7

[A]Results were expressed as the mean of triplicates ± standard deviation (S.D.).
[B]Total phenolic content was expressed as mg gallic acid equivalents (GAE) in 1 g dried extract ± S.D.
[C]Total flavonoid content was expressed as mg quercetin equivalents (QE) in 1 g dried extract ± S.D.
[D]Total proanthocyanidin content was expressed as mg epigallocatechin gallate equivalents (EGCG-E) in 1 g dried extract ± S.D.

Table 2 *In vitro* antioxidant activities of 80% MeOH extract of *B. crataegina* fruit (BCFE)[A]

	DPPH radical scavenging activity[B]	Superoxide radical scavenging activity[C]	FRAP[D]	CUPRAC[E]	β-carotene bleaching assay[F]	TOAC[G]	TEAC[H]
BCFE	405 ± 11.6	9.04 ± 0.92	0.76 ± 0.03	56.3 ± 0.17	77 ± 2.2	86.69 ± 4.62	198 ± 5.6
BHT*	133 ± 6.4		3.02 ± 0.07		96 ± 2.6		
Gallic acid		0.18 ± 0.01					

[A]Results were expressed as the averages of triplicates ± standard deviation (S.D.), [B]IC_{50}, expressed in µg/mL, [C]IC_{50}, expressed in mg/mL, [D]Ferric reducing antioxidant power was expressed as mM $FeSO_4$ equivalents in 1 g material, [E]Copper reducing antioxidant capacity was expressed as mg ascorbic acid equivalents in 1 g material, [F]The results of β-carotene bleaching assay was given as % in 1 mg/mL extract or reference compound, [G]Total antioxidant capacity was expressed as mg ascorbic acid equivalents in 1 g material, [H]Trolox equivalent antioxidant capacity was expressed as µM Trolox equivalent in 1 g material, *Butylated hydroxy toluene.

the DNA integrity. The DNA integrity of HeLa cells was identified by using the comet assay and expressed in terms of tail % intensity. As shown in Figure 1, the mean tail % intensity was significantly increased in each tested concentrations with the exception of 0.05 mg/mL (p < 0.05) under the treatment duration of 2 hours. These results indicate a negative effect of BCFE on the DNA integrity of HeLa cells. On the other hand, the mean tail % intensity values were completely changed under the treatment duration of 24 hours. The mean tail % intensity value was sharply increased at the concentration of 0.05 mg/mL and even the mean tail % intensity value of the positive control (50 µM H_2O_2) was exceeded at the

concentration of 4 mg/mL as shown in Figure 2. However, the mean tail % intensity values determined for the concentrations of 0.001 and 0.01 mg/mL were decreased to the control level. Apparently, the damaged DNA was repaired in 24 hour. These results indicate an adaptive cellular response in HeLa cells at these two concentrations of BCFE.

The viability of lymphocytes varied between 93.75% and 100% within the tested concentrations are shown in Figure 3. The genotoxic effect of BCFE was determined also in human peripheral blood lymphocytes. The DNA damage started to occur at 2 mg/mL with a significantly increased (p < 0.05) mean tail % intensity value. The

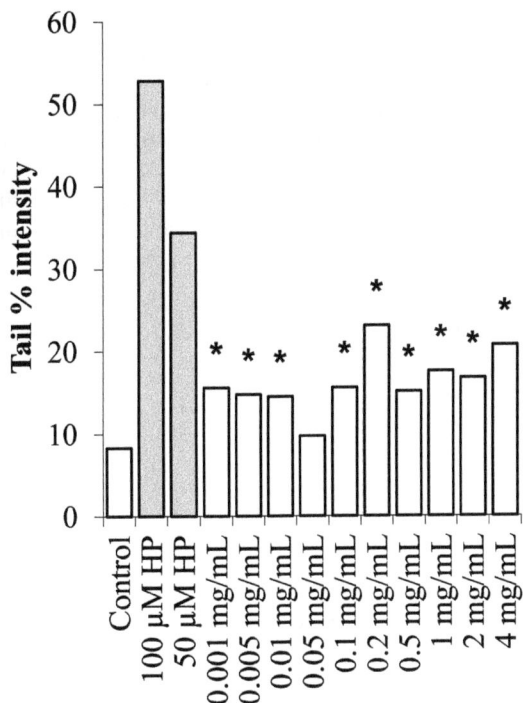

Figure 1 The DNA integrity of HeLa cells treated with increasing concentrations of BCFE for 2 hours. *The tail % intensity was significantly increased when compared with the control (p < 0.05). Black bars representing the positive controls.

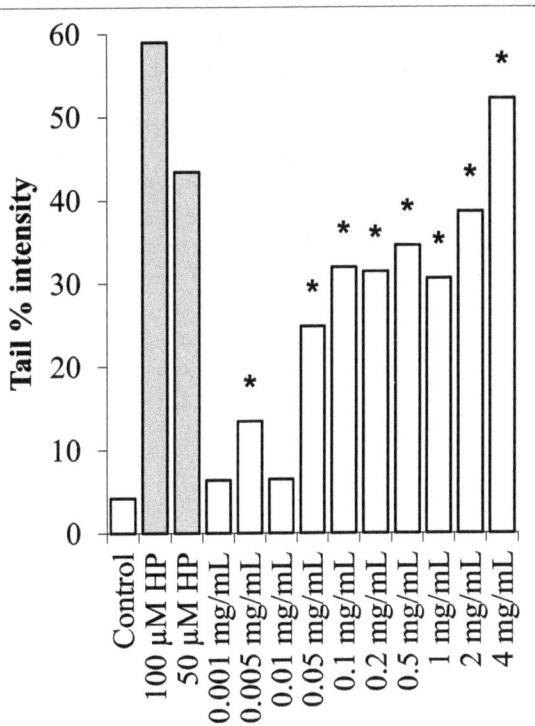

Figure 2 The DNA integrity of HeLa cells treated with increasing concentrations of BCFE for 24 hours. *The tail % intensity was significantly increased when compared with the control (p < 0.05). Black bars representing the positive controls.

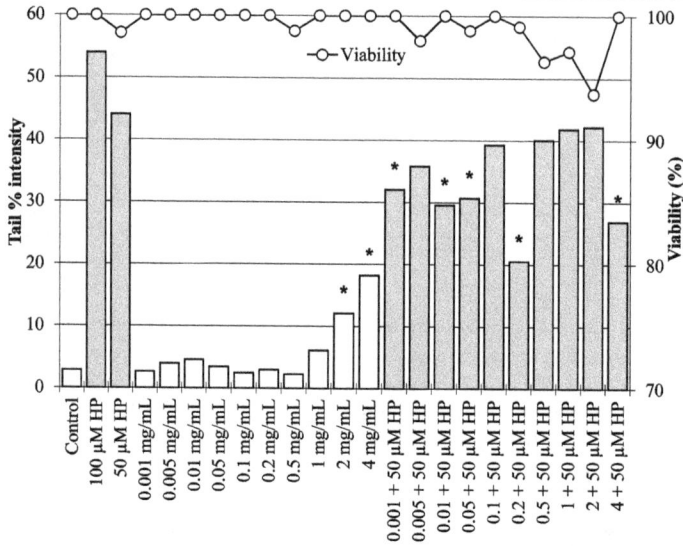

Figure 3 Dose-dependent effects of BCFE on the DNA integrity of human peripheral blood lymphocytes. The H₂O₂ (50 and 100 μM) treated lymphocytes are the controls for the combined treatments (black bars). The white and black bars represent the mean tail % intensity values determined after the treatment period of 2 hours. *Significantly different from the related control. The viability of lymphocytes varied between 93.75% and 100% within the tested concentrations.

mean tail % intensity values at the lower concentrations were not statistically different from the mean tail % intensity value of the control. In other words, the DNA integrity of lymphocytes was not affected by BCFE at the concentration of 1 mg/mL or lower.

Interestingly, the results obtained in HeLa cells and lymphocytes were not comparable to each other. Although, HeLa cells and lymphocytes were treated with the same concentrations of BCFE for the same period of time (2 hours), HeLa cells were more vulnerable to the components in BCFE as shown in Figure 1. Apparently,

human peripheral blood lymphocytes are more resistant to the in BCFE.

The influence of H_2O_2 (50 μM) on the DNA integrity of lymphocytes treated with increasing concentrations of BCFE was investigated within the study. Accordingly, the DNA damage generated by 50 μM H_2O_2 was significantly decreased in lymphocytes previously treated with BCFE at concentrations of 0.001, 0.01, 0.05, 0.2, and 4 mg/mL (Figure 3). BCFE has clearly ameliorate the H_2O_2 mediated DNA damage in lymphocytes at the above mentioned concentrations. In other words, BCFE

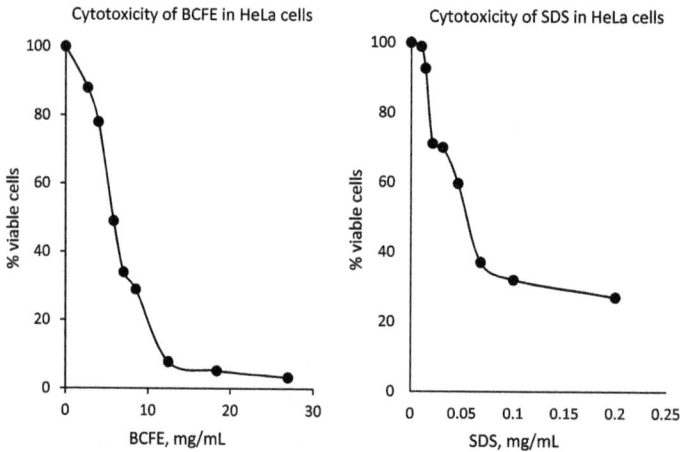

Figure 4 The cytotoxic effects of BCFE and SDS (positive control). The IC₅₀ values of BCFE and SDS were 4.98 mg/mL and 0.055 mg/mL, respectively.

might be protective against oxidative DNA damage. This protective effect might be a reflection of the induced DNA repair or the antioxidant capacity of polyphenolic compounds in BCFE [21]. On the other hand, the DNA damage of lymphocytes was significantly induced with BCFE at 4 mg/mL. In spite of this genotoxic effect at 4 mg/mL, the H_2O_2 (50 μM) induced oxidative DNA damage was significantly reduced at the same extract concentration.

The results obtained in NRU cytotoxicity tests were used to identify the IC_{50} value of the BCFE in HeLa cells. Accordingly, the computed IC_{50} values of BCFE and SDS (positive control) were 4.98 mg/mL and 0.055 mg/mL, respectively (Figure 4).

Conclusions

In conclusion, the present study has revealed that BCFE possesses potent total antioxidant activity, scavenging stable radicals like DPPH, prevent ferric induced oxidative stress and has a good activity against lipid peroxidation. Also, the BCFE can be a potent protective nutrient against oxidative DNA damage. However, it should be considered that the results of *in vitro* antioxidant assays may sometimes conflict with the results obtained from *in vivo* models. Therefore, in order to ascertain the role of dietary antioxidants fully, *in vivo* tests are incredibly necessary.

Competing interests

We declare that there is no competing financial interest for any author of this article, whether actual or potential.

Authors' contributions

MC carried out phytochemical screening of the extract and measurement of *in vitro* antioxidant activity. He is also participated in design of study, analysis and interpretation of data and revising the manuscript. HS participated in coordination and drafted the manuscript. She also carried out interpretation of data and statistical analysis. EC carried out preparation of fruit extract and helped in phytochemical screening and measurement of *in vitro* antioxidant activity of the extract. AÜ, ÖCÜ and YD carried out evaluation of genotoxicity and cytotoxicity. They also helped acquisition and interpretation of data. AA and EY have given final approval of the version to be published. All authors read and approved the final manuscript.

Author details

[1]Faculty of Pharmacy, Department of Toxicology, Yeditepe University, 34755 Atasehir, Istanbul, Turkey. [2]Faculty of Pharmacy, Department of Pharmacognosy, Yeditepe University, 34755 Atasehir, Istanbul, Turkey. [3]Faculty of Pharmacy, Department of Toxicology, Ankara University, 06100 Tandoğan, Ankara, Turkey.

References

1. Zovko-Koncic M, Kremer D, Karlovic K, Kosalec I. Evaluation of antioxidant activities and phenolic content of *Berberis vulgaris* L. and *Berberis croatica* Horvat. Food Chem Toxicol. 2010;48:2176–80.
2. Rouhani S, Salehi N, Kamalinejad M, Zayeri F. Efficacy of *Berberis vulgaris* aqueous extract on viability of *Echinococcus granulosus* protoscolices. J Invest Surg. 2013;26:347–51.
3. Kim M, Cho KO, Shin MS, Lee JM, Cho HS, Kim CJ, et al. Berberine prevents nigrostriatal dopaminergic neuronal loss and suppresses hippocampal apoptosis in mice with Parkinson's disease. Int J Mol Med. 2014;33:870–8.
4. Sezik E, Yesilada E, Tabata M, Honda G, Takaishi Y, Fujita T, et al. Traditional medicine in Turkey VIII. Folk medicine in east anatolia; Erzurum, Erzíncan, Ağri, Kars, Iğdir provinces. Econ Bot. 1997;51:195–211.
5. Yesilada E, Kupeli E. *Berberis crataegina* DC. root exhibits potent anti-inflammatory, analgesic and febrifuge effects in mice and rats. J Ethnopharmacol. 2002;79:237–48.
6. Ardestani SB, Sahari MA, Barzegar M, Abbasi S. Some Physicochemical Properties of Iranian Native Barberry Fruits (abi and poloei): *Berberis integerrima* and *Berberis vulgaris*. J Food Pharm Sci. 2013;1:60–7.
7. Ivanovska N, Philipov S. Study on the anti-inflammatory action of *Berberis vulgaris* root extract, alkaloid fractions and pure alkaloids. Int J Immunopharmacol. 1996;18:553–61.
8. Kupeli E, Kosar M, Yesilada E, Baser KHC. A comparative study on the anti-inflammatory, antinociceptive and antipyretic effects of isoquinoline alkaloids from the fruits of Turkish *Berberis* species. Life Sci. 2002;72:645–57.
9. Yesilada E. Biodiversity in Turkish Folk Medicine. In: Sener B, editor. Biodiversity: Biomolecular aspects of biodiversity and innovative utilization. London: Kluwer Academic/Plenum Publishers; 2002. p. 119–35.
10. Kohen R, Nyska A. Oxidation of biological systems: oxidative stress phenomena, antioxidants, redox reactions, and methods for their quantification. Toxicol Pathol. 2002;30:620–50.
11. Apel K, Hirt H. Reactive oxygen species: metabolism, oxidative stress, and signal transduction. Annu Rev Plant Biol. 2004;55:373–99.
12. Sun L, Zhang J, Lu X, Zhang L, Zhang Y. Evaluation to the antioxidant activity of total flavonoids extract from persimmon (*Diospyros kaki* L.) leaves. Food Chem Toxicol. 2011;49:2689–96.
13. Celep E, Aydin A, Kirmizibekmez H, Yesilada E. Appraisal of *in vitro* and *in vivo* antioxidant activity potential of cornelian cherry leaves. Food Chem Toxicol. 2013;62:448–55.
14. Hanachi P, Kua S, Asmah R, Motalleb G, Fauziah O. Cytotoxic effect of *Berberis vulgaris* fruit extract on the proliferation of human liver cancer cell line (HepG2) and its antioxidant properties. Int J Cancer Res. 2006;2:1–9.
15. Celep E, Aydin A, Yesilada E. A comparative study on the *in vitro* antioxidant potentials of three edible fruits: cornelian cherry, Japanese persimmon and cherry laurel. Food Chem Toxicol. 2012;50:3329–35.
16. Üstündağ A, Simsek K, Ay H, Dundar K, Suzen S, Aydin A, et al. DNA integrity in patients undergoing hyperbaric oxygen (HBO) therapy. Toxicol In Vitro. 2012;26:1209–15.
17. Duydu Y, Basaran N, Üstündağ A, Aydin S, Undeger U, Ataman OY, et al. Assessment of DNA integrity (COMET assay) in sperm cells of boron-exposed workers. Arch Toxicol. 2012;86:27–35.
18. National Institute of Health. Guidance document on using *in vitro* data to estimate *in vivo* starting doses for acute toxicity. NIH Publication 2001 No. 01-4500. 2001.
19. Gundogdu M. Determination of antioxidant capacities and biochemical compounds of *Berberis vulgaris* L. fruits. Adv Environ Biol. 2013;7:344–8.
20. Kukula-Koch W, Aligiannis N, Halabalaki M, Skaltsounis AL, Glowniak K, Kalpoutzakis E. Influence of extraction procedures on phenolic content and antioxidant activity of Cretan barberry herb. Food Chem. 2013;138:406–13.
21. Ruiz A, Hermosin-Gutierrez I, Mardones C, Vergara C, Herlitz E, Vega M, et al. Polyphenols and antioxidant activity of calafate (*Berberis microphylla*) fruits and other native berries from Southern Chile. J Agric Food Chem. 2010;2010(58):6081–9.
22. Silva JP, Gomes AC, Coutinho OP. Oxidative DNA damage protection and repair by polyphenolic compounds in PC12 cells. Eur J Pharmacol. 2008;601:50–60.
23. Akbulut, Calısır S, Marakoglu T, Coklar H. Some Physicomechanical and nutritional properties of barberry (*Berberis vulgaris* L.) fruits. J Food Process Eng. 2009;32:497–511.

20

Saffron as an antidote or a protective agent against natural or chemical toxicities

Bibi Marjan Razavi[1] and Hossein Hosseinzadeh[2*]

Abstract

Saffron (*Crocus sativus*) is an extensively used food additive for its color and taste. Since ancient times this plant has been introduced as a marvelous medicine throughout the world. The wide spectrum of saffron pharmacological activities is related to its major constituents including crocin, crocetin and safranal. Based on several studies, saffron and its active ingredients have been used as an antioxidant, antiinflammatory and antinociceptive, antidepressant, antitussive, anticonvulsant, memory enhancer, hypotensive and anticancer. According to the literatures, saffron has remarkable therapeutic effects. The protective effects of saffron and its main constituents in different tissues including brain, heart, liver, kidney and lung have been reported against some toxic materials either natural or chemical toxins in animal studies.

In this review article, we have summarized different in vitro and animal studies in scientific databases which investigate the antidotal and protective effects of saffron and its major components against natural toxins and chemical-induced toxicities. Due to the lake of human studies, further investigations are required to ascertain the efficacy of saffron as an antidote or a protective agent in human intoxication.

Keywords: Saffron, *Crocus sativus* L, Crocin, Crocetin, Safranal, Antidote, Protective, Natural toxin, Chemical toxin

Background

Crocus sativus L., is a perennial herb which belongs to the Iridaceae family and is cultivated in Azerbaijan, France, Greece, India, Iran, Italy, Spain, China, Morocco, Turkey, Egypt, and Mexico [1]. Saffron, the dried stigma of the *C. sativus*, has been extensively used as a spice and food colorant because of its color and taste [2].

Saffron contains more than 150 chemicals agents [3]. Among which three main components of saffron are responsible for its pharmacological effects including: crocins, the principle coloring agent (mono and diglycosyl esters of a polyene dicarboxylic acid, named crocetin) [4], the glycoside picrocrocin which is a precursor of safranal and responsible for its bitter taste and safranal, a monoterpen aldehyde which is the deglycosylated form of picrocrocin and is responsible for the characteristic aroma of saffron [5,6].

In folk medicine, saffron has been believed to have several properties such as antispasmodic, eupeptic, anticatarrhal, nerve sedative, carminative, diaphoretic, expectorant, stimulant, stomachic and aphrodisiac [7,8]. Moreover, modern pharmacological studies have demonstrated that saffron and its constituents have a wide spectrum of activities including antioxidant [9], anticonvulsant [10-12], antidepressants and anxiolytics [13-16], antinociceptive and anti-inflammatory [17,18], memory enhancers [19-21], antitussive [22], reducing withdrawal syndrome [23], improving male erectile dysfunction [24], hypotensive [25-27], anticancer [28,29] and anti-solar [30,31].

Furthermore according to the literature, the protective effects of saffron as well as its active components in different tissues including brain [32], heart [33], liver [34], kidney [35], lung [36] and etc have been reported against some toxic materials.

Methods

In this review article, we have discussed different studies in scientific databases including Scopus, MEDLINE and Web of Science databases and local references, which investigate the antidotal and protective effects of saffron

* Correspondence: hosseinzadehh@mums.ac.ir
[2]Pharmaceutical Research Center, Department of Pharmacodynamy and Toxicology, School of Pharmacy, Mashhad University of Medical Sciences, Mashhad, Iran
Full list of author information is available at the end of the article

and its major components against natural toxins and chemical-induced toxicity. Studies were identified through electronic databases from their inception up to October 2014. The keywords for the search were: *Crocus sativus*, saffron, crocin, safranal, crocetin, antidote, natural toxin, chemical toxin and protective effects.

Natural toxins

Documents have been shown saffron and its main components exhibit antidotal effects against some natural toxins including snake venoms [37], aflatoxins [38], lipopolysaccharides (LPS) [39] and 3-nitropropionic acid (3- NP) [40]. These effects might be due to their antioxidant [41], anti-inflammatory [37] and antiapoptotic [37] effects (Table 1).

Snake venoms

It is established that crocin could neutralize oxidative stress and hematological complications induced by viper venoms. The pre-incubation of crocin with venom (1:10; venom: crocin, w/w) at 37°C for 10 min), suppressed the venom-induced oxidative stress, hematological alteration and pro inflammatory cytokine levels in Swiss albino male mice [41]. Furthermore, the inhibitory effect of crocin on viper venom-induced platelet and neutrophil apoptosis has been shown in other studies [37,42].

Crocin ameliorated the *Vipera russelli* venom-induced apoptotic events such as the generation of endogenous ROS, mobilization of intracellular calcium, depolarization of mitochondrial membrane, cytochrome c release, caspase activation, phosphatidylserine externalization and DNA damage [37,42].

Lipopolysaccharide (LPS)

Based on the documents, saffron active constituents could suppress LPS-(endotoxin derived from gram-negative bacteria) induced mice lung injury [39], distributed intravascular coagulation in rabbits (DIC) [43] and LPS-stimulated RAW 264.7 macrophages [44].

Briefly, crocetin (50 and 100 mg/kg, gavage) could reduce the LPS-induced lung edema and histological changes, increased LPS impaired SOD activity, and decreased lung MPO activity. Moreover, crocetin significantly attenuated LPS-induced mRNA and the protein expressions of IL-6, MCP-1, TNF-α, phospho-IκB expression and NF-κB activity [39].

Another study revealed crocetin could improve DIC related haemostatic indices impaired by endotoxin including platelet blood counts, blood plasma fibrinogen and protein C concentration in rabbits [43].

In addition, in vitro studies showed that crocin suppressed the LPS-stimulated expression of iNOS by inducing

Table 1 Antidotal effects of saffron and its main constituents against natural toxins

Toxin	In vitro/In vivo	Constituents	Results	Ref. NO
Snake venom	Swiss albino male mice	Crocin	Suppression of oxidative stress, hematological alteration and pro inflammatory cytokine levels	[37]
Snake venom	Isolated platelet	Crocin	Inhibition of oxidative stress and platelet apoptosis	[41]
Snake venom	Isolated neutrophils	Crocin	Inhibition of oxidative stress and neutrophil apoptosis	[42]
AflatoxinB1	Male Wistar rats	Crocetin (0.1 mg/day/rat)	Reduction of AST, ALT, AIP, and γ-GGT, Elevation of GSH, Reduction of the formation of hepatic AFB₁-DNA adducts	[38]
AflatoxinB1	Female Sprague-Dawley rats	Crocin dyes (50 mg/kg/day, 3 days)	Reduction of AST, ALT, AIP, γ-GGT and LDH	[47]
Lipopolysaccharide	mice	Crocetin (50 and 100 mg/kg, gavage) for 24 hr	Reduction of lung edema, Increase in SOD, Decrease in MPO, Attenuation of mRNA and protein expressions of IL-6, MCP-1, TNF-α, P-IκB and NF-κB	[39]
Lipopolysaccharide	RAW 264.7 macrophages	Crocin	Suppression of iNOS induction of HO-1 expression via Ca2+/calmodulin-CAMK4-PI3K/Akt-Nrf2	[45]
Lipopolysaccharide	Rabbit	Crocetin	Improve of DIC-related haemostatic indices such as platelet blood counts, blood plasma fibrinogen and protein C concentration, Amelioration of DIC-associated disease and fibrin deposition in the glomeruli	[43]
Lipopolysaccharide	RAW 264.7 macrophages	Crocin	Inhibition of the PGE(2) products, Prevention of NF-kappaB p50 and p65 subunits	[44]
3-nitropropionic acid	Isolated striatal synaptosomes	Saffron extract (1 mg/kg/day, for 5 days, IP.)	Decrease of lipid peroxidation, Improve of mitochondrial function	[40]

HO-1 expression via Ca^{2+}/calmodulin-dependent protein kinase 4 -PI3K/Akt-Nrf2 signaling cascades [45].

In another study, crocin inhibited the prostaglandin E2 products in LPS-stimulated RAW 264.7. Furthermore, crocin prevented the nuclear translocation of the NF-kappa B p50 and p65 subunits [44].

Mycotoxins
Aflatoxin B1 (AFB1)
AFB1 is an aflatoxin produced by *Aspergillus flavus* and *Aspergillus parasiticus* [46]. Crocetin and crocin were found to possess protective effects against AFTB1 hapatotoxicity and AFTB1 DNA adducts via the reduction of hepatic injury markers (AST, ALT, ALP and γ-GGT) and elevations of hepatic glutathione (GSH) and activities of GST and GSH-Px in animal models [38,47].

Nitropropionic acid (3-NPA)
3-NPA is a fungal toxin which is known to affect mito-chondria and subsequently leads to ATP depletion and causes neurotoxicity [40]. The protective effect of saffron extract in striatal synaptosomes isolated from the brain of rats exposed to the mitochondrial toxin 3-NPA has been reported. 3-NPA-(20 mg/kg/day, for 3 days, IP.), induced a significant increase in lipid peroxidation and decreased the mitochondrial function in synaptosomal fractions. However, saffron extract (1 mg/kg/day, for 5 days, IP.) de-creased lipid peroxidation and improved mitochondrial function through antioxidant property [40].

Chemical-induced toxicity
Protective effects of saffron against chemical-induced hepatotoxicity
Based on the evidences from animal studies, saffron has ability to possess protective effects against hepatotoxicity induced by some materials including beryllium chloride (BeCl2) [48], aluminum chloride (AlCl3) [49], carbon tetrachloride (CCl4) [50], acetaminophen [51], cyclophos-phamide [52], diazinon (DZN) [34] and paraquate (PQ) [53] through modulation of antioxidant enzymes [49,52], improvement in structural liver damages [51], reduction in markers of hepatic injury such as AST, ALT, ALP, LDH, GGT, lipid and protein oxidation [48,50-52], alleviation of apoptosis [34], increase in GSH [48] and improvement in lipid dysregulation through ERK1/2 pathway [54].

Metals
Beryllium (Be) BeCl2 is a highly toxic material which ac-cumulates in different tissues after absorption. Oral intake through drinking water is a common route of human exposure to Be. Furthermore, workers are exposed to Be containing dusts during the crushing and grinding of ores, and during the processing of Be metal and alloys [55].

It is documented that crocin (200 mg/kg, for 7 con-secutive days with BeCl2 or 7 consecutive days before BeCl2, IP.), reduced BeCl2-(86 mg/kg, orally for 5 consecutive days) induced liver toxicity. The increase in MDA and LDH levels, decrease in GSH content and haematological parameters induced by BeCl2 were mo-dulated by crocin [48].

Aluminum (Al)
Aluminum (Al) is the third most abundant element in nature [56]. It is a constituent of cooking utensils, medi-cines, deodorants, and food additives. The sources of Al include corn, yellow cheese, salt, herbs, spices, tea, cos-metics, cookwares, and containers [57].

Shati et al. (2010) revealed saffron and honey mini-mized the toxic effect of $AlCl_3$ in the liver by alleviating its disruptive effect on the biochemical and molecular levels. A significant increase in the cholesterol levels, tri-glycerides, GGT, ALT, AST, ALP, lipid peroxidation, and glucose were observed in the $AlCl_3$ group. However, co treatment of $AlCl_3$ with saffron and honey improved the disrupted liver biochemical markers and alleviated the increase of lipid peroxidation [49].

Acetaminophen
Acetaminophen (N-acetyl-p-aminophenol) is a widely used drug as an analgesic and antipyretic (Ahmad, 2010). It is a known hepatotoxic in overdose [58]. Omidi et al. (2014) showed that 20 mg/kg of *C. sativus* petals hydroal-coholic extract ameliorated acetaminophen-induced acute liver injury in rats through reducing the levels of AST, ALT and bilirubin, and increased the total protein and albumin. Cell swelling, severe inflammation and necrosis were observed in acetaminophen exposed rats; however in saffron treated rats only mild hepatocyte degeneration was seen [51].

Carbon tetrachloride (CCl4)
CCl4 is a solvent which causes liver toxicity by many roots of administration (oral, inhalation, and parenteral exposures) [50]. It has been shown that CCl4-induced fatty degeneration and vacuole formation and increased the levels of ALT and AST in plasma. The aqueous and ethanolic extracts of *C. sativus* stigmas and petals signifi-cantly decreased these impairments [50].

Cyclophosphamide
Cyclophosphamide is an alkylating agent commonly used as a chemotherapeutic and immunosuppressive drug [59]. A study by Jnaneshwari et al. (2013) exhibited the protec-tive efficacy of crocin against hepatotoxicity induced by cyclophosphamide in Wistar rats. Crocin (10 mg/kg for 6 days, orally) after the administration of a single dose of cyclophosphamide (150 mg/kg, IP.), significantly improved

hepatic and antioxidant enzymes, lipid and protein oxidation [52]. Another study showed crocetin significantly elevated GST activity both in the bladder and the liver of mice treated with cyclophosphamide [60].

Pesticides

Paraquat It was reported that paraquat (PQ 5 mM), a widely used herbicide, increased leakage of LDH and ALT in rat primary hepatocytes and crocetin (10, 20 µM) significantly suppressed the hepatotoxicity [53].

Diazinon (DZN) DZN is an organophosphate insecticide. In addition to the acetyl cholinesterase inhibition, it can damage tissues via oxidative stress [61]. Lari et al. (2013) indicated that crocin reduced DZN- induced hepatotoxicity through suppression the increase in MDA and attenuation the activation of caspases and reduction the Bax/Bcl-2 ratio [34].

Protective effects of saffron against chemical-induced cardiovascular toxicity

The protective effects of saffron and its active constituents have been shown against DZN (an organophosphate insecticide) [33], doxorubicin (an antitumor agent) [62] and isoproterenol-(a synthetic non-selective β adrenoceptor

agonist) [63] induced cardiac toxicity in previous studies through several mechanisms including modulation of cardiac hemodynamic [63], histopathological and ultrastructural impairments [63], improvement in cardiac markers such as CK-MB [33,64], alleviation of lipid peroxidation [33], suppression of genes involved in cardiac apoptosis and anti-inflammatory effects [33].

Diazinon (DZN)

It was reported that DZN-(15 mg/kg, gavage, for 28 days) induced vascular toxicity which may be due to oxidative stress and not to a cholinergic mechanism [65]. Crocin (20 mg/kg, IP., for 28 days) improved toxic effects of DZN via reducing lipid peroxidation and restoring altered contractile and relaxant responses in rat aorta [65]. In addition concurrent administration of crocin and DZN could restore the effects of subchronic DZN administration on systolic blood pressure and heart rate in rats [66]. Besides antioxidant effects, a research has been shown that crocin exhibited protective effects against DZN-induced mitochondrial-mediated apoptosis in heart tissue of rat following subchronic exposure [33] (Figure 1). Furthermore, it was reported the aqueous extract of *C. sativus* (saffron) stigma and its main components, crocin and safranal, prevented DZN-induced

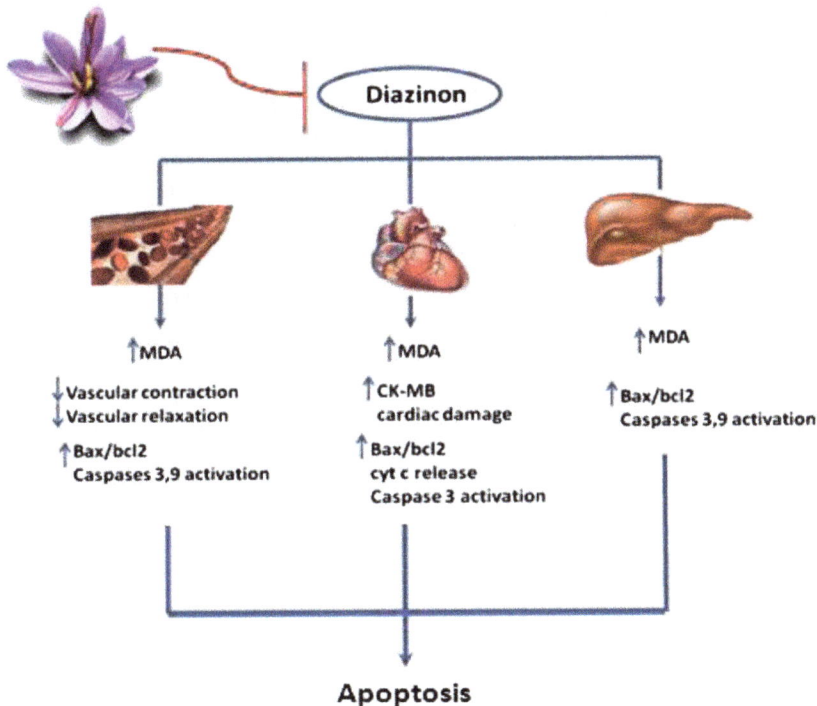

Figure 1 Schematic mechanistic description of saffron against toxicity induced by DZN.

enzymes elevation and some specific biomarkers including, CK-MB, TNF-a, 8-iso-prostaglandin F2a and soluble protein-100β in rats [67,68].

Isoproterenol

Mehdizadeh et al. (2013) demonstrated saffron or safranal could reduce histopathological damages as well as lipid peroxidation in rat heart tissues and also decreased CK-MB and LDH activities in serum induced by isoproterenol [64]. Similar study showed crocin (20 mg/kg/day) may have cardioprotective effects in isoproterenol-induced cardiac toxicity via modulation hemodynamic, antioxidant, histopathological and ultrastructural impairments [63].

Doxorubicin

Doxorubicin is an anthracycline antibiotic which is used as an antitumor agent [69]. It is well known that anthracyclines can induce cardiotoxicity by releasing ROS [62].

To evaluate the effect of saffron against acute myocardium injury by anthracyclines, the model of an isolated rabbit heart was used. ROS was generated by electrolysis of the perfused heart solution and/or generated by perfusion with 30 μM doxorubicin in the presence and absence of 10 μg/ml saffron extracts. ROS generated by two models affects cardiovascular function; it decreased ventricular pressure, heart rate and coronary flow and increased lipid peroxidation while SOD activity decreased. The myocardial architecture was also altered by ROS. Saffron perfused during electrolysis could trap ROS and significantly improved myocardial function [62].

Protective effects of saffron against chemical-induced genotoxicity

Antitumors

It was proved saffron extract could protect against some antitumor agents including cisplatin [70,71], cyclophosphamide [70,71], mitomycin-C [70,71], and methyl methanesulfonate (MMS) [72] in animals via modulation of lipid peroxidation, antioxidants and detoxification systems [70]. Saffron (20, 40 and 80 mg/kg) was orally administered to mice for 5 days prior to these antitumor agents. A significant reduction in lipid peroxidation with an increase in the liver enzymatic (SOD, CAT, GST, GPx) and non-enzymatic antioxidants (GSH) were observed in saffron pretreated animals. Moreover saffron significantly inhibited antitumor drugs-induced cellular DNA damage (strand breaks) as revealed by decreased comet tail length, tail moment and DNA percentage in the tail [70,71].

Hosseinzadeh et al (2007 and 2008) reported the effect of aqueous extract of C. sativus stigmas, crocin and safranal on MMS-(120 mg/Kg, IP.) induced DNA damage in different mice organs using the comet assay. The MMS-induced DNA damage (increase in the % tail DNA) (80 mg/Kg) was decreased in some tissues including kidney, lung and spleen in C. sativus stigmas aqueous extract, crocin and safranal pretreated mice [72,73].

Paraquat (PQ)

Crocetin also decreased genotoxicity induced by PQ. In this study oxyradical generated by PQ caused DNA damage which was evaluated with unscheduled DNA synthesis in rat primary hepatocytes [53].

Protective effects of saffron against chemical-induced pulmonary toxicity

Benzo[a]pyrene

Benzo[a]pyrene is a polycyclic aromatic hydrocarbon isolated from coal tar [36]. It can interact with lipids of membrane and consequently produces free radicals [36]. A study showed that single dose of benzo[a]pyrene (100 mg/kg, IP) could increase the level of ROS and lipid peroxides in lung mitochondria, and reduced the levels of membrane ATPase, GSH and lung mitochondrial enzymes in mice. Furthermore, the level of 8-Hydroxy-2-deoxyguanosine (8-OHdG) in lung DNA of mice was induced by benzo[a]pyrene. Crocetin (20 mg/kg, IP.) protected the structural and functional impairment of lung mitochondria induced by benzo[a]pyrene following 18 weeks treatment (starting from 4th to 22nd week) after the first dose of benzo[a]pyrene [36].

Protective effects of saffron against chemical-induced neurotoxicity

Aluminum

Aluminum is the third most abundant element in nature [36]. It is an accepted neurotoxin implicated in the pathogenesis of neurodegenerative diseases [32]. Linardaki et al. (2013) reported Al intake (50 mg/kg/day in the drinking water for 5 weeks) could cause memory impairment, increase of brain MDA and reduction of GSH content, significant reduction of AChE and BuChE activity, activation of brain MAO isoforms and inhibition of cerebellar MAO-B in mice. Although co-administration with saffron extract (60 mg/kg/day, for the last 6 days, IP.) had no effect on cognitive performance, it reversed significantly the Al-induced changes in MAO activity and the levels of MDA and GSH.

Another study revealed 40 mg/kg/day of AlC1$_3$ for 90 days caused a decrease in the AChE activity and enzymatic antioxidant activities in both cerebral hemisphere and cerebellum of rats. Moreover, the expression of A Disintegrin and Metalloprotease, AChE, P53, Bcl-2 and interleukins (IL-4 and IL-12) genes in AlCl$_3$ group was changed. Saffron aqueous extract (200 mg/kg/day) attenuated the neurotoxic effects of AlC1$_3$ [74].

Acrylamide (ACR)

ACR, is an industrial potent neurotoxic agent in human and animals that has been recently found in carbohydrate rich foods cooked at high temperatures [75]. The effect of crocin, on ACR-induced cytotoxicity was evaluated using PC12 cells. The pretreatment of cells with 10-50 μM crocin significantly attenuated ACR cytotoxicity in a dose-dependent manner. Crocin inhibited the down regulation of Bcl-2 and the up regulation of Bax and decreased apoptosis in treated cells. Also, crocin inhibited ROS generation in cells exposed to ACR [76].

Protective effects of saffron against chemical-induced nephro-or uro-toxicity
Antitumors

Cisplatin is an antitumor agent which induces nephrotoxicity via oxidative stress [77]. Naghizadeh et al. (2008) showed blood urea, creatinine, urinary glucose, protein concentrations and oxidative stress markers in crocin treated groups (100, 200 and 400 mg/kg, IP., for 4 consecutive days) were significantly lower than those of cisplatin (5 mg/kg). Cisplatin caused damage in S3 segment of proximal tubules, whereas no damage was observed in crocin treated rats [77].

Moreover, the administration of cysteine and vitamin E, C. sativus and Nigella sativa together with cisplatin partly reversed the kidney enzymes impairments induced by cisplatin [78].

Another study revealed crocetin (50 mg/kg) modulated the release of chloroacteldehyde, a urotoxic metabolite of cyclophosphamide in the urine of mice [60].

Antibiotics

The nephroprotective activity of saffron against gentamicin and ceftazidime-induced nephrotoxicity has been shown [79-81]. Gentamicin and/or ceftazidime caused histological changes as well as significant decrease in the body weights and urine output along with increase in protein and blood urea, serum creatinine, ESR, renal tissue levels of MDA and kidney weights in comparison with control rats. These changes were prevented by saffron [81].

Hexachlorobutadiene

Hexachlorobutadiene, is a potent nephrotoxic in rodents, which can cause degeneration, necrosis and regeneration in renal tubular epithelial cells [82]. Boroushaki et al. (2007) revealed that safranal (0.25 and 0.5ml/kg), has a protective effect against nephrotoxicity induced by hexachlorobutadiene in rats [82].

Cadmium

Cadmium (Cd) is an extremely toxic heavy metal used in industry. It is known to cause serious environmental and health effects including damage to renal and testis [83]. Asadi et al. (2014) showed that cadmium reduced sperm count, motility and vitality in comparison to control group. Saffron improved sperm parameters [84].

Protective effects of saffron against chemical-induced hematological toxicity
Diazinon (DZN)

Hariri et al. (2011) showed that vitamin E, safranal (0.025 and 0.05 ml/kg) and crocin (50 mg/kg) restored the reduction of red blood cells, hemoglobin and hematocrit induced by diazinon. These agents also prevented the reduction in platelets and the increase in reticulocytes. Vitamin E, crocin and safranal did not inhibit the effect of diazinon on RBC cholinesterase activity [85].

Protective effects of saffron against chemical-induced embryo toxicity

It is indicated that saffron aqueous extract (200 mg/kg) treated animals revealed improvement in maternal weight gain, embryolethality and bone ossification impaired by administration of AlCL$_3$ (200 mg/kg) during the embryogenesis (6th to 15th day of gestation) period [86]. Although saffron's usage in pregnancy can have some complication on the embryo. A study showed that high concentrations of the aqueous extract of saffron (0.2%) can produce embryonic abnormalities [87]. Moreover Moallem et al. (2013) reported crocin or safranal can induce embryonic malformations when administered in pregnant mice as evidenced by decrease in length and weight of fetuses and induction of minor skeletal malformations, mandible and calvaria malformations, and growth retardation [68].

Saffron as a protective agent against its constituent

It was also shown that saffron could act as an antidote against its toxic constituent [88]. Safranal, the main component of C. sativus essential oil, is thought to be responsible for the unique odor of saffron [5,6]. Safranal has been shown protective effects against some drug- and chemical- induced toxicity [73,79,82,85]. However, this constituent itself also exhibited side effects [89]. According to Iranian Traditional Medicine (ITM), the usage of whole plant may reduce some adverse effects induced by plant containing toxic ingredients [90]. A study by Ziaee et al (2014) showed that the aqueous extract of saffron stigma could reduce the toxicity of safranal [88]. It was found that the co-treatment of safranal and saffron significantly reduced the mortality rate induced by safranal and improved significantly all toxic effects of safranal on biochemical parameters in acute and subacute toxicities. Therefore, the consumption of saffron as a whole plant could be considered as a valuable method to reduce safranal toxicity [88].

Conclusions

In this review article, the different in vitro and animal studies summarized in order to discover the efficacy of saffron and its active constituents in protection against toxicities induced by natural or chemical toxins in different tissues.

According to the results of several important investigations, saffron and its active components act as an antidote in different intoxications induced by natural toxins including snakebites, mycotoxins and endotoxins.

Furthermore it is established saffron could act as an antidote for its constituent, safranal, which has more toxicity than the other constituents presented in saffron. Metals (Al, Be and cadmium), pesticides (DZN and PQ), acrylamide, benzo[a]pyrene and CCL4 are some examples of environmental and/or industrial chemical toxins which saffron could protect different tissues such as brain, cardiovascular, lung, kidney and liver against their toxicities. It is also documented this plant with wonderful power of therapeutic effects, exhibits protective effects against some chemical drugs such as antitumors (cisplatin, doxurobicin, cyclophosphamide and mitomycin), antibiotics (gentamycin and ceftazidime), analgesics (acetaminophen) which have organ toxicities especially in overdose. Some mechanisms including antioxidant, the modulation of cardiac, renal and liver enzymes, improvement in antioxidant defense systems, and the inhibition of apoptosis are involved in saffron antidotal effects.

In conclusion, based on the current review, saffron has an extensive spectrum of protective properties against toxicities induced by either natural or chemical toxins. As these findings have not yet been verified by clinical trials on humans, to establish the antidotal effects of saffron in human intoxications, human trials should be carried out.

Abbreviations

AST: Aspartate transaminase; ALT: Alanine transaminase; ALP: Alkaline phosphatase; γ-GGT: Gamma glutamyl transpeptidase; GST: Glutathione transpeptidase; GSH-Px: Glutathione peroxidase; LDH: Lactate dehydrogenase; CK-MB: Creatine kinase MB; ROS: Reactive oxygen species; SOD: Superoxide dismutase; CAT: Catalase; AChE: Acetylcholinesterase; BuChE: Butyrylcholinesterase; MAO: Monoamine oxidase; DIC: Disseminated intravascular coagulation; MPO: Myeloperoxidase; 3NPA: 3-Nitropropionic acid; IL-6: Interleukin-6; MCP-1: Macrophage chemo attractant protein-1; TNF-α: Tumor necrosis factor-α; iNOS: Inducible nitric oxide synthase; HO-1: Heme oxigenase-1.

Competing interests

The authors declare that they have no competing interests.

Authors' contributions

BR collected data and drafted the manuscript. HH gave the idea, designed and supervised the study, and edited the manuscript. Both authors read and approved the final manuscript.

Author details

[1]Targeted Drug Delivery Research Center, Department of Pharmacodynamy and Toxicology, School of Pharmacy, Mashhad University of Medical Sciences, Mashhad, Iran. [2]Pharmaceutical Research Center, Department of Pharmacodynamy and Toxicology, School of Pharmacy, Mashhad University of Medical Sciences, Mashhad, Iran.

References

1. Xue X. Cultivation of Crocus sativus. Zhong Yao Tong Bao. 1982;7:3.
2. Winterhalter P, Straubinger M. Saffron—renewed interest in an ancient spice. Food Rev Int. 2000;16:39–59.
3. Bathaie SZ, Mousavi SZ. New applications and mechanisms of action of saffron and its important ingredients. Crit Rev Food Sci Nutr. 2010;50:761–86.
4. Alavizadeh S, Hosseinzadeh H. Bioactivity assessment and toxicity of crocin: a Comprehensive Review. Food Chem Toxicol. 2014;64:65–80.
5. Abdullaev FI. Biological effects of saffron. Biofactors. 1993;4:83–6.
6. Rezaee R, Hosseinzadeh H. Safranal: from an aromatic natural product to a rewarding pharmacological agent. Iran J Basic Med Sci. 2013;16:12–26.
7. Moghaddasi M. Saffron chemicals and medicine usage. J Med Plants Res. 2010;4:427–30.
8. Hosseinzadeh H, Nassiri-Asl M. Avicenna's (Ibn sina) the canon of medicine and saffron (Crocus sativus): a review. Phytother Res. 2013;27:475–83.
9. Hosseinzadeh H, Shamsaie F, Mehri S. Antioxidant activity of aqueous and ethanolic extracts of Crocus sativus L. stigma and its bioactive constituents crocin and safranal. Pharmacogn Mag. 2010;5:419–24.
10. Hosseinzadeh H, Khosravan V. Anticonvulsant effects of aqueous and ethanolic extracts of Crocus sativus L. stigmas in mice. Arch Iran Med. 2002;5:44–7.
11. Hosseinzadeh H, Talebzadeh F. Anticonvulsant evaluation of safranal and crocin from Crocus sativus in mice. Fitoterapia. 2005;76:722–4.
12. Hosseinzadeh H, Sadeghnia H. Protective effect of safranal on pentylenetetrazol-induced seizures in the rat: involvement of GABAergic and opioids systems. Phytomedicine. 2007;14:256–62.
13. Hosseinzadeh H, Karimi G, Niapoor M. Antidepressant effect of Crocus sativus L. stigma extracts and their constituents, crocin and safranal, in mice. J Med Plants. 2004;3:48–58.
14. Hosseinzadeh H, Noraei N. Anxiolytic and hypnotic effect of Crocus sativus aqueous extract and its constituents, crocin and saftanal, in mice. Phytother Res. 2009;26:768–74.
15. Ghasemi T, Abnous K, Vahdati F, Mehri S, Razavi BM, Hosseinzadeh H. Antidepressant effect of Crocus sativus aqueous extract and its effect on CREB, BDNF, and VGF transcript and protein levels in Rat hippocampus. Drug Res. 2014, [Epub ahead of print].
16. Vahdati Hassani F, Naseri V, Razavi B, Mehri S, Abnous K, Hosseinzadeh H. Antidepressant effects of crocin and its effects on transcript and protein levels of CREB, BDNF, and VGF in rat hippocampus. Daru. 2014;8:22.
17. Hosseinzadeh H, Younesi MH. Antinociceptive and anti-inflammatory effects of Crocus sativus L. stigma and petal extracts in mice. BMC Pharmacol. 2002;2:7.
18. Hosseinzadeh H, Shariaty VM. Anti-nociceptive effect of safranal, a constituent of Crocus sativus (saffron), in mice. Pharmacologyonline. 2007;2:498–503.
19. Abe K, Saito H. Effects of saffron extract and its constituent crocin on learning behaviour and long-term potentiation. Phytother Res. 2000;14:149–52.
20. Hosseinzadeh H, Ziaei T. Effects of Crocus sativus stigma extract and its constituents, crocin and safranal, on intact memory and scopolamine-induced learning deficits in rats performing the Morris water maze task. J Med Plants. 2006;5:40-50+60.
21. Hosseinzadeh H, Sadeghnia H, Abbasi Ghaeni F, Motamedshariaty V, Mohajeri S. Effects of saffron (Crocus sativus L.) and its active constituent, crocin, on recognition and spatial memory after chronic cerebral hypoperfusion in rats. Phytother Res. 2012;10:1002.
22. Hosseinzadeh H, Ghenaati J. Evaluation of the antitussive effect of stigma and petals of saffron (Crocus sativus) and its components, safranal and crocin in guinea pigs. Fitoterapia. 2006;77:446–8.
23. Hosseinzadeh H, Jahanian Z. Effect of Crocus sativus L. (saffron) stigma and its constituents, crocin and safranal, on morphine withdrawal syndrome in mice. Phytother Res. 2010;24:726–30.
24. Shamsa A, Hosseinzadeh H, Molaei M, Shakeri MT, Rajabi O. Evaluation of Crocus sativus L. (saffron) on male erectile dysfunction: a pilot study. Phytomedicine. 2009;16:690–3.
25. Imenshahidi M, Hosseinzadeh H, Javadpour Y. Hypotensive effect of aqueous saffron extract (Crocus sativus L.) and its constituents, safranal and crocin, in normotensive and hypertensive rats. Phytother Res. 2010;24:990–4.
26. Imenshahidi M, Razavi BM, Faal A, Gholampoor A, Mousavi SM, Hosseinzadeh H. The effect of chronic administration of saffron (Crocus sativus) stigma aqueous

extract on systolic blood pressure in rats. Jundishapur J Nat Pharm Prod. 2013;8:175–9.

27. Imenshahidi M, Razavi BM, Faal A, Gholampoor A, Mousavi SM, Hosseinzadeh H. Effects of chronic crocin treatment on desoxycorticosterone acetate (doca)-salt hypertensive rats. Iran J Basic Med Sci. 2014;17:9–13.

28. Hosseinzadeh H, Behravan J, Ramezani M, Ajgan K. Anti-tumor and cytotoxic evaluation of saffron of Crocus sativus L. stigma and petal extracts using brine shrimp and potato disc assays. J Med Plants. 2005;4:59–65.

29. Aung HH, Wang CZ, Ni M, Fishbein A, Mehendale SR, Xie JT, et al. Crocin from Crocus sativus possesses significant anti-proliferation effects on human colorectal cancer cells. Exp Oncol. 2007;29:175–80.

30. Golmohammadzadeh S, Jaafari MR, Hosseinzadeh H. Does saffron have antisolar and moisturizing effects? Iran J Pharm Res. 2010;9:133–40.

31. Golmohammadzadeh S, Imani F, Hosseinzadeh H, Jaafari MR. Preparation, characterization and evaluation of sun protective and moisturizing effects of nanoliposomes containing safranal. Iran J Basic Med Sci. 2011;14:521–33.

32. Linardaki ZI, Orkoula MG, Kokkosis AG, Lamari FN, Margarity M. Investigation of the neuroprotective action of saffron (Crocus sativus L.) in aluminum-exposed adult mice through behavioral and neurobiochemical assessment. Food Chem Toxicol. 2013;52:163–70.

33. Razavi B, Hosseinzadeh H, Movassaghi A, Imenshahidi M, Abnous K. Protective effect of crocin on diazinon induced cardiotoxicity in subcronic exposure. Chem boil inter. 2013;25:547–55.

34. Lari P, Abnous K, Imenshahidi M, Rashedinia M, Razavi M, Hosseinzadeh H. Evaluation of diazinon-induced hepatotoxicity and protective effects of crocin. Toxicol Ind Health. 2015;31:367–76.

35. Bandegi AR, Rashidypour A, Vafaei AA, Ghadrdoost A. Protective effects of Crocus Sativus L. extract and crocin against chronic-stress induced oxidative damage of brain, liver and kidneys in rats. Pharm Bull. 2014;4:493–9.

36. Venkatraman M, Konga D, Peramaiyan R, Ganapathy E, Dhanapal S. Reduction of mitochondrial oxidative damage and improved mitochondrial efficiency by administration of crocetin against benzo[a]pyrene induced experimental animals. Biol Pharm Bull. 2008;31:1639–45.

37. Santhosh MS, Thushara RM, Hemshekhar M, Sunitha K, Devaraja S, Kemparaju K, et al. Alleviation of viper venom induced platelet apoptosis by crocin (Crocus sativus): implications for thrombocytopenia in viper bites. J Thromb Thrombolysis. 2013; 1-9.

38. Lin JK, Wang CJ. Protection of crocin dyes on the acute hepatic damage induced by aflatoxin B1 and dimethylnitrosamine in rats. Carcinogenesis. 1986;7:595–9.

39. Yang R, Yang L, Shen X, Cheng W, Zhao B, Hamid Ali K, et al. Suppression of NF-κB pathway by crocetin contributes to attenuation of lipopolysaccharide-induced acute lung injury in mice. Eur J Pharmacol. 2012;674:391–6.

40. Urrutia EC, Riverón-Negrete L, Abdullaev F, Del-Angel DS, Martínez NLH, Cruz MEG, et al. Saffron extract ameliorates oxidative damage and mitochondrial dysfunction in the rat brain. Acta Hortic. 2007;739:359–66.

41. Santhosh SM, Hemshekhar M, Thushara RM, Devaraja S, Kemparaju K, Girish KS. Vipera russelli venom-induced oxidative stress and hematological alterations: amelioration by crocin a dietary colorant. Cell Biochem Function. 2013;31:41–50.

42. Santhosh MS, Sundaram MS, Sunitha K, Jnaneshwari S, Devaraja S, Kemparaju K, et al. Propensity of crocin to offset Vipera russelli venom induced oxidative stress mediated neutrophil apoptosis: a biochemical insight. Cytotechnology. 2014, [Epub ahead of print].

43. Tsantarliotou MP, Markala D, Kazakos G, Sapanidou V, Lavrentiadou S, Zervos I, et al. Crocetin administration ameliorates endotoxin-induced disseminated intravascular coagulation in rabbits. Blood Coagul Fibrinolysis. 2013;24:305–10.

44. Xu GL, Li G, Ma HP, Zhong H, Liu F, Ao GZ. Preventive effect of crocin in inflamed animals and in LPS-challenged RAW 264.7 cells. J Agric Food Chem. 2009;57:8325–30.

45. Kim JH, Park GY, Bang SY, Park SY, Bae SK, Kim Y. Crocin suppresses LPS-stimulated expression of inducible nitric Oxide synthase by upregulation of heme oxygenase-1 via calcium/calmodulin-dependent protein kinase 4. Mediators Inflamm. 2014;2014:728709.

46. Koehler P, Hanlin R, Beraha L. Production of aflatoxins B1 and G1 by Aspergillus flavus and Aspergillus parasiticus isolated from market pecans. Appl microbiol. 1975;30:581–3.

47. Wang CJ, Shiow SJ, Lin JK. Effects of crocetin on the hepatotoxicity and hepatic DNA binding of aflatoxin B1 in rats. Carcinogenesis. 1991;12:459–62.

48. El-Beshbishy HA, Hassan MH, Aly H, Doghish A, Alghaithy A. Crocin "saffron"protects against beryllium chloride toxicity in rats through diminution of oxidative stress and enhancing gene expression of antioxidant enzymes. Ecotoxicol Env Safety. 2012;83:47–54.

49. Shati A, Alamri S. Role of saffron (Crocus sativus L.) and honey syrup on aluminium induced hepatotoxicity. Saudi Med J. 2010;31:1106–13.

50. Iranshahi M, Khoshangosht M, Mohammadkhani Z, Karimi G. Protective effects of aqueous and ethanolic extract of saffron stigma and petal on liver toxicity induced by carbon tetrachloride in mice. Pharmacologyonline. 2011;1:203–12.

51. Omidi A, Riahinia N, Montazer Torbati M, Behdani M. Hepatoprotective effect of Crocus sativus (saffron) petals extract against acetaminophen toxicity in male Wistar rats. Avicenna J Phytome. 2014;4:330–6.

52. Jnaneshwaria S, Hemshekhara M, Santhosha S, Sunithaa K, Thusharaa R, Thirunavukkarasub C, et al. Crocin, a dietary colorant mitigates cyclophosphamide-induced organ toxicity by modulating antioxidant status and inflammatory cytokines. J Pharm Pharmacol. 2013;65:604–14.

53. Tseng TH, Chu CY, Huang JM, Shiow SJ, Wang CJ. Crocetin protects against oxidative damage in rat primary hepatocytes. Cancer Lett. 1995;97:61–7.

54. Lari P, Rashedinia M, Abnous K, Hosseinzadeh H. Crocin improves lipid dysregulation in subacute diazinon exposure through ERK1/2 pathway in rat liver. Drug Res. 2014;64:301–5.

55. Deubner DC, Lowney YW, Paustenbach DJ, Warmerdam J. Contribution of incidental exposure pathways to total beryllium exposure. ApplOccup Environ Hyg. 2011;16:568–78.

56. Verstraeten SV, Aimo L, Oteiza PI. Aluminium and lead: molecular mechanisms of brain toxicity. Arch Toxicol. 2008;82:789–802.

57. Yokel R. The toxicology of aluminum in the brain: a review. Neurotoxicology. 2000;21:813–28.

58. Larson A, Polson J, Fontana R. Acetaminophen-induced acute liver failure: results of a united states multicenter, prospective study. Hepatology. 2005;42:1364–72.

59. Huttunen K, Raunio H, Rautio J. Prodrugs–from serendipity to rational design. Pharmacol Rev. 2011;63:750–71.

60. Nair SC, Panikkar KR, Parthod RK. Protective effects of crocetin on the bladder toxicity induced by cyclophosphamide. Cancer Biother. 1993;8:339–44.

61. Akturk O, Demirin H, Sutcu R, Yilmaz N, Koylu H, Altuntas I. The effects of diazinon on lipid peroxidation and antioxidant enzymes in rat heart and ameliorating role of vitamin E and vitamin C. Cell Biol Toxicol. 2006;22:455–61.

62. Chahine N, Hanna J, Makhlouf H, Duca L, Martiny L, Chahine R. Protective effect of saffron extract against doxorubicin cardiotoxicity in isolated rabbit heart. Pharm Biol. 2013;51:1564–71.

63. Goyal SN, Arora S, Sharma AK, Joshi S, Ray R, Bhatia J, et al. Preventive effect of crocin of Crocus sativus on hemodynamic, biochemical, histopathological and ultrastructural alterations in isoproterenol-induced cardiotoxicity in rats. Phytomedicine. 2010;17:227–32.

64. Mehdizadeh R, Parizadeh M-R, Khooei A-R, Mehri S, Hosseinzadeh H. Cardioprotective effect of saffron extract and safranal in isoproterenol-induced myocardial infarction in wistar rats. Iran J Basic Med Sci. 2013;16:56–63.

65. Razavi B, Hosseinzadeh H, Abnous K, Imenshahidi M. Protective effect of crocin on diazinon induced vascular toxicity in subchronic exposure in rat aorta ex-vivo. Drug Chem Toxicol. 2014;37:378–830.

66. Razavi M, Hosseinzadeh H, Abnous K, Motamedshariaty V, Imenshahidi M. Crocin restores hypotensive effect of subchronic administration of diazinon in rats. Iran J Basic Med Sci. 2013;16:64–72.

67. Hariri A, Moallem S, Mahmoudi M, Memar B, Hosseinzadeh H. Sub-acute effects of diazinon on biochemical indices and specific biomarkers in rats: protective effects of crocin and safranal. Food Chem Toxicol. 2010;48:2803–8.

68. Moallem S, Afshar M, Etemad L, Razavi B,Hosseinzadeh H. Evaluation of teratogenic effects of crocin and safranal, active ingredients of saffron, in mice. Toxicol Ind Health. 2013, [Epub ahead of print]

69. Tacar O, Sriamornsak P, Dass C. Doxorubicin: an update on anticancer molecular action, toxicity and novel drug delivery systems. J Pharm Pharmacol. 2013;65:157–70.

70. Premkumar K, Abraham SK, Santhiya ST, Ramesh A. Protective effects of saffron (Crocus sativus Linn.) on genotoxins-induced oxidative stress in Swiss albino mice. Phytother Res. 2003;17:614–7.

71. Premkumar K, Thirunavukkarasu C, Abraham SK, Santhiya ST, Ramesh A. Protective effect of saffron (Crocus sativus L.) aqueous extract against genetic damage induced by anti-tumor agents in mice. Human Exp Toxicol. 2006;25:79–84.

72. Hosseinzadeh H, Abootorabi A, Sadeghnia HR. Protective effect of *Crocus sativus* stigma extract and crocin (trans-crocin 4) on methyl methanesulfonate-induced DNA damage in mice organs. DNA Cell Biol. 2008;27:657–64.

73. Hosseinzadeh H, Sadeghnia HR. Effect of safranal, a constituent of *Crocus sativus* (saffron), on methyl methanesulfonate (MMS)-induced DNA damage in mouse organs: an alkaline single-cell gel electrophoresis (comet) assay. DNA Cell Biol. 2007;26:841–6.

74. Elsaid FG, Shati AA, Hafez EE. The protective role of *coffea arabica* L. and *crocus sativus* L. against the neurotoxicity induced by chronic administration of aluminium chloride. J Pharmacol Toxicol. 2011;6:647–63.

75. Manna F, Abdel-Wahhab M, Ahmed H, Park M. Protective role for *Panax ginseng* extract standardized with ginsenoside Rg3 against acrylamide induced neurotoxicity in rats. J Appl Toxicol. 2006;26:198–206.

76. Mehri S, Abnous K, Mousavi S, Motamed Shariaty V, Hosseinzadeh H. Neuroprotective effect of crocin on acrylamide-induced cytotoxicity in PC12 cells. Cell Mol Neurobiol. 2012;32:227–35.

77. Naghizadeh B, Boroushaki MT, Mashhadian NV, Mansouri SMT. Protective effects of crocin against cisplatin-induced acute renal failure and oxidative stress in rats. Iran Biomed J. 2008;12:93–100.

78. El Daly ES. Protective effect of cysteine and vitamin E, *Crocus sativus* and *Nigella sativa* extracts on cisplatin-induced toxicity in rats. J Pharm Belg. 1998;53:85–93.

79. Boroushaki MT, Sadeghnia HR. Protective effect of safranal against gentamicin-induced nephrotoxicity in rat. Iran J Med Sci. 2009;34:285–8.

80. Ajami M, Eghtesadi S, Pazoki-toroudi HR, Habibey R, Ebrahimi SA. Effect of *crocus sativus* on gentamicin induced nephrotoxicity. Biol Res. 2010;43:83–90.

81. Dhar MH, Shah KU, Ghongane BB, RANE SR. Nephroprotective activity of *crocus sativus* extract against gentamicin and/or ceftazidime - Induced nephrotoxicity in rats. Inter J Pharm Bio Sci. 2013;4:864–P70.

82. Boroushaki MT, Mofidpour H, Sadeghnia H. Protective effect of safranal against hexachlorobutadiene-induced nephrotoxicity in rat. Iran J Med Sci. 2007;32:173–6.

83. Nolan C, Shaikh Z. An evaluation of tissue metallothionein and genetic resistance to cadmium toxicity in mice. Toxicol Appl Pharmacol. 1986;85:135–44.

84. Asadi MH, Zafari F, Sarveazad A, Abbasi M, Safa M, Koruji M, et al. Saffron improves epididymal sperm parameters in rats exposed to cadmium. Nephro-Urol Month. 2014;6:e12125.

85. Hariri A, Moallem S, Mahmoudi M, Hosseinzadeh H. The effect of crocin and safranal, constituents of saffron, against subacute effect of diazinon on hematological and genotoxicity indices in rats. Phytomedicine. 2011;18:499–504.

86. Hussein HH, Mahmoud OM. Effects of maternal administration of aluminum chloride on the development of the skeletal system of albino rat fetuses - protective role of saffron. Eur J Anat. 2013;17:63–71.

87. Tafazoli M, Kermani T, Saadatjoo A. Effects of saffron on abortion and its side effects on mice balb/c. OFOGH-E-DANESH. 2004;10:53–6.

88. Ziaee T, Razavi B, Hosseinzadeh H. Saffron reduced toxic effects of its constituent, safranal, in acute and subacute toxicities in rats. Jundishapur J Nat Pharm Prod. 2014;9:3–8.

89. Hosseinzadeh H, Sadeghi Shakib S, Khadem Sameni A, Taghiabadi E. Acute and subacute toxicity of safranal, a constituent of saffron, in mice and rats. Iran J Pharm Res. 2013;12:93–9.

90. Mirheydar H. Herbal information: application of herbs in prevention and treatment of deseases. Tehran, IR (Iran): Islamic culture press centre; 2001.

21

Anti-hyperlipidemic and anti-atherosclerotic effects of *Pinus eldarica* Medw. nut in hypercholesterolemic rabbits

Hasan Fallah Huseini[1], Maryam Sotoudeh Anvari[2], Yaser Tajallizadeh khoob[3], Shahram Rabbani[4], Farshad Sharifi[5], Seyed Masoud Arzaghi[5] and Hossein Fakhrzadeh[5*]

Abstract

Background: Previous studies suggest that chemical constituents present in *Pinus eldarica* Medw (*P. eldarica*) nut possess antioxidant properties that may positively influence lipid profile.
The present study was conducted to evaluate the efficacy of *P. eldarica* nut on the experimental atherosclerosis development in hypercholesterolemic rabbits.

Methods: Forty male 6 months old white New Zealand rabbits (1.8–2 kg) were randomly assigned into five equal groups. One group was kept as control (normal) group, fed on standard rabbit diet and other 4 groups were fed on high cholesterol diet (HCD). Out of four HCD groups one group was kept as control (HCD) and other three groups were treated with different doses (50, 100 and 200 mg/kg/day) of *P. eldarica* nut for 8 weeks. Percentage of aortic wall area changes as indication of atherosclerosis development and fasting blood cholesterol, LDL, HDL and triglyceride levels were determined in all groups.

Results: The results indicate that fasting blood cholesterol and aortic atherosclerotic involvements in 200 mg/kg/day and 100 mg/kg/day *P. eldarica* nut extract treated groups significantly decreased as compared to the high cholesterol-diet control group.

Conclusion: *P. eldarica* nut lowers blood cholesterol level and aortic atherosclerotic involvement in hypercholesterolemic rabbits.

Keywords: *Pinus eldarica* nut, Rabbits, Atherosclerosis, Hypercholesterolemia

Introduction

Atherosclerotic vascular disease is a major cause of morbidity and mortality worldwide [1]. Dyslipidemia is a crucial risk factor for atherosclerosis and oxidative stress following free radical-mediated oxidation of low-density lipoproteins is associated with progression of atherogenesis and its vascular complications [2–4]. In the search for plant foods that provide cardiovascular benefits, nuts have recently enticed attention. Among nuts, the Iranian pine, *Pinus eldarica* Medw (*P. eldarica*) nuts are used as food. *P. eldarica* belongs to the botanical family pinaceae

and naturally grows in the Transcaucasian region between Europe and Asia, and it is also spread in Iran, Afghanistan and Pakistan [5, 6].

In Russia and the Central Asian countries the *P. eldarica* needles, buds, resin and nuts have been widely used in traditional medicine for the treatment of bronchial asthma, and various skin diseases [7, 8]. Several components such as β-caryophyllene, α-pinene, longifolene, α-humulene, δ-3-carene and β-pinene with antioxidant properties have been reported in the *P. eldarica* nut oil [9].

In our previous study high concentrations of total polyphenols and fatty acids have been detected in *P. eldarica* nut as indication of its antioxidant properties [10]. Experimental studies strongly support the efficacy of polyphenols and unsaturated fatty acids in the treatment of chronic diseases including cardiovascular disorders

* Correspondence: Fakhrzad@tums.ac.ir
[5]Elderly Health Research Center, Endocrinology and Metabolism Population Sciences Institute, Tehran University of Medical Sciences, 4th floor, No 4, Ostad Nejatollahi Street, Engelab Avenue, Tehran, Iran
Full list of author information is available at the end of the article

[11–14]. The present study was conducted to evaluate the possible anti-hypercholesterolemic and anti-atherosclerotic effects of *P. eldarica* nut in hypercholesterolemic rabbits.

Methods

Chemicals

Methanol, phosphoric acid, chloroform, acetonitril and sodium chloride were purchased from Merck Company (India) nn. Ethyl acetate was purchased from Sinopharm Chemical Reagent Company (China). Polyphenol standards: (+) - catechin, (–) - epicatechin, Gallic acid, vanillic acid, *para* coumaric acid, ferullic acid, *ortho* coumaric acid and tyrosol were purchased from Sigma-Aldrich Corporation (Germany). Cholesterol powder was purchased from Solvay Duphar Co., Belgium.

Plant material

P. eldarica cones were collected from Chitgar Forest Park (West of Tehran). The cones were collected between June and July of 2010. The plant was identified by M. Ahvazi and herbarium specimen was preserved in the herbarium of Medicinal Plants Institute (ACECR) with Herbarium code of 689. *P. eldarica* cones were dried in a dark place at room temperature. The nuts were removed from cones and grounded to powder by grinder.

Plant extract

The hydroalcholic extract of *P. eldarica* nut powder was prepared using 70 % ethanol in water, using percolation method at room temperature. The powdered plant material was soaked initially in a solvent in a percolator and then sufficient amount of the solvent was added to cover material and kept for 24 h with occasional stirring. Then the outlet of the percolator was opened and the liquid contained therein was allowed to drip slowly. The procedure was repeated twice and the combined extractions were clarified by filtration and concentrated to dryness on rotary evaporator at a maximum of 40 °C temperature and under reduced pressure.

Polyphenol determination

The polyphenol content of *P. eldarica* nut was determined by the High-performance liquid chromatography (HPLC) method developed by Dogan et al. [15]. In brief a standard solution was prepared by dissolving 10 mg of (+) catechin (sigma), epicatechin (sigma), and other phenolic compounds in 10 ml methanol and diluting this solution with methanol HPLC grade. The range of concentration was between 50 and 1000 µg/ml and standard curve was linear ($R^2 \geq 0.998$). Then 20 µL of sample solution was injected to the HPLC and the chromatogram was recorded at 280 nm. First, 20 µl of standard solution was injected and the chromatogram was

recorded at 280 nm. Next, we compared the area of the peaks in standard and sample chromatograms and calculated the amount of polyphenols in *P. eldarica*. Total phenol was computed from measurement of individually detected phenols [16].

Animals and diet

Forty male 6-month-old white New Zealand rabbits (1.8–2 kg) were purchased from Razi Research Institute, Karaj, Iran. High cholesterol diet (HCD) was prepared by adding of 1 g cholesterol powder and 3 g corn oil to 96 g of standard laboratory food.

General procedures

Rabbits were housed individually in cages in temperature-controlled room (24 °C) under a 12-h light/dark cycle with free access to food and water in the Animal Research Center of Institute of Medicinal Plants. The experimental protocol was approved by the Iranian Institutional Animal Ethics Committee and was conducted according to the Iranian Institutional Animal Care Guidelines for the use and care of experimental animal, drug, dose, and treatment schedule.

After a 2-week adaptation period, rabbits were randomly assigned to five equal groups: control (normal) group fed on standard a diet, HCD control group fed on HCD (1 % cholesterol), and three groups fed on HCD and treated with *P. eldarica* nut in three different doses (50, 100 and 200 mg/kg/day). The extract in the dosages of 50, 100, 200 mg was mixed with little amount of rabbit pellets and fed orally one hour before feeding. The whole experiment lasted 8 weeks. Upon termination of the study biochemical analysis of serum lipids and pathological evaluation of aortas were performed.

Biochemical analysis

At the end of the study, the overnight fasting blood sample was taken from marginal ear veins for lipid analysis. Fasting blood cholesterol (Cho) LDL, HDL and triglyceride (TG) levels in sera were measured using enzyme assay kits (Pars Azmun Co., Iran).

Pathological analysis

At the end of the study, rabbits were killed by chloroform (overdose) and their aortas were separated up to diaphragm. The aortas were then divided into the proximal, middle, and distal segments. The aortic specimens were dehydrated in a graded series of alcohol xylene and embedded in paraffin for light microscopic examination. From each paraffin block, four sections of 4 mm^2 were cut and stained with hematoxylin and eosin. All sections were evaluated microscopically for fatty streak, foam cells, extracellular lipid core, as atheromatous plaque elements. The degree of vascular injury and atherosclerosis was

Table 1 Percent of polyphenols in *P. eldarica* nut mean ± SD [16]

Polyphenols	Percent
Catechin	10.1 ± 0.18
Epicatechin	10.3 ± 0.18
Gallic acid	1.6 ± 0.09
P. coumaric acid	1.4 ± 0.12
Ferulic acid	1.7 ± 0.21
O. coumaric acid	0.12 ± 0.02
Tyrosol	29.1 ± 0.08
Dimers of catechin and epicatechin	7.5 ± 1.06
Unknown	38.18 ± 0.28
Total phenols (ppm)	483 ± 27

quantitatively measured based on lesion area (on scale of mm^2) with use of a color image analyzer (E200; Nikon, Tokyo, Japan) [17]. Both the surgeon and the pathologist were blinded to the control and experiment groups.

Statistical analysis

All values are expressed as means ± SE. Data were analyzed by one way ANOVA, and all differences were inspected by Duncan's multiple test. Differences were considered to be significant at $p < 0.05$.

Results

The polyphenol content of the *P. eldarica* nut is presented in Table 1. Considering this method more than 8 polyphenols were identified in *P. eldarica* nut in which catechin, epicatechin and tyrosol were highest in concentration.

Results show that feeding the rabbits for 8 weeks with HCD leads to a significant increase in their blood serum total cholesterol, LDL-C and to a lesser extent in TG levels. Results indicate that serum total cholesterol and LDL-C levels significantly decrease in the groups treated with 200 mg/kg/day and 100 mg/kg/day of *P. eldarica* compared to the control group; although it is of note that all of the aortic samples from HCD-fed rabbits showed some degree of atherogenesis and none of them were normal. There were no significant changes in fasting blood TG and HDL-C levels in *P. eldarica* treated groups compared to control group (Table 2) (Fig. 1).

Morphological changes of the aortic wall atherosclerotic involvement are shown in Fig. 1. The aortic wall area percent in groups treated with 200 mg/kg/day and 100 mg/kg/day *P. eldarica* nut decreased significantly compared to the control group (Table 2).

Discussion

The results suggest that *P. eldarica* nut extract reduced total cholesterol, LDL-C and extent of aortic atherosclerotic involvement in hypercholesterolemic rabbits. The mechanism underlying inhibition of aortic atherosclerotic progression by *P. eldarica* nut extract may not be solely due to its lipid lowering effect, as the levels of serum total cholesterol and LDL-C were remarkably higher in cholesterol-fed rabbits than in normal ones. Other mechanisms may also play a role for such effect. Increases in serum cholesterol and LDL-C and consequent oxidation of LDL-C are essential steps for development of atherosclerotic plaques [2]. In fact formation of oxidatively-modified LDL-C is the first step of atherogenesis in so-called "oxidation hypothesis" [17].

Table 2 The fasting blood parameters and aortic wall area percent (mm^2) after 8 weeks of high cholesterol diet (HCD) fed rabbits treated with *P. eldarica* nut extract at dosages of 50, 100, 200 mg/kg compared with high control HCD fed rabbits (mean ± SD)

Groups	Triglyceride (mg/dl)	Cholesterol (mg/dl)	LDL (mg/dl)	HDL (mg/dl)	Aortic wall area percent (mm^2)	Percent of aortic wall area changes
Control (normal)	60.4 ± 15.8	31.4 ± 4.5	9.2 ± 4.7	13.2 ± 3.2	0.247 ± 0.032	
Control (HCD)	91.2 ± 48.9	1545.6 ± 510.6	1060.6 ± 360.5	113.4 ± 55.8	0.296 ± 0.049	16.55↑ Compared with control (normal)
	$P = 0.218*$	$P = 0.003*$	$P = 0.016*$	$P = 0.003*$	$P = 0.005*$	
P. eldarica nut extract 50 mg/kg	93.6 ± 31.2	1253.0 ± 578.0	834.4 ± 201.2	87.6 ± 17.7	0.276 ± 0.048	6.76↓ compared with control (HCD)
	$P = 0.929**$	$P = 0.421**$	$P = 0.544**$	$P = 0.351**$	$P = 0.350**$	
P. eldarica nut extract 100 mg/kg	102.2 ± 37.7	834.4 ± 201.2	552.4 ± 158.2	90.2 ± 15.9	0.261 ± 0.038	11.83↓ compared with control (HCD)
	$P = 0.700**$	$P = 0.020**$	$P = 0.034**$	$P = 0.410**$	$P = 0.048**$	
P. eldarica nut extract 200 mg/kg	108.8 ± 28.0	710.4 ± 448.0	438.4 ± 292.2	99.4 ± 11.8	0.259 ± 0.042	12.50↓compared with control (HCD)
	$P = 0.505**$	$P = 0.025**$	$P = 0.020**$	$P = 0.47**0$	$P = 0.032**$	

$P < 0.05$ was considered as statistically significant
*compared with control (normal) group
**compared with control (HCD) group

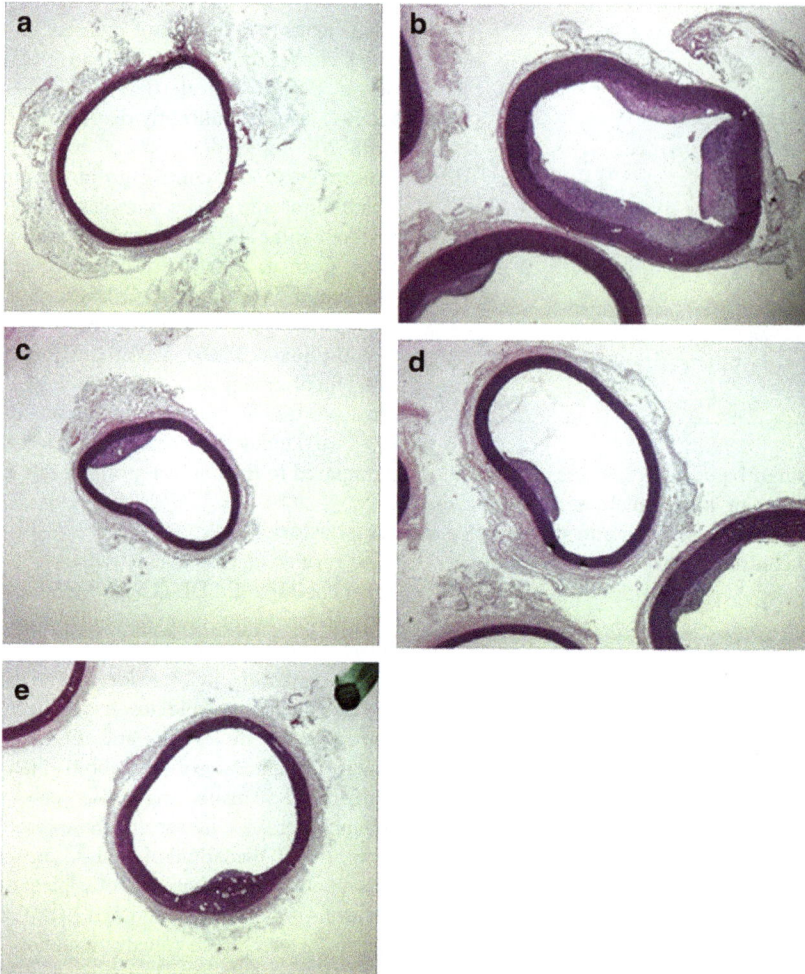

Fig. 1 Morphological changes of the aortic wall atherosclerotic involvement. **a** Normal rabbits fed on standard laboratory diet, **b** Rabbits fed on HCD; **c** Rabbits fed on HCD and treated with 50 mg/kg of *P. eldarica*; **d** Rabbits fed on HCD and treated with 100 mg/kg of *P. eldarica*; **e** Rabbits fed on HCD and treated with 200 mg/kg of *P. eldarica*

Moreover it has been shown that susceptibility of LDL-C to oxidation independently correlates with the extent of atherosclerosis [18]. It is now established that inhibition of oxidative stress and lipid oxidation could have beneficial effects on regression of atherogenesis [19]. *P. eldarica* nuts contain high concentrations of polyphenols and flavonoids (Table 1) [10]. Several data suggested that, flavonoids improve dyslipidemia, inhibit low-density lipoprotein cholesterol oxidation and protect vascular endothelium against oxidative damage [20–22]. Furthermore, catechin and epicatechin which are found in high concentrations in *P. eldarica* nuts are also main chemical constituent of other Pinus species barks such as French matitime pine bark extract (pycnogenol) [23]. Several studies have shown the beneficial effects of pycnogenol for health to be mainly due to its antioxidant

properties and consequent excellent free radical scavenging function [24–26]. In addition other components such as tyrosol with antioxidant properties which are present in high concentrations in *P. eldarica* nuts may directly or indirectly influence lipoprotein and cellular metabolism against atherogenesis [10, 27].

On the other hand, the observed anti-atherogenic effects of *P. eldarica* nut in the rabbits may also be in part due to appreciable amounts of essential oils such as α-pinene, β-pinene and β-caryophyllene present in this nut [9]. The antioxidant properties of α-pinene, β-pinene and β-caryophyllene are reported in other studies [28]. Of note the limitations of this study were lack of determination of the essential oil components and antioxidant properties of *P. eldarica* nut extract. To our knowledge this is the first trial on the anti-atherosclerotic and hypolipidemic effects of *P. eldarica* extracts on hyper-cholesterolemic rabbits. In a similar study we also have recently shown the beneficial effects of *Pinus eldarica* nut extract on blood glucose and cholesterol levels in hypercholesterolemic alloxan-induced diabetic rats [29]. As *P. eldarica* nuts are usually safe and used as food, further investigation of their clinical efficacy in the treatment of hypercholesterolemia is suggested.

Competing interests

The authors declare that they have no competing interests.

Authors' contributions

HFH performed the field trial and preparation of the manuscript, MSA performed the pathological analysis, YTk contributed in preparing the research proposal, SR prepared aortic specimens for pathological analysis, FS performed the statistical analysis, SMA contributed in the field trial and laboratory analysis, HF was the principle investigator who conceived the idea and prepared the research proposal and helped in the preparation of the manuscript. All authors read and approved the final manuscript.

Acknowledgements

This research was supported by a grant from the Endocrinology and Metabolism Research Institute, Tehran University of Medical Sciences Tehran, Iran and the Institute of Medicinal Plants (ACECR), Karaj.

Author details

[1]Medicinal Plants Research Center, Institute of Medicinal Plants, ACECR, Karaj, Iran. [2]Clinical and Surgical Pathology Department Tehran Heart Center, Tehran University of Medical Sciences, Tehran, Iran. [3]Endocrinology and Metabolism Research Center, Endocrinology and Metabolism Clinical Sciences Institute, Tehran University of Medical Sciences, Tehran, Iran. [4]Experimental Research Center, Tehran Heart Center, Tehran University of Medical Sciences, Tehran, Iran. [5]Elderly Health Research Center, Endocrinology and Metabolism Population Sciences Institute, Tehran University of Medical Sciences, 4th floor, No 4, Ostad Nejatollahi Street, Engelab Avenue, Tehran, Iran.

References

1. Finegold JA, Asaria P, Francis DP. Mortality from ischaemic heart disease by country, region, and age: statistics from World Health Organisation and United Nations. Int J Cardiol. 2012;168(2):934–45.

2. Badimon L, Vilahur G. LDL-cholesterol versus HDL-cholesterol in the atherosclerotic plaque: inflammatory resolution versus thrombotic chaos. Ann N Y Acad Sci. 2012;1254:18–32.

3. Stocker R, Keaney Jr JF. Role of oxidative modifications in atherosclerosis. Physiol Rev. 2004;84(4):1381–478.

4. Chen K, Keaney Jr JF. Evolving concepts of oxidative stress and reactive oxygen species in cardiovascular disease. Curr Atheroscler Rep. 2012;14(5):476–83.

5. Zargary A. Medicinal plants. 5th ed. Tehran: Tehran University Press; 1996. p. 9–12.

6. Mozaffarian W. Tree and shrubs of Iran. 1st ed. Tehran Iran: Farhang Moaser Press; 1983. p. 563–5.

7. Mamedov N, Craker LE. Medicinal plants used for the treatment of bronchial asthma in Russia and Central Asia. J Herbs Spices Med Plants. 2001;8:91–117.

8. Mamedov N, Gardner Z, Craker LE. Medicinal plants used in Russia and Central Asia for the treatment of selected skin conditions. J Herbs Spices Med Plants. 2005;11:191–222.

9. Afsharypour S, Sanaty F. Essential oil constituents of leaves and fruits of Pinus eldarica Medw. J Essent Oil Res. 2005;17:327–8.

10. Sadeghi Afjeh M, Fallah Huseini H, Tajalizadekhoob Y, Mirarefin M, Sharifi F, Taheri E, et al. Determination of phenolic compounds in Pinus eldarica by HPLC. J Med Plant Res. 2014;49:23–33.

11. Pandey KB, Rizvi SI. Plant polyphenols as dietary antioxidants in human health and disease. Oxid Med Cell Longev. 2009;2(5):270–8.

12. Pandey KB, Rizvi SI. Current understanding of dietary polyphenols and their role in health and disease. Curr Nutr Food Sci. 2009;5(4):249–63.

13. Tavakoli R, Mohadjerani M, Hosseinzadeh R, Tajbakhsh M, Naqinezhad A. Essential-oil and fatty-acid composition, and antioxidant activity of extracts of Ficaria kochii. Chem Biodivers. 2012;9(12):2732–41.

14. Causey JL. Korean pine nut fatty acids induce satiety-producing hormone release in overweight human volunteers, American Chemical Society National Meeting & Exposition. 2006. p. 26–30.

15. Dogan S, Diken ME, Dogan M. Antioxidant, phenolic and protein contents of some medicinal plants. J Med Plant Res. 2010;4:2566–73.

16. Sadeghi Afjeh M, Fallah Huseini H, Tajallizadekhoob Y, Mirarefin M, Taheri E, Saeednia S, et al. Determination of phenolic compounds in Pinus Eldarica by HPLC. J Med Plant Res. 2014;13(49):22–33.

17. Kumar V, Abbas AK, Fausto N. Pathologic basis of disease. 7th ed. Philadelphia: Saunders; 2005. p. 25–6.

18. Regnström J, Nilsson J, Tornvall P, Landou C, Hamsten A. Susceptibility to low- density-lipoprotein oxidation and coronary atherosclerosis in man. Lancet. 1992;339:1183–6.

19. Heinecke JW. Oxidants and antioxidants in the pathogenesis of atherosclerosis: implications for the oxidised low density lipoprotein hypothesis. Atheroscler. 1998;141:1–15.

20. Loke WM, Proudfoot JM, Hodgson JM, McKinley AJ, Hime N, Magat M, et al. Specific dietary polyphenols attenuate atherosclerosis in apolipoprotein E-knockout mice by alleviating inflammation and endothelial dysfunction. Arterioscler Thromb Vasc Biol. 2010;30(4):749–57.

21. Martin S, Andriantsitohaina R. Cellular mechanism of vasculo-protection induced by polyphenols on the endothelium. Ann Cardiol Angeiol (Paris). 2002;51(6):304–15.

22. Mulvihill EE, Huff MW. Antiatherogenic properties of flavonoids: implications for cardiovascular health. Can J Cardiol. 2010;26:17A–21.

23. Yesli-Celiktas O, Ganzera M, Akgun I, Sevimli C, Korkmaz KS, Bedir E. Determination of polyphenolic constituents and biological activities of bark extracts from different Pinus species. J Sci Food Agric. 2009;89(8):1339–45.

24. Rohdewald P. A review of the French maritime pine bark extract (Pycnogenol), a herbal medication with a diverse pharmacology. Int J Clin Pharmacol Ther. 2002;40:158–68.

25. Sato M, Yamada Y, Matsuoka H, Nakashima S, Kamiya T, Ikeguchi M, et al. Dietary pine bark extract inhibit atherosclerotic lesion development in male Apo-E-deficient mice by lowering the serum cholesterol level. Biosci Biotechnol Biochem. 2009;73:1314–7.

26. Maritim A, Dene BA, Sanders RA, Watkins JB. Effects of Pycnogenol treatment on oxidative stress in streptozotocin-induced diabetic rats. J Biochem Mol Toxicol. 2003;17:193–9.

27. Giovannini C, Straface E, Modesti D, Coni E, Cantafora A, De Vincenzi M, et al. Tyrosol, the major olive oil biophenol, protects against oxidized-LDL-induced injury in Caco-2 cells. J Nutr. 1999;129(7):1269–77.

28. Miguel MG. Antioxidant and anti-inflammatory activities of essential oils: a short review. Molecules. 2010;15(12):9252–87.

29. Fallah Huseini H, Mehrzadi S, Ghaznavi H, Tajallizadehkhoob Y, Fakhrzadeh H. Effects of pinus eldarica medw: nut extract on blood glucose and cholesterol levels in hypercholesterolemic alloxan-induced diabetic rats. J Med Plant Res. 2013;1(45):68–74.

22

Potential therapeutic effect of *Allium cepa* L. and quercetin in a murine model of *Blomia tropicalis* induced asthma

Tatiane Teixeira Oliveira[1], Keina Maciele Campos[1], Ana Tereza Cerqueira-Lima[1], Tamires Cana Brasil Carneiro[1], Eudes da Silva Velozo[2], Ingrid Christie Alexandrino Ribeiro Melo[3], Eugênia Abrantes Figueiredo[3], Eduardo de Jesus Oliveira[3], Darizy Flávia Silva Amorim de Vasconcelos[1], Lain Carlos Pontes-de-Carvalho[4], Neuza Maria Alcântara-Neves[1] and Camila Alexandrina Figueiredo[1*]

Abstract

Background: Asthma is an inflammatory condition characterized by airway hyperresponsiveness and chronic inflammation. The resolution of inflammation is an essential process to treat this condition. In this study we investigated the effect of *Allium cepa* L. extract (AcE) and quercetin (Qt) on cytokine and on smooth muscle contraction *in vitro* and its therapeutic potential in a murine model of asthma.

Methods: AcE was obtained by maceration of *Allium cepa* L. and it was standardized in terms of quercetin concentration using high performance liquid chromatography (HPLC). *In vitro*, using AcE 10, 100 or 1000 μg/ml or Qt 3.5, 7.5, 15 μg/ml, we measured the concentration of cytokines in spleen cell culture supernatants, and the ability to relax tracheal smooth muscle from A/J mice. *In vivo*, *Blomia tropicalis* (BT)-sensitized A/J mice were treated with AcE 100, 1000 mg/kg or 30 mg/kg Qt. We measured cell influx in bronchoalveolar lavage (BAL), eosinophil peroxidase (EPO) in lungs, serum levels of Bt-specific IgE, cytokines levels in BAL, and lung histology.

Results: We observed a reduction in the production of inflammatory cytokines, a relaxation of tracheal rings, and a reduction in total number of cells in BAL and EPO in lungs by treatment with AcE or Qt.

Conclusion: AcE and Qt have potential as antiasthmatic drugs, as they possess both immunomodulatory and bronchodilatory properties.

Keywords: Natural product, Asthma, *Blomia tropicalis*, *Allium* cepa L., Quercetin

Background

Asthma is an inflammatory condition characterized by airway hyperresponsiveness, mucus cell hyperplasia, inflammatory cell infiltration and reversible bronchoconstriction, which may progress to airway remodeling with fibrosis and an increase in smooth muscle reactivity [1-4]. In allergic asthma, exposure to allergens causes an imbalance between the T helper type (Th) 1 and Th2 responses. Cytokines produced by the Th2-type CD4 + T cells (interleukin (IL-4, IL-5, IL-13) in asthma have a central role in orchestrating the inflammatory response.

Strong support for this T-cell-centric paradigm has been enriched by the identification of Treg cells with the capacity to control both Th1 and Th2 responses [5]. The synthesis and release of IL-4 (which stimulates B cells to synthesize IgE), IL-13 (which stimulates mucus production) and IL-5 (which is necessary for eosinophilic infiltration to the lung tissue) increase vascular permeability and chemotaxis, which amplify the inflammatory response. Additionally, activated mast cells are able during an allergen challenge to release several inflammatory and bronchoconstrictor mediators [6,7].

The prevalence of asthma continues to rise worldwide [8], and treatment of asthma faces many challenges, including under diagnosis, access to care, ability of healthcare workers to manage asthma, education of healthcare

* Correspondence: cavfigueiredo@gmail.com
[1]Instituto de Ciências da Saúde, Universidade Federal da Bahia, Salvador, Bahia, Brazil
Full list of author information is available at the end of the article

providers and patients, and availability and affordability of inhaled therapy [9]. Treatment with inhaled steroids and bronchodilators often results in good control of symptoms [10]. However, the treatment for patients with severe asthma with uncontrolled and frequent exacerbations still contributes to morbidity and mortality of asthma in all age groups and remains a challenge [11,12]. The safety concerns and the obstacles for the asthmatic patients justify continued efforts to find new alternative therapies [13].

Historically, herbal medicine has been studied in asthma treatment, and some of the drugs currently used to treat this disease such as the inhaled corticosteroids, sympatho-mimetics, anti-cholinergics, methylxanthines and cro-mones have origins in herbal treatments [14]. Thus, our group performed an ethnopharmacological survey [15], and one of the herbs described was Allium cepa L., commonly used to treat inflammatory conditions such as asthma [16,17].

Several plant-derived secondary metabolites have been shown to interfere directly with molecules and mechanisms, such as the mediation of inflammatory responses and activity of second messengers, as well as the expression of transcription factors and key pro-inflammatory molecules [18]. The main compounds found in Allium cepa L. extract (AcE) are the flavonoids such as quercetin, which are natural phenolic compounds present in fruits and vegetables, exhibiting many pharmacological properties such as its anti-inflammatory and antioxidant effects [17,19-21]. Along with flavanols, the major bioactive constituents in Allium cepa L. are sulfurous compounds. In previous studies, using mass spectrometry for direct analysis of volatile sulfurous compounds has described the presence of propanethiol, dipropyl disulfide and thiosulfinates [22-24]. The sulfoxides, which are responsible for the onion flavor and odor, might also be responsible in part for the onion biological activity of different Allium spp. species. The propanethiol is suggested to be the main source of the characteristic onion odor [23,24].

In previous studies, the anti-allergic potential of the extracts of Allium cepa L. [16,17] and its flavonoid quercetin [18,19,25] has been reported using a mouse model of ovalbumin (OVA)-induced asthma. This study is the first which was conducted using extracts of Allium cepa L. (AcE) and quercetin treatment in murine model of allergic airway disease induced by the sensitization to the clinically relevant aeroallergen Blomia tropicalis mite. This mite is a major house dust mite in dust worldwide [26]. In addition, it has been shown that flavonoids, typically found in Allium cepa, have a relaxing effect on the smooth muscle of isolated trachea and may have bronchodilator effect [25,27,28].

Thus, the objective of this study was to assess the therapeutic potential (anti-inflammatory and bronchodilator) of the methanolic extract of Allium cepa L. (AcE) and its flavonoid quercetin (Qt) in a murine model of respiratory allergy to Blomia tropicalis mite.

Methods

Animals

A/J mice aged 5–7 weeks (20–25 g), females, were from the Fundação Oswaldo Cruz, Bahia, Brazil. Five animals per group were used in each experiment. Mice were housed in controlled temperature and humidity environment with 12-hour light–dark cycles, and had free access to food and water. The experimental procedures were approved by the Ethical Committee for Use of Experimental Animals of the Faculdade de Odontologia, Universidade Federal da Bahia, Brazil (protocol number: 02/09).

Sensitization and challenge of mice with Blomia tropicalis (Bt-sensitized mice)

A B. tropicalis extract was obtained as previously described [15]. The experimental model of allergy to B. tropicalis (Bt) dust mite was used as previously described [29]. The animals were sensitized with subcutaneous injections of Bt (100 μg of protein) adsorbed to 4 mg/ml of $Al(OH)_3$ in saline on days 0 and 7, and 1 day after the last sensitization the animals received four intranasal challenges with Bt (10 μg/instilation) every other day. Animals were euthanized with intraperitoneal injections of xilazine and ketamine (40 mg/kg/body weight), 24 hours after the last challenge. A schematic diagram of the sensitization and allergen challenge schedule is shown in Figure 1.

Preparation of the Allium cepa L. extract and obtaining of quercetin

A methanolic extract was obtained by maceration of Allium cepa L. previously peeled and cut in a closed container containing 1000 ml of 99.8% methyl alcohol (CH_3OH) during 7 days at room temperature. Subsequently, we proceeded to filtration of the extractive liquid, which then was rota-evaporated at a temperature of 60–70°C in a thermostatic bath. This concentration process was repeated three times. The AcE was dried in the oven and then maintained at −20°C until use.

The flavonoid quercetin [2-(3, 4-dihydroxyphenyl)-3, 5, 7-trihydroxy-4H-1-benzopyran-4-one, 3, 3′, 4′, 5, 6 - entahydroxyflavone] was obtained commercially (98% purity) from Sigma-Aldrich® (St. Louis, MA, USA).

In vitro, different concentrations of AcE—10 μg/ml (AcE_{10}), 100 μg/ml (AcE_{100}), or 1000 μg/ml (AcE_{1000}), and Qt—3.5 μg/ml ($Qt_{3.5}$), 7.5 μg/ml ($Qt_{7.5}$) or 15 μg/ml (Qt_{15}) were tested. In vivo, the tested groups were animals sensitized to Bt and daily treated orally with AcE containing 100 mg/kg (AcE_{100}) and 1000 mg/kg (AcE_{1000}) or 30 mg/kg Qt (Qt_{30}) dissolved in saline (vehicle) from the 8th to the 14th day of the experimental

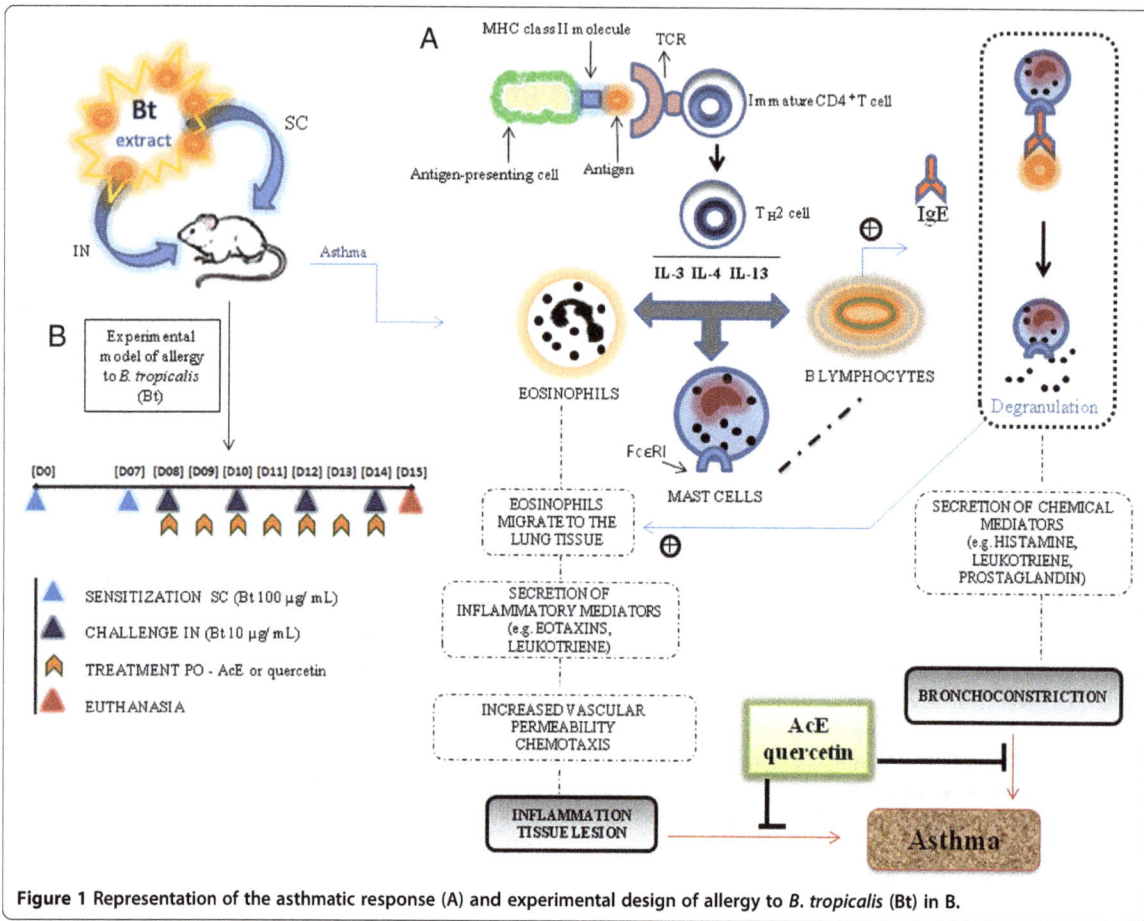

Figure 1 Representation of the asthmatic response (A) and experimental design of allergy to *B. tropicalis* (Bt) in B.

protocol and one hour after the intranasal challenges with Bt. Mice receiving the following treatments were studied: non-sensitized and vehicle-treated mice (negative control group); Bt, Bt-sensitized mice and vehicle-treated mice (positive control group); Bt/AcE$_{100}$, Bt-sensitized and AcE$_{100}$-treated mice; Bt/AcE$_{1000}$, Bt-sensitized and AcE$_{1000}$-treated mice; Bt/Qt, Bt-sensitized and Qt$_{30}$-treated mice (tested groups).

Standardization of *Allium cepa* L. extract

The major flavonoid found in *Allium cepa* L. is quercetin [30,31]. The AcE was standardized in terms of quercetin concentration by high performance liquid chromatography, with ultraviolet light detection at 250 nm, using a C-18 column (150×4.6 mm ID, 5 μm particle size, Thermo Scientific) and a C-18 pre-column (Phenomenex, Torrance, USA). The mobile phase consisted of 0.1% aqueous formic acid (A) and methanol (B) at a flow rate of 1.0 ml/min. The following gradient elution method was used for separation: 5% to 90% of B in A in 30 min. The injection volume was 20 μL and quercetin calibration curves were in the range of 5 to 100 μg/ml.

Cell viability assay

Cell viability after *in vitro* exposure to AcE and Qt was determined using the MTT assay. Spleen cells were seeded at a density of 5×10^5 cells/well in 96-well plate and were then exposed to AcE and Qt diluted in RPMI. After 48 hours of incubation, the viability of the cells was evaluated by using FCS-free medium containing 1 mg/ml of 3-[4, 5-dimethylthiazol-2-yl]-2, 5 diphenyltetrazoliumbromide (MTT, Sigma). After 4 hours of incubation at 37°C, the medium was discarded and the formazan blue dissolved with DMSO. The optical density (OD) was measured at 540 nm. The percentage of viable cells was calculated by defining the cell viability without treatment as 100%.

In vitro cytokine production by spleen cells

Levels of IL-4, IL-5 and IL-13 T-helper (Th) type 2 cytokines in splenocytes cultures were evaluated. According to the method described by Bezerra-Santos [32], splenocytes from Bt-sensitized mice were washed twice in RPMI medium by centrifugation at $200 \times g$ for 10 min. The obtained pellet was resuspended in RPMI medium supplemented with 200 mM l-glutamine, 100 units/ml penicillin, 100 μg/ml streptomycin, 5β-mercaptoethanol and 10% fetal calf serum (Gibco, Pisley, UK). Viable cells number was determined in a hemocytometer by exclusion using trypan blue. The spleen cells were plated in 96-well flat-bottomed tissue culture plates (Costar, Cambridge, MA, USA) at a density of 5×10^5 cells/well. The cells were treated with non-cytotoxic concentrations of AcE or Qt and stimulated with 5 μg/ml of pokeweed (PWM) (Sigma Aldrich, Saint Louis, MA, USA). The cells were incubated at 37°C in a humidified atmosphere of 5% CO_2 for 48 hours. Supernatants of the cell cultures were collected and analyzed by enzyme-linked immunosorbent assay (ELISA) for IL-4, IL-5 and IL-13 cytokine concentrations (BD Pharmingen, San Diego, CA, USA).

In vitro airway smooth muscle relaxation

AJ mice were euthanized and the trachea was rapidly removed. The trachea was cleared of loose connective tissue and divided into 2 rings of 2 mm, containing on average three to four cartilage bands. The rings were suspended on metal rods, attached to a force transducer (FORT10 WPI, Sarasota, USA) and placed in tanks for isolated organ with Krebs-bicarbonate solution (composition in mM: NaCl 119, $NaHCO_3$ 25, $CaCl_2 \times H_2O$ 1.6, KCl 4.7, KH_2PO_4 1.2, $MgSO_4 \times 7H_2O$ 1.2 and glucose 11.1), aerated with a carbogen mixture (95% O_2 and 5% CO_2) and maintained at 37°C. After the stabilization period (1 hour at 0.5 g), the rings were contracted with 10 μM of carbachol (Cch; Sigma, St Louis, MA, USA) to assess the contractile state of the tissue and to evaluate the presence of functional epithelium. The rings, after reaching a plateau of contractile state, were stimulated with bradykinin (Bk; Sigma, St Louis, MA, USA) (10^{-6} M). The rings were again contracted with Cch (10 μM) and cumulatively increasing concentrations of AcE or Qt were added. Concentration response curve was constructed and data were analyzed. Additionally, the tracheal rings were previously exposed to IL-13 in culture as described previously [33] to evaluate the effects of AcE or Qt on the hyper-responsive airway smooth muscle. The rings were placed individually in each well of a 48-well plate and incubated at 37°C in the presence or absence of IL-13 (10 ng/ml, 24 hours; BD Pharmingen, San Diego, CA, USA) in supplemented Dulbecco's modified Eagle's medium (containing 25 mM D-glucose, 1 mM sodium pyruvate, 100 U/ml penicillin, 100 μg/ml streptomycin, 0.2 M L-glutamine, 2.5 μg/ml Fungizone, and 0.1% w/v bovine serum albumin) (Sigma, St Louis, MA, USA) for 24 hours. Cumulative concentration-response curves to Cch after incubation in the absence or presence of IL-13 was built to analyze the hyper-reactivity of smooth muscle. After that, concentration-response curved for AcE or Qt was built.

Collection of bronchoalveolar lavage (BAL) fluid and cell counting

The trachea of the euthanized mice were canulated and BAL fluid was obtained by three successive aspirations (total volume 1.5 ml) via tracheal cannulation of phosphate buffered saline, pH 7.4 (PBS) containing 1% of bovine serum albumin (Sigma-Aldrich St. Louis, MA, USA). Total number of leukocytes in the BAL was determined using Trypan blue and differential cell counts for eosinophils were performed by using Wright-stained cytospin preparations. Differential counts of eosinophils of at least 100 cells were made in a blind fashion in accordance with standard morphologic protocol. The concentrations of IL-4, IL-5 and IL-13 in BAL were quantified by ELISA, as recommended by the manufacturer (BD Pharmingen, San Diego, CA, USA).

Eosinophil peroxidase (EPO) activity in lung

The cell suspensions from mouse lungs were frozen and thawed three times in liquid nitrogen. After centrifugation at 4°C for 10 min at 1000 g, the cell lysates were placed into wells of 96-well plates, followed by the addition of the chromogen and substrate solution (1.5 mmol/L of o-phenylenediamine and 6.6 mmol/L of H_2O_2 in 0.05 mol/L Tris–HCl, pH 8.0). After 30 minutes room temperature, the reaction was stopped with the addition of 0.2 mol/L citric acid, and the absorbance of the sample determined at 492 nm in an ELISA reader.

Measurement of serum levels of Bt-specific IgE

Anti-Bt IgE antibody levels from mice were determined by indirect ELISA. 96-well micro titer high-binding plate (Costar, Cambridge, MA, USA) were coated with Bt (100 μg/well) overnight (at 4°C). The serum samples were added and the plates were incubated again. Biotin-conjugated IgE anti-mouse (BD Pharmingen, San Diego, CA, USA) were added to the wells and incubated during 1 hour at room temperature (RT). A solution of avidin-horseradish peroxidase (BD Pharmingen, San Diego, CA, USA) was then added to each well for 30 minutes. After that, a solution containing 3, 3′, 5, 5′-tetramethylbenzidine and hydrogen peroxide (BD Pharmingen, San Diego, CA, USA) was added and incubated during additional 30 minutes (at RT). The reaction was stopped with 4 M sulfuric acid. Between all steps the wells were washed 3 times with PBS containing 0.05% Tween 20 (PBS-T). The absorbance of each sample was determined at 492 nm in an ELISA reader.

Lung histology

The analyses the histopathological changes and the degree of inflammation in peribronchiolar and perivascular regions were performed. The lungs were perfused, via the heart right ventricle, to remove residual blood, and immersed in 10% (v/v) formaldehyde (Sigma-Aldrich St. Louis, MA, USA). The tissue was dehydrated, embedded in paraffin and cut in 5 μm sections. The slides were stained with hematoxylin-eosin (HE) for inflammatory cell infiltration and were then stained with periodic acid-Schiff (PAS) for the evaluation of mucus production, under light microscopy with 40× magnification.

Statistical analysis

Multiple comparisons were performed by one-way analysis of variance (ANOVA) and Tukey's post-test (for data with normal distribution). Data were expressed as mean ± standard error of the mean. Differences in p values ≤0.05 were considered statistically significant. Each experiment was repeated at least twice.

Results

Quercetin is present in the methanolic extract of *Allium cepa* L

The chromatogram of the methanolic extract of AcE (Figure 2A) and a quercetin standard solution (Figure 2B)

demonstrated the separation of a compound in the methanolic extract with the same retention time of Qt in the standard sample (Figure 2A and B). The calculated average percentage of Qt in the AcE extract is 2.5% (based on peak area).

Effect of AcE and Qt on cell viability and cytokine levels in spleen cells culture

The non-cytotoxic concentrations of AcE and Qt used were determined by MTT assay. As can be seen in Figure 3A, none of the evaluated concentrations were toxic for spleen cells (AcE: 1000–10 μg/ml and Qt: 15–3.75 μg/ml). The production of Th2 cytokines, including IL-4, IL-5, and IL-13 by PWM-stimulated splenocytes from Bt-sensitized mice was increased in comparison to that by PWM-non-stimulated splenocytes from Bt-sensitized mice (p < 0.001). IL-4 (Figure 3B), IL-5 (Figure 3C), and IL-13 (Figure 3D) levels were significantly lower in the culture supernatants

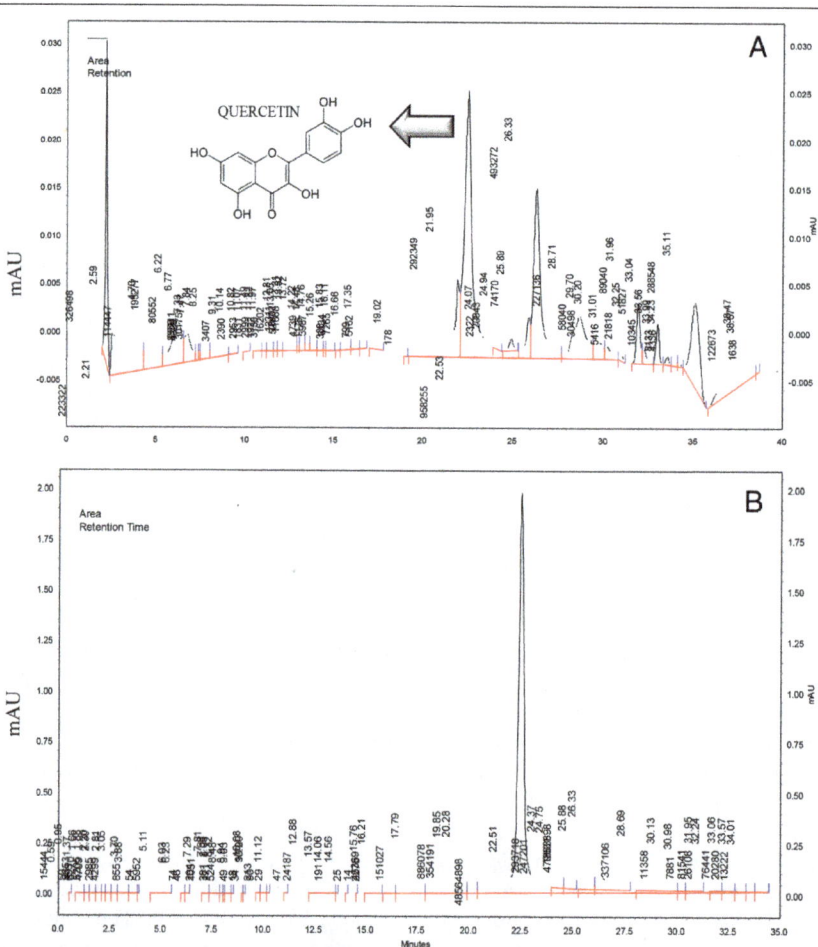

Figure 2 Chromatogram of samples subjected to high performance liquid chromatography. (A) Chromatogram of *Allium cepa* L. methanol extract. **(B)** Chromatogram of quercetin. Retention times of 22.51 minutes are shown above peaks in **(A)** and **(B)**.

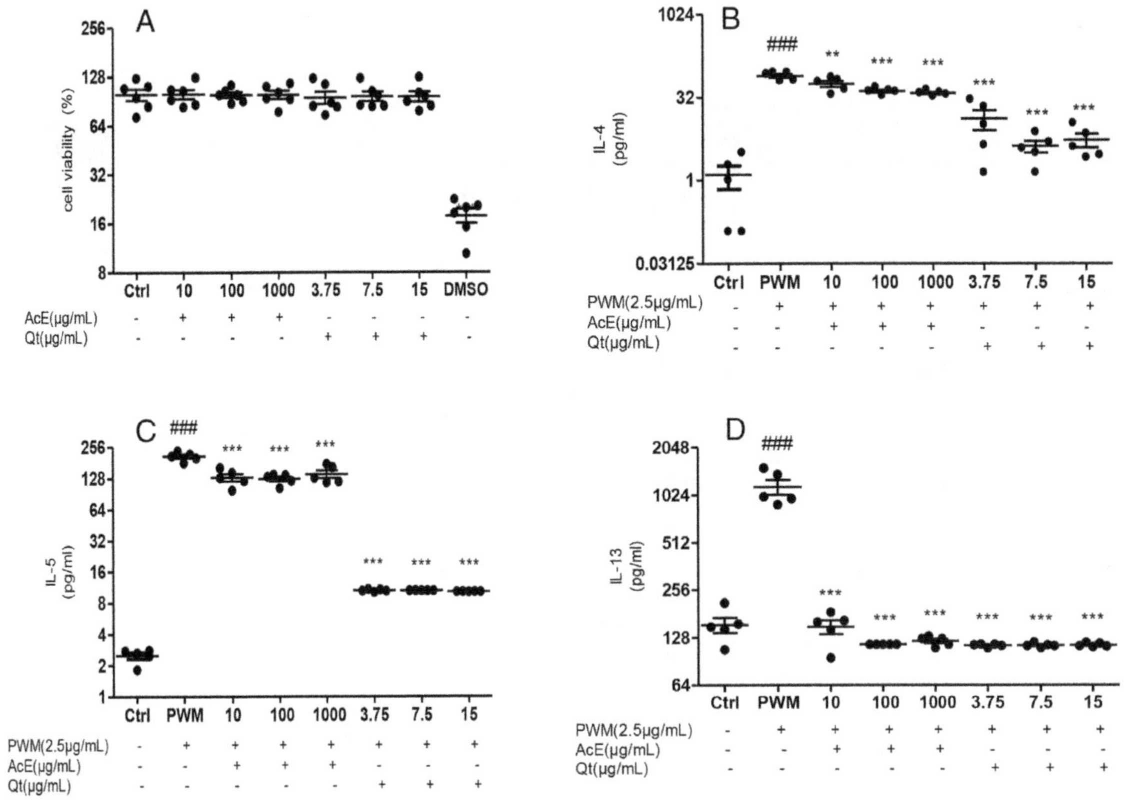

Figure 3 Effect of the in vitro treatment with AcE or Qt on cell viability (A) and on the levels of IL-4 (B), IL-5 (C) and IL-13 (D). The following groups were presented: splenocytes supernatant from animals Bt-sensitized without stimulation (control), stimulated with PWM (PWM) and stimulated with PWM and exposed to different concentrations of AcE (10 µg/ml, 100 µg/ml or 1000 µg/ml) or Qt (3.75 µg/ml, 7.5 µg/ml, or 15 µg/ml). Values represent mean ± SEM (n = 5, per group). [###]$p < 0.001$ vs. control, and [***]$p < 0.001$, [**]$p < 0.01$ vs. PWM group (one-way ANOVA followed by Tukey's test).

of splenocytes from PWM-stimulated mice that had been treated with AcE or Qt, when compared to the control group.

Effect of AcE and Qt on airway smooth muscle contractility

As can be seen in Figure 4(A and C), the cumulative addition of AcE (1, 3, 10, 30, 10^2, and 3×10^2 µg/ml) and Qt (10^{-8}, 10^{-7}, 10^{-6}, 10^{-5}, 10^{-4}, and 10^{-3} M), respectively, induced a transient relaxing effect, in a concentration-dependent manner, with the values of CE50 = 7.1 (1.8 – 27.4) mg/ml and CE50 = 8.9 (4.8 – 16.2) × 10^{-5} M for AcE and Qt, respectively. The data set may be seen in Figure 4 (B and D), which shows an ACE concentration-response curve. The percentage of the maximum relaxation (Emax) induced by AcE was Emax = 47.2 ± 7.0 (%), and induced by Qt was Emax = 84.0 ± 13.1 (%).

Additionally, in our in vitro model of hyper-reactivity using IL-13, murine tracheal rings that were incubated overnight with IL-13 (10 ng/ml) increased the constrictor responses to Cch but without changes in pharmacological

potency (Emax = 0.84 ± 0.08 (%); pD2 = 6.8 ± 0.1091) when compared with non-treated rings Emax = 0.55 ± 0.04 (%); pD2 = 6.4 ± 0.1887 (Figure 4E). Moreover, a reduction in intensity of smooth muscle contraction in the absence or presence of IL-13 with different concentrations of AcE (CE50 = 0.075 (0.011-0.5) Emax = 25.14 ± 5.52 (%)) or Qt (pD2 = 4.6 ± 0.07 Emax = 104.42 ± 2.94 (%) was observed (Figure 4F and G). However, the efficacy and potency of the tested drugs in hyper-reactive tracheal rings (sensitized with IL-13) were not altered when the drugs were tested in normal rings, not sensitized with IL-13.

Effect of AcE or Qt on cell influx in BAL fluid and on EPO levels in lungs

We examined changes in total cell numbers in the BAL fluid to determine the effects of AcE or Qt on experimental respiratory allergy. The BAL cellularity was estimated by counting the cells recruited to the BAL fluid 48 h after the last challenge. In relation to the control group, Bt-sensitized mice displayed a significant increase in total cell numbers (p < 0.01). However, in Bt-sensitized mice, the

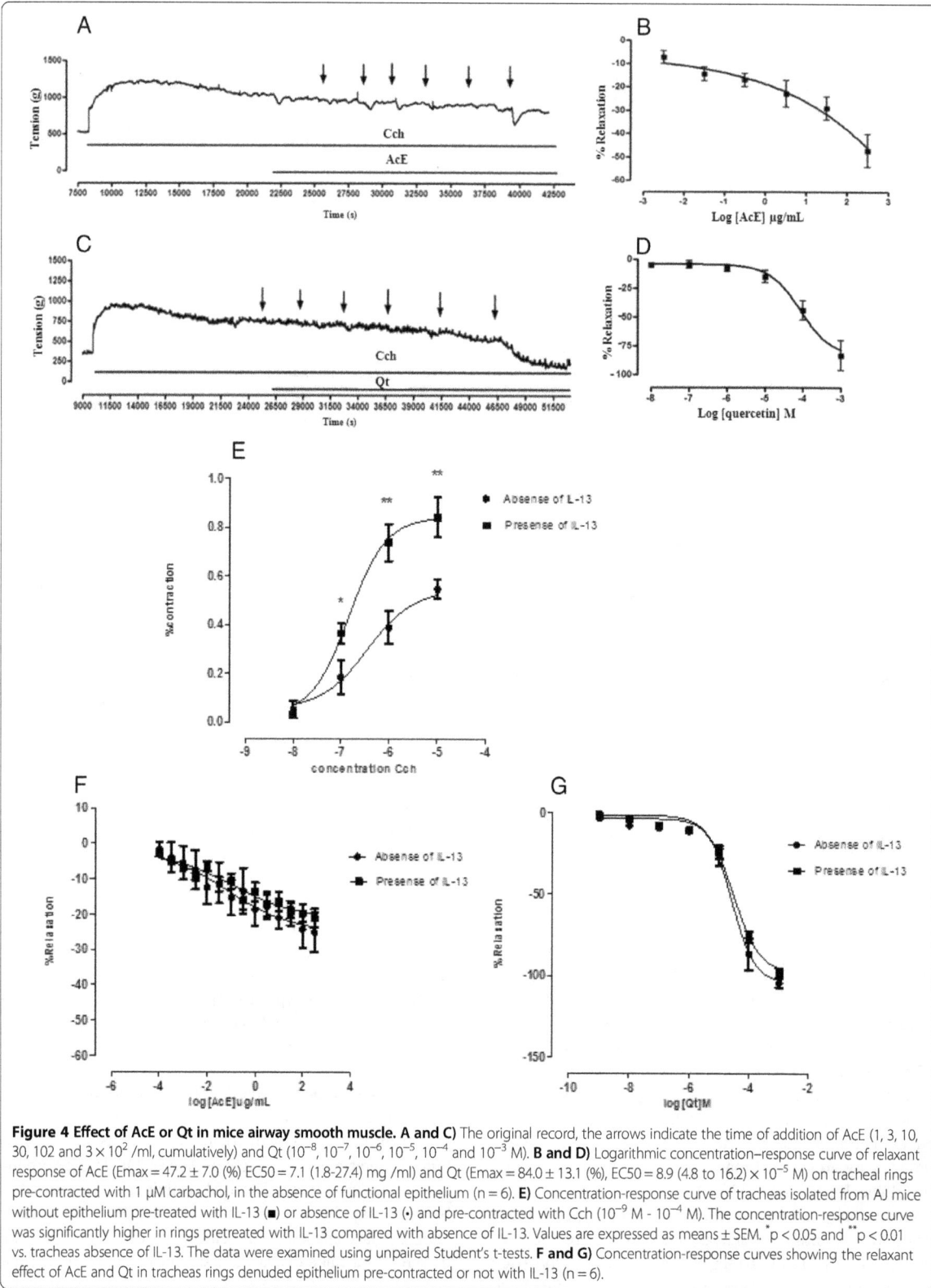

Figure 4 Effect of AcE or Qt in mice airway smooth muscle. A and C) The original record, the arrows indicate the time of addition of AcE (1, 3, 10, 30, 102 and 3×10^2 /ml, cumulatively) and Qt (10^{-8}, 10^{-7}, 10^{-6}, 10^{-5}, 10^{-4} and 10^{-3} M). **B and D)** Logarithmic concentration–response curve of relaxant response of AcE (Emax = 47.2 ± 7.0 (%) EC50 = 7.1 (1.8-27.4) mg /ml) and Qt (Emax = 84.0 ± 13.1 (%), EC50 = 8.9 (4.8 to 16.2) × 10^{-5} M) on tracheal rings pre-contracted with 1 µM carbachol, in the absence of functional epithelium (n = 6). **E)** Concentration-response curve of tracheas isolated from AJ mice without epithelium pre-treated with IL-13 (■) or absence of IL-13 (•) and pre-contracted with Cch (10^{-9} M - 10^{-4} M). The concentration-response curve was significantly higher in rings pretreated with IL-13 compared with absence of IL-13. Values are expressed as means ± SEM. *p < 0.05 and **p < 0.01 vs. tracheas absence of IL-13. The data were examined using unpaired Student's t-tests. **F and G)** Concentration-response curves showing the relaxant effect of AcE and Qt in tracheas rings denuded epithelium pre-contracted or not with IL-13 (n = 6).

treatment with AcE_{100} ($p < 0.05$), AcE_{1000} ($p < 0.01$) or Qt_{30} ($p < 0.05$) decreased the total number of cells in relation to untreated Bt-sensitized mice (Figure 5A). Additionally, the lung tissue was collected 48 hours after the final Bt challenge and EPO activity were measured. The EPO levels from lung tissue of Bt-sensitized mice were increased in relation to control group ($p < 0.001$). The mice from Bt-sensitized group and treated with AcE_{100} ($p < 0.001$) or AcE_{1000} ($p < 0.001$) had significantly lower EPO levels after respiratory allergy induction. No effect in EPO levels was observed in mice treated with Qt_{30} (Figure 5B).

Effect of treatment with AcE or Qt on inflammatory cell infiltration and amount of mucus in lungs

Because AcE or Qt inhibits inflammatory cell recruitment into the lung tissue and EPO levels in lungs, we examined the histology of lung tissue. In Bt-induced asthmatic lung tissue, we observed a marked infiltration of inflammatory cells into the perivascular and the peribronchiolar regions (Figure 6A-E), and airway mucus hypersecretion (Figure 6F-J) compared with the normal tissue. Cell infiltration and mucus hypersecretion in lungs of Bt-sensitized were attenuated by treatment with AcE when compared with the level seen in Bt-sensitized mice, as shown in Figure 6.

Effect of treatment with AcE or Qt on cytokine levels in BAL fluid

To determine whether AcE or Qt influenced the generation of a Th2-type immune response, cytokine concentrations in BAL fluid (IL-4, IL-5 and IL-13) were measured by ELISA 24 hours after the last challenge. As shown in Figure 7, Bt-sensitized animals had significantly higher IL-4 ($p < 0.01$), IL-5 ($p < 0.01$) and IL-13 ($p < 0.05$) levels in the BAL fluid than control mice. In Bt-sensitized mice the treatment with AcE or Qt significantly decreased IL-4 and IL-5 levels ($p < 0.05$) when compared with the levels seen in the

Bt-sensitized group. The oral treatment with AcE did not affect the levels of IL-13 in the BAL of Bt-sensitized mice.

Effect of treatment with AcE or Qt on serum levels of Bt-specific IgE antibodies

The cross-linking of allergen-specific IgE on the surface of mast cells upon allergen challenge is relevant to the initiation of the early asthmatic reaction. The serum levels of Bt-specific IgE were measured 24 hours after the last challenge. We observed that sensitization and challenge with Bt resulted in increased serum levels of Bt-specific IgE when compared with non-sensitized animals ($p < 0.001$). The treatment of sensitized mice with AcE or Qt did not reduce significantly Bt-specific IgE (Figure 8).

Discussion

The chronic inflammatory response to allergens on allergic asthma is characterized by eosinophilia, airway hyperresponsiveness (AHR) and increased mucus production. The actions of inflammatory cells in airways are tightly regulated by a network of Th2 cytokines, such as IL (interleukin)-4, IL-5, and IL-13 [34]. The present study was conducted using a murine model of allergic airway disease induced by *Blomia tropicalis* mite that was previously characterized by our research group [29]. Previous studies show that once Bt sensitization induced cells infiltration to the lungs, increased EPO activity and high amounts of Bt-specific IgE were obsrved. All these were associated to a Th2-type cytokine profile (with the production of IL-5, IL-13 and IL-4), which is important for the development and maintenance of the Th2 response characteristic of asthma [29,15]. The resolution of inflammation is fundamental to the return of normal physiological parameters. In this study we observed that *Allium cepa* L. and quercetin were associated to anti-inflammatory and bronchodilator activities in an airway inflammation murine model of asthma. As previously described [29], the total BAL cell numbers were increased in Bt-sensitized mice.

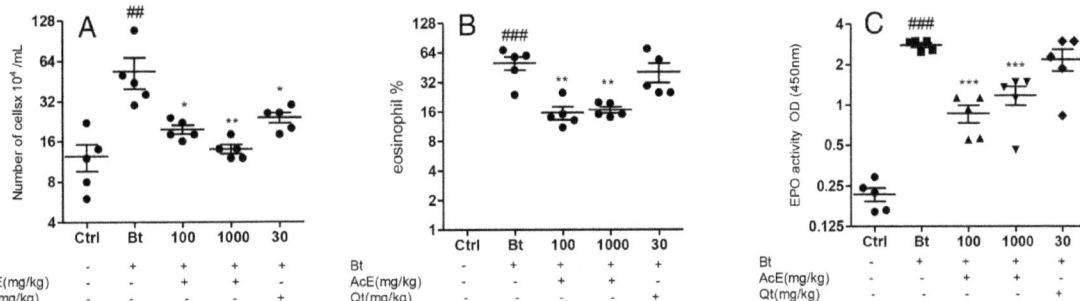

Figure 5 Effect of AcE or Qt on the levels of total cells in the BAL and on EPO in lungs. Effect of the treatment with AcE or Qt on the level of **A)** total cells counting **B)** eosinophilia in the BAL and **C)** eosinophil peroxidase (EPO) activity in lung tissue. Control (Ctrl); Bt-sensitized animals (Bt); and Bt-sensitized, AcE (100 or 1000 mg/kg) or Qt (30 mg/kg) treated mice. Values represent mean ± SEM (n = 5, per group). $^{##}p < 0.01$; $^{###}p < 0.001$ vs. control; $^{*}p < 0.05$; $^{**}p < 0.01$; $^{***}p < 0.001$ vs. Bt group (one-way ANOVA followed by Tukey's test).

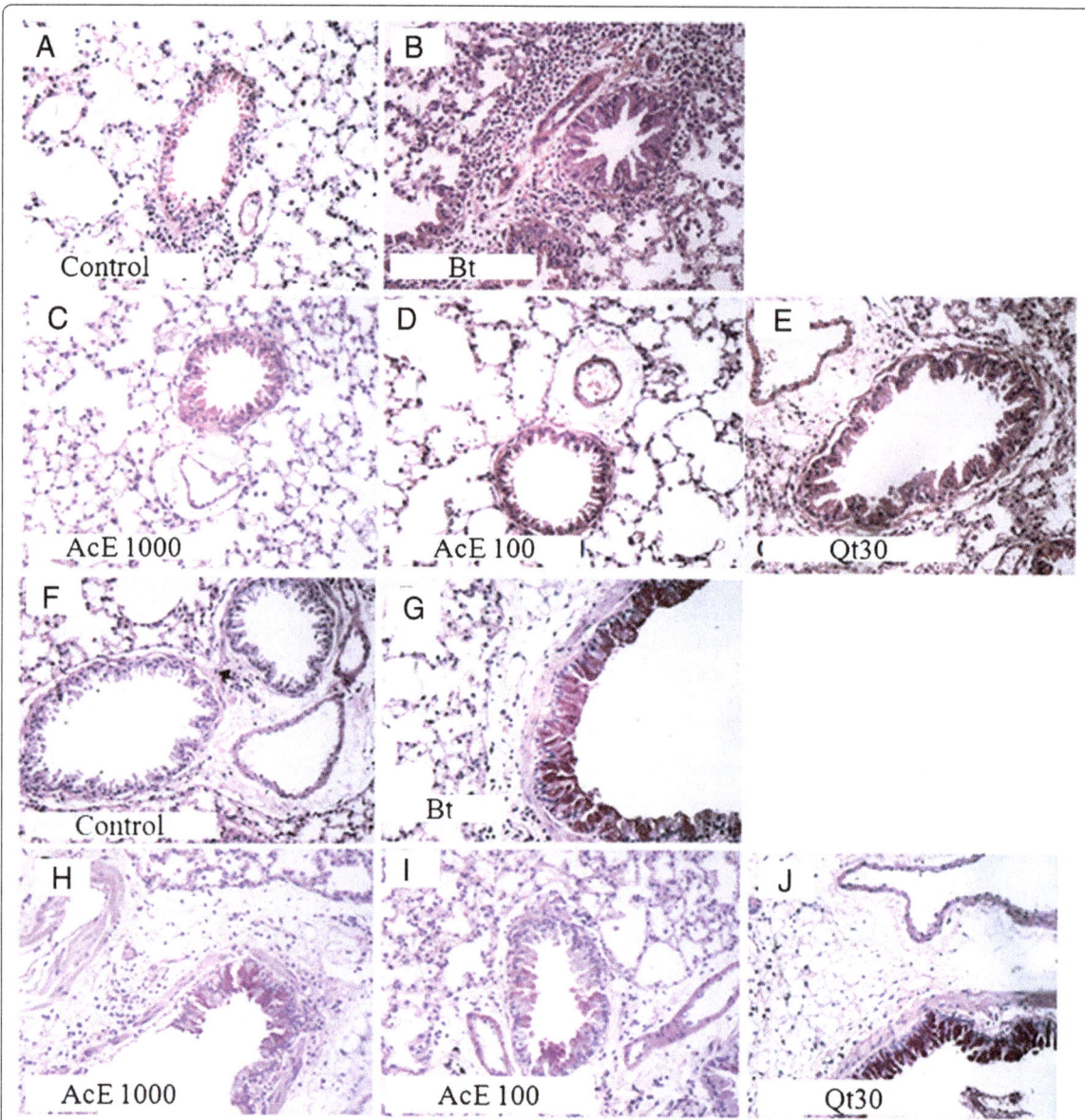

Figure 6 Effect of the treatment with AcE or Qt on celular infiltration and mucus production in lung tissues. Sections were stained with hematoxylin-eosin (magnification × 400) **(A-E)** and sections were stained with periodic acid-Schiff (magnification × 400) **(F-J)**. **(A and F)** Lung section from a control, saline-treated mice; **(B and G)** Lung section from a Bt-sensitized, saline-treated mice; **(C and H)** Lung section from a Bt-sensitized, AcE 100 mg/kg treated mice; **(D and I)** Lung section from a Bt-sensitized, AcE 1000 mg/kg treated mice; **(E and J)** Lung section from a Bt-sensitized, Qt 30 mg/kg treated mice.

Additionally, there was a statistically significant decrease in total cell numbers in the groups of Bt-sensitized animals treated with AcE_{10}, AcE_{1000}, or Qt_{30}. Drugs that modulate the recruitment of eosinophils and their activation may be important in reducing lung inflammation in asthma [35,29,36]. AcE and Qt when administered to allergic mice induce a decrease in total cellularity in BAL, a parameter required to suppress eosinophil degranulation.

Despite the fact that Qt_{30} did not significantly modulate EPO in the lung, the Bt-sensitized mice treated with AcE_{100} or AcE_{1000} had significantly lower EPO levels than untreated Bt-sensitized control mice, suggesting that a substance other than Qt is mediating this effect in AcE.

Previous studies in humans have shown that the addition of anti-IL-5 monoclonal antibody on asthma therapy significantly accelerated apoptosis of eosinophils, thereby

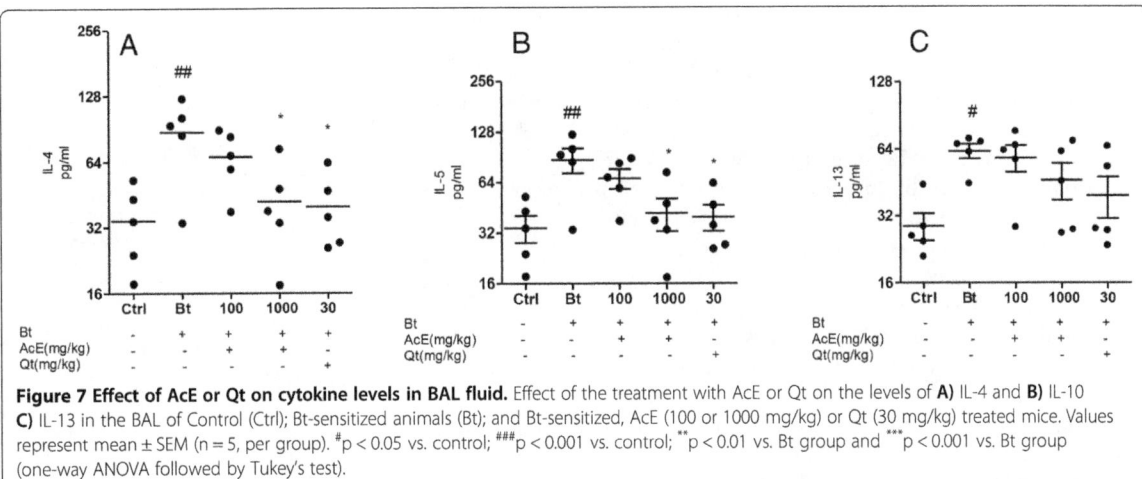

Figure 7 Effect of AcE or Qt on cytokine levels in BAL fluid. Effect of the treatment with AcE or Qt on the levels of **A)** IL-4 and **B)** IL-10 **C)** IL-13 in the BAL of Control (Ctrl); Bt-sensitized animals (Bt); and Bt-sensitized, AcE (100 or 1000 mg/kg) or Qt (30 mg/kg) treated mice. Values represent mean ± SEM (n = 5, per group). $^{\#}p < 0.05$ vs. control; $^{\#\#\#}p < 0.001$ vs. control; $^{**}p < 0.01$ vs. Bt group and $^{***}p < 0.001$ vs. Bt group (one-way ANOVA followed by Tukey's test).

decreasing pulmonary eosinophilia [37]. In this study, we could observe a significant reduction of IL-5, accompanied by a significant decrease in eosinophil peroxidase in the lungs of sensitized mice treated with Bt and AcE.

AcE and Qt had a statistically significant inhibitory effect on IL-4 and IL-5 levels in the BAL fluid of mice treated with AcE$_{100}$ and Qt$_{30}$. Despite the modulation of IL-13 *in vitro*, a similar effect could not be observed *in vivo*. AcE and Qt suppressed the secretion of IL-4, IL-5 and IL-13 by spleen cells stimulated with PWM. This fact reinforces the importance of *in vivo* studies to elucidate the mechanisms involved in drug activities.

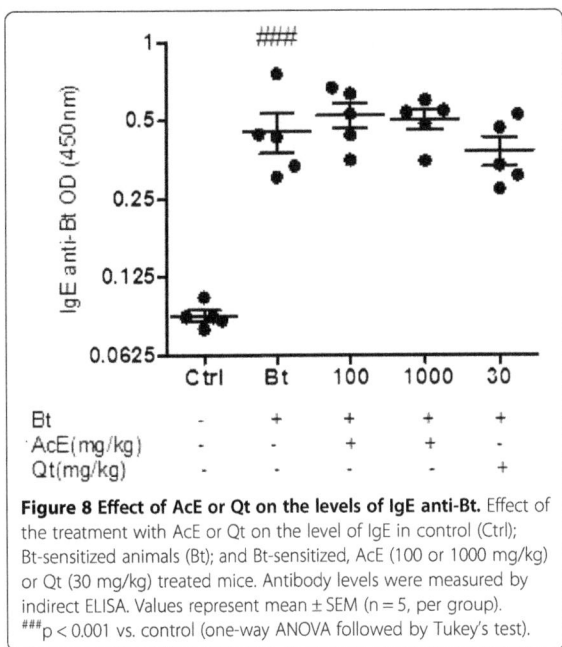

Figure 8 Effect of AcE or Qt on the levels of IgE anti-Bt. Effect of the treatment with AcE or Qt on the level of IgE in control (Ctrl); Bt-sensitized animals (Bt); and Bt-sensitized, AcE (100 or 1000 mg/kg) or Qt (30 mg/kg) treated mice. Antibody levels were measured by indirect ELISA. Values represent mean ± SEM (n = 5, per group). $^{\#\#\#}p < 0.001$ vs. control (one-way ANOVA followed by Tukey's test).

IL-4 along with IL-5 modulates eosinophil activation to stimulate B cells, IgE production, and mast cell degranulation [38] and their reduction, has been shown in this study, could be involved in the modulation of symptoms of allergic disease.

IL-13 also plays important role in allergic asthma [33,34], such as eosinophilic lung infiltration and mucus hypersecretion [39,40], which could be observed in our allergic mice. As there was no significant modulation of IL −13 by the tested drugs, we believe that in this work, as well as in other prior work, mucus is strongly connected to increased levels of IL-13 on asthmatic mice [40]. Nevertheless, AcE (AcE$_{100}$) was able to decrease the amount of mucus in the lungs of treated and Bt-sensitized mice. This effect was not observed with Qt$_{30}$.

Regarding IgE levels, no reduction on antibody titers were observed. These results may be related to the lack of a modulating effect on IL-13, which in addition to IL-4, is an important regulator of IgE production. Another hypothesis to explain the absence of effect on IgE levels is related to the short duration of our acute model, which may not be suitable for evaluating humoral responses, considering the necessary time for the variation in certain cytokine levels to reflect on serum antibody concentrations.

The interaction between the allergen and IgE present on mast cells plays a critical role in allergic inflammation. IgE cross-linking on mast cells leads to the release of histamine, prostaglandin (PG) D2 and leukotrienes, which results in smooth muscle contraction, mucous secretion and vasodilatation [41,42]. In previous studies [25,27,28], the therapeutic potential of flavonoids in isolated trachea was investigated. In this study it was observed that both AcE and Qt exerted a relaxing activity on the smooth muscle of isolated murine trachea precontracted with Cch. Additionally, our study supports the findings that interleukin-13 has been implicated as a key cytokine in smooth muscle hyperreactivity on asthma, since we demonstrated an increased contractility in response to Cch in airway smooth muscle induced by IL-13 [33]. Significant changes in Emax were observed, indicating that IL-13 seemed to increase smooth muscle contractility and cause hyperreactivity at the level of contractions. However the bronchodilatory potential of AcE or Qt is not selective for IL-13-induced hyperactivity pathway, as there was no difference between their effect on hyperreactive smooth muscle (IL-13- sensitized) and their effect on normal smooth muscle.

This study corroborates other previous studies on the anti-inflammatory and antiallergic properties of *Allium cepa* L. and quercetin [16-19,25], which might be linked to the ability of AcE an quercetin in down-modulate inflammatory processes through different signaling pathways such as NF-κB [43-45]. On the other hand, some authors discuss allergic reaction to onion. In such previous studies regarding onion hypersensitivity, authors reported patients producing IgE as well as cell-mediated mechanisms against plant lipid transfer proteins (LTPs) [46]. These are a group of highly-conserved proteins found in higher plant tissues [47]. The hypersensitivity to onion has been described as a cause of asthma induced by handling of onions. However, few publications in the literature report allergic reactions due to onion ingestion despite its wide use [48]. No toxic effect was found in animals exposed to AcE in the present study (data not shown).

AcE displayed a greater efficacy when compared to Qt, as it was able to regulate a greater amount of the parameters evaluated. This research corroborates with previous studies of natural products, which state that better biological responses can be achieved by the additive or synergistic effects of different compounds from an extract [49]. However, further studies are required in order to elucidate the cellular and molecular mechanisms by which AcE performs its action and to determine what substances are present in AcE in addition to quercetin, that contribute to the observed biological responses.

Conclusions

The results obtained in this work provide the first evidence that *Allium cepa* L. may have an anti-allergic effect more intense than Qt, and may be a future target for new molecules to treat allergic asthma. Our work may also validate and explain the long-held traditional use of this species by folk Brazilian medicine to treat asthma. This work also opens new perspectives in the context of elucidating the cellular and molecular mechanisms involved in the mechanism of action of *Allium cepa* L. as a way to enable clinical trials to evaluate its efficacy in humans.

Competing interests
The authors declare that they have no competing interests.

Authors' contributions
TTO- Collaboration in vitro and vivo experiments, statistical analysis, interpretation of data, draft of the manuscript and revising. KMC- Collaboration in *in vitro* and *in vivo* experiments, statistical analysis, interpretation of data, draft of the manuscript. ANCL- Collaboration in *in vivo* experiments and revising the manuscript. TCBC- Collaboration in *in vitro* experiments and revising the manuscript. ESV- study design and AcE supervised the extract production. ICARM and EAF- standardization of the extract in terms of quercetin concentration by high performance liquid chromatography (HPLC). EJO- Study design, standardization of the extract in terms of quercetin concentration by high performance liquid chromatography (HPLC), draft of the manuscript and final review. DFSAV-Collaboration in *in vitro* experiments, draft of the manuscript and revising the manuscript. LPC- study design, draft of the manuscript and revising the manuscript. NMAN- study design, draft the manuscript and revising the manuscript. CAF- study design, interpretation of data, draft the manuscript and revising the manuscript. All authors read and approved the final manuscript.

Acknowledgments
The authors want to thank the Brazilian agencies FAPESB, CNPq and CAPES for financial support.

Author details
[1]Instituto de Ciências da Saúde, Universidade Federal da Bahia, Salvador, Bahia, Brazil. [2]Faculdade de Farmácia, Universidade Federal da Bahia, Salvador, Bahia, Brazil. [3]Centro de Biotecnologia, Universidade Federal da Paraíba, João Pessoa, Paraíba, Brazil. [4]Centro de Pesquisas Gonçalo Moniz, Fundação Oswaldo Cruz, Salvador, Bahia, Brazil.

References
1. Hogg JC. Pathology of asthma. J Allergy Clin Immunol. 1993;92:1–5.
2. Holgate S, Smith N, Massanari M, Jimenez P. Effects of omalizumab on markers of inflammation in patients with allergic asthma. Allergy. 2009;64(12):1728–36.
3. Lougheed MD, Olajos-Clow JG. Asthma care pathways in the emergency department. Curr Opin Allergy Clin Immunol. 2010;10(3):181–7.
4. Deckers J, Branco Madeira F, Hammad H. Innate immune cells in asthma. Trends Immunol. 2013;34(11):540–7.
5. Illi S, Depner M, Genuneit J, Horak E, Loss G, Strunz-Lehner C, et al. Protection from childhood asthma and allergy in Alpine farm environments-the GABRIEL Advanced Studies. J Allergy Clin Immunol. 2012;129:1470–7.
6. Barnes PJ. Theophylline: new perspectives for an old drug. Am J Respir Crit Care Med. 2003;167(6):813–8.
7. Nauta AJ, Engels F, Knippels LM, Garssen J, Nijkamp FP, Redegeld FA. Mechanisms of allergy and asthma. Eur J Pharmacol. 2008;585(2–3):354–60.
8. Lee SI. Prevalence of childhood asthma in Korea: international study of asthma and allergies in childhood. Allergy Asthma Immunol Res. 2010;2(2):61–4.
9. Zar HJ, Levin ME. Challenges in treating pediatric asthma in developing countries. Paediatr Drugs. 2012;14:353–9.
10. Kew KM, Karner C, Mindus SM, Ferrara G. Combination formoterol and budesonide as maintenance and reliever therapy versus combination inhaler maintenance for chronic asthma in adults and children. Cochrane Database Syst Rev. 2013;12:CD009019.
11. Hashimoto S, Bel EH. Current treatment of severe asthma. Clin Exp Allergy. 2012;42(5):693–705.
12. Busse W. Asthma diagnosis and treatment: filling in the information gaps. J Allergy Clin Immunol. 2011;128:740–50.
13. Martinez FD, Vercelli D. Asthma. Lancet. 2013;382(9901):1360–72.
14. Mullane K. The increasing challenge of discovering asthma drugs. Biochem Pharmacol. 2011;82(6):586–99.
15. Costa RS, Brasil TC, Santos CJ, Santos DB, Barreto ML, Alcântara-Neves NM, et al. Natural products used for asthma treatment in children living in Salvador-BA, Brazil. Rev Bras Farmacogn. 2010;20:594–9.
16. Dorsch W, Wagner H, Bayer T, Fessler B, Hein G, Ring J, et al. Anti-asthmatic effects of onions. Alk(en)ylsulfinothioic acid alk(en)yl-esters inhibit histamine release, leukotriene and thromboxane biosynthesis in vitro and counteract PAF and allergen-induced bronchial obstruction *in vivo*. Biochem Pharmacol. 1988;1;37(23):4479–86.

17. Kaiser P, Youssouf MS, Tasduq SA, Singh S, Sharma SC, Singh GD, et al. Anti-allergic effects of herbal product from *Allium cepa* (bulb). J Med Food. 2009;12(2):374–82.

18. Rogerio AP, Kanashiro A, Fontanari C, da Silva EV, Lucisano-Valim YM, Soares EG, et al. Anti-inflammatory activity of quercetin and isoquercitrin in experimental murine allergic asthma. Inflamm Res. 2007;56(10):402–8.

19. Park HJ, Lee CM, Jung ID, Lee JS, Jeong YI, Chang JH, et al. Quercetin regulates Th1/Th2 balance in a murine model of asthma. Int Immunopharmacol. 2009;9(3):261–7.

20. Elberry AA, Mufti S, Al-Maghrabi J, Abdel Sattar E, Ghareib SA, Mosli HA, et al. Immunomodulatory effect of red onion (Allium cepa Linn) scale extract on experimentally induced atypical prostatic hyperplasia in Wistar rats. Mediators Inflamm. 2014;2014:640746.

21. Guo C, Hou GQ, Li XD, Xia X, Liu DX, Huang DY, et al. Quercetin triggers apoptosis of lipopolysaccharide (LPS)- induced osteoclast and inhibits bone resorption in RAW 264.7 cells. Cell Physiol Biochem. 2012;30(1):123–36.

22. Kubec R, Cody RB, Dane AJ, Musah RA, Schraml J, Vattekkatte A, et al. Applications of direct analysis in real time-mass spectrometry (DART-MS) in Allium chemistry. (Z)-butanethial S-oxide and 1-butenyl thiosulfinates and their S-(E)-1-butenylcysteine S-oxide precursor from Allium siculum. J Agric Food Chem. 2010;58(2):121–8.

23. Løkke MM, Edelenbos M, Larsen E, Feilberg A. Investigation of volatiles emitted from freshly cut onions (Allium cepa L.) by real time proton-transfer reaction-mass spectrometry (PTR-MS). Sensors (Basel). 2012;12(12):16060–76.

24. Colina-Coca C, González-Peña D, Vega E, de Ancos B, Sánchez-Moreno C. Novel approach for the determination of volatile compounds in processed onion by headspace gas chromatography–mass spectrometry (HS GC-MS). Talanta. 2013;103:137–44.

25. Joskova M, Franova S, Sadlonova V. Acute bronchodilator effect of quercetin in experimental allergic asthma. Bratisl Lek Listy. 2011;112(1):9–12.

26. Fernández-Caldas E, Puerta L, Caraballo L. Mites and allergy. Chem Immunol Allergy. 2014;100:234–42.

27. Capasso R, Aviello G, Romano B, Atorino G, Pagano E, Borrelli F. Inhibitory effect of quercetin on rat trachea contractility in vitro. J Pharm Pharmacol. 2009;61(1):115–9.

28. Fernandez J, Reyes R, Ponce H, Oropeza M, Vancalsteren MR, Jankowski C, et al. Isoquercitrin from Argemone platyceras inhibits carbachol and leukotriene D4-induced contraction in guinea-pig airways. Eur J Pharmacol. 2005;522(1–3):108–15.

29. Baqueiro T, Russo M, Silva VM, Meirelles T, Oliveira PR, Gomes E, et al. Respiratory allergy to Blomia tropicalis: immune response in four syngeneic mouse strains and assessment of a low allergen-dose, short-term experimental model. Respir Res. 2010;1:11:51.

30. Ly TN, Hazama C, Shimoyamada M, Ando H, Kato K, Yamauchi R. Antioxidative compounds from the outer scales of onion. J Agric Food Chem. 2005;53(21):8183–9.

31. Lee J, Mitchell AE. Quercetin and isorhamnetin glycosides in onion (*Allium cepa* L.): varietal comparison, physical distribution, coproduct evaluation, and long-term storage stability. J Agric Food Chem. 2011;59(3):857–63.

32. Bezerra-Santos CR, Balestiari FM, Rossi-Bergmann B, Peçanha LM, Piuvezam MR. Cissampelos sympodialis Eichl. (Menispermaceae): oral treatment decreases IgE levels and induces a Th1-skewed cytokine production in ovalbumin-sensitized mice. J Ethnopharmaco. 2004;95(2–3):191–7.

33. Farghaly HS, Blagbrough IS, Medina-Tato DA, Watson ML. Interleukin13 increases contractility of murine tracheal smooth muscle by a phosphoinositide 3-kinase p110 delta-dependent mechanism. Mol Pharmacol. 2008;73(5):1530–7.

34. Walter DM, McIntire JJ, Berry G, McKenzie AN, Donaldson DD, DeKruyff RH, et al. Critical role for IL-13 in the development of allergen-induced airway hyperreactivity. J Immunol. 2001;167(8):4668–75.

35. Baatjes AJ, Sehmi R, Saito H, Cyr MM, Dorman SC, Inman MD, et al. Anti-allergic therapies: effects on eosinophil progenitors. Pharmacol Ther. 2002;95(1):63–72.

36. Cerqueira-Lima AT, Alcântara-Neves NM, de-Carvalho LC, Costa RS, Barbosa-Filho JM, Piuvezam M, et al. Effects of Cissampelos sympodialis Eichl. and its alkaloid, warifteine, in an experimental model of respiratory allergy to Blomia tropicalis. Curr Drug Targets. 2010;11(11):1458–67.

37. Simon HU, Yousefi S, Schranz C, Schapowal A, Bachert C, Blaser K. Direct demonstration of delayed eosinophil apoptosis as a mechanism causing tissue eosinophilia. J Immunol. 1997;158(8):3902–8.

38. Galli SJ, Tsai M. IgE and mast cells in allergic disease. Nat Med. 2012;18(5):693–704.

39. Wynn TA. IL-13 effector functions. Annu Rev Immunol. 2013;21:425–56.

40. Kibe A, Inoue H, Fukuyama S, Machida K, Matsumoto K, Koto H, et al. Differential regulation by glucocorticoid of interleukin-13-induced eosinophilia, hyperresponsiveness, and goblet cell hyperplasia in mouse airways. Am J Respir Crit Care Med. 2003;167(1):50–6.

41. Bateman ED, Hurd SS, Barnes PJ, Bousquet J, Drazen JM, FitzGerald M, et al. Global strategy for asthma management and prevention: GINA executive summary. Eur Respir J. 2008;31(1):143–78.

42. Hamid Q, Tulic M. Immunobiology of asthma. Annu Rev Physiol. 2009;71:489–507.

43. Yamaguchi M, Weitzmann MN. Quercetin, a potent suppressor of NF-κB and Smad activation in osteoblasts. Int J Mol Med. 2011;28(4):521–5.

44. Tang CH, Huang TH, Chang CS, Fu WM, Yang RS. Water solution of onion crude powder inhibits RANKL-induced osteoclastogenesis through ERK, p38 and NF-kappab pathways. Osteoporos Int. 2009;20(1):93–103.

45. Wattel A, Kamel S, Prouillet C, Petit JP, Lorget F, Offord E, et al. Flavonoid quercetin decreases osteoclastic differentiation induced by RANKL via a mechanism involving NF kappa B and AP-1. J Cell Biochem. 2004;92(2):285–95.

46. Valdivieso R, Subiza J, Varela-Losada S, Subiza JL, Narganes MJ, Martinez-Cocera C, et al. Bronchial asthma, rhinoconjunctivitis, and contact dermatitis caused by onion. J Allergy Clin Immunol. 1994;94(5):928–30.

47. Asero R, Mistrello G, Roncarolo D, Amato S. Relationship between peach lipid transfer protein specific IgE levels and hypersensitivity to non-Roseaceae vegetable foods in patients allergic to lipid transfer protein. Ann Allergy Asthma Immunol. 2004;92(2):268–72.

48. Enrique E, Malek T, De Mateo JA, Castelló J, Lombardero M, Barber D, et al. Involvement of lipid transfer protein in onion allergy. Ann Allergy Asthma Immunol. 2007;98(2):202.

49. Jaki BU, Franzblau SG, Chadwick LR, Lankin DC, Zhang F, Wang Y, et al. Purity-activity relationships of natural products: the case of anti-TB active ursolic acid. J Nat Prod. 2008;71(10):1742–8.

23

Preventive effects of *phenylethanol glycosides* from *Cistanche tubulosa* on bovine serum albumin-induced hepatic fibrosis in rats

Shu-Ping You[1], Jun Zhao[2,3], Long Ma[1], Mukaram Tudimat[1], Shi-Lei Zhang[1] and Tao Liu[1*]

Abstract

Background: *Cistanche tubulosa* is a traditional Chinese herbal medicine that is widely used for regulating immunity. Phenyl ethanol glycosides (CPhGs) from this plant are the primarily efficacious materials. This aim of this study was to evaluate the preventive and therapeutic effects of CPhGs on BSA-induced hepatic fibrosis in rats and related molecular mechanisms involving hepatic stellate cells. Biejiarangan (BJRG), another traditional Chinese herbal medicine, was used as a positive control.

Methods: In in vivo experiments, 75 SD rats were randomly divided into 6 groups: normal (distilled water-treated), model (BSA-treated), positive drug (BSA-treated + BJRG 600 mg/kg/day), and BSA-treated + CPhGs (125, 250, and 500 mg/kg/day) groups. The liver and spleen indices, serum levels of aspartate aminotransferase (AST), alanine aminotransferase (ALT), hexadecenoic acid (HA), laminin (LN), type III procollagen (PCIII), type IV collagen (IV-C), hydroxyproline (Hyp), and transforming growth factor β_1 (TGF-β_1) were measured in rat livers. Histopathological grades for liver fibrosis were assessed for each group using H&E and Masson's trichrome staining. The expression of TGF-β_1, collagen I (Col-I) and collagen III (Col-III) were determined by an immunohistochemical staining method. These effects were further evaluated in vitro by determining expression levels of NF-κB p65 and Col-I by quantitative real-time PCR analyses. Col-I protein expression was also examined by western blotting.

Results: All dose groups (125, 250, and 500 mg/kg/day) of CPhGs significantly reduced the liver and spleen index, decreased ALT, AST, HA, LN, PCIII, IV-C serum levels, TGF-β_1 content ($P < 0.01$, $P < 0.01$, and $P < 0.01$), and Hyp content. CPhGs also markedly alleviated the swelling of liver cells and effectively prevented hepatocyte necrosis and inflammatory cell infiltration. Immunohistochemical results showed that CPhGs significantly reduced the expression of TGF-β_1 ($P < 0.01$, $P < 0.01$, and $P < 0.01$), Col- I, and Col-III. The in vitro effects of CPhGs (100, 75, 50, and 25 ug/ml) on HSC-T6 showed that CPhGs significantly reduced mRNA expression of NF-κB p65 and Col-I, and CPhGs also downregulated Col-I protein expression.

Conclusions: CPhGs have a significant anti-hepatic fibrosis effect, and may be used as hepatoprotective agents for treatment of hepatic fibrosis.

Keywords: Hepatic fibrosis, Cistanche tubulosas, Phenylethanol glycoside, Chemokine BSA, Prevention and therapy

* Correspondence: xjmult@163.com
[1]Department of Toxicology, School of Public Health, Xinjiang Medical University, No. 393 Xinyi Road, Urumqi 830011Xinjiang Uyghur Autonomous Region, China
Full list of author information is available at the end of the article

Background

Hepatic fibrosis is a wound healing response to severe liver injury that occurs in the pathogenesis of chronic hepatitis induced by various factors. These factors are viral infection, alcohol abuse, cholestasis, and metabolic and autoimmune diseases [1–3]. Progressive accumulation of extracellular matrix (ECM) and decreased remodeling disrupt the normal architecture of the liver, resulting in hepatic fibrosis [4]. Hepatic fibrosis is critical in chronic liver disease, and often develops into irreversible cirrhosis and carcinogenesis. At present, there are no methods or effective drugs for the treatment of hepatic fibrosis. Therefore, it is urgent to find an anti-hepatic fibrosis drug that will attenuate the progression of liver injury to fibrosis and cancer.

Cistanche tubulosa W (of the family Orobanchaceae) is a parasitic plant that is widely grown in the southern region of Xinjiang in China [5]. People usually use it to invigorate the kidneys, nourish the blood, relax the bowel, and delay senescence. It is officially listed in the Chinese Pharmacopoeia [6]. *C. tubulosa* contains a variety of active components. These include phenyl ethanol glycosides (CPhGs), iridoids, and polysaccharides. As one of many active components in *C. tubulosa*, CPhGs have exhibited convincing antioxidant, anti-fatigue, neuroprotective, and anti-inflammory effects in both in vivo and in vitro studies [7]. In recent years, it has been reported that CPhGs have hepatoprotective effects. Potential mechanisms underlying these effects are scavenging of free radicals, protection of hepatic membranes, immunoregulation, inhibition of apoptosis, inhibition of the expression of HBsAg and HBeAg, and inhibition of HBV DNA replication and others [8–11]. However, few studies in the literature address the anti-hepatic fibrosis effect of GPhCs. Therefore, this study aimed to investigate the anti-hepatic fibrosis effect of GPhCs by using a model of bovine serum albumin (BSA) induced hepatic fibrosis in rats. Related molecular mechanisms were investigated in HSC-T6 cells.

Methods

Chemicals and reagents

A Hydroxyproline kit (Alkaline hydrolysis) (Lot: 20140616) was purchased from Nanjing Jiancheng Bio-engineering Institute (China). Rat TGF-β_1 sandwich ELISA kits (Lot: 238240615) was purchased from Lianke Biotech Co., Ltd. (China). Rabbit Anti-Collagen I antibody (Lot: 140619), Rabbit Anti-Collagen III antibody (Lot: 980788 W), and Rabbit Anti-TGF-β_1 antibody (Lot: 140619) were provided by Beijing Biosynthesis Biotechnology Co., LTD (China). Enclosed with normal sheep serum (working fluid) (Lot: WP141214), PV-6000 (Lot: WK141225), and DAB kit (Lot: K136621D) were purchased from Zhongshan Golden Bridge Bio-tech

Co., Ltd. (China). Detection of primary antibodies was performed by using 2. Antibody solution (Alk-Phos. Conjugated, Anti-rabbit) and 2. Antibody solution (Alk-Phos. Conjugated, Anti-mouse) (lot: 272387) purchased from Invitrogen company (USA).

Bovine serum albumin (BSA) (Lot: SLBG8239V) was purchased from Sigma (USA). Before use, BSA was prepared at 18 g/L in normal saline, the bacteria removed by filtration, and BSA stored at 4 °C. Freund's incomplete adjuvant containing 1 g of lipid from sheep hair (Lot: AF0220LA14, Shanghai yuanye Bio-Technology Co., Ltd. (China,) was mixed with 2 g liquid paraffin (Lot: 20130815, Tianjin Fuyu Fine Chemical Co., Ltd. (China,), sterilized in a steam autoclave, and stored at 4 °C . The positive drug BJRG was obtained as Biejiarangan tablets from Inner Mongolia Furui Medical Science Co., Ltd. (China). BJRG drug stocks were prepared by dissolving BJRG tablets in distilled water at a concentration of 600 mg/kg.

Plant materials

C. tubulosa (Orobanchaceae family) was purchased from the Minfeng region of Xinjiang of China. The material was authenticated by researcher Jun Zhao, Key Laboratory for Uighur Medicine, Institute of Materia Medica of Xinjiang. Voucher specimens were deposited in the Institute of Materia Medica of Xinjiang.

Preparation of CPhGs

Dried and sliced rhizomes of *C. tubulosa* (6.0 kg) were consecutively extracted under reflux three times with 70 % ethanol, and the solvent was removed to yield the ethanol extract. Ethanol extracts were purified by using AB-8 resin to obtain the phenyl ethanol glycosides (CPhGs). Stock solutions of CPhGs used for different dose groups in animal studies (500 mg/kg, 250 mg/kg, and 125 mg/kg, respectively) were dissolved in 0.5 % (5 g/L) carboxymethyl cellulose (sodium salt).

Quantification of CPhGs

The contents of two components (echinacoside and acteoside) in the CPhGs were determined by HPLC using a previously reported method (Zhang et al. 2004) [12]. HPLC was performed by using a Shimadzu LC-10A HPLC equipped with a UV detector. The HPLC column was a Phenomenex Gemini ODS column (250 × 4.6 mm, 5 μm). The isocratic mobile phase consisted of methanol-acetonitrile-1 % acetic acid (15:10:75, v/v/v). Elution was for 40 min and the flow rate was kept at 0.6 mL/min. Column temperature was kept constant at 30 °C. UV detection was at 334 nm.

Animals and HSC-T6 cell line

[Grade SPF] healthy adult male Sprague–Dawley (SD) rats (180–220 g) were purchased from Xinjiang Medical University Animal Center, License No.: SCXK (New) 2011–0004. Rats were fed specific-pathogen free (SPF) chow. All of the procedures related to the animal experiments were approved by the Animal Ethics Committee of First Affiliated Hospital of Xinjiang Medical University. Rats were housed in cages under controlled environmental conditions (25 °C and a 12 h light/dark cycle) and had free access to standard rat pellet food and tap water. Rats were acclimated before treatment.

An immortalized rat hepatic stellate cell line, HSC-T6, was obtained from Wuhan Procell Gene Bio-technology Co., LTD. (Wuhan, China). HSC-T6 cells were cultured in Dulbecco's Modified Eagle's Medium (High Glucose) (DMEM, Beijing, China) supplemented with 10 % fetal bovine serum (Gibco, South America), 100 IU/ml penicillin and 100 μg/ml streptomycin (Beijing, China) in a humidified incubator at 37 °C with 5 % CO_2.

BSA-induced liver injury and treatments

Seventy-five SD rats were randomly divided into six groups: Normal (distilled water-treated), model (BSA-treated), positive drug (BSA-treated + BJRG 600 mg/kg/day), and BSA-treated + CPhGs (125, 250, 500 mg/kg/day) groups. BSA-treated + CPhGs (125, 250, 500 mg/kg/day) groups had 13 rats in each group, and other group had 12 rats in each group. The BSA-induced liver injury model is divided into primary sensitization followed by immunological attack) [13]. Except for the normal group, the other groups were administered multiple subcutaneous injections with 0.5 ml (9 mg/ml) BSA Freund' incomplete adjuvant on day $_1$, day $_{15}$, day $_{22}$, day $_{29}$, and day $_{36}$ for primary sensitization. Seven days after the fifth injection, blood was obtained through the rat retinal vein plexus and tested for serum albumin antibodies. BSA antibody in rat serum was detected by a double agar diffusion method. The attack injection was performed by administering 0.4 ml of BSA in normal saline was through the caudal vein in BSA antibody-positive rats twice a week for ten times. The concentrations and times of injections were 5.00, 5.50, 6.00, 6.50, 7.00, 7.50, 8.50, 9.00, 9.50 and 10.00 g/L at day $_{46}$, day $_{50}$, day $_{53}$, day $_{57}$, day $_{60}$, day $_{64}$, day $_{67}$, day$_{71}$, day $_{74}$ and day $_{78}$, respectively. In the normal group, normal saline was used for immunological primary (sensitization) and secondary (attack) injections instead of BSA, and other conditions were the same as those in the model group.

The normal group was orally administered distilled water with dose 10 ml/kg/day. The model group was orally administered 10 ml/kg/day 0.5 % CMC-Na solution. The positive drug group was orally administered 600 mg/kg/day BJRG. The BSA-treated + CPhGs (125,

250, and 500 mg/kg/day) groups were orally administered 125, 250, and 500 mg/kg/day CPhGs, respectively. Daily dosing rats continued for two weeks after the last injection.

After the experimental period, rats were fasted for 12 h prior to 10 % chloral hydrate and then immediately euthanized.. Serum samples were collected from each rat and immediately used. Livers were harvested for two purposes: (1) preservation in liquid nitrogen for Hyp kits and (2) fixation in 10 % formaldehyde for histological and immunohistochemical examinations. The entire duration of the animal studies was 93 days.

Liver and spleen indices

The liver and spleen were dissected by laparotomy and washed with 4 °C normal saline. After absorbing excess water with filter paper, the liver and spleen were weighed to calculate the corresponding indices: Relative organ weight = organ mass (g)/individual body mass (g) × 100 % [14].

Analysis of markers of liver fibrosis

The protective effect of CPhGs against BSA-induced liver injury was evaluated by measuring ALT and AST (Mindray automatic biochemical analyzer,A086A0182). The development of liver fibrosis and effects of treatment were determined by examining HA, LN, PC III, and IV-C (Chemiluminescence analyzer,TaiGeKeXin, MP2808).

Hyp content and TGF-β_1 analysis

The level of Hyp in liver tissue was determined by a spectrophotometric method according to the kit's instructions. The level of Hyp was expressed as Hyp (μg)/protein (mg). Hyp (μg/mg) = (Measured $_{OD}$- blank $_{OD}$)/(standard $_{OD}$- blank $_{OD}$) × 5 (μg/ml) × 10/tissue wet weight (ml/mg). The hepatic concentration of TGF-β_1 was detected by using ELISA kits according to the manufacturer's instructions. The inhibitory effect of CPhGs on fibrosis was confirmed by the expression levels of TGF-β_1.

Histopathological examination

The liver tissue in the same part of the left lobe was resected and fixed in 10 % formaldehyde solution. Tissues were stained with conventional H&E and Masson's trichrome staining to observe histopathological changes under a light microscope. Expression of collagen type I, collagen type III, and TGF-β_1 in liver tissues was analyzed by immunohistochemical staining [15].

Semi-quantitative immunohistochemistry was performed according to reported methods [16, 17]. The following classifications were used for TGF-β_1 positive cells: "-" indicates almost no expression, 2^0 = l; "+" indicates positive cells individually gathered in the lesion area, 2^1 = 2; "++" indicates positive cells in small groups gathered around the lesion area, $2^2 = 4$; "+++" indicates dispersed positive cells expressed, as $2^3 = 8$. The results represent a hierarchical integration. The collagen type I and collagen type III chromogenic degree and scope were converted into CRI for statistical analysis (chromogenic degree × chromogenic range). The chromogenic degree is divided into weak "+", moderate "++" and strong "+++". The chromogenic range is divided into: "+", its chromogenic range < view 1/4; "++", its chromogenic range of vision/4-2/4; "+++", its chromogenic range of vision 2/4-3/4; "++++", its chromogenic range > 3/4. Blinded scoring was performed by two people where "+" is 1; "++" is 2, "+++" is 3, and "++++" is 4. Three microscope observational fields (magnification × 200) were randomly selected for each section, with the average level of the samples used as a semi quantitative level.

Cell experiments

HSC-T6 cells were plated in a 96-well plate. Initially, cells were cultured with DMEM containing 10 % FBS for 48 h. The medium was then replaced with DMEM without FBS to starve the cells for 12 h. The cells were then cultured with DMEM that contained 5.0 ng/mL TGF-β_1 (without FBS) for 24 h. Finally, different concentrations of CPhGs (100ug/ml, 50ug/ml, and 25ug/ml), acteoside (6 ug/ml, 3 ug/ml, and 1.5 ug/ml), and echinacoside (500ug/ml, 250ug/ml, and 125ug/ml) were carried out in the plate in qudruplicate wells and incubated for 48 h.

Real-time PCR analysis

The mRNA expression level of NF-κB, p65, and collagen I were determined by real-time PCR. To determine mRNA expressions in HSC-T6 cells, the cells (4×10^5 cells) were seeded in six-well plates with 3 mL DMEM with 10 % FBS and incubated overnight at 37 °C and 5 % CO_2, after which the cell culture media were changed to serum-free DMEM. Next, CPhGs (100 ug/ml, 50 ug/ml, and 25 ug/ml), acteoside (6 ug/ml, 3 ug/ml, and 1.5 ug/ml), and echinacoside (500 ug/ml, 250 ug/ml, and 125 ug/ml) were added to the wells. After 48 h of incubation with CPhGs or monomeric compositions, total RNA was extracted using TRIzol reagent (Invitrogen, USA) and agitated vigorously with chloroform for 15 s. After sitting at room temperature for 3 min, the lysate was centrifuged at $12,000 \times g$ for 15 min at 4 °C. RNA in the aqueous phase was precipitated with isopropanol, and the upper aqueous phase was transferred to a new microcentrifuge tube. RNA was precipitated by adding 0.75 % ethanol, after which the microcentrifuge tube and centrifuged at $12,000 \times g$ at 4 °C for no more than 5 min. The supernatant was removed and the RNA was dried at room temperature for 5–10 min. Specific sets of primers (Sangon, Shanghai, China) that were used for

amplification of rat β-actin [GenBank: NM_031144.3], Collagen I [GenBank: NM_ 053304.1], and NF-κB p65 [GenBank: NM_199267.2] genes were designed using Batch Primer 3. The forward (fw) and reverse (rv) primers were as follows: Collagen I (fw: GGA GAG AGC ATG ACC GAT GG, rv: GGG ACT TCT TGA GGT TGC CA), NF-κB p65 (fw: CAT ACG CTG ACC CTA GCC TG, rv: TTT CTT CAA TCC GGT GGC GA), β-actin (fw: TAA GGC CAA CCG TGA AAA GAT G, rv: AGA GGC ATA CAG GGA CAA CAC A). Results were normalized to the mRNA of the housekeeping gene β-actin as an internal control and are presented as relative mRNA levels.

Reactions were performed with 8 μL iQ SYBR Green Supermix, 1 μL 10 pM primer pair, 8.5 μL distilled water, and 2.5 μL cDNA. Each polymerase chain reaction was performed under the following conditions: 95 °C for 3 min, then 40 cycles of 10 s at 95 °C, 30 s at 55 °C, and 10 s at 55 °C – 95 °C for extension, followed by a single fluorescence measurement. The final results were described with the relative values ($2^{-\Delta\Delta Ct}$). Calculation and analysis were performed by the iQ5 Real Time PCR Detection System.

Western blot analysis

Collagen I (Abcam, Cambridge, UK, Art No: ab34710) protein expression levels were determined by Western blotting [with β-actin (Lot: 60008-1-lg; Proteintech, China) as a housekeeping control. Whole cell extracts were prepared using Radioimmunoprecipitation assay (RIPA) (Thermo Scientific, USA) buffer with 1 % Halt protease inhibitor cocktail (Thermo Scientific, USA) and 1 % Halt phosphatase inhibitor cocktails (Thermo Scientific, USA). The protein concentration was measured and quantified by the Bradford method [18]. Protein (10–50 ug) was separated on a 10 % SDS-PAGE gel and transferred to PVDF membranes (Millipore, USA). Membranes were blocked for 1 h at room temperature with 5 % BSA, and the primary antibodies (Anti-Collagen I antibody, 1:200 dilution or mouse mAb of β-actin, 1:5000 dilution) were incubated at 4 °C overnight. The corresponding Alk-Phos. conjugated secondary antibodies were incubated at room temperature. Finally, the membranes were washed three times with 1 × Tris–HCl saline with 0.1 % Tween 20, and signals were scanned and visualized by GEL DOC XR Imaging System (Bio-Rad). Densitometric analysis was performed on the proteins of interest and normalized to β-actin by GEL DOC Image Studio software (Bio-Rad). β-actin was used as the internal control.

Statistical analysis

The Shapiro-Wilk normality test and Levene's variance homogeneity test were applied to verify normality and homogeneity of variance. Analysis of variance (ANOVA) followed by Tukey's post hoc test was used to identify statistical differences in homogeneous, normally distributed data. The Kruskal-Wallis non-parametric test was used to analyze data not normally distributed or homogeneous. Results were expressed as mean ± SD. Significance was set at $P < 0.05$. All data were analyzed by SPSS 16.0 software (Xinjiang Medical University).

Results

Quantitative determination of CPhGs

CPhGs in *C. tubulosa* contains two phenylethyl alcohol glycosides, echinacoside and acteoside, and their contents in the CPhGs were determined by HPLC analysis (Fig. 1) to be 42.71 ± 0.42 % and 14.27 ± 0.18 %, respectively.

Liver and spleen indices

As Table 1 was shown, the liver and spleen indices of the model group were elevated significantly [$P < 0.01$, $P < 0.05$]. The liver and spleen indices of the positive drug BJRG and CPhGs at different dose groups were significantly reduced compared with the model group [$P_{Liver} = 0.004$, $P_{Liver} = 0.003$, $P_{Liver} = 0.004$, $P_{Liver} = 0.005$; $P_{Spleen} = 0.017$, $P_{Spleen} = 0.027$, $P_{Spleen} = 0.024$, $P_{Spleen} = 0.070$, respectively]. The liver and spleen indices were lower than those of the model group.

Effects of CPhGs on ALT, AST activities and liver fibrosis markers

In the present study, the serum levels of the hepatic enzymes AST and ALT were significantly increased in the model group, reflecting hepatocellular damage in BSA-induced liver fibrosis rats. However, the experiments

Table 1 Effects of CPhGs on the liver and spleen indices of hepatic fibrosis rats

Group	Dose (mg/kg/day)	n	Liver index (%)	Spleen index (%)
Normal	—	12	$2.21 \pm 0.077^{**}$	$0.15 \pm 0.010^{**}$
Model	—	11	2.65 ± 0.245	0.19 ± 0.025
BJRG	600	10	$2.21 \pm 0.253^{**}$	$0.17 \pm 0.013^{*}$
CPhGs	500	12	$2.32 \pm 0.153^{**}$	$0.16 \pm 0.025^{*}$
	250	9	$2.40 \pm 0.150^{**}$	$0.16 \pm 0.017^{*}$
	125	10	$2.39 \pm 0.103^{**}$	0.16 ± 0.033

Values are expressed as mean ± SD, n = Survival number of animals
$^{*}P < 0.05$, Compared with the model group; $^{**}P < 0.01$, Compared with the model group

showed that treatment with BJRG (600 mg/kg) and CPhGs (125, 250, and 500 mg/kg) significantly reduced AST [$P_{AST} < 0.001$, $P_{AST} < 0.001$, $P_{AST} < 0.001$, $P_{AST} < 0.001$, respectively] and ALT [$P_{ALT} = 0.117$, $P_{ALT} = 0.139$, $P_{ALT} = 0.189$, $P_{ALT} = 0.255$, respectively] levels in hepatic fibrosis rats. (Table 2).

The levels of HA, LN, PC and IV-C in model rats were significantly increased [$P_{HA} < 0.001$, $P_{LN} < 0.001$, $P_{PCIII} = 0.002$, $P_{IV-C} < 0.001$, respectively]. Compared with the model group, the levels of HA [$P_{HA} = 0.009$, $P_{HA} = 0.007$, $P_{HA} = 0.009$, $P_{HA} = 0.023$, respectively], LN [$P_{LN} = 0.011$, $P_{LN} = 0.004$, $P_{LN} = 0.026$, $P_{LN} = 0.069$, respectively], PC III [$P_{PCIII} = 0.006$, $P_{PCIII} = 0.067$, $P_{PCIII} = 0.136$, $P_{PCIII} = 0.296$, respectively], and IV-C [$P_{IV-C} < 0.001$, $P_{IV-C} < 0.001$, $P_{IV-C} < 0.001$, $P_{IV-C} < 0.001$, respectively] in rats were markedly decreased by BJRG (600 mg/kg) and CPhGs at different dose groups (125, 250, and 500 mg/kg) (Table 3).

Hyp content and TGF-β_1

Collagen content was also detected by measuring Hyp levels in liver tissue. As shown in Table 4, the mean Hyp

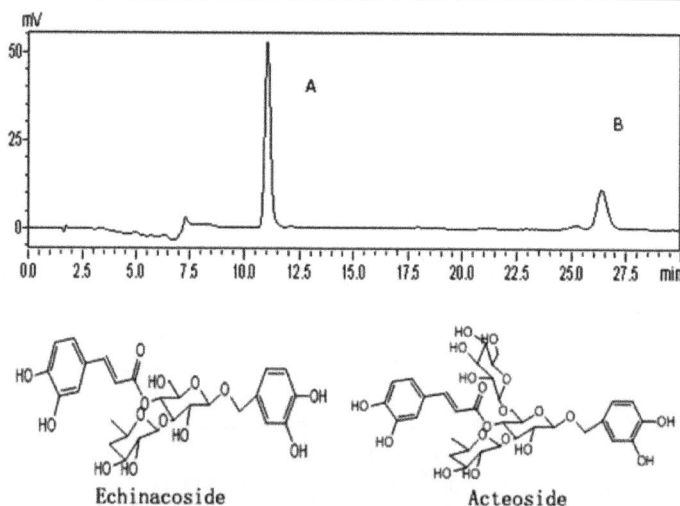

Fig. 1 The HPLC analysis of CPhGs and two phenylethyl alcohol glycosides, echinacoside and acteoside

Table 2 Effects of CPhGs on the serum AST, ALT activities of hepatic fibrosis rats

Group	Dose (mg/kg/day)	n	ALT (U/L)	AST (U/L)
Normal	—	12	$38.12 \pm 2.789^{**}$	$77.82 \pm 16.675^{**}$
Model	—	11	46.26 ± 6.904	173.27 ± 27.389
BJRG	600	10	39.68 ± 6.716	$104.65 \pm 8.891^{**}$
CPhGs	500	12	39.69 ± 7.048	$105.23 \pm 8.865^{**}$
	250	9	39.98 ± 5.476	$106.60 \pm 20.270^{**}$
	125	10	40.95 ± 3.920	$119.72 \pm 25.368^{**}$

Values are expressed as mean ± SD, n = Survival number of animals
$^{**}P < 0.01$, Compared with the model group

Table 4 Effects of CPhGs on the Hyp content and TGF-β_1 of hepatic fibrosis rats

Group	Dose (mg/kg/day)	n	Hyp (µg/mg)	TGF-β_1 (ng/ml)
Normal	—	12	$125.61 \pm 57.118^{*}$	$16.58 \pm 2.814^{**}$
Model	—	11	196.70 ± 82.545	31.24 ± 6.726
BJRG	600	10	129.57 ± 36.806	$20.16 \pm 4.638^{**}$
CPhGs	500	12	132.77 ± 50.705	$21.75 \pm 3.711^{**}$
	250	9	134.99 ± 64.824	$22.93 \pm 3.576^{**}$
	125	10	139.14 ± 41.352	$23.03 \pm 4.212^{**}$

Values are expressed as mean ± SD, n = Survival number of animals
$^{*}P < 0.05$, Compared with the model group; $^{**}P < 0.01$, Compared with the model group

level in the model group was significantly higher than the normal group, but it was markedly decreased in the BJRG group and the different CPhGs dose groups.

The hepatic concentration of TGF-β_1 of the model group in rats was significantly increased [$P < 0.001$]. Compared with the model group, TGF-β_1 levels of the positive drug and the different CPhGs dose groups were markedly decreased [$P_{\text{TGF-}\beta1} < 0.001$, $P_{\text{TGF-}\beta1} < 0.001$, $P_{\text{TGF-}\beta1} < 0.001$, $P_{\text{TGF-}\beta1} < 0.001$, respectively]. The results are summarized in Table 4.

Histopathological examination
Observations of normal liver tissue sections stained with H&E and Masson's trichrome exhibit distinct hepatic lobules and hepatic sinusoids. The liver tissue structure in the model rats was disordered, and the liver tissue and hepatic sinusoids were replaced by a large amount of connective tissue. However, more normal cytoarchitechture and less connective tissue were detected in the treatment group than those in the model group.

H&E staining
In the normal group, hepatic lobule structural integrity without abnormal portal areas and hepatic sinusoids was observed. The hepatic cords were arranged in an orderly fashion, with the core round and clear. The nuclei are located in the central of the cell, with abundant cytoplasm. Only the portal area has a small amount of fibrous tissue (Fig. 2a).

In the model group, the lobular structure was severely damaged. Liver cells showed mild watery degeneration, mostly ballooning degeneration and/or fatty degeneration. The formation of inflammatory cell infiltration, extensive fibrous tissue hyperplasia, the formation of a large number of fibrous septum, split lobules, and significant liver cells proliferation were also observed. These observations confirmed the success of the establishment of the rat immune injury animal model of hepatic fibrosis (Fig. 2b).

Compared with the model group, there was reduction in inflammatory cell infiltration in the different CPhGs. Also observed were less necrosis and fatty degeneration of liver cells as well as alleviation of fibrosis. CPhGs significantly mitigated the pathology of BSA-induced hepatic fibrosis in rats, alleviated the swelling of liver cells, and effectively prevented hepatocyte necrosis and inflammatory cells infiltration, suggesting that CPhGs exert protective effect on BSA -induced rat hepatic fibrosis. (Fig. 2c–f).

Masson's trichrome staining
In the normal group, the liver tissue was normal. The hepatic portal area showed a small amount of blue collagen fibers, and the liver tissue was normally structured (Fig. 3a). Compared with the liver tissue of the normal group, fibrous tissue proliferated by the central leaflet and expanded into the liver parenchyma. Collagen fibers extended and linked and

Table 3 Effects of CPhGs on the serum HA, LN, PCIII, IV-C activities of hepatic fibrosis rats

Group	Dose (mg/kg/day)	n	HA (mg/l)	LN (mg/l)	PCIII (mg/l)	IV-C (mg/l)
Normal	—	12	$98.67 \pm 15.798^{**}$	$21.27 \pm 3.003^{**}$	$12.69 \pm 6.525^{**}$	$1.99 \pm 0.691^{**}$
Model	—	11	116.08 ± 7.683	29.38 ± 4.716	33.87 ± 16.336	8.10 ± 0.369
BJRG	600	10	$106.85 \pm 7.650^{**}$	$23.35 \pm 3.106^{*}$	21.09 ± 7.113	$2.16 \pm 0.603^{**}$
CPhGs	500	12	$104.97 \pm 9.139^{**}$	$23.91 \pm 5.945^{*}$	23.58 ± 8.815	$2.52 \pm 0.464^{**}$
	250	9	$106.19 \pm 6.250^{**}$	$24.12 \pm 3.593^{*}$	24.07 ± 11.859	$3.10 \pm 0.692^{**}$
	125	10	$108.11 \pm 8.261^{*}$	25.41 ± 4.925	21.79 ± 7.877	$3.39 \pm 0.980^{**}$

Values are expressed as mean ± SD, n = Survival number of animals
$^{*}P < 0.05$, Compared with the model group; $^{**}P < 0.01$, Compared with the model group

enveloped the entire lobule and surrounded the central vein. These effects, along with hepatocyte fibrosis, lobular structural damage, periportal fibrosis, and pseudolobule formation (Fig. 3b) provided evidence that the model was established.

Compared with the model group, the collagen fibers in the positive drug control group were mildly extended outward from the peripheral portal area (Fig. 3c). Compared with the model group, the collagen fibers in the different CPhGs dose groups were significantly reduced, fiber proliferation was inhibited, and proliferation of fibrous tissue within the liver parenchyma significantly reduced. These results suggested that CPhGs protected rats from BSA-induced hepatic fibrosis (Fig. 3d–f).

Immunohistochemical staining
Importantly, the expression of collagen type I and collagen type III play essential roles in the development of hepatic fibrosis, and their generation and deposition in the liver tissue could serve as an important determinant of the anti-hepatic fibrosis efficacy. The results are summarized in Table 5.

Collagen type I
The normal group expressed collagen type I mainly in blood vessels and the portal area. The model group highly expressed collagen type I vascular fibrosis in portal areas. In the space of Disse, collagen type I staining was observed a streaks or as a patchy distribution. Collagen encased fibrous septa to form pseudolobule. In these experiments, fewer fibrous septa were formed for BJRJ (600 mg/kg) and different dose groups of CPhGs s (125, 250, and 500 mg/kg) [$P_{Col\ I}$ = 0.002, $P_{Col\ I}$ = 0.001, $P_{Col\ I}$ = 0.023, and $P_{Col\ I}$ = 0.044, respectively]. The semiquantitative results revealed that the expression of their collagen type I was significantly lower compared with the model group (Fig. 4).

Collagen type III
Collagen type III was weakly expressed in the normal group, and peripheral areas surrounding the portal and hepatic veins displayed a small amount of fine yellow instead of continuous fibers (Fig. 5a). In the model group, collagen fibers exhibited wide and thick cords, indicating strong expression, mainly located in the portal and fibrous tissue areas (Fig. 5b).

Collagen fibers of BJRJ (600 mg/kg) and different dose groups of CPhGs (125, 250, and 500 mg/kg) were filamentous and distributed around the central vein and portal areas. Compared with the model group, the collagen fibers were significantly reduced, staining was pale and thin, and immunohistochemical staining was weakly positive (Fig. 5c–f). These semi quantitative results show that the positively expressed cells in the positive and different dose groups [$P_{Col\ III}$ = 0.015, $P_{Col\ III}$ = 0.001, $P_{Col\ III}$ = 0.010, and $P_{Col\ III}$ = 0.037, respectively] were different from those in the model group.

TGF-β_1
There was little expression ofTGF-β_1 in normal rat liver cells. Expression was limited to a small number of interstitial cells (Fig. 6a). In the model group, TGF-β_1 expression was widely distributed in the portal area, fibrous spaces, hepatic stellate cells, inflammatory cells, the sinusoidal wall and cytoplasm. Aparticular portal area exhibited a strongly positive expression with brownish yellow staining (Fig. 6b).

There was a small amount of expression in the portal area and fibrous septa of BJRJ (600 mg/kg) and different dose groups of CPhGs (125, 250, and 500 mg/kg). The extent of positive staining in these groups was significantly reduced compared with that of the model group. Staining in the interstitial cells in the fibrous septa and the cytoplasm of inflammatory cells was decreased (Fig. 6c–f). Semi quantitative results revealed that BJRJ and different dose groups of CPhGs [$P_{TGF-\beta1}$ = 0.001, $P_{TGF-\beta1}$ < 0.001, $P_{TGF-\beta1}$ = 0.009, $P_{TGF-\beta1}$ = 0.004, respectively] were significant compared with the model group.

As mentioned earlier in the article, TGF-β_1 is an important cytokine in the pathophysiology of liver

Table 5 The immunohistochemical staining intensity of *Collagen type I, Collagen type III and TGF-β1* i n BSA-induced hepatic fibrosis rats

Group	Dose (mg/kg/day)	n	Collagen type I				Collagen type III				TGF-β1			
			+	++	+++	++++	+	++	+++	++++	-	+	++	+++
Normal	—	12	11	1	0	0	10	2	0	0	12	0	0	0
Model	—	11	0	1	1	9	0	1	2	8	0	1	1	9
BJRG	600	10	2	4	4	0	2	4	3	1	2	5	3	0
CPhGs	500	12	3	5	3	1	4	4	3	1	3	6	2	1
	250	9	1	4	3	1	2	4	2	1	1	5	2	1
	125	10	1	5	1	3	1	5	3	1	2	4	3	1
Total		64	18	20	12	14	19	20	13	12	20	21	11	12

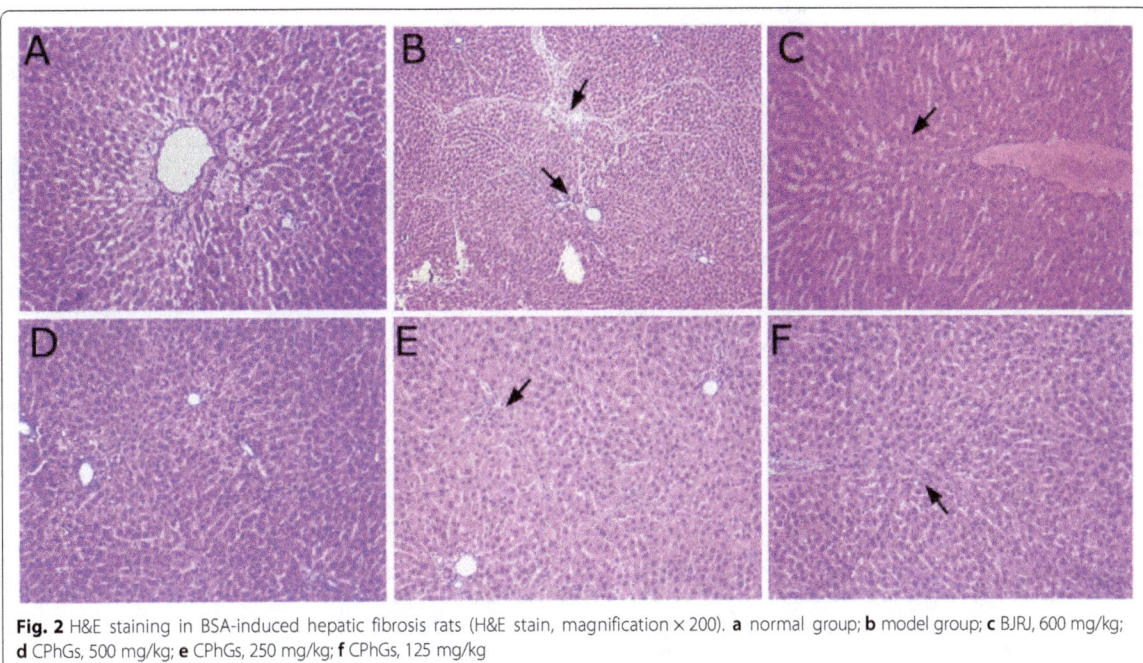

Fig. 2 H&E staining in BSA-induced hepatic fibrosis rats (H&E stain, magnification × 200). **a** normal group; **b** model group; **c** BJRJ, 600 mg/kg; **d** CPhGs, 500 mg/kg; **e** CPhGs, 250 mg/kg; **f** CPhGs, 125 mg/kg

fibrosis, stimulating the production of extracellular matrix [19]. We showed that the level of TGF-β_1 increased in the model group in a manner consistent with the severity of liver fibrosis. The expression levels of TGF-β_1 in liver were consistent with serum TGF-β_1 levels. This indicates that CPhGs can significantly reduce liver fibrosis due to TGF-β_1 expression by participating in the synthesis and degradation of ECM.

The expression of collagen type I, collagen type III, and TGF-β_1 can detect the pathological process of hepatic fibrosis. Their expression levels in the treatment

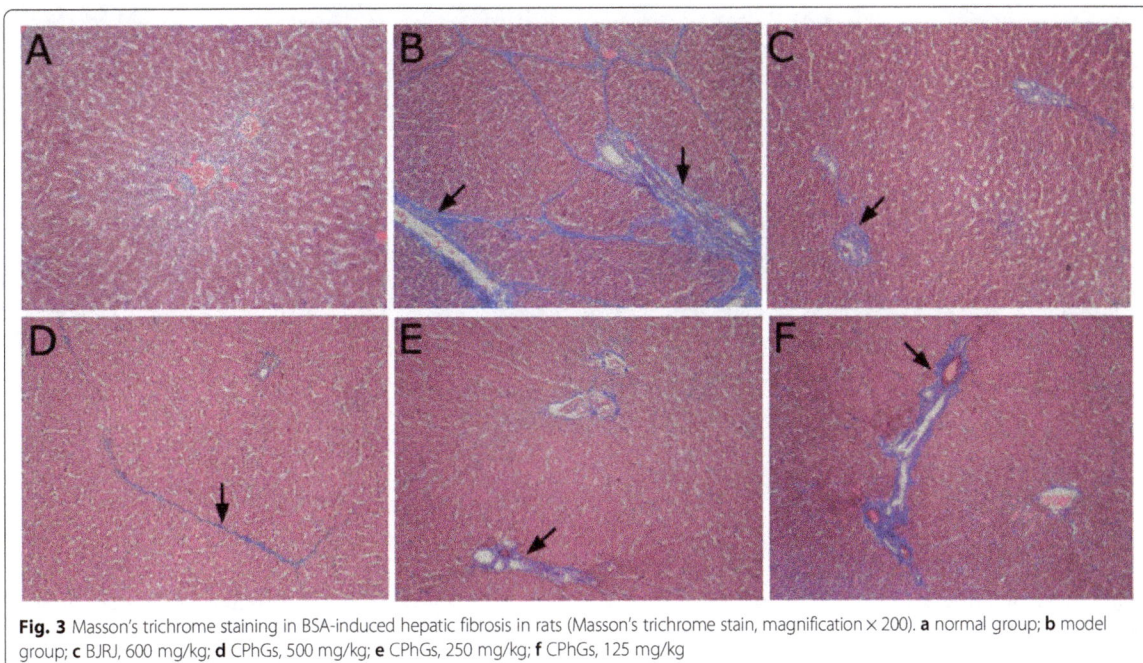

Fig. 3 Masson's trichrome staining in BSA-induced hepatic fibrosis in rats (Masson's trichrome stain, magnification × 200). **a** normal group; **b** model group; **c** BJRJ, 600 mg/kg; **d** CPhGs, 500 mg/kg; **e** CPhGs, 250 mg/kg; **f** CPhGs, 125 mg/kg

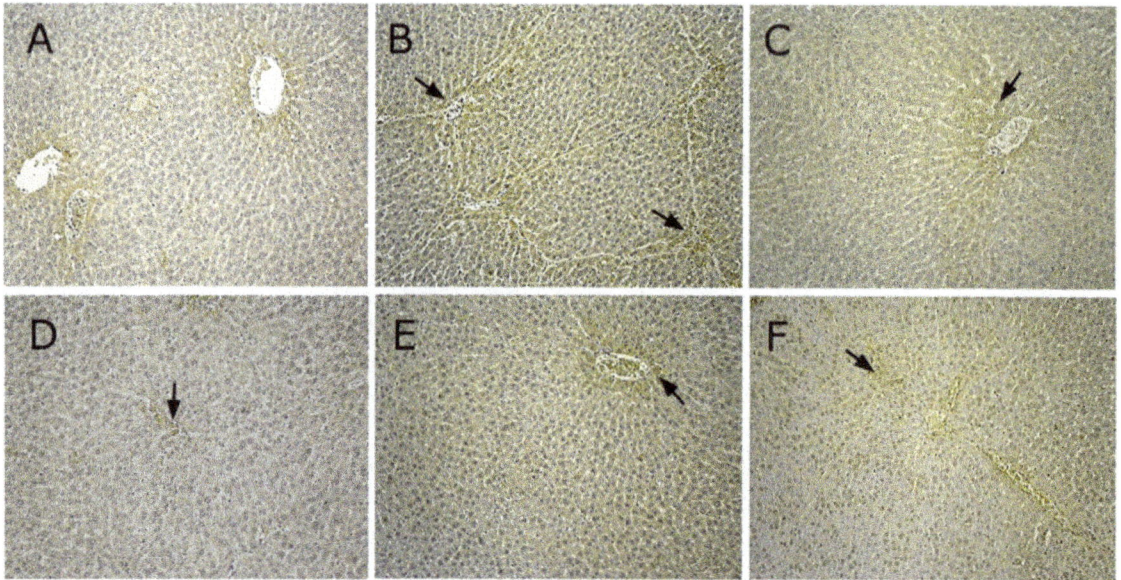

Fig. 4 Expression of collagen type I in BSA-induced hepatic fibrosis in rats (immunohistochemical staining, magnification × 200). **a** normal group; **b** model group; **c** positive group; **d** CPhGs high dose group; **e** CPhGs middle dose group; **f** CPhGs low dose group

groups were significantly decreased, and illustrated that CPhGs can improve collagenase activity, maintaining the dynamic equilibrium of liver ECM synthesis and degradation, thus delaying and preventing the formation of liver fibrosis.

NF-κB p65 and collagen I expression after drug intervention in HSC-T6 cells

In order to characterize signals of hepatic fibrosis, two key regulatory genes in the liver were determined via RT-PCR assay. The data showed that tHSC-T6

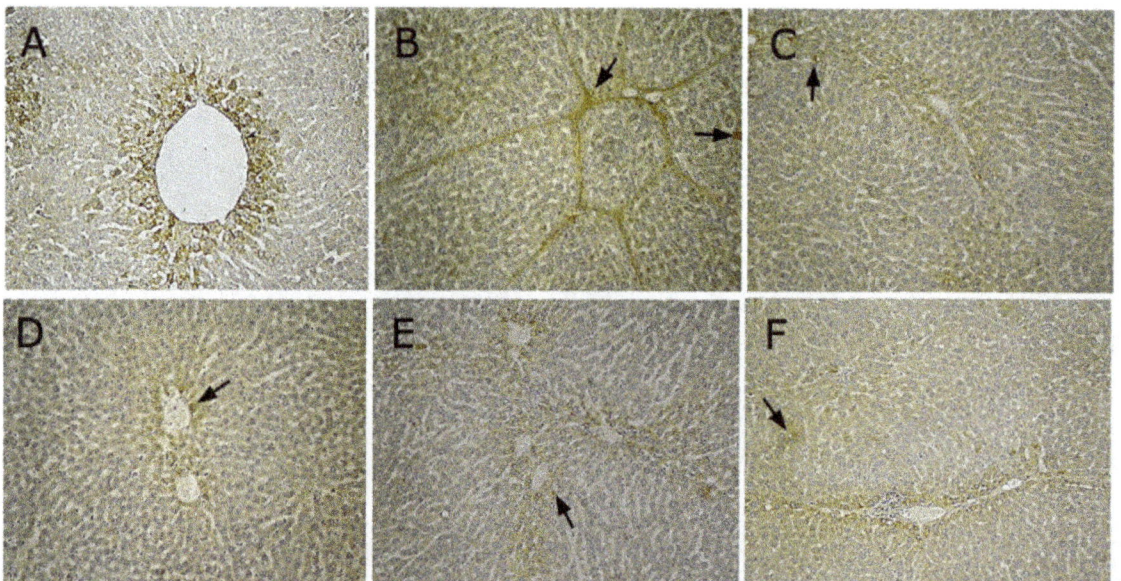

Fig. 5 Expression of collagen type III in BSA-induced hepatic fibrosis in rats (immunohistochemical staining, magnification × 200). **a** normal group; **b** model group; **c** positive group; **d** CPhGs high dose group (500 mg/kg); **e** CPhGs middle dose group (250 mg/kg); **f** CPhGs low dose group (125 mg/kg)

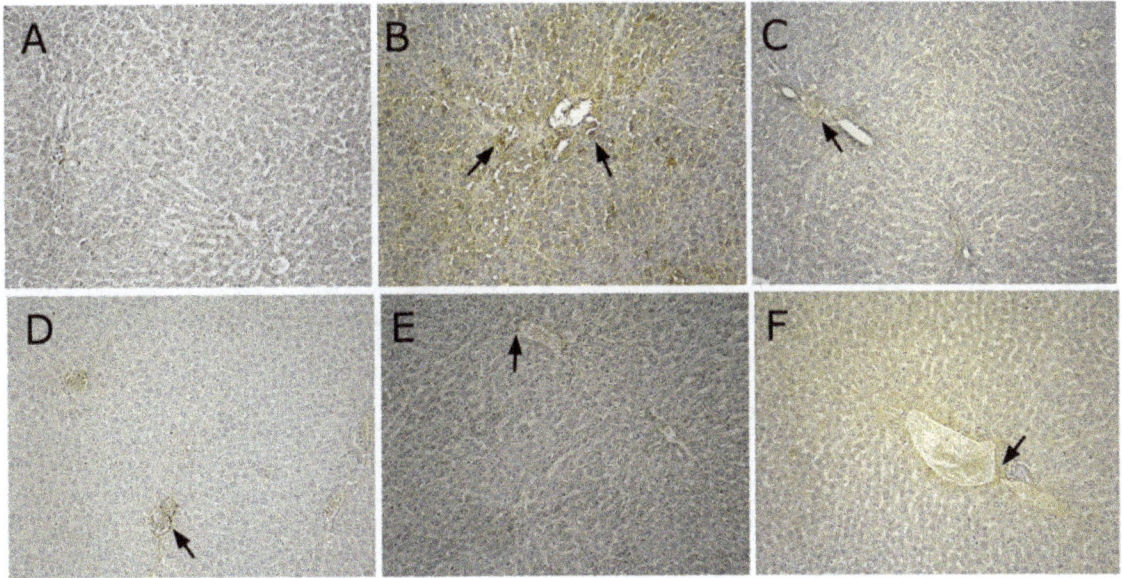

Fig. 6 Expression of TGF-β_1 in BSA-induced hepatic fibrosis in rats (immunohistochemical staining, magnification × 200). **a** normal group; **b** model group; **c** positive group; **d** CPhGs high dose group (500 mg/kg); **e** CPhGs middle dose group (250 mg/kg); **f** CPhGs low dose group (120 mg/kg)

cells from the control group had lower levels of NF-κB and collagen type I mRNA. Conversely, TGF-β_1 induced HSC-T6 cells to markedly upregulate NF-κB ($P < 0.01$) and Col-I ($P < 0.01$) mRNA, with levels higher than those in the control group. In the presence of different concentrations of CPhGs , the results of NF-κB p65 [$P_{\text{NF-}\kappa\text{B}} = 0.001$ for 100 ug/ml, $P_{\text{NF-}\kappa\text{B}} = 0.002$ for 75 ug/ml, $P_{\text{NF-}\kappa\text{B}} = 0.007$ for 50 ug/ml, and $P_{\text{NF-}\kappa\text{B}} = 0.012$ for 25 ug/ml, respectively] and Col-I [$P_{\text{Col-I}} = 0.006$, $P_{\text{Col-I}} = 0.009$, $P_{\text{Col-I}} =$

0.014, $P_{\text{Col-I}} = 0.019$, respectively] showed reduced expressions of these mRNAs (Fig. 7).

Western blot analysis of collagen I levels after drug intervention in HSC-T6 cells

Figure 8 shows the collagen I protein expression levels in HSC-T6 cells of the different experimental groups. The collagen I protein expression level was significantly decreased in the various dose groups of CPhGs (100 ug/

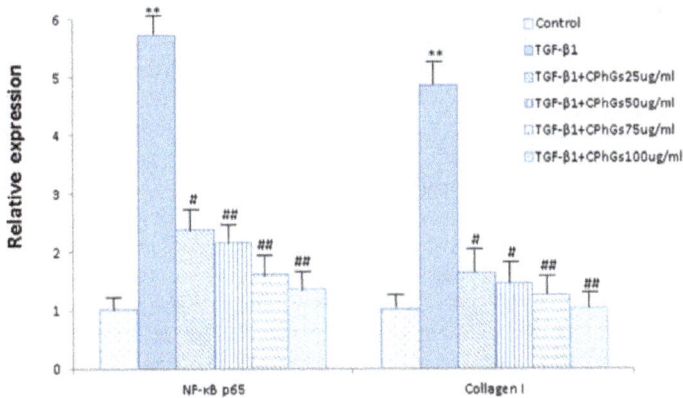

Fig. 7 CPhGs down-regulated the expressions of NF-κB and collagen I mRNA in HSC-T6 cells (RT-PCR assay). Data were analyzed via one-way ANOVA followed by Bonferroni post-tests. Results are expressed as the mean ± SE. Notes the following: **$P < 0.01$ *vs.* control group; #$P < 0.05$ *vs.* TGF-β_1 induced; ##$P < 0.01$ *vs.* TGF-β_1 induced

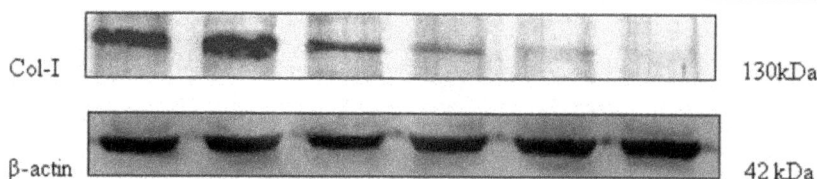

Fig. 8 Collagen I protein expression. Protein samples were subjected to electro-transfer to a PVDF membrane, incubated with primary antibodies and anti-rabbit secondary antibodies conjugated with AP. Lane 1: normal; lane 2: TGF-β_1 (5.0 ng/mL); lane 3: TGF-β_1 + CPhGs (25ug/ml); lane 4: TGF-β_1 + CPhGs (50 ug/ml); lane 5: TGF-β_1 + CPhGs (75ug/ml); lane 6: TGF-β_1 + CPhGs (100ug/ml)

ml, 75 ug/ml, 50 ug/ml, and 25 ug/ml) compared with the TGF-β_1 group.

Discussion

CPhGs is a phenylethanoid glycoside isolated and purified from rhizome of Cistanche, which is used as a traditional Chinese herbal medicine. In recent years, CPhGs had been shown to possess powerful ability to prevent liver injuries [20]. Therefore, we aimed to investigate whether CPhGs have inhibitory effects on hepatitis fibrosis by BSA induced hepatic fibrosis in rats. BJRG is commonly used as therapeutic drug for hepatic fibrosis in China. It is made from turtle shell. *Radix paeoniae rubra, Cordyceps sinensis, Radix isatidis*, and etc. have the effects of replenishing Qi and blood, relieving fatigue, softening nodes. In addition, previous studies show that it has the obvious function of blocking early liver fibrosis, inhibiting proliferation of fat storing cells, and reducing collagen synthesis [21]. Therefore, BJRG was used as a positive drug in this study.

The pathological changes of hepatic fibrosis in rats induced by BSA injections are similar to those in human portal cirrhosis [22]. CPhGs dose-dependently alleviated the degree of liver fibrosis and inhibited HSC transformation into myofibroblast-like cells, reduced the elevated levels of serum ALT, AST, HA, LN, CIV, TGF-β1 and the liver index, and markedly suppressed expression of collagen I, collagen III and TGF-β1 in liver tissue.

The stages of hepatic fibrosis are correlated with the serum levels of HA, LN and IV-C, which as markers may play a role in detecting the degree of hepatic fibrosis [23]. It has been reported that HA is the major resource of extracellular matrix. IV-C as the essential element of the basement membrane will be synthesized abundantly and deposit heavily in the earlier phases liver cirrhosis. The serum levels of LN and IV-C are the indexes of the turnover rate of the basement membrane and show the degree of fibrosis in the portal area and sinusoidal capillaries [24]. PC III is a marker in the diagnosis of hepatic fibrosis and early cirrhosis, but its sensitivity and specificity are not high, and there is no significant difference between the various stages of

fibrosis in many references [24, 25]. This study obtained a similar result.

In addition, the H&E and Masson's trichrome stained section observations exhibit normal liver tissues with distinct hepatic lobules and hepatic sinusoids. The liver tissue structure in the model group was disordered, and the liver tissue and hepatic sinusoid were replaced by a large amount of connective tissue. However, significantly improvement was observed in the treatment groups compared with the model group.

Importantly, collagen type I and collagen type III expression play essential roles in the development of hepatic fibrosis, the blocking of which can prevent and treat hepatic fibrosis. Therefore, the generation and deposition in the liver tissue of collagen type I and collagen type III could serve as an important determinant of anti-hepatic fibrosis efficacy. TGF-β_1 is also an important profibrogenic cytokine in liver injury and it is biologically active with multiple pharmacological actions [26]. A balance among these actions is required to maintain tissue homeostasis. The aberrant expression of TGF-β_1 is involved in the pathogenesis of liver diseases [27, 28]. It is known that TGF-β_1 is a crucial cytokine that is involved in the early stages of liver fibrosis. Oxidative stress triggers TGF-β_1, resulting in the latter stimulating ECM production and deposition [29]. Therefore, one of the effective strategies to produce anti-hepatic fibrosis drug is to identify anti-TGF-β_1 agents. Immunohistochemical analysis showed that the expressions of collagen type I, collagen type III and TGF-β_1 could detect the pathological process of hepatic fibrosis. The expressions of the collagen type I, collagen type III and TGF-β_1 in the treatment groups are decreased, which were significantly lower in the high dose CPhGs treatment group in particular, and suggested that CPhGs is an effective collagen type I, collagen type III and TGF-β1 inhibitor. Presumably, CPhGs can improve collagenase activity, maintaining the dynamic equilibrium of ECM synthesis and degradation, thus delaying and preventing the formation of liver fibrosis.

CPhGs not only could ameliorate BSA-induced hepatic fibrosis in rats, but also might be associated with inhibiting the activation of HSC in vitro. HSC activation is thought to represent the crucial step of fibrogenesis. In this study, the results illustrated that administration of CPhGs from 25 to 100 ug/ml remarkably attenuated the decreased NF-κB p65, collagen I mRNA expression, and collagen I protein expression in HSC.

NF-κB plays an important role in modulating the immune response to infection or stimuli [30]. Buildup of NF-κB in liver cells can result in the recruitment of inflammatory cytokines/mediators, thus inducing fibrosis development [31, 32]. Moreover, collagen is also a sensitive index that reflects the fibrosis level and accounts for about 50 % of the total protein in fibrous liver [33]. As a result, we postulated that the molecular mechanism against hepatofibrosis is linked to CPhGs-mediated inactivation of NF-κB expression, in which the benefit contributes to synergistic roles of attenuating immunotoxicity and inflammation stress in BSA-lesioned liver tissue, further correcting dysmetabolism to ameliorate liver functions.

Conclusions

In conclusion, our studies indicate that CPhGs significantly attenuate the extent of hepatic fibrosis induced by BSA in rats. Its mechanism may at least partially be due to the inhibitory effect of CPhGs on the composition of ECM and stimulation of the degradation of ECM, and/or by directly inhibition of the synthesis of collagen type I, collagen type III and the expression of TGF-β_1. Therefore, we expected that CPhGs can be used in health care products or in clinical medications for prevention of human liver fibrosis. Future studies are required to establish the efficacy of CPhGs as a potent anti-hepatic fibrosis drug.

Abbreviations

CPhGs: Phenylethanol glycosides from cistanche; BSA: Bovine serum albumin; HSC-T6: Hepatic stellate cells; Hyp: Hydroxyproline; BJRG: Compound Biejiarangan tablets; TGF-β_1: Transforming growth factor β_1; ALT: Alanine aminotransferase; AST: Aspartate aminotransferase; HA: Hyaluronic acid; LN: Laminin; PC III: Type III precollagen; IV-C: Type IV collagen; NF-κB: Nuclear factor kappa-light-chain-enhancer of activated B cells; RT-PCR: Reverse transcriptase polymerase chain reaction; SDS-PAGE: Sodium dodecyl sulfate polyacrylamide gel electrophoresis.

Competing interests

The authors declare that they have no competing interests.

Authors' contributions

TL, JZ, SPY, LM, MT and SLZ conceived and designed the experiments. SPY, TL and JZ analyzed the data. SPY and JZ wrote the manuscript. TL, LM and JZ reviewed the manuscript. All authors read and approved the final manuscript.

Acknowledgment

This research was supported by National Natural Science Foundation of China (81260624) . The authors would like to express their sincere thanks to Professor Tao Liu for his suggested improvements for the writing of this paper.

Author details

¹Department of Toxicology, School of Public Health, Xinjiang Medical University, No. 393 Xinyi Road, Urumqi 830011Xinjiang Uyghur Autonomous Region, China. ²Key Laboratory for Uighur Medicine, Institute of Materia Medica of Xinjiang, Urumqi 830004, China. ³No. 140 Xinhua South Road, Tianshan District, Urumqi 830000Xinjiang Uyghur Autonomous Region, China.

References

1. Cohen-Naftaly M, Friedman SL. Current status of novel antifibrotic therapies in patients with chronic liver disease. Ther Adv Gastroenterol. 2011;4(6):391–417.
2. Puche JE, Saiman Y, Fiedman SL. Hepatic stellate cells and liver fibrosis. Compr Physiol. 2013;3(4):1473–92.
3. Hernandez-Gea V, Friedman SL. Pathogenesis of liver fibrosis. Annu Rev Pathol. 2011;6:425–56.
4. Sohrabpour AA, Mohamadnejad M, Malekzadeh R. Review article: the reversibility of cirrhosis. Aliment Pharmacol Ther. 2012;36(9):824–32.
5. Raven PH, Zhang LB, Ventenat O. Chinese academy of sciences. 23rd ed. China: Editorial Committee of Flora of China; 2013. p. 1–16.
6. Chinese Pharmacopoeia Commission of Sanitary Ministry of People's Republic of China. Chinese pharmacopoeia, Part 1. China: Chemical Industry Publishing House; 2010. p. 126.
7. Yan GH, Tian JH, Long BW, Li N. Research progress of phenylethanol glycosides from Cistanche tubulosa. Central South Pharm. 2012;10:692–5.
8. Li J, Huang D, He L. Effect of roucongrong (Herba Cistanches Deserticolae) on reproductive toxicity in mice induced by glycoside of Leigongteng (Radix et Rhizoma Tripterygii). J Tradit Chin Med. 2014;34(3):324–32.
9. Xing Y, Liao J, Tang Y, Zhang P, Tan C, Ni H, et al. ACE and platelet aggregation inhibitors from Tamarix hohenackeri Bunge (host plant of Herba Cistanches) growing in Xinjiang. Pharmacogn Mag. 2014;10(38):111–7.
10. Jia Y, Guan Q, Jiang Y, Salh B, Guo Y, Tu P, et al. Amelioration of dextran sulphate sodium-induced colitis in mice by echinacoside-enriched extract of Cistanche tubulosa. Phytother Res. 2014;28(1):110–9.
11. Wong HS, Ko KM. Herba Cistanches stimulates cellular glutathione redox cycling by reactive oxygen species generated from mitochondrial respiration in H9c2 cardiomyocytes. Pharm Biol. 2013;51(1):64–73.
12. Zhang SJ, Liu L, Yu JY. A RP: A RP-HPLC method for simultaneous determination of echinacoside and acteoside in Herbe Cistanches. Chin Pharm J 2004; 39(10): 740-741.
13. Zhu QG, Fang BW, Zhu QN, Wu HS, Fu QL. The study of the immunity liver fibrosis animal model induced by bovine serum albumin. Chin J Pathol. 1993;22:121–2.
14. Qin DM, Wen ZP, Nie YR, Yao GM. Effect of cichorium glandulosum extracts on CCl4-induced hepatic fibrosis. Iran Red Crescent Med J. 2013;15, e10908.
15. Niu HM, Zeng DQ, Long CL, Peng YH, Wang YH, Luo JF, et al. Clerodane diterpenoids and prenylated flavonoids from Dodonaea viscosa. J Asian Nat Prod Res. 2010;12(1):7–14.
16. Li WW, Song XW, Wang HW, Shen BS, Wang QC. Correlation of NF-κB and pathological staging of liver fibrosis in patients with chronic hepatitis B. Chin J Immunol. 2013;29(3):251–4.
17. Zhang GL, Shi XF, Ran CQ, Xu M, Zhu ZJ. Effects of total saponins of panax notoginseng against liver fibrosis in rats. Acta Academiae Medicinae Militaris Tertiae. 2007;29:2212–4.
18. Rossi O, Maggiore L, Necci F, Koberling O, MacLennan CA, et al. Comparison of colorimetric assays with quantitative amino acid analysis for protein quantification of generalized modules for membrane antigens (GMMA). Mol Biotechnol. 2015;57(1):84–93.
19. Dang SS, Li YP. Advances in understanding the role of transforming growth factor-β1 in the pathogenesis of liver fibrosis. Shijie Huaren Xiaohua Zazhi. 2010;18:1631–6.
20. Zhao J, Liu T, Ma L, Yan M, Zhao Y, Gu Z, et al. Protective effect of acteoside on immunological liver injury induced by Bacillus Calmette-Guerin plus lipopolysaccharide. Planta Med. 2009;75(14):1463–9.
21. Yang FR, Fang BW, Lou JS. Effects of Fufang Biejia Ruangan pills on hepatic fibrosis in vivo and in vitro. World J Gastroenterol. 2013;19(32):5326–33.
22. Liu P, Fang BW, Liu C. The role of transforming growth factor β1 and its receptor in immunological induced liver fibrogenesis in rats and effect of cordyceps polysaccharide on them. Chin J Hepatol. 1998;6:232–3.
23. Xu GG, Luo CY, Wu SM, Wang CL. The relationship between staging of hepatic fibrosis and the levels of serum biochemistry. HBPD INT. 2002;1:246–8.

24. Liu J, Wang JY, Lu Y. Serum fibrosis markers in diagnosing liver fibrosis. Chin J Intern Med. 2006;145:475–7.

25. Li CZ, Wan MB, Zeng MD, Mao YM, Fan ZP, Cao AP, et al. A preliminary study of the combination of noninvasive parameters in the diagnosis of liver fibrosis. Chin J Hepatol. 2001;9:261–3.

26. Chen YL, Li ZY. The relationship between TGF-β1, PDGF-BB, CTGF and chronic hepatitis B with fibrosis. Chin J Diffic Compl Cas. 2010;9:19–20.

27. Sferra R, Vetuschi A, Catitti V, Ammanniti S, Pompili S, Melideo D, et al. Boswellia serrata and Salvia miltiorrhiza extracts reduce DMN-induced hepatic fibrosis in mice by TGF-beta1 downregulation. Eur Rev Med Pharmacol Sci. 2012;16(11):1484–98.

28. Liu L, Li XM, Chen L, Feng Q, Xu LL, Hu YY, et al. The effect of Gypenosides on TGF-β1/Smad pathway in liver fibrosis induced by carbon tetrachloride in rats. Intern J Integr Med. 2013;1:1–6.

29. Zhang BJ, Xu D, Guo Y, Ping J, Chen LB, Wang H. Protection by an anti-oxidant mechanism of berberine against rat liver fibrosis induced by multiple hepatotoxic factors. Clin Exp Pharmacol Physiol. 2008;35(3):303–9.

30. Tornatore L, Thotakura AK, Bennett J, Moretti M, Franzoso G. The nuclear factor kappa B signaling pathway: integrating metabolism with inflammation. Trends Cell Biol. 2012;22(11):557–66.

31. Luedde T, Schwabe RF. NF-κB in the liver–linking injury, fibrosis and hepatocellular carcinoma. Nat Rev Gastroenterol Hepatol. 2011;8(2):108–18.

32. Petrasek J, Csak T, Szabo G. Toll-like receptors in liver disease. Adv Clin Chem. 2013;59:155–201.

33. Wang Y, Cheng M, Zhang B, Nie F, Jiang H. Dietary supplementation of blueberry juice enhances hepatic expression of metallothionein and attenuates liver fibrosis in rats. PLoS One. 2013;8, e58659.

24

Ionic liquid phase microextraction combined with fluorescence spectrometry for preconcentration and quantitation of carvedilol in pharmaceutical preparations and biological media

Mohsen Zeeb* and Behrooz Mirza

Abstract

Background: Carvedilol belongs to a group of medicines termed non-selective beta-adrenergic blocking agents. In the presented approach, a practical and environmentally friendly microextraction method based on the application of ionic liquids (ILs) was followed by fluorescence spectrometry for trace determination of carvedilol in pharmaceutical and biological media.

Methods: A rapid and simple ionic liquid phase microextraction was utilized for preconcentration and extraction of carvedilol. A hydrophobic ionic liquid (IL) was applied as a microextraction solvent. In order to disperse the IL through the aqueous media and extract the analyte of interest, IL was injected into the sample solution and a proper temperature was applied and then for aggregating the IL-phase, the sample was cooled in an ice water-bath. The aqueous media was centrifuged and IL-phase collected at the bottom of the test tube was introduced to the micro-cell of spectrofluorimeter, in order to determine the concentration of the enriched analyte.

Results: Main parameters affecting the accuracy and precision of the proposed approach were investigated and optimized values were obtained. A linear response range of 10–250 µg l^{-1} and a limit of detection (LOD) of 1.7 µg l^{-1} were obtained.

Conclusion: Finally, the presented method was utilized for trace determination of carvedilol in commercial pharmaceutical preparations and biological media.

Keywords: Carvedilol, Hydrophobic ionic liquid, Spectrofluorimetry, Real samples

Background

Carvedilol belongs to a group of medicines termed non-selective beta-adrenergic blocking agents (Figure 1). This drug is useful in treatment of congestive heart failure. In addition, carvedilol is applied to treat high blood pressure (hypertension) and for prevention of heart attacks [1,2].

In order to assay the presence of carvedilol in pharmaceutical and biological samples, some analytical approaches including chromatography [3-6], spectrophotometery [7], electrochemistry [8,9] and fluorimetry [10] have been developed. These methods suffer form some limitations including poor sensitivity, high cost of analysis, unsuitable selectivity and high time of analysis. One of the best choices for overcoming the mentioned problems is the combination of a practical sample enrichment method with analytical instruments.

In recent years, analytical chemists have developed some practical liquid phase microextraction methods and among these sample pretreatment methods, dispersive liquid-liquid microextraction (DLLME) has received much attention [11,12]. Unfortunately, one of the most important disadvantages of these microextraction methods is the usage of toxic solvents as the extraction solvent such as $CHCl_3$, CCl_4 and etc. In order to remove these toxic materials from microextraction procedures, ionic liquids (ILs) are the best choice. ILs offer many

* Correspondence: Zeeb.mohsen@gmail.com
Department of Applied Chemistry, Faculty of science, Islamic Azad University, South Tehran Branch, Tehran, Iran

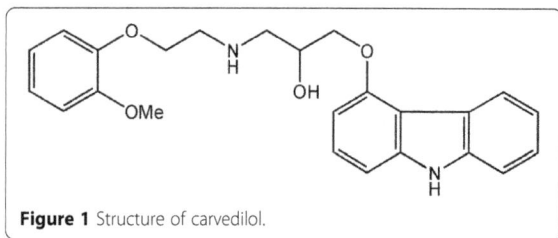

Figure 1 Structure of carvedilol.

advantages such as low vapor pressure, tunable solubility, desire thermal stability and etc. [13].

In recent years, some microextraction methods based on the application of ILs such as ionic liquid-based dispersive liquid-liquid microextraction (IL-DLLME) [14-16], ionic liquid cold-induced aggregation dispersive liquid-liquid microextraction (IL-CIA-DLLME) [17-19], ionic Liquid-based ultrasound-assisted in situ solvent formation microextraction [20], temperature-controlled ionic liquid dispersive liquid phase microextraction (TCIL-DLPME) [21], etc. have been introduced.

Solubility of ILs depends on the aqueous media temperature; hence it is possible to control the solubility of ILs by changing the temperature. In the presented ionic liquid phase microextraction, in order to disperse the IL-phase into the sample solution and increase the extraction recovery, a high temperature was applied. For collecting the IL-phase, sample solution was cooled and centrifuged.

Our previous studies revealed that the solubility of ILs depends on ionic strength of aqueous media, which has a negative influence on reproducibility and accuracy [18,19]. For solving this problem, a common ion of IL was introduced to the aqueous media. As a result, the solubility of IL phase was not affected by variations of ionic strength, and reproducible volume of enriched phase was obtained.

Some analytical instrument such as spectrofluorimetry offer many advantages such as proper sensitivity, selectivity, cost of analysis, speed of quantitative measurements and etc. In addition, by coupling a microextraction method with fluorescence spectrometry and due to the proper selectivity of this analytical technique, it is avoided the need of employing a high performance separation instrumental for pretreatment of biological samples prior to measurement.

As a part of our continuing efforts for quantitation of drugs using combination of new and benign sample enrichment methods with inexpensive, selective and sensitive analytical instrument [18,21], herein, for the first time a practical and environmentally friendly microextraction method based on the application of ILs was followed with spectrofluorimetry for trace determination of carvedilol in real samples. All variable were evaluated in details and optimized values were obtained.

Material and methods

Instrumentation

Detection of fluorescence signals were performed using a Perkin-Elmer LS 50 spectrofluorimeter. This instrument was equipped with xenon discharge lamp, and quartz micro-cell with a volume of 100 µl. Excitation and emission slits were fixed at 15 nm. In order to perform microextraction and optimization steps, a centrifuge from Hettich (Tuttlingen, Germany), a pH-meter, an adjustable sampler (10–100 µL) and a 1 ml syringe was prepared.

Reagents and materials

Analytical-reagent grade of 1-Hexyl-3-methylimidazolium hexafluorophosphate [Hmim][PF$_6$], acetone, acetonitrile, methanol, ethanol, HCl, NaOH and sodium hexafluorophosphate (NaPF$_6$) were obtained from Merck (Darmstadt, Germany). A working solution of NaPF$_6$ (250 mg ml^{-1}) was prepared. For preparing stock solution of carvedilol (1000 mg l^{-1}) (Fluka, Switzerland), proper amount of this drug was dissolved in methanol and diluted with ultra pure water. Standard solutions were prepared by dilution of the stock solution with ultra pure water. Tablets containing 12.5 mg and 25 mg carvedilol were purchased from a local pharmacy.

Sample pretreatment procedure

In this sample pretreatment method, ten milliliters of sample solution (10–250 µg l^{-1} of carvedilol) was transferred to a centrifuge tube. The pH of the solution was adjusted at 9. Afterwards, 60 mg of 1-Hexyl-3-methylimidazolium hexafluorophosphate [Hmim][PF$_6$] ionic liquid and 0.7 ml of hexafluorophosphate (NaPF$_6$) (250 mg ml^{-1}) was injected into the aqueous sample solution. After mixing the extractor with sample solution, the resultant solution was transferred into a hot water batch equipped with a thermostat. The temperature of the water batch was fixed at 50°C for 4 min. Under driving the temperature, IL-phase was dissolved and dispersed through the aqueous media. In order to aggregate the IL-phase, the sample was cooled at 0°C for 7 min. In order to collect the enriched phase, sample solution was centrifuged (6 min, 4000 r.p.m). After removing the aqueous media, the enriched phase was diluted with ethanol to 200 µl and transferred into the micro-cell of the spectrofluorimeter. Finally, quantitation of carvedilol was performed. Schematic diagram of the designed method is shown in Figure 2.

Preparation of pharmaceutical preparations, human urine and human plasma

To obtain pharmaceutical solutions for quantification, eight carvedilol tablets containing 12.5 or 25 mg drug were powdered, mixed and weighted. Required amount of the resultant material containing 10 mg carvedilol

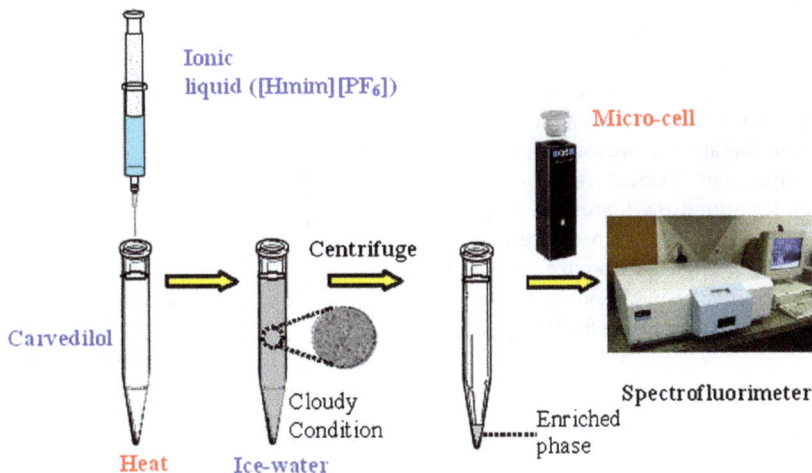

Figure 2 Schematic diagram of the proposed method.

was dissolved in methanol with signification. After filtration, the solution was transferred into a 100 ml volumetric vessel and diluted with ultra pure water. In order to set the concentration of carvedilol within the linear response range, further dilution was performed.

For preparing human plasma samples, different concentrations of carvedilol were added to one milliliter of human plasma. After this step, the real sample was deproteinized using 5 ml of acetonitrile. After centrifugation (12 min, 4000 r.p.m), 2.0 ml of the upper phase (clear condition) was diluted with ultra pure water and 10.0 ml of the obtained sample was utilized for quantitation.

In order to prepare human urine samples, ten milliliters of urine were centrifuged (5 min, 4000 r.p.m). Then, 2.0 ml of the upper clear phase was placed in centrifuge test tube and different amount of carvedilol was added to

this and diluted to 10.0 ml. Finally, the defined quantitation procedure was performed.

Results and discussion

In recent work, a simple and benign sample pretreatment method based on the application of ILs was combined with fluorescence spectrometry for enrichment and determination carvedilol in real samples. Main parameters affecting the accuracy and precision of the proposed approach were investigated and optimized values were obtained.

Fluorescence spectra properties and linear dynamic range

Native Fluorescence intensities of molecules with π-electron and cyclic structure are relatively high. As a result, measurement of fluorescence intensity provides a

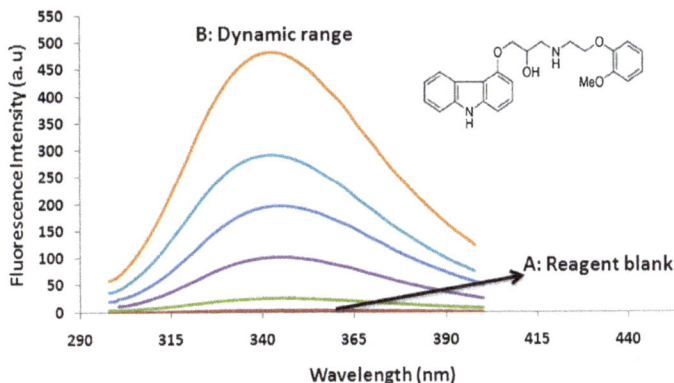

Figure 3 Fluorescence spectra of reagent blank and carvedilol. (A) Fluorescence spectrum of reagent blank after applying microextraction procedure. (B) Fluorescence spectra of carvedilol within linear dynamic range (10, 50, 100, 150, 250 µg l^{-1}) after applying microextraction procedure. Applied parameters: sample volume 10 ml; IL 60 mg; NaPF$_6$ 175 mg; pH 9; temperature 50°C; λ_{ex} 285 ± 5 nm; λ_{em} 345 ± 5 nm.

practical tool for sensitive quantitative analysis. After applying the designed microextraction procedure, fluorescence spectra of carvedilol (100 μg l^{-1}) was recorded (Figure 3). In this study, emission peaks were recorded at 345 ± 5 nm (excitation wave length was fixed at 285 ± 5 nm).

In order to evaluate the spectra properties of reagent blank, sample pretreatment method was performed without analyte of interest and the fluorescence spectra were recorded at 345 ± 5 nm. No main measurable influence of reagent blank on the quantitative analysis of carvedilol was observed. As a result, these excitation and emission wavelengths were selected for further quantitation of carvedilol.

Kind of ionic liquid

Based on the results obtained in our previous studies [18,19], three factors must be considered, in order to select a proper IL: (a) the density of IL as the extraction solvent must be higher than aqueous media, (b) IL must illustrate a desire hydrophobicity, (c) IL must be liquid and (d) these ionic material must be inexpensive. ILs with imidazolium scaffold which contain Cl$^-$, BF$_4^-$ and CF$_3$SO$_3^-$ show hydrophilic properties and those contain PF$_6^-$ and (CF$_3$SO$_2$)$_2$ N$^-$ show hydrophobic properties.

According to these factors, [Hmim][PF$_6$] was used as an optimum microextraction solvent in all tests.

Optimization of diluting solvent

The viscosity of ionic liquids is relatively high; hence their direct transfer into the micro-cell of spectrofluorimeter for analyzing carvedilol is difficult. As a result, enriched-phase was conditioned and diluted. For this goal, some conditioner solvents such as methanol, ethanol, acetonitrile and acetone were evaluated as the diluting solvent. The obtained data showed that reproducible and sensitive

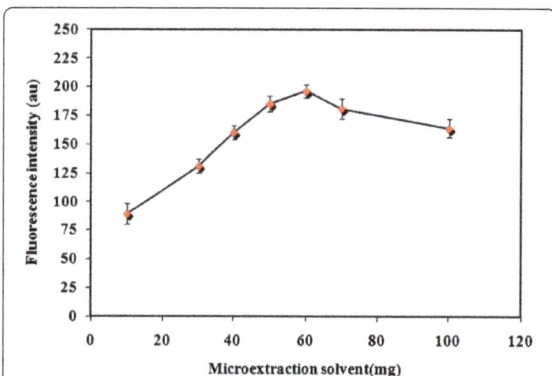

Figure 5 Effect of PF$_6^-$ Applied parameters: Carvedilol concentration 100 μg l^{-1}; Sample volume 10 ml; IL 60 mg; pH 9; temperature 50°C; λ_{ex} 285 ± 5 nm; λ_{em} 345 ± 5 nm. Indicated analytical signals are the average of three independent measurements and error bars correspond to their standard deviations.

signals were obtained in using ethanol as a conditioner agent. Due to the better data stability and ethanol environmental safety (less toxicity), this organic solvent was preferred and used in all experiments.

Optimization of IL amount

As it was mentioned, in this microextraction procedure, IL was applied as the microextraction phase. In this kind of sample pretreatment method, one of the major parameters affecting the performance is the amount of IL. This parameter has a significant effect on the reproducibility and sensitivity. In order to optimize the amount of extraction solvent, this parameter was tested within the range of 10–100 mg (Figure 4). Stable and sensitive fluorescence signals were obtained at 60 mg and this value was used for the rest of the work.

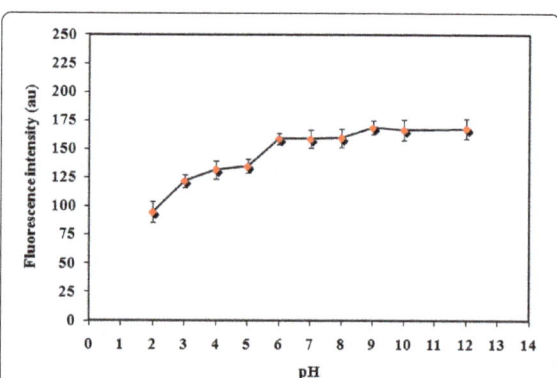

Figure 4 Effect of IL as the microextraction phase. Applied parameters: Carvedilol concentration 100 μg l^{-1}; sample volume 10 ml; NaPF$_6$ 175 mg; pH 9; temperature 50°C; λ_{ex} 285 ± 5 nm; λ_{em} 345 ± 5 nm. Indicated analytical signals are the average of three independent measurements and error bars correspond to their standard deviations.

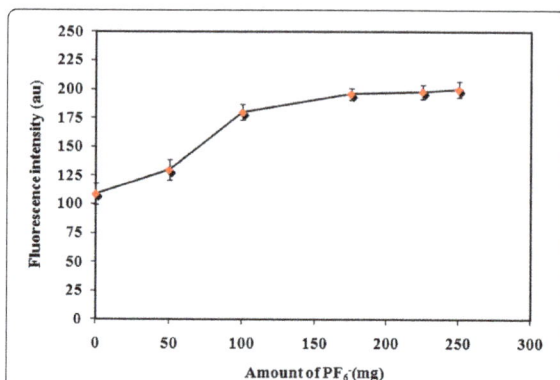

Figure 6 Effect of pH. Applied parameters: Carvedilol concentration 100 μg l^{-1}; sample volume 10 ml; IL 60 mg; NaPF$_6$ 175 mg; temperature 50°C; λ_{ex} 285 ± 5 nm; λ_{em} 345 ± 5 nm. Indicated analytical signals are the average of three independent measurements and error bars correspond to their standard deviations.

Table 1 Analytical characteristics of the presented work

Analytical factor	Values
Linear analytical response range ($\mu g \, l^{-1}$)	10-250
Correlation coefficient (R^2)	0.9980
LOD[a] ($\mu g \, l^{-1}$)	1.7
RSD[b] (%) (n = 4) ($C_{carvedilol} = 100 \, \mu g \, l^{-1}$)	3.8
PF[c]	50
Sample volume (mL)	10

[a]Limit of detection.
[b]Relative standard deviation.
[c]The ratio of diluted settled phase volume to aqueous volume gives the preconcentration factor (PF).

Table 3 Results of recoveries of spiked biological samples

Sample	Carvedilol added ($\mu g \, l^{-1}$)	Carvedilol found ($\mu g \, l^{-1}$)[a]	RSD (%)	Recovery (%)
Urine	50	53.2	6.1	106.4
	100	98.3	5.9	98.3
	150	146.1	3.8	97.4
Plasma	50	44.6	5.6	89.2
	100	107.3	7.1	107.3
	150	154.8	4.2	103.2

[a]Average of four independent measurements.

Optimization of PF$_6^-$ amount and ionic strength

As it was demonstrated in our previous works [18,19], dissolving a common ion of IL like PF$_6^-$, significantly reduce the solubility of IL. This act improves the extraction performance of carvedilol and provides better analytical sensitivity. Effect of this parameter was examined in the range of 0–250 mg (see Figure 5). A value of 175 mg was selected as an optimum value, in order to obtain proper signal stability and reproducibility.

One of the most important parameters which affects on the extraction performance is ionic strength of the aqueous media. An increase in ionic strength causes a considerable increase in solubility of IL. As a result, the volume of the settled phase depends on the salt content of the sample solution. This phenomenon has a negative influence on the stability of analytical data. Fortunately, presence of PF$_6^-$ (as a common ion) solves this problem and fixes the volume of the enrich phase. The effect of ionic strength was studied within the range of 0–40% (w/v) using NaNO$_3$ as an electrolyte. In the studied range, no significant influence on fluorescence signal was observed.

Table 2 Comparison of the proposed methodology with reported methods

Method	Sample	LOD ($\mu g \, l^{-1}$)	LR ($\mu g \, l^{-1}$)	Reference
DLLME-HPLC[a]	Human Urine, Human Plasma	4, 14	50-750, 20-1000	[6]
SPE-CE[b]	Human Urine	50	50-500	[23]
Synchronous fluorimetry	Pharmaceutical preparations	1	5-100	[24]
LLE-HPLC[c]	Human serum	2.5	5-500	[25]
Ionic liquid phase microextraction-spectrofluorimetry	Human Urine, Human Plasma, Pharmaceutical preparations	1.7	10-250	This work

[a]Dispersive liquid-liquid microextraction.
[b]Solid phase extraction-capillary electrophoresis.
[c]Liquid-liquid extraction.

Optimization of pH

In the case of microextraction of molecules like carvedilol, which have ionizable property, pH of the aqueous media reveals a significant role. In order to obtain the highest extraction efficiency, the uncharged condition of carvedilol must be prevalent (pK$_a$ value of carvedilol is 7.97) [22]. The effect of sample pH on the analytical sensitivity and reproducibility was tested within the range of 2–12 (Figure 6). In the recent experiments, HCl and NaOH were used for adjusting the pH. Based on the results obtained in this study, in order to obtain a compromise between sensitivity and reproducibility, pH 9 was selected for further experiments.

Influence of temperature

In this microextraction procedure, IL-phase is dispersed into the aqueous media under increasing the temperature. The effect of this parameter was evaluated in the range of 25–80°C. Finally, a temperature of 50°C was used as an optimum value. In order to collect the IL-phase after extraction, the sample solution must be cooled. For the recent goal, the aqueous media was placed in ice-water bath and kept at 0°C for 7 min.

Interference study

For studying the possible interferences coming form other compounds, which exist in real samples, some ions and compounds were subjected to the recent combined methodology. In this investigation, the effect of 100-fold of K$^+$, Na$^+$, Mg$^+$, F$^-$, Cl$^-$ NO$_3^-$, SO$_4^{2-}$, glucose, urea, lactic acid, sucrose, ascorbic acid and fructose as the interfering or quenching agents on the determination of

Table 4 Analysis of carvedilol tablets by the present work and the reported method (5)

Claimed (mg/tablet)	Proposed method (mg)[a]	Reported method (mg)[a]	Error (%)[b]	Error (%)[c]
12.5	12.3 (±0.5)	12.6 (±0.4)	−1.6	−2.9
25	25.5 (±1.0)	25.7 (±1.1)	+2.0	−0.7

[a]Values in parenthesis give the standard deviation based on four determinations.
[b]Error against the tablet value.
[c]Error against the reported method.

carvedilol (100 µg L^{-1}) was evaluated. No change in signals over than 4.5% was observed.

Analytical figures of merits

Linear analytical response range was defined by analyzing standard solutions of carvedilol. The obtained results revealed that analytical responses are linear from 10 to 250 µg l^{-1}. Other analytical figures of merits obtained by the ionic liquid phase microextraction-spectrofluorimetry are shown in Table 1. Limit of detection (LOD) was determined using a conventional equation, LOD = ks$_{bl}$/m. This equation is resulted from the equation showed below:

$$S_m = S_{bl} + ks_{bl}$$
$$S_m = mc_m + S_{bl}$$
$$c_m = \frac{S_m - S_{bl}}{m} = \frac{ks_{bl}}{m}$$

S_m, S_{bl}, s_{bl}, K, m and C_m show the minimum distinguishable analytical signal, average of blank analytical signal, blank standard deviation, constant value equal with 3 (confidence level of 95%), calibration graph slope and detection limit, respectively. Using this way, a value of 1.7 µg l^{-1} carvedilol was achieved. In order to determine the relative standard deviation (RSD), four 100 µg l^{-1} of carvedilol was subjected to the designed methodology and finally a value of 3.8% was obtained.

Comparison with reported methods

In order to show the analytical advantages of the proposed method for the quantitation of carvedilol, some details were compared with reported methods in literature, and these results are shown in Table 2. As it can be seen, considerable LOD and relatively wide dynamic range were obtained. In addition, in most of the reported methods, tedious sample pretreatment procedures, toxic solvents and expensive analytical instrument have been used for quantification. In contrast, in the proposed method, a rapid, benign and simple ionic liquid phase microextraction was utilized for preconcentration and extraction of carvedilol. No hazardous material was used in this sample pre-treatment method. In addition, an inexpensive and sensitive analytical instrument was applied for quantitation.

Analysis of carvedilol in real samples

In order to demonstrate the analytical application of the presented technique, real samples including human urine and human plasma were spiked with different amounts of carvedilol and analyzed. Results of this investigation are shown in Table 3. At it can be seen, the averages of recoveries are placed in the range of 97.4-106.2% (urine) and 89.2-107.3% (plasma). It can be concluded that in the case of accuracy and reproducibility,

satisfactory results were obtained. In the next step, some commercial pharmaceutical formulations involving carvedilol capsules and tablets were subjected to the designed method, in order to determine concentration of carvedilol (Table 4). The results obtained with the present work were compared with a reported method [5]. These data reveal the practical analytical application of the proposed method for analyzing the analyte of interest in pharmaceutical preparations.

Conclusion

A rapid, benign and simple ionic liquid phase microextraction was utilized for preconcentration and extraction of carvedilol. The enriched-phase was introduced to spectrofluorimeter for quantitation of carvedilol. No toxic and hazardous material was used in this sample pre-treatment method. In addition, an inexpensive and sensitive analytical instrument was applied for quantitative measurements. Finally, the combined methodology was successfully applied for quantitation of carvedilol in real samples.

Competing interests
The authors declare that they have no competing interests.

Authors' contributions
All authors contributed equally. Both authors read and approved the final manuscript.

Acknowledgment
Support of this investigation by the Islamic Azad University Tehran south branch through grant is gratefully acknowledged.

References
1. Packer M, Colicci WS, Sacker-Bernstein JD. Placebo-controlled study of the effects of carvedilol in patients with moderate to severe heart failure, the PRECISE trial. Circulation. 1996;94:2793–9.
2. Bristow MR, Gilbert EM, Abraham WT, Adams KF, Fowler MB, Hershberger RE, et al. Carvedilol produces dose related improvements in left ventricular function and survival in subjects with chronic heart failure. Circulation. 1996;94:2807–16.
3. Hokama N, Hobara N, Kameya H, Ohshiro S, Sakanashi M. Rapid and simple micro-determination of carvedilol in rat plasma by high performance liquid chromatography. J Chromatogr, B. 1999;732:233–8.
4. Machida M, Watanabe M, Takechi S, Kakinoki S, Nomura A. Measurement of carvedilol in plasma by high-performance liquid chromatography with electrochemical detection. J Chromatogr, B. 2003;798:187–91.
5. Zarghi A, Foroutan SM, Shafaati A, Khoddam A. Quantification of carvedilol in human plasma by liquid chromatography using fluorescence detection: application in pharmacokinetic studies. J Pharm Biomed Anal. 2007;44:250–3.
6. Zamani-Kalajahi M, Fazeli-Bakhtiyari R, Amiri M, Golmohammadi A, Afrasiabi A, Khoubnasabjafari M, et al. Analysis of losartan and carvedilol in urine and plasma samples using a dispersive liquid–liquid microextraction isocratic HPLC–UV method. Bioanalysis. 2012;4:2805–21.
7. Cardoso SG, Ieqqli CV, Pomblum SC. Spectrophotometric determination of carvedilol in pharmaceutical formulations through charge-transfer and ion-pair complexation reactions. Pharmazie. 2007;62:34–7.
8. Radi A, Elmogy T. Differential pulse voltammetric determination of carvedilol in tablets dosage form using glassy carbon electrode. II Farmaco. 2005;60:43–6.

9. Soleymanpour A, Ghasemian M. Chemically modified carbon paste sensor for the potentiometric determination of carvedilol in pharmaceutical and biological media. Measurement. 2015;59:14–20.

10. Silva RA, Wang CC, Fernandez LP, Masi AN. Flow injection spectrofluorimetric determination of carvedilol mediated by micelles. Talanta. 2008;76:166–71.

11. Zeeb M, Ganjali MR, Norouzi P. Dispersive liquid-liquid microextraction followed by spectrofluorimetry as a simple and accurate technique for determination of thiamine (vitamin B_1). Michrochim Acta. 2010;168:317–24.

12. Bidari A, Jahromi EZ, Assadi Y, Hosseini MRM. Monitoring of selenium in water samples using dispersive liquid-liquid microextraction followed by iridium-modified tube graphite furnace atomic absorption spectrometry. Microchem J. 2007;87:6–12.

13. Zeeb M, Ganjali MR, Norouzi P, Kalaei MR. Separation and preconcentration system based on microextraction with ionic liquid for determination of copper in water and food samples by stopped-flow injection spectrofluorimetry. Food Chem Toxicol. 2011;49:1086–91.

14. Yao C, Anderson JL. Dispersive liquid-liquid microextraction using an in situ metathesis reaction to form an ionic liquid extraction phase for the preconcentration of aromatic compounds from water. Anal Bioanal Chem. 2009;395:1491–502.

15. Yao C, Li T, Wu P, Pitner WR, Anderson JL. Selective extraction of emerging contaminants from water samples by dispersive liquid-liquid microextraction using functionalized ionic liquids. J Chromatogr A. 2011;1218:1556–66.

16. Gharehbaghi M, Shemirani F, Baghdadi M. Dispersive liquid-liquid microextraction based on ionic liquid and spectrophotometric determination of mercury in water samples. Int J Environ Anal Chem. 2009;89:21–33.

17. Zeeb M, Sadeghi M. Modified ionic liquid cold-induced aggregation dispersive liquid-liquid microextraction followed by atomic absorption spectrometry for trace determination of zinc in water and food samples. Microchim Acta. 2011;175:159–65.

18. Zeeb M, Ganjali MR, Norouzi P. Modified ionic liquid cold-induced aggregation dispersive liquid-liquid microextraction combined with spectrofluorimetry for trace determination of ofloxacin in pharmaceutical and biological samples. Daru. 2011;19:446–54.

19. Zeeb M, Ganjali MR, Norouzi P. Preconcentration and Trace Determination of Chromium Using Modified Ionic Liquid Cold-Induced Aggregation Dispersive Liquid-Liquid Microextraction: Application to Different Water and Food Samples. Food Anal Method. 2013;6:1398–406.

20. Zeeb M, Mirza B, Zare-Dorabei R, Farahani H. Ionic Liquid-based Ultrasound-Assisted In Situ Solvent Formation Microextraction Combined with Electrothermal Atomic Absorption Spectrometry as a Practical Method for Preconcentration and Trace Determination of Vanadium in Water and Food Samples. Food Anal Method. 2014;7:1783–90.

21. Zeeb M, Tayebi-Jamil P, Berenjian A, Ganjali MR, Talei BOMR. Quantitative analysis of piroxicam using temperature controlled ionic liquid dispersive liquid phase microextraction followed by stopped-flow injection spectrofluorimetry. Daru. 2013;6:1398–406.

22. Stojanovic J, Vladimirov S, Marinkovic V, Velickovic D, Sibinovic P. Monitoring of the photochemical stability of carvedilol and its degradation products by the RP-HPLC method. J Serb Chem Soc. 2007;72:37–44.

23. Mazzarino M, De La Torre X, Mazzei F, Botre F. Rapid screening of beta-adrenergic agents and related compounds in human urine for anti-doping purpose using capillary electrophoresis with dynamic coating. J Sep Sci. 2009;32:3562–70.

24. Xiao Y, Wang HU, Han J. Simultaneous determination of carvedilol and ampicillin sodium by synchronous fluorimetry. Spectrochim Acta, Part A. 2005;61:567–73.

25. Gannu R, Yamsani VV, Rao YM. New RP-HPLC method with UV-detection for the determination of carvedilol in human serum. J Liq Chromatogr Rel Technol. 2007;30:1677–85.

25

Comparative Pharmacokinetics of three major bioactive components in rats after oral administration of Typhae Pollen-Trogopterus Feces drug pair before and after compatibility

Huiting Zeng[1,2,3], Ping Xue[1,2,3], Shulan Su[1,2,3,4]*, Xiaochen Huang[1,2,3], Erxin Shang[1,2,3], Jianming Guo[1,2,3], Dawei Qian[1,2,3], Yuping Tang[1,2,3] and Jin-ao Duan[1,2,3,4]*

Abstract

Background: Typhae Pollen (TP) and Trogopterus Feces (TF) are well-known traditional medicine in china which widely used for thousands of years as drug pair called Shixiao San for treatment of blood stasis syndrome, specially shown great efficacy in gynecological disease. Typhaneoside, vanillic acid and *p*-coumaric acid are the main bioactive components of Typhae Pollen. This study was carried out for comparing the pharmacokinetic profile of these three major bioactive components in rats after oral administration of Typhae Pollen-Trogopterus Feces (TP-TF) drug pair before and after compatibility.

Methods: A sensitive and rapid UPLC-TQ/MS method has been developed for simultaneous quantification of the three main bioactive compounds in blood at different time points after oral administration of Typhae Pollen (TP) and the combination with Trogopterus Feces (TF).

Results: There were significant differences of C_{max}, T_{max}, $T_{1/2}$ and $AUC_{0\sim t}$ for three bioactive compounds among the groups, for typhaneoside with the most highest plasma concentration of 370.86 ± 315.71 ng/mL and more longer T_{max} in TP-TF co-decoction group (C_M); for vanillic acid, TP-TF co-decoction group (C_M) had a good absorption with C_{max} (3870.99 ± 2527.99 ng/mL) and T_{max} (1.47 ± 3.20 h); for *p*-coumaric acid, it had similar pharmacokinetic characteristics with vanillic acid.

Conclusions: The three bioactive components in Typhae Pollen (TP) were simultaneously determined by UPLC-TQ/MS and had a good absorption in rat plasma after the combination with Trogopterus Feces (TF).

Keywords: Typhae Pollen-Trogopterus Feces drug pair, Typhaneoside, Vanillic acid, *p*-coumaric acid, Pharmacokinetic, UPLC-TQ/MS

* Correspondence: sushulan1974@163.com; duanja@163.com
[1]Jiangsu Key Laboratory for High Technology Research of TCM Formulae, Nanjing University of Chinese Medicine, Nanjing 210023, China
Full list of author information is available at the end of the article

Background

Blood stasis (BS) is considered as a familiar type of clinical symptoms and signs in Traditional Chinese Medicine (TCM) for thousands of years, which is the underlying pathology of many disease processes according to TCM theory. Generally speaking, Blood stasis (BS) refers to retarded blood flow and it is often associated with disruption of heart Qi (vital energy), thus giving rise to a series of hematological disorders such as congestion, hemorrhage, thrombosis, local ischemia (microclots) and even tissue changes [1, 2]. It mainly manifested as pain, lassitude, bleeding, chills and fever, bruise, muscle tension, and some dark blue signs like black rim of eyes [3], women's blood stasis mostly for gynecology diseases for instance of dysmenorrhea, menoxenia, uterine fibroids in clinic [4].

The drug pair of Typhae Pollen and Trogopterus Feces which we named it for Shixiao San originally came from the *Classified Materia Medica* in volume twenty-two *jinxiao fang*, which was written by Shen-wei Tang in Song dynasty of ancient china [5]. As described in early publications, Typhae Pollen-Trogopterus Feces drug pair is famous for its remarkable and reliable therapeutic actions in a multitude diseases caused by blood stasis such as hyperlipidemia, atherosclerosis, thrombosis, stroke, angina pectoris and gynecological diseases by means of promoting blood circulation and removing stasis [6–8]. Typhae Pollen, known as Puhuang in Chinese is the dry pollen of typhaceae plant *Typha angustifolia* L., *Typha orientalis* Presl., and all species of the genus *Typha* [9]. Recent pharmacological study indicated that Typhae Pollen is proved to possess quite a few of biological activities including inducing uterine contractions, antioxidant, anti-inflammation, wound healing, and etc. [10–12], which owes to the main active ingredients among them like flavonoids, steroids, fatty acids, etc. [13]. Typhaneoside, vanillic acid and *p*-coumaric acid are just the three major bioactive components consist in Typhae Pollen due to their high content and significant bioactivities. Trogopterus feces also called Wulingzhi originally recorded in the *Kaibao Bencao*, and it is the dry feces of *Trogopterus xanthipes* Milne-Edwards (Petauristidae) [14]. It has been reported that the main chemical constituents including terpenoids [15], phenolic acids, sterols, aliphatics, fatty acids, and flavonoids are commonly used in the inhibition of tumor formation, inducing tumor cell apoptosis, antioxidant, reducing antithrombin levels, cytotoxic activity, immunity enhancement, anti-inflammatory activities, etc. [16, 17].

Drug pair, as is less known at abroad, it is the unique combination of two relatively fixed drugs based on theory of TCM in clinic, which nowadays have played a key role increasingly in the development of TCM and captured researcher's attention for the most fundamental and the simplest form of Chinese drug formulae [18, 19]. As the basic composition units of Chinese drug compatibility, reducing the toxicity and increasing the efficacy of drugs are supposed to be the basis of its efficiency [20]. With an increasing number of researches on drug pairs, works about the possible modes of actions for some famous pairs have obtained a certain achievement, just like Danggui Buxue Decoction (Astragali Radix and Angelicae sinensis Radix) [21] and Taoren-Honghua (Persicae Semen and Carthami Flos) herb pair [22]. More recent study suggested that how the synergistic effects of drug pairs come into being not only by changing the constitution or content of bioactive compounds but also regulating its absorption, distribution, metabolism and excretion (ADME) [23, 24].

According to the previous report, there are numerous studies about Typhae Pollen-Trogopterus Feces drug pair in each aspect while hardly any about the compatibility mechanism of it. Here, based on our early investigations [25, 26], the ultra-performance liquid chromatography coupled with a triple quadrupole electrospray tandem mass spectrometry (UPLC-TQ/MS) method has been performed to compare the pharmacokinetic profile of three major bioactive components including typhaneoside, vanillic acid and *p*-coumaric acid among Typhae Pollen-Trogopterus Feces drug pair before and after compatibility. Achievements of this study were desired to provide beneficial scientific information for revealing the reasonable compatibility of this drug pair and better understanding about its *in vivo* behavior mechanism.

Methods

Chemicals, reagents and materials

The reference standards of typhaneoside (111573–200603), vanillic acid (110776–200602), *p*-coumaric acid (D-032-120603) and diphenhydramine hydrochloride as internal standards (IS, 130356–200503) were purchased from the National Institute for the Control of Pharmaceutical and Biological Products (Beijing, China), the chemical structures of them are showed in Fig. 1.

Acetonitrile and methanol were of HPLC grade and obtained from Jiangsu Hanbon Science and Technology Co., Ltd. (China) and Tedia (Fairfield, USA), respectively. Formic acid was analytical grade from Merck (Darmstadt, Germany). Ultra-pure water was purified by an EPED super purification system (China). All other reagents were of analytical grade.

Typhae Pollen and Trogopterus Feces were purchased from Nanjing Chinese and Western Pharmaceutical Co., Ltd., and authenticated by the corresponding author. They were within the qualitative and quantitative stipulation of Chinese Pharmacopoeia. The voucher specimens (No.NJUTCM-20090118 for Typhae Pollen and No.NJUTCM-20090119 for Trogopterus Feces) were

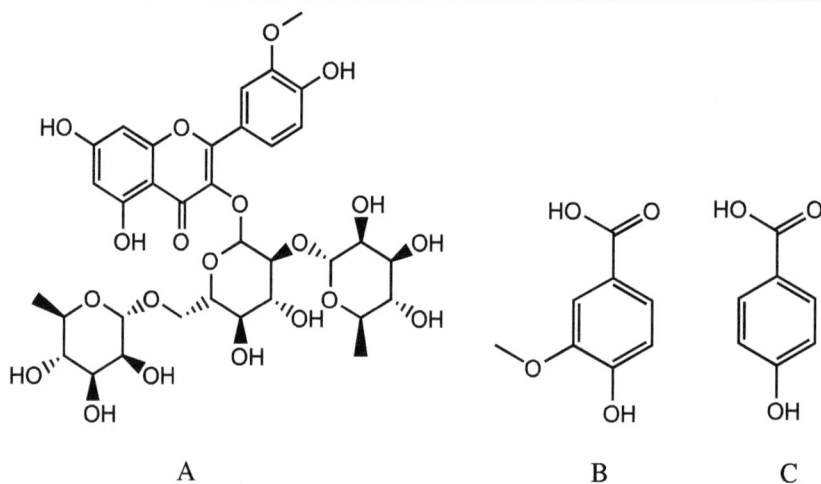

Fig. 1 Chemical structures of the reference substances (A. typhaneoside; B. vanillic acid; C. p-coumaric acid)

deposited at the herbarium in Nanjing University of Chinese Medicine, China.

Apparatus and UPLC-TQ/MS conditions

ACQUITY^{TM} UPLC system, XevoTM TQ mass spectrometry system (Waters Corp., Milford, MA, USA); EPED ultrapure water machine (Nanjing, China); Sartorius BT1250 electronic balance (Sartorius Scientific Instruments Corporation, Beijing, China); CENTRIVAP centrifuge enrichment apparatus (Labconco); ML303 electronic balance (Mettler Toledo Instruments Co., Ltd. Shanghai, China); TDL-80-2B centrifuge (Beckman Coulter, Inc.).

An ACQUITY UPLC BEH C_{18} column (2.1 mm × 100 mm, 1.7 μm, Waters Corp., Milford, MA, USA) was applied and the column temperature was maintained at 35 °C. The mobile phase was composed of A (0.1 % aqueous formic acid) and B (acetonitrile) using a gradient elution of 5–10 % B at 0–1 min, 10–30 % B at 1–6 min, 30–40 % B at 6–7 min, 40–95 % B at 7–8 min, 95–5 % B at 8–9 min, 95 % B at 9–10 min with a flow rate set at 0.4 mL/min. The auto-sampler was conditioned at 4 °C and the injection volume was 5 μL.

Mass spectrometry detection was performed by using a Xevo Triple Quadrupole MS (Waters Corp., Milford, MA) equipped with an electrospray ionization source (ESI). The ESI source was set in positive ionization mode. The scanning mode was set multiple reaction monitoring (MRM) mode. Parameters set in the source were as follows: the capillary voltage at 1 kV; sampling cone voltage of 30 V; source temperature 15 °C; desolvation temperature 550 °C; dwell time was automatically set by MassLynx (Waters Corp., Milford, MA, USA). The cone voltage and collision energy optimized for each analyte and selected values are given in Table 1.

Preparation of calibration standards and quality control (QC) samples

The mixture of standard stock solution containing above three compounds were prepared in methanol and giving a final concentrations of 28.2 μg/mL for typhaneoside, 25.7 μg/mL for vanillic acid, and 26.5 μg/mL for p-coumaric acid, respectively. The mixture stock solution was serially diluted with methanol to provide working standard solutions of desired concentration of 0.282 mg/mL for typhaneoside, 0.257 mg/mL for vanillic acid, and 0.265 mg/mL for p-coumaric acid, respectively. The IS stock solution were also prepared in methanol for diphenhydramine hydrochloride (IS) of 1.04 μg/mL.

Calibration standards and quality control (QC) samples were prepared as following: the mixture of standard working solution was diluted into eight different concentration gradients, and given the final concentration of 0.142 ~ 7100 ng/mL for typhaneoside, 0.104 ~ 5200 ng/mL for vanillic acid, 0.102 ~ 5100 ng/mL for p-coumaric acid. Quality control (QC) samples at low, middle and high concentrations were 3.55, 71.0, 710 ng/mL for typhaneoside, 2.60, 52.0, 260 ng/mL for vanillic acid and 2.55, 51.0, 255 ng/mL for p-coumaric acid. All solutions were stored at 4 °C and brought to room temperature before use. QC samples were stored at –20 °C before analysis.

Preparation of drug extraction and sample solutions

The raw materials of Typhae Pollen (200 g) for single extract and Typhae Pollen–Trogopterus Feces (200 g + 200 g) for co-decoction (two drugs decoct together) and mixed decoction (two drugs decoct separately and then mix) was accurately weighed, extracted with boiling

Table 1 The optimum mass spectrometry conditions for three compounds and IS

Analytes	Ionizationmode	MRM transitions (precursor-product)	Cone voltage (V)	Collision energy (eV)
Typhaneoside	ES$^+$	$771.0319 \rightarrow 317.0719$	18	26
Vanillic Acid	ES$^+$	$168.8404 \rightarrow 65.1300$	16	20
P-coumaric Acid	ES$^+$	$164.8404 \rightarrow 91.0910$	16	26
Diphenhydramine Hydrochloride	ES$^+$	$256.2127 \rightarrow 167.1291$	12	16

water (1:10) for 2 h, and then extracted with boiling water (1:8) for 2 h. The filtrates were combined and solvent was removed under reduced pressure in a rotary evaporator to reach a certain volume at the ratio of 1:1 (w/w, weight of all constituting drugs and the extract filtrates) for the TP single drug extraction; 2:1 for the TP-TF co-decoction and TP-TF mixed decoction. The contents of three compounds measured quantitatively by UPLC were 167.73, 168.37, 153.32 μg/mL for typhaneoside; 51.83, 48.67, 45.02 μg/mL for vanillic acid and 36.62, 35.67, 33.12 μg/mL for p-coumaric acid in single extract, co-decoction and mixed decoction, respectively.

A 200 μL aliquot of plasma sample was added with 10 μL diphenhydramine hydrochloride working solution and 600 μL of methanol. After vortex for 2 min and centrifugation at 13,000 rpm for 10 min, the supernatant was transferred to another 1.5 mL tube and concentrated in the centrifuge enrichment apparatus at 37 °C.

Finally, each residue was reconstituted in 200 μL 70 % methanol, then vortexed for 3 min and centrifuged at 13,000 rpm for 10 min. 5 μL of supernatant was injected into the UPLC-TQ/MS system for analysis.

Validation of the HPLC method
Specificity, linearity and LLOQ
The specificity of the method was evaluated by comparing chromatograms of blank plasma sample, blank plasma sample spiked with reference standards and internal standards, and plasma sample after oral administration of Typhae Pollen-Trogopterus Feces co-decoction for 30 min.

The linearity of each calibration curve was determined by plotting the peak area ratio (Y) of analytes to corresponding IS versus the nominal concentration (X) of analytes with weighted ($1/X^2$) least square linear regression. The lower limit of quantification (LLOQ) was determined as the lowest concentration with a signal-to-noise (S/N) ratio of 10.

Precision and accuracy
Accuracy and intra- and inter-day precision of the established method were evaluated by QC samples at low, medium and high concentrations (six samples for each)

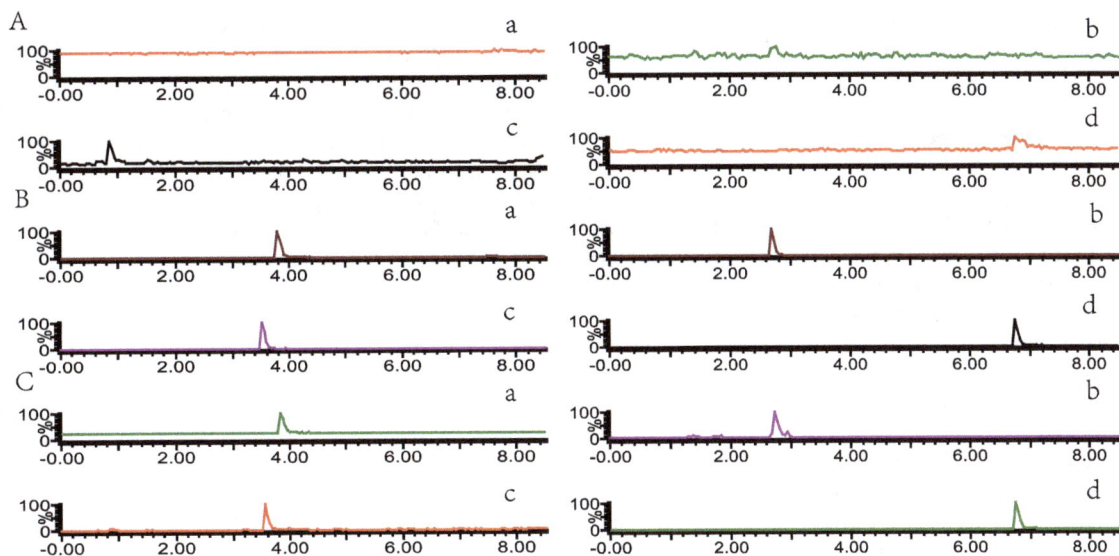

Fig. 2 Representative MRM chromatograms of the three components in rats: A. blank plasma. B. blank plasma samples spiked with reference standards and internal standards. C. plasma sample after oral administration of Typhae Pollen- Trogopterus Feces co-decoction for 30 min. Note: a. typhaneoside; b. vanillic acid;c. p-coumaric acid; d. diphenhydramine hydrochloride

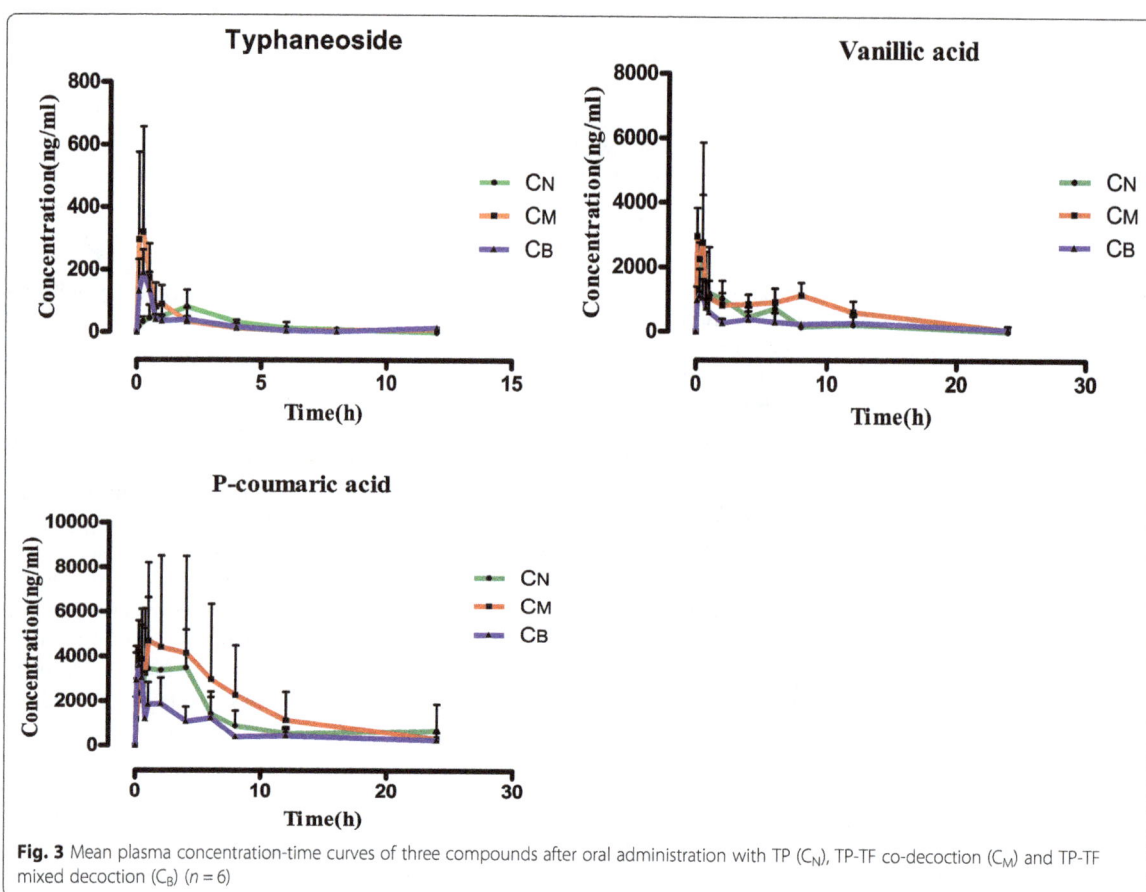

Fig. 3 Mean plasma concentration-time curves of three compounds after oral administration with TP (C_N), TP-TF co-decoction (C_M) and TP-TF mixed decoction (C_B) ($n = 6$)

on 3 consecutive validation days. The precision expressed by relative standard deviation (RSD%), and the accuracy by relative percentage error (%).

Extraction recovery, matrix effect and stability

The extraction recoveries of analytes were determined by comparing the peak responses of three QC samples (six samples for each) in the post-extraction spiked samples to that acquired from pre-extraction spiked samples at equivalent concentrations. The matrix effect was evaluated by comparing the peak responses of samples where the extracted matrix was spiked with standard solutions to those obtained from neat standard solutions at equivalent concentrations.

The stability of the analytes in rat plasma was assessed by analyzing QC samples at three concentration levels (six samples for each) under different condition. Three QC samples were tested for pre-treatment, post-treatment and three freeze-thaw cycles at room temperature for 12 h, refrigerated (4 °C) for 24 h and repeatedly frozen and thawed for three times at –80 °C, respectively.

Pharmacokinetic studies

All experiments were performed on female Sprague–Dawley (SD) rats, weighing 220–250 g, obtained from Shanghai Slac Laboratory Animal Co., Ltd. (Shanghai, China). They were kept in plastic cages at 22 ± 2 °C and a relative humidity of 50–65 %, with free access to pellet food and water on a 12 h light/dark cycle. Animal welfare and experimental procedures strictly conformed to the Guide for the Care and Use of Laboratory Animals [27] and the related ethics regulations of Nanjing University of Chinese Medicine.

For pharmacokinetic studies, the SD rats were divided into four groups randomly ($n = 6$ per group), and housed with unlimited access to food before the experiment while water available. Each group except the control group was oral administration of TP (C_N) single drug decoction, TP-TF co-decoction (C_M) and TP-TF mixed decoction (C_B) at a dosage of 5 g/kg, 10 g/kg, 10 g/kg body weight, respectively. Blood samples (0.5 mL) were collected at certain time points and placed at a 1.5 mL tube before oral (0 min) and after oral (5, 15, 30, 45, 60, 120, 240, 360, 480, 720 and 1440 min) administration. Afterwards all the blood samples were centrifuged at

13,000 rpm for 10 min and stored at −80 °C until analysis.

Results and discussion

Validation of the quantitative analysis

Fig. 2 shows the typical MRM chromatograms of blank plasma sample, blank plasma sample spiked with reference standards and internal standards, and plasma sample after oral administration of Typhae Pollen-Trogopterus Feces co-decoction for 30 min. No interference peaks were observed at the retention times of analytes and IS in any plasma that used for analysis, the method presented good specificity.

The linear regression equation, correlation coefficient and LLOQ for typhaneoside, vanillic acid and p-coumaric acid in rat plasma samples are shown in Additional file 1. The calibration curves exhibited good linearity with correlation coefficients (r) and the LLOQ were sufficient for pharmacokinetic studies of these analytes.

Intra-day, inter-day accuracy and precision of the three compounds in rat plasma samples are presented in Additional file 2, which showed the method with good accuracy and precision. All the results were found to be within the accepted variable limits.

Extraction recoveries and matrix effect of the three compounds were evaluated by analyzing QC samples at low, medium and high concentrations with six replicates. As the results are shown in Additional file 3, the mean recovery of the analytes was within 70 to 91 % (RSD was less than 11). The corresponding matrix effect ranged from 76 to 106 % (RSD was less than 9).

The stability of the analytes in rat plasma samples was evaluated under different conditions. Deviations for the peak area of the three components were within 15 %, which indicated good stability under the experimental conditions.

Pharmacokinetic study

The mean plasma concentration-time profiles of typhaneoside, vanillic acid and p-coumaric acid were determined after oral administration with different compatibility of Typhae Pollen-Trogopterus Feces drug pair in rats, the concentration-time curves are presents in Fig. 3, and the noncompartment model pharmacokinetic parameters including maximum plasma concentration (C_{max}), time to reach the maximum concentrations (T_{max}), half-time ($T_{1/2}$), area under concentration-time curve ($AUC_{0 \sim t}$) are summarized in Table 2.

From the datas, it indicated that typhaneoside, vanillic acid and p-coumaric acid could be detected immediately by UPLC-TQ/MS, which revealed superior absorption of the three compounds, and significant differences existed among three different compatibilities, all comparing to the control group with TP single drug extraction by t-test. For typhaneoside, the peak plasma concentration (C_{max}) was 370.86 ± 315.71 ng/mL ($P < 0.05$) in TP-TF co-decoction group (C_M) and 214.32 ± 73.72 ng/mL ($P < 0.01$) in TP-TF mixed decoction group (C_B), it was significantly higher than TP single drug extraction (C_N), though in the previous report it was described as a low bioavailability [28]. What's more, the time to reach maximum concentrations (T_{max}) were 0.24 ± 0.15 h ($P < 0.05$) for TP-TF co-decoction group (C_M) and 0.21 ± 0.08 h for TP-TF mixed decoction group (C_B), which implies highly uptake of this compound in rats plasma.

As a kind of common compound in many Chinese medicines, vanillic acid in TP-TF co-decoction group (C_M) had a good absorption after oral administration for the C_{max} was 3870.99 ± 2527.99 ng/mL and T_{max} was 1.47 ± 3.20 h. In TP-TF mixed decoction group (C_B) the

Table 2 Noncompartment model pharmacokinetic parameters of the three compounds after oral administration with extracts ($n = 6$)

Compounds	Pharmacokinetic parameters	TP	TP-TF co-decoction	TP-TF mixed decoction
Typhaneoside	C_{max} (ng/mL)	76.39 ± 53.21	$370.86 \pm 315.71^{*}$	$214.32 \pm 73.72^{**}$
	T_{max} (h)	2.95 ± 2.88	$0.24 \pm 0.15^{*}$	0.21 ± 0.08
	$T_{1/2}$ (h)	3.35 ± 2.58	1.91 ± 1.26	1.37 ± 0.54
	$AUC_{0 \sim t}$ (ng/h/mL)	268.31 ± 167.71	333.46 ± 191.84	275.62 ± 206.06
Vanillic acid	C_{max} (ng/mL)	2211.68 ± 1187.17	3870.99 ± 2527.99	1447.29 ± 500.99
	T_{max} (h)	1.25 ± 0.71	1.47 ± 3.20	$0.17 \pm 0.09^{**}$
	$T_{1/2}$ (h)	3.69 ± 0.87	11.25 ± 13.61	8.88 ± 3.76
	$AUC_{0 \sim t}$ (ng/h/mL)	10445.53 ± 4148.68	14137.57 ± 4540.37	6193.78 ± 4499.17
P-coumaric acid	C_{max} (ng/mL)	4901.39 ± 1887.30	5110.22 ± 3671.26	4189.45 ± 844.37
	T_{max} (h)	1.08 ± 1.67	1.42 ± 1.39	0.46 ± 0.40
	$T_{1/2}$ (h)	3.67 ± 1.82	10.08 ± 7.86	10.08 ± 10.23
	$AUC_{0 \sim t}$ (ng/h/mL)	36881.01 ± 25783.25	41512.56 ± 41763.28	17689.11 ± 3882.21

$^{*}P < 0.05$, $^{**}P < 0.01$ versus TP sole administration

C_{max} was 1447.29 ± 500.99 ng/mL and T_{max} 0.17 ± 0.09 h ($P < 0.01$). In addition, it is not difficult to find that T_{max} and $T_{1/2}$ in co-decoction group (C_M) were longer than the two others, and double peak phenomenon was observed at the same time, it probably attribute to the enterohepatic circulation in drug metabolism or the interactivity in Typhae pollen-Trogopterus Feces drug pair. Similarly as vanillic acid, p-coumaric acid was also absorbed well, C_{max} was 5110.22 ± 3671.26 ng/mL in TP-TF co-decoction group (C_M) in addition to its T_{max} was somewhat longer. It may be in virtue of its hydrolyzed diffusion *in vivo* after oral administration with decoction [29], and we can see double peaks clearly on the concentration-time curves, all these hypothesis need further investigations.

When making comparison between TP-TF co-decoction group (C_M) and TP-TF mixed decoction group (C_B), C_{max} and $AUC_{0\sim t}$ of the three active ingredients in TP-TF co-decoction group (C_M) are higher than TP-TF mixed decoction group (C_B). It proved that the absorption was increased after compatibility and the duration of drug action was prolonged for $T_{1/2}$ of the three compounds in TP-TF co-decoction group (C_M) were longer than TP-TF mixed decoction group (C_B). Generally speaking, the TP-TF co-decoction group (C_M) showed more advantages of bioavailability for bioactive components.

The results indicated that after Typhae Pollen and Trogopterus Feces used in combination as a drug pair, the three bioactive compounds typhaneoside, vanillic acid and p-coumaric acid were well absorbed and slowly eliminated in rats, thus to enhance and prolong clinical efficacy, which may be due to the synergic action between Typhae Pollen and Trogopterus Feces. According to traditional Chinese medicine theory, the compatibility mechanisms of drug pairs are not only arbitrary plus of two drugs but also the regularity of active components *in vivo* [30]. When Typhae Pollen combined with Trogopterus Feces, the dissolution of chemical ingredients were increased [31], followed by the good absorption of three components in TP. We speculated that it's probably the volatile components in TF which enhanced the absorption of the three components in TP [32, 33]. Furthermore the higher uptake and slower elimination of three compounds in TP by drug pair administration were related to the interaction between drugs mediated by transport proteins, metabolic enzymes, or plasma protein binding, etc. The compatibility mechanism of TP-TF still deserves further research.

Conclusion

In this paper, the simple, rapid and sensitive UPLC-TQ/MS method was successfully applied to detect three bioactive components in Typhae Pollen before and after the

combination with Trogopterus Feces simultaneously. It was the first study to report about the pharmacokinetic parameters of typhaneoside, vanillic acid and p-coumaric acid in TP-TF after oral administration. Results indicated that the three compounds have better absorption and slower elimination after Typhae Pollen and Trogopterus Feces combination. The *in vivo* changes of three main active substances was helpful for finding the compatibility principles of TP-TF and clarifying its rational compatibility, thus for better clinical application and research about relative TCM formulas.

Additional files

Additional file 1: The regression equations, correlation coefficient, linear ranges and LLOQ of three analytes ($n = 6$). (DOC 21 kb)

Additional file 2: Intra-day, inter-day accuracy and precision of three analytes ($n = 6$). (DOC 21 kb)

Additional file 3: Recoveries and matrix effects of three analytes ($n = 6$). (DOC 21 kb)

Abbreviations
TP: Typhae Pollen; TF: Trogopterus Feces; C_N: TP single extract group; C_M: TP–TF co-decoction group; C_B: TP–TF mixed decoction group; BS: Blood stasis; TCM: Traditional Chinese Medicine; ADME: Absorption, distribution, metabolism and excretion; UPLC-TQ/MS: Ultra-performance liquid chromatography coupled with a triple quadrupole electrospray tandem mass spectrometry; ESI: Electrospray ionization source; MRM: Multiple reaction monitoring; QC: Quality control; LLOQ: Lower limit of quantification; SD: Sprague–Dawley.

Competing interests
The authors declare that they have no competing interest.

Authors' contribution
HTZ performed the experiments, analyzed the data and drafted the manuscript. PX, XCH and JMG assisted in carrying out experiments. JAD, YPT and SLS participated in the conception and design of the study. EXS and DWQ performed the statistical analysis and revised the manuscript. All authors read and approved the final version of the manuscript.

Acknowledgements
This work was supported by the Key Research Project in Basic Science of Jiangsu College and University (No. 11KJA360002; 12KJA360002) and the National Natural Science Foundation of China (No. 81373889; 81102898; 81102885). This work was also supported by the Construction Project for Jiangsu Key Laboratory for High Technology Research of TCM Formulae (BM2010576; BK2010561), and supported by Program for Excellent Talents in School of Pharmacy of Nanjing University of Chinese Medicine (15ZYXET-2), and a project funded by the Priority Academic Program Development of Jiangsu Higher Education Institutions (ysxk-2014) and the Construction Project for Jiangsu Collaborative Innovation Center of Chinese Medicinal Resources Industrialization. This work was also supported by 2013 Program for New Century Excellent Talents by the Ministry of Education (Grant NCET-13-0873), 333 High-level Talents Training Project Funded by Jiangsu Province, and Six Talents Project Funded by Jiangsu Province (2012-YY-010).

Author details
[1]Jiangsu Key Laboratory for High Technology Research of TCM Formulae, Nanjing University of Chinese Medicine, Nanjing 210023, China. [2]Jiangsu Collaborative Innovation Center of Chinese Medicinal Resources Industrialization, Nanjing University of Chinese Medicine, Nanjing 210023, China. [3]National and Local Collaborative Engineering Center of Chinese Medicinal Resources Industrialization and Formulae Innovative Medicine, Nanjing University of Chinese Medicine, Nanjing 210023, China. [4]Jiangsu Key

Laboratory for TCM Formulae Research, Nanjing University of Chinese Medicine, Nanjing 210046, People's Republic of China.

References

1. Park B, Yun KJ, Jung J, You S, Lee JA, Choi J, et al. Conceptualization and utilization of blood stasis syndrome among doctors of Korean medicine: results of a web-based survey. Am J Eransl Res. 2014;6(6):857–68.

2. Zhao XJ, Zhang Y, Meng XL, Yin PY, Deng C, Chen J, et al. Effect of a traditional Chinese medicine preparation Xindi soft capsule on rat model of acute blood stasis: a urinary metabonomics study based onliquid chromatography–mass spectrometry. J Chromatogr B. 2008;873(2):151–8.

3. Park YJ, Yang DH, Lee JM, Park YB. Development of a valid and reliable blood stasis questionnaire and its relationship to heart rate variability. Complement Ther Med. 2013;21(6):633–40.

4. Su SL, Cui WX, Duan JA, Hua YQ, Guo JM, Shang EX, et al. UHPLC-MS Simultaneous determination and pharmacokinetic study of three aromatic acids and one monoterpene in rat plasma after oral administration of Shaofu Zhuyu Decoction. Am J Chin Med. 2013;41(3):697–715.

5. Zhou W, Su SL, Duan JA, Tao WW. The association analysis of shixiaosan's traditional utility and modern research. Chin Trad Plant Med. 2009;31(10):1602–4.

6. Zhang P, Xia XH, Li Q. The effects of anti-thrombosis and thrombolysis of diferent solvent extract of shixiaosan. China Pharm. 2003;12(3):44–5.

7. Wang XF, Zhao X, Gu LQ, Zhang YY, Bi KS, Chen XH. Discrimination of aqueous and vinegary extracts of Shixiao San using metabolomics coupled with multivariate data analysis and evaluation of anti-hyperlipidemic effect. Asi J Pharm Sci. 2014;9(1):17–26.

8. Zhou W, Su SL, Liu P, Hua YQ, Duan JA. Effects of promoting blood circulation to remove blood stasis of Puhuang-Wulingzhi drug pair in Shaofu Zhuyu Decoction. Chin J Exp Tradit Med Form. 2010;16(6):179–83.

9. Chen PD, Liu SJ, Dai GL, Xie LY, Xu J, Zhou L, et al. Determination of typhaneoside in rat plasma by liquid chromatography–tandem mass spectrometry. J Pharm Biomed Anal. 2012;70:636–9.

10. Lee BC, Park HM, Sims HS, Kim GS, Gu SH, Oh MJ. Biological activity and chemical analysis of cattail pollens. J Agric Sci. 2009;36(2):185–97.

11. Sun B, Sun GB, Xiao J, Chen RC, Wang X, Wu Y, et al. Isorhamnetin inhibits H_2O_2-induced activation of the intrinsic apoptotic pathway in H9c2 cardiomyocytes through scavenging reactive oxygen species and ERK inactivation. J Cell Biochem. 2012;113(2):473–85.

12. Peterson JJ, Dwyer JT, Jacques PF, McCullough ML. Associations between flavonoids and cardiovascular disease incidence or mortality in European and US populations. Nutr Rev. 2012;70(9):491–508.

13. Gallardo-Williams MT, Geiger CL, Pidala JA, Martin DF. Essential fatty acids and phenolic acids from extracts and leachates of southern cattail (Typha domingensis P.). Phytochemistry. 2002;59(3):305–8.

14. Yang NY, Tao WW, Zhu M, Duan JA, Zhang JG. Two new isopimarane diterpenes from the feces of Trogopterus xanthipes. Fitoterapia. 2010;81(5):381–4.

15. Zhao J, Zhu HJ, Zhou XJ, Yang TH, Wang YY, Su J, et al. Diterpenoids from the feces of Trogopterus xanthipes. J Nat Prod. 2010;73(5):865–9.

16. Yang NY, Tao WW, Duan JA. Antithrombotic flavonoids from the faeces of Trogopterus xanthipes. Nat Prod Res. 2010;24(19):1843–9.

17. Baek S, Xia X, Min BS, Park C, Shim SH. Trogopterins A-C: Three new neolignans from feces of Trogopterus xanthipes. Beilstein J Org Chem. 2014;10:2955–62.

18. Wang SP, Hu YY, Tan W, Wu X, Chen RE, Cao JL, et al. Compatibility art of traditional Chinese medicine: From the perspective of herb pairs. J Ethnopharmacol. 2012;143(2):412–23.

19. Guo YP, Lin LG, Wang YT. Chemistry and pharmacology of the herb pair *Flos Lonicerae japonicae-Forsythiae fructus*. Chin Med. 2015;10:16.

20. Chen L, Yang J, Davey AK, Chen YX, Wang JP, Liu XQ. Effects of diammonium glycyrrhizinate on the pharmacokinetics of aconitine in rats and the potential mechanism. Xenobiotica. 2009;39(12):955–63.

21. Shi XQ, Tang YP, Zhu HX, Li WX, Li ZH, Li W, et al. Comparative tissue distribution profiles of five major bioactive components in normal and blood deficiency rats after oral administration of Danggui Buxue Decoction by UPLC-TQ/MS. J Pharm Biomed Anal. 2014;88:207–15.

22. Liu L, Duan JA, Tang YP, Guo JM, Yang NY, Ma HY, et al. Taoren–Honghua herb pair and its main components promoting blood circulation through influencing on hemorheology, plasma coagulation and platelet aggregation. J Ethnopharmacol. 2012;139(2):381–7.

23. Gilbert B, Alves LF. Synergy in plant medicines. Curr Med Chem. 2003;10(1):13–20.

24. Ung CY, Li H, Cao ZW, Li YX, Chen YZ. Are herb-pairs of traditional Chinese medicine distinguishable from others? Pattern analysis and artificial intelligence classification study of traditionally defined herbal properties. J Ethnopharmacol. 2007;111(2):371–7.

25. Su SL, Hua YQ, Duan JA, Zhou W, Shang EX, Tang YP. Inhibitory effects of active fraction and its main components of Shaofu Zhuyu Decoction on uterus contraction. Am J Chin Med. 2010;38(4):777–87.

26. Zhou W, Su SL, Duan JA, Guo JM, Qian DW, Shang EX, et al. Characterization of the active constituents in Shixiao San using bioactivity evaluation followed by UPLC-QTOF and Markerlynx analysis. Molecules. 2010;15(9):6217–30.

27. National Research Council. Guide for the care and use of laboratory animals. Washington, D.C: National Academies Press; 2011.

28. Huang XC, Su SL, Cui WX, Liu P, Duan JA, Guo JM, et al. Simultaneous determination of paeoniflorin, albiflorin, ferulic acid, tetrahydropalmatine, protopine, typhaneoside, senkyunolide I in Beagle dogs plasma by UPLC–MS/MS and its application to a pharmacokinetic study after Oral Administration of Shaofu Zhuyu Decoction. J Chromatogr B. 2014;962:75–81.

29. Liu K, Yan LQ, Yao GC, Guo XJ. Estimation of p-coumaric acid as metabolite of E-6-O-p-coumaroyl scandoside methyl ester in rat plasma by HPLC and its application to a pharmacokinetic study. J Chromatogr B. 2006;831(1–2):303–6.

30. Bi XL, Gong MR, Di LQ. Review on prescription compatibility of Shaoyao Gancao Decoction and reflection on pharmacokinetic compatibility mechanism of traditional Chinese medicine prescription based on *in vivo* drug interaction of main efficacious components. Evid Based Complement Alternat Med. 2014; Article ID 208129, 8 pages.

31. Su SL, Xue P, Ouyang Z, Zhou W, Duan JA. Study on antiplatelet and antithrombin activitives and effective components variation of Puhuang-Wulingzhi before and after compatibility. Zhongguo Zhong Yao Za Zhi. 2015; 40(16):3187–93.

32. Cheng M, Yang LX, Yang LJ, Feng XF, Wang HJ. GC-MS analysis on volatile components of wild Trogopterus Faeces from Laishui county of Hebei province. Zhongguo Zhong Yao Za Zhi. 2011;36(24):3480–3.

33. Qi JP, Sun MJ, Ping QE, Zhuang J, Li JR, Peddie F, et al. The Mechanisms for enhanced oral absorption of hydroxysafflor yellow A by Chuanxiong volatile oil. Planta Med. 2010;76(8):786–92.

26

Effects of phloretin on oxidative and inflammatory reaction in rat model of cecal ligation and puncture induced sepsis

Mehdi Aliomrani[1,2], Mohammad Reza Sepand[1,2], Hamid Reza Mirzaei[3], Ali Reza kazemi[1,2], Saeid Nekonam[4] and Omid Sabzevari[5,2*]

Abstract

Background: Sepsis is a debilitating systemic disease and described as a severe and irregular systemic inflammatory reaction syndrome (SIRS) against infection. We employed CLP (Cecal Ligation and Puncture) model in rats to investigate anti-inflammatory and antioxidant effects of phloretin, as a natural antioxidant agent, and its protective effect on liver tissue damage caused by sepsis.

Methods: Male Wistar albino rats were randomly divided into three groups: sham group, CLP induced sepsis group and phloretin treated CLP group. Sepsis was induced by CLP method. 50 mmol/kg Phloretin was administered intraperitoneally in two equal doses immediately after surgery.

Results: It was observed that blood urea nitrogen (BUN) and tumor necrosis factor alpha (TNF-α) levels were dramatically increased in the CLP induced sepsis group (43.88 ± 1.905 mg/dl, 37.63 ± 1.92, respectively) when compared to the sham group. Moreover, tissue Glutathione (GSH) and liver nuclear factor κB (NF-κB p65) transcription factor values were higher in CLP induced sepsis group. This elevation was considerably reduced in the phloretin treated CLP group. No significant differences were observed in serum creatinine and creatinine phosphokinase levels.

Conclusions: The present study suggested that phloretin, as a natural protective agent, act against tissue damages introduced following the experimental sepsis induced model, likely caused by free oxygen radicals.

Keywords: Phloretin, Sepsis, NF-κB, TNF- α, Oxidative stress, Antioxidants

Background

Sepsis is a common and expensive condition especially in the elderly, which is associated with a very high mortality rate (40 to 60 %) [1, 2]. In spite of advances in critical care treatment of the disease such as invasive surgical therapy and chemotherapy, and better understanding of its pathophysiology, the fatal frequency has not changed significantly over the past 35 years, even in developed countries. Sepsis is described as a severe and irregular systemic inflammatory reaction syndrome (SIRS) against infection [3]. Bacterial lipopolysaccharide

endotoxins trigger macrophages and enhance the release of pro-inflammatory cytokines, hence play a pivotal role in the development of systemic inflammatory response. Free oxygen radicals are among important mediators responsible for the inflammatory response. They disrupt cell membranes by rising lipid peroxidation, inhibit ATP synthesis in the mitochondria, and may lead to oxidative damage to DNA and proteins [4].

The systemic inflammatory stress response such as sepsis, septic shock, and multiple organ dysfunction syndromes are conditions of severity and deterioration of essential organ function [5, 6]. It has been documented that a relation exists between oxidative stress and peritoneal sepsis [7]. Antioxidant agents might counter the toxicity of reactive oxygen species and reactive nitrogen species [8, 9], thus free radical ablation might be

* Correspondence: omid@tums.ac.ir
[5]Drug design and discovery Research Centre, Tehran University of Medical Sciences, Tehran, Iran
[2]Department of Pharmacology and Toxicology, Faculty of Pharmacy, Tehran University of Medical Sciences, P. O. Box, 1417614411, Tehran, Iran
Full list of author information is available at the end of the article

complementary in the clinical management of sepsis-induced multiple organ failures [10].

Secondary plant metabolites are a vast group of chemicals that are synthesized from carbohydrates, fatty acids and amino acids [11]. Flavonoids are polyphenolic compounds in a natural manner and represent one of the most extensive ingredients in fruits, vegetables, nuts, tea and coffee [11], as well as in herbal medicine [12]. Flavonoids are made up of flavones, flavonols, flavanones, chalcones, anthocyanins, and isoflavones. Flavonoids are well known for their role as an anti-inflammatory and antioxidant agents and shown to have health encouraging, chemopreventive, and disease-preventing characteristics [13, 14].

Chalcones contain 2 benzene rings which are bound together by an unsaturated carboxyl group. They are the secondary metabolite of plants with a chemical structure similar to curcumin [15]. By now, chalcones proven to have many therapeutic characteristics such as antifungal, anti-leishmania, anti-bacterial, anti-malarial and chemopreventive activities, in which part of these properties disclosed to antioxidant activity and chelating the metallic ions [16, 17]. Phloretin is a dihydrogen chalcone flavonoid which primarily extracted from apple [18]. Many studies have demonstrated the pharmacophore responsible region for the anti oxidative activity of phloretin [19, 20]. However, no detailed investigation has described the role of phloretin in sepsis induced by CLP model. This study was designed to investigate protective effect of phloretin against sepsis-induced oxidative organ damage using biochemical parameters, such as nuclear factor kappa-light-chain-enhancer of activated B cells (NF-κB), tumor necrosis factor–alpha (TNF-α) and tissue glutathione (GSH) levels as well as the histopathological examination of liver tissues.

Methods
Chemicals
2′, 4′, 6′, 4 Tetrahrdroxydihydrochalcone (phloretin) was obtained from Sigma-Aldrich Company (St. Louis, MO, USA). All solvents including ethanol, tween 80 and DMSO were supplied by Merck Company (Darmstadt, Germany). TNF-α assay kit were purchased from Biosource Europe, S.A. (Nivelles, Belgium). P65 NF-κB transcription factor kit was obtained from Cayman chemical (USA).

Animals
Animal experiments were carried on in the light of the protocol of Ministry of Health & Medical Education Convention for the Protection of vertebrate animals used for experimental and other scientific goals, and the protocol was accepted by the Ethics Committee of the Tehran University of Medicine Sciences (TUMS), Tehran, Iran.

Male Wistar albino rats, weighing 200-250 g, were included in the study. The rats were kept in a temperature controlled (22 ± 1 °C) room with a 12:12 h alternating light/dark cycle in Animal Care Center, Faculty of Pharmacy, TUMS.

Cecal Ligation and Puncture (CLP) as a sepsis model
General anesthesia was applied to the rats using ketamine HCl (100 mg/kg) and xylazine HCl (10 mg/kg) via intraperitoneal route. The subjects were immobilized on the operation table in the supine position and the abdominal skin was shaved totally, and laparotomy was carried out through a 2 cm midline incision. Poly microbial sepsis was induced by the CLP technique described previously [21]. The cecum was isolated through laparotomy, and the ascending colon was gently touched downward to fill the cecum with feces. The cecum was ligated below the ileocecal valve using 3.0 silk thread, and the ventral side was perforated twice using No.21 gauge needle to let fecal contents spread into the peritoneum. Then, the abdomen was closed with two layers continuous suture using 3.0 silk thread. Rats were resuscitated with normal saline (1 ml/100 g body weight given subcutaneously) at the end of the operation. In the sham group, the cecum was explored but CLP was not applied. The rats were monitored in room temperature of 22 °C, with controlled humidity and light and allowed standard food and drinking water till 12 h after the operation. All the rats were sacrificed 24 h after operation.

Experimental protocol
The rats were randomly subdivided into 4 groups of 7 rats. Group I (Sham group): operative procedure was applied, but cecal ligation perforation was not performed. Group II (CLP group): sepsis was induced using the cecal ligation and perforation (CLP) method. Group III (Phloretin group): sepsis was induced using the CLP method and 50 mmol/kg phloretin was administered via the intraperitoneal route in two equal doses immediately after surgery and at the post-operative 12th hour and finally, control group which peritoneally received dimethyl sulfoxide as phloretin solvent [15, 22].

Blood collection and determination of biochemical parameters
Blood samples collected through a cardiac puncture, centrifuged at 1000 g for 5 min and serum was separated. The samples were then transferred into Eppendorf tubes and stored at 4 °C within 1 h after collection for biochemical assay according to the instructions provided by the manufacturers.

Serum creatinine concentration was measured using Jaffe method [21]. The rest of serum was stored at -70 °C for further analysis. BUN and creatine phosphokinase (CPK) were determined by UV method using auto analyzer (COBAS Integra C111; Roche Diagnostics, Switzerland).

Measurement of serum TNF-α level

Serum level of TNF-α, as an inflammatory cytokine, was assayed according to the manufacturer's instruction using an enzyme-linked immunosorbent assay (ELISA) kit from BioSource Europe. The concentration of TNF-α was calculated from the standard curve and results were presented as pg/ml.

Immunoassay of NF-κB P65

To investigate liver NF-κB activity, p65 Transcription Factor Assay kit (Cayman chemical) was employed. NF-κB activity was measured calorimetrically according to the manufacturer's instructions. For preparation of hepatic cells nuclear fraction, frozen liver tissue was homogenized in lysis buffer with 2 % Triton X-100 and aprotinin, and centrifuged at 1000 g for 5 min. The pellet was then resuspended in 5 ml ice-cold 1X Nuclear extraction PBS/Phosphatase inhibitor solution and centrifuged at 300xg for 5 min at 4 °C, and the aliquot of the nuclear extract was used for the measurement. Total proteins were quantified by Lowry's method (Lowry et al. 1951). Briefly, 10 μl of samples were added to the appropriate well that contained its relevant complete transcription factor buffer (CTFB). The plate was incubated overnight at 4 °C, and the wells were washed with 1x washing buffer five times. Primary antibody was then added to the appropriate well, and the plate was incubated for 1 h at 37 °C. Subsequently, the horseradish peroxidase (HRP) linked secondary antibody was added and the plate was incubated for 30 min at 37 °C. Following addition of the substrate, plates were incubated for 45 min at room temperature, the reaction was stopped and samples were measured spectrophotometerically at 450 nm. Each phosphoprotein absorbance was corrected by the negative control and was normalized by its relevant NF-κB p65 absorbance.

Tissue GSH level

The level of GSH was determined by the method explained previously by Sedlak and Lindsay [22]. This assay is based on the production of yellow color when 5, 5-dithionitrobisbenzoic acid (DTNB) is added to compounds containing sulphydryl groups. The liver tissue was homogenized in 0.02 M EDTA and mixed for 10–15 min with an equal volume of 10 % TCA. It was then centrifuged at 10,000 g for 10 min. 1 ml of the supernatant was mixed with 0.5 ml of Ellman's reagents (19.8 mg of DTNB in 100 ml of 0.1 % sodium nitrate) and 3 ml of phosphate buffer (0.2 M, pH 8.0). The absorbance was immediately recorded at 412 nm on a spectrophotometer. Results were expressed as μmol GSH/g tissue [23].

Histopathological examination

Liver tissues were fixed in a 10 % formalin solution. They were washed with PBS buffer overnight and were slowly dehydrated by crossing through the solutions by enhancing the concentrations of alcohol. Subsequently, the tissue samples were placed in paraffin and were fixed in blocks. Then sections with 5-6 μm thickness were obtained from the tissue samples placed on slides. Finally, slides were stained by hematoxylin-eosin and examined under a light microscope (Olympus BHX51; Tokyo, Japan) at X40 magnification.

Statistical analysis

Statistical analysis was performed using a GraphPad Prism 3.0 (GraphPad Software, San Diego; CA; USA). Data were evaluated by one-way analysis of variance (ANOVA) and Tukey's test was used for pairwise comparisons. All data were expressed as means ± SEM. Values of $p \leq 0.05$ were considered as statistically significant.

Results

Blood Urea Nitrogen (BUN)

Our findings showed that cecal ligation and puncture caused a significant increase in serum BUN level (43.88 ± 1.905 mg/dl) compared with the sham group (26.17 ± 2.303), $p < 0.01$. Following treatment with phloretin (CLP + P), serum BUN levels were decreased (31.77 ± 1.514 mg/dl), in comparison with CLP group ($p < 0.01$), Fig. 1a.

Serum creatinine level (Scr)

Serum creatinine mildly increased in CLP group (0.670 ± 0.017) in comparison with the sham group (0.575 ± 0.027). There were no significant differences in serum creatinine level between phloretin treated (0.646 ± 0.023) and untreated control group ($p < 0.05$), Fig. 1b.

Serum Creatine Phosphokinase (CPK)

The serum CPK level was not changed significantly when compared to the sham group, Fig. 1c.

Serum TNF-α levels

TNF-α levels were dramatically increased in CLP operated group (37.63 ± 1.92) when compared to the sham group (10.69 ± 1.03), $p < 0.05$. This rise was significantly abolished following phloretin treatment (29.14 ± 2.29) $p < 0.05$, Fig. 2.

Liver NF-κB level

The protective effect of phloretin on liver NF-κB level is shown in Fig. 3. In CLP group, the liver NF-κB level was significantly elevated (more than two-fold) in comparison

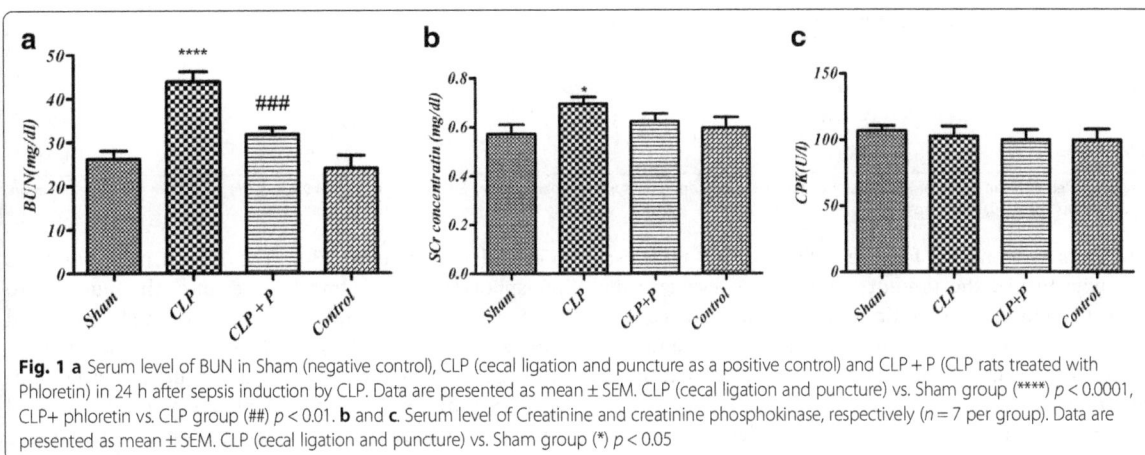

Fig. 1 a Serum level of BUN in Sham (negative control), CLP (cecal ligation and puncture as a positive control) and CLP + P (CLP rats treated with Phloretin) in 24 h after sepsis induction by CLP. Data are presented as mean ± SEM. CLP (cecal ligation and puncture) vs. Sham group (****) $p < 0.0001$, CLP+ phloretin vs. CLP group (##) $p < 0.01$. **b** and **c**. Serum level of Creatinine and creatinine phosphokinase, respectively ($n = 7$ per group). Data are presented as mean ± SEM. CLP (cecal ligation and puncture) vs. Sham group (*) $p < 0.05$

with the sham group ($p < 0.05$), whereas the elevation was significantly reduced in the phloretin treated group.

Tissue Glutathione (GSH) levels

Sepsis caused a significant decrease (p ≤0.01–p ≤0.0001) in GSH levels in liver, kidney, heart and lung tissues in comparison to the sham group. Phloretin treatment significantly ($p < 0.05$) restored the GSH level (Table 1).

Histopathological findings

Histological examinations were carried out by a pathologist and pathological events were scored semi-quantitatively. Slides were stained with hematoxylin-eosin and vascular change, local necrosis, hepatocytes morphology, presence and severity of poly morphonuclear leukocytes (PMNL) were considered in the histopathological sections of the liver tissue.

Normal sinusoids and hepatocytes were noticed in the hepatic parenchyma of the sham group, Fig. 4a. Within sepsis group, serious sinusoidal duct dilation and vascular obstruction, and damaged hepatocytes with many cytoplasmic vacuoles were seen. Moreover, increased number of Kupffer cells and liver dead cells (LDC) were found, Fig. 4b. Meanwhile, treatment with phloretin improved sinusoidal duct dilation, vascular blockage, and hepatocytes morphology. In addition, phloretin decreased the foam like cells near the lobular central vein, Fig. 4c.

Discussion

Sepsis is described as a severe and irregular systemic inflammatory reaction syndrome (SIRS) against infection, and free oxygen radicals are among important

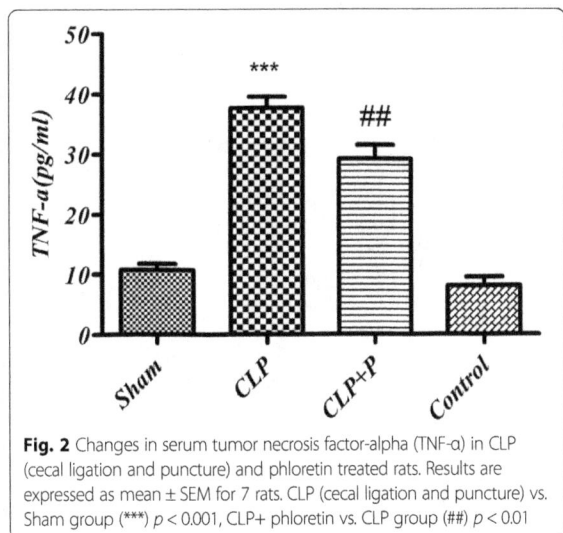

Fig. 2 Changes in serum tumor necrosis factor-alpha (TNF-α) in CLP (cecal ligation and puncture) and phloretin treated rats. Results are expressed as mean ± SEM for 7 rats. CLP (cecal ligation and puncture) vs. Sham group (***) $p < 0.001$, CLP+ phloretin vs. CLP group (##) $p < 0.01$

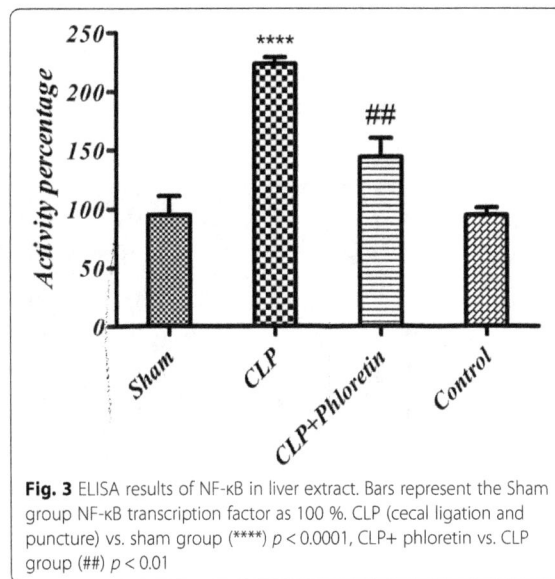

Fig. 3 ELISA results of NF-κB in liver extract. Bars represent the Sham group NF-κB transcription factor as 100 %. CLP (cecal ligation and puncture) vs. sham group (****) $p < 0.0001$, CLP+ phloretin vs. CLP group (##) $p < 0.01$

Table 1 Tissue glutathione level (μmol/g) in septic rats treated with phloretin

Groups	Liver	Kidney	Lung	Heart
Sham	7.08 ± 0.15	5.38 ± 0.09	7.82 ± 0.5	6.38 ± 0.29
CLP	$4.87 \pm 0.24^{***}$	$3.94 \pm 0.27^{***}$	$6.07 \pm 0.14^{***}$	$4.94 \pm 0.32^{****}$
CLP + Phloretin	$6.08 \pm 0.11^{###}$	$4.93 \pm 0.17^{##}$	$7.02 \pm 0.82^{##}$	$4.81 \pm 0.13^{##}$

Data presented as Mean ± SEM of 7 samples. CLP (Cecal Ligation and puncture) compared to the Sham group. (***) $p < 0.001$, (****) $p < 0.0001$ and CLP+ phloretin vs. CLP group (##) $p < 0.01$, (###) $p < 0.001$

mediators responsible for the inflammatory response. The objective of the present study was to evaluate the protective effect of phloretin against sepsis-induced oxidative organ damage using biochemical parameters, tissue GSH level and histopathological examination of liver tissue.

CLP caused a sharp increase in serum levels of TNF-α in comparison to the sham group ($p < 0.001$). TNF-α is pro-inflammatory cytokine produced by stimulated macrophages [24]. In sepsis, cytokines like TNF-α, interleukin-1 beta (IL-1β) and IL-6 which are released after infection, play an important role in the inflammatory process [25]. Triggering inflammation by high levels of TNF-α may lead to tissue damage and, if not treated, to sepsis or death [26]. Serum levels of TNF-α were significantly suppressed following phloretin treatment as compared to the untreated CLP group ($p < 0.001$). Phloretin is an effective antioxidant for inhibiting the peroxidation of nitroso anions and lipids, and it has antitumor functions [27]. In an animal model, it was demonstrated that phloretin protect hepatocytes against oxidative stress through the ERK_2/Nrf_2 pathway and GCL expression [28]. Moreover, it was observed that phloretin has significantly decreased levels of NO, TNF-α, PGE_2, iNOS and COX-2 in LPS-stimulated RAW264.7 cells [29].

In CLP group, the liver NF-κB transcription factor level was significantly elevated (more than two-fold) in comparison to the sham group ($p < 0.05$). NF-κB is a protein complex with DNA transcription regulatory effect. NF-κB is a heterodimer and primarily composed of p50 and p65 subunits [30]. The NF-κB p65 subunit is phosphorylated and translocated into the nucleus to bind promoter of inflammatory-associated gene and expression inflammatory cytokines and Mediators [31]. It is activated by multiple signals, including tissue damage, oxidative stress, pro-inflammatory cytokines, and pathogen associated molecular patterns, that induce inhibition of kK (IkK) phosphorylation. Stimulated IkK discharge NF-κB from its cytoplasmic retainer, an inhibitor of κB, facilitating its translocation to the nucleus. NF-κB binds to distinct DNA sequences to increase transcription of genes encoding significant inflammatory mediators [32]. Binding of NF-κB to DNA, transcription of TNF-α and iNOS are obvious in inflammatory diseases [32–35]. It was observed that phloretin inhibited phosphorylation in MAPK pathways by suppressing NF-κB p65 proteins nuclear translocation in macrophages [29].

Although the exact mechanism of phloretin action remains unclear, a large body of evidence suggests that phloretin exhibits anti-oxidant properties and may be used as an anti-inflammatory agent [29, 36, 37]. Phloretin prevented inflammation process by reducing liver NF-κB level ($p < 0.01$). It is believed that phloretin is responsible for NF-κB activation mainly via IkK phosphorylation. The IkK phosphorylation inhibits IkK activity which may lead to κB attachment to DNA sequences. The following gene expression has been documented in vitro in inflammatory and vascular cells provoked with LPS, staphylococcal enterotoxin A, TNF-α, or IL-1β, and

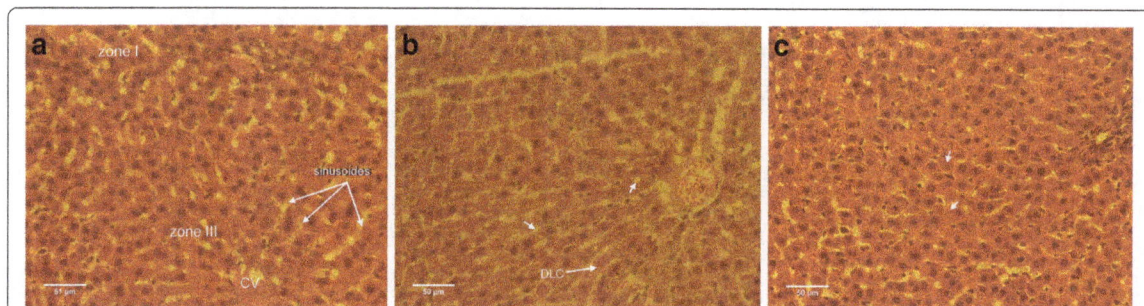

Fig. 4 Liver tissue sections are shown. **a**: in the sham group, central vein, normal sinusoids and hepatocytes with regular morphology are seen. **b**: through sepsis group, enormous vascular obstruction, extreme cytoplasmic vacuoles (→), sinusoidal duct dilation, damaged hepatocytes and stimulated Kupffer cells are observed. **c**: in the sepsis group treated with phloretin, mildly damaged hepatocytes (→), moderate vascular obstruction and sinusoidal duct dilatation are noted. Hepatic parenchyma slides were stained with hematoxylin-eosin, original magnification: X400

in vivo in models of inflammatory disease [38]. A relation between sepsis and NF-κB activation has been reflected in several cell culture and animal studies [38]. Oxidative stress regulates NF-κB activation, and the manifest of such stress has been demonstrated in sufferers from sepsis. Previously it was reported that phloretin possess anti-inflammatory properties due to inhibition of nucleus NF-κB translocation and suppression of mitogen-activated protein kinase (MAPK) signaling pathway proteins phosphorylation in human keratinocytes [37, 39]. It is more likely that an increase in NF-κB and, therefore, up-regulation of cytokines, will happen in these patients [38]. This is in collaboration with our findings of more than two-fold increase in NF-κB transcription factor levels (P <0.05) which was significantly decreased by phloretin treatment (p < 0.001).

Creatinine level was measured 24 h after sepsis induction and a mild increase in untreated CLP group (0.670 ± 0.017) was observed in comparison with the sham group (0.575 ± 0.027). Creatinine is a byproduct of creatine phosphate in breakdown muscles. Serum creatinine is an important marker of kidney function which is excreted unchanged. In addition, there were no significant differences in serum creatinine phosphokinase level between treated and untreated groups level (p < 0.05). Phloretin significantly decreased BUN in comparison to the untreated CLP group. BUN is a good marker for renal damage in cases of decreased Glomerular Filtration Rate (GFR) (suggestive of renal failure).

There is a relation between oxidative stress and peritoneal sepsis [7]. There are several defense mechanisms against the toxic effects of free oxygen radicals. GSH is a natural antioxidant defense system which is found in high concentrations in all cells and in epithelial surface fluid. GSH shows a protective effect by neutralizing free radicals and reactive oxygen intermediates [40, 41]. It is well understood that a wide group of natural products such as plant polyphenols and flavonoids have anti-inflammatory and anti oxidative properties [42, 43]. Polyphenols are the most available dietary antioxidants. A large body of evidence strongly suggests a contribution of polyphenols to the prevention of life threatening disease such as cancers, diabetes mellitus, osteoporosis and cardiovascular [44, 45]. Based on meta-analyses and associated epidemiological studies, polyphenols as secondary plants metabolites are considerably involved in biological defense against ultraviolet radiation or pathogens aggression [46–49]. Flavonoid is a general term for flavanones, flavanols, flavones, chalcones and anthocyanins [50]. Beside antioxidant activity, certain polyphenols possess a potent anticarcinogenic activity through enzyme modulation, upregulation of gap junction communication, gene expression, apoptosis and P-glycoprotein activation in cell culture and animal models [51–53].

Phloretin treatment was able to protect animals against sepsis-induced oxidative tissue damage and maintained GSH levels in hepatic, renal, heart and respiratory tissues in comparison to the untreated sepsis group (p < 0.01). It was previously demonstrated that phloretin increases GSH level and HO-1 expression in carbon tetrachloride-induced rat hepatotoxicity [28]. Reduced glutathione as the main source of sulfhydryl pool is well known to be a crucial scavenger of free radicals in the cell [24, 26]. The non-protein sulphydryls binds to a diverse group of electrophilic radicals and metabolites [54]. It has been suggested that antioxidants which save GSH content, may restore the cellular defense mechanisms, inhibit lipid peroxidation and thus provide cellular protection against the oxidative tissue damage. Previously it showed that phloretin has biological and anti-infective activity with beneficial effect on inflammatory bowel diseases (IBD) as well as anti-oxidative charactrisitcs and inhibition of Escherichia coli O157:H7 biofilm formation without harming beneficial commensal E. coli biofilms [15, 55–58]. In addition, phloretin (24 μM) May also be involved in lipid peroxidation and oxidative stress inhibition in cell culture [54].

Erkel et al. showed that dihydrochalcone aglycone phloretin significantly blocked pro-inflammatory gene expression and decreased IL-8, IP-10 and NF-κB promoter signal transduction in a dose-dependent manner. Furthermore, the apple juice critically hinder the expression of NF-κB regulated pro-inflammatory genes (IL-1β, CXCL9, TNF-α), inflammatory-related enzymes (CYP3A4, COX-2), and transcription factors (STAT1, IRF1) in LPS/IFN-γ provoked MonoMac6 cells without significant influence on the expression of house-keeping genes [37]. Phloretin exhibited anti-inflammatory effects through decreasing IL-6, IL-8, intercellular adhesion molecule (ICAM)-1 production and mRNA expression in TNF-α stimulated HaCaT human cells [39]. Furthermore, neuroprotective effects of phloretin has been demonstrated thorough Nrf2 pathway activation and oxidative stress suppression in rat [36].

Conclusion

The present study evidenced strong anti-oxidant and anti-inflammatory effects of phloretin against tissue damage from CLP-induced sepsis, likely caused by free oxygen radicals. Thus, it will open a new window for the possibility of clinical application of phloretin in severe conditions such as sepsis. However, further studies required to highlight the exact underlying mechanisms of the observed protective effect. As our knowledge improves in this field, therapeutic targeting would be possible in several disorders.

Competing interests
The authors declare that they have no competing interests.

Authors' contributions
MA participated in the design of the study, acquisition of data, statistical analysis and drafted the manuscript. MRS participated in the design of the study and performed the statistical analysis. HM carried out the immunoassays. ARK participated in coordination and helped to analytical assays. SN carried out the histopathological examinations and drafted the manuscript. OS have been involved in study design, analysis and interpretation of data and revising the manuscript critically for important intellectual content. All authors read and approved the final manuscript.

Acknowledgment
This study was supported by a grant (Project No. 17164) from Tehran University of Medical Sciences, Tehran, Iran.

Author details
[1]Toxicology and Poisoning Research Centre, Tehran University of Medical Sciences, Tehran, Iran. [2]Department of Pharmacology and Toxicology, Faculty of Pharmacy, Tehran University of Medical Sciences, P. O. Box, 1417614411, Tehran, Iran. [3]Department of Immunology, Faculty of Medicine, Tehran University of Medical Sciences, Tehran, Iran. [4]Department of Anatomy, Faculty of Medicine, Tehran University of Medical Sciences, Tehran, Iran. [5]Drug design and discovery Research Centre, Tehran University of Medical Sciences, Tehran, Iran.

References
1. Dejager L, Pinheiro I, Dejonckheere E, Libert C. Cecal ligation and puncture: the gold standard model for polymicrobial sepsis. Trends Microbiol. 2011; 19(4):198–208.
2. Angus DC, Linde-Zwirble WT, Lidicker J, Clermont G, Carcillo J, Pinsky MR. Epidemiology of severe sepsis in the United States: analysis of incidence, outcome, and associated costs of care. Crit Care Med. 2001;29(7):1303–10.
3. Hinshaw LB. Sepsis/septic shock: participation of the microcirculation: an abbreviated review. Crit Care Med. 1996;24(6):1072–8.
4. Bostanoglu A, Bostanoglu S, Erverdi N, Hamamcı O, Özgen G, Dursun A, et al. The role of oxygen free radicals in an experimental sepsis model. Turkish J Gastroenterol. 1999;10:427–31.
5. Lever A, Mackenzie I. Sepsis: definition, epidemiology, and diagnosis. BMJ. 2007;335(7625):879–83.
6. Annane D, Bellissant E, Cavaillon J-M. Septic shock. Lancet. 2005;365(9453): 63–78.
7. Koksal G, Sayilgan C, Aydin S, Oz H, Uzun H. Correlation of plasma and tissue oxidative stresses in intra-abdominal sepsis. J Surg Res. 2004;122(2): 180–3.
8. Lee Y, Chou Y. Antioxidant profiles in full term and preterm neonates. Chang Gung Med J. 2005;28(12):846.
9. Razavi-Azarkhiavi K, Ali-Omrani M, Solgi R, Bagheri P, Haji-Noormohammadi M, Amani N, et al. Silymarin alleviates bleomycin-induced pulmonary toxicity and lipid peroxidation in mice. Pharm Biol. 2014;52(10):1267–71.
10. García JJ, Reiter RJ, Guerrero JM, Escames G, Yu BP, Oh CS, et al. Melatonin prevents changes in microsomal membrane fluidity during induced lipid peroxidation. FEBS Lett. 1997;408(3):297–300.
11. Hollman P, Katan M. Absorption, metabolism and health effects of dietary flavonoids in man. Biomed Pharmacother. 1997;51(8):305–10.
12. Moon YJ, Wang X, Morris ME. Dietary flavonoids: effects on xenobiotic and carcinogen metabolism. Toxicol In Vitro. 2006;20(2):187–210.
13. Nijveldt RJ, Van Nood E, Van Hoorn DE, Boelens PG, Van Norren K, Van Leeuwen PA. Flavonoids: a review of probable mechanisms of action and potential applications. Am J Clin Nut. 2001;74(4):418–25.
14. Sabzevari O, Galati G, Moridani MY, Siraki A, O'Brien PJ. Molecular cytotoxic mechanisms of anticancer hydroxychalcones. Chem Biol Intract. 2004;148(1): 57–67.
15. Lee J-H, Regmi SC, Kim J-A, Cho MH, Yun H, Lee C-S, et al. Apple flavonoid phloretin inhibits Escherichia coli O157: H7 biofilm formation and ameliorates colon inflammation in rats. Infect Immun. 2011;79(12):4819–27.
16. Hsieh H-K, Lee T-H, Wang J-P, Wang J-J, Lin C-N. Synthesis and anti-inflammatory effect of chalcones and related compounds. Pharm Res. 1998; 15(1):39–46.
17. Natanzi E, Reza A, Mahmoudian S, Minaeie B, Sabzevari O. Hepatoprotective activity of phloretin and hydroxychalcones against Acetaminophen Induced hepatotoxicity in mice. Iran J Pharm Res. 2011;7(2):89–97.
18. Zuo A, Yanying Y, Li J, Binbin X, Xiongying Y, Yan Q, et al. Study on the relation of structure and antioxidant activity of isorhamnetin, quercetin, phloretin, silybin and phloretin isonicotinyl hydrazone. Free Radic Res. 2011; 1(4):39–47.
19. Rezk BM, Haenen GR, van der Vijgh WJ, Bast A. The antioxidant activity of phloretin: the disclosure of a new antioxidant pharmacophore in flavonoids. Biochem Biophys Re Commun. 2002;295(1):9–13.
20. Nakamura Y, Watanabe S, Miyake N, Kohno H, Osawa T. Dihydrochalcones: evaluation as novel radical scavenging antioxidants. J Agric Food Chem. 2003;51(11):3309–12.
21. Fujimura N, Sumita S, Narimatsu E, Nakayama Y, Shitinohe Y, Namiki A. Effects of isoproterenol on diaphragmatic contractility in septic peritonitis. Am J Respir Crit Care Med. 2000;161(2):440–6.
22. Monge P, Solheim E, Scheline R. Dihydrochalcone metabolism in the rat: phloretin. Xenobiotica. 1984;14(12):917–24.
23. Allameh A, Razavi-Azarkhiavi K, Mohsenifar A, Jamali-Zavarei M. Effect of acute ethanol treatment on biochemical and histopathological factors in rat liver in an experimental sepsis model. Pathol Res Pract. 2012;208(6):331–7.
24. Ross D. Glutathione, free radicals and chemotherapeutic agents: mechanisms of free-radical induced toxicity and glutathione-dependent protection. Pharmacol Ther. 1988;37(2):231–49.
25. GİRİŞGİN S, ERAYMAN İ, ERDEM S. The effect of N-acetyl cysteine on serum glutathione, TNF-α and tissue malondialdehyde levels in the treatment of sepsis. Ulus Travma Acil Cerrahi Derg. 2011;17(4):293–7.
26. Shaw S, Herbert V, Colman N, Jayatilleke E. Effect of ethanol-generated free radicals on gastric intrinsic factor and glutathione. Alcohol. 1990;7(2):153–7.
27. Kim MS, Kwon JY, Kang NJ, Lee KW, Lee HJ. Phloretin Induces Apoptosis in H-Ras MCF10A Human Breast Tumor Cells through the Activation of p53 via JNK and p38 Mitogen-Activated Protein Kinase Signaling. Ann N Y Acad Sci. 2009;1171(1):479–83.
28. Yang Y-C, Lii C-K, Lin A-H, Yeh Y-W, Yao H-T, Li C-C, et al. Induction of glutathione synthesis and heme oxygenase 1 by the flavonoids butein and phloretin is mediated through the ERK/Nrf2 pathway and protects against oxidative stress. Free Radic Biol Med. 2011;51(11):2073–81.
29. Chang W-T, Huang W-C, Liou C-J. Evaluation of the anti-inflammatory effects of phloretin and phlorizin in lipopolysaccharide-stimulated mouse macrophages. Food Chem. 2012;134(2):972–9.
30. Yang L, Boldin MP, Yu Y, Liu CS, Ea C-K, Ramakrishnan P, et al. miR-146a controls the resolution of T cell responses in mice. J Exp Med. 2012;209(9): 1655–70.
31. Olefsky JM, Glass CK. Macrophages, inflammation, and insulin resistance. Annu Rev Physiol. 2010;72:219–46.
32. Liu SF, Malik AB. NF-κB activation as a pathological mechanism of septic shock and inflammation. Am J Physiol Lung Cell Mol Physiol. 2006;290(4):L622–L45.
33. Higdon J. An evidence-based approach to dietary phytochemicals. Thieme Publ., New York/Stuttgart; 2007. p. 238.
34. Shapiro H, Singer P, Halpern Z, Bruck R. Polyphenols in the treatment of inflammatory bowel disease and acute pancreatitis. Gut. 2007;56(3):426–36.
35. Surh Y-J, Kundu JK, Na H-K, Lee J-S. Redox-sensitive transcription factors as prime targets for chemoprevention with anti-inflammatory and antioxidative phytochemicals. J Nutr. 2005;135(12):2993S–3001S.
36. Liu Y, Zhang L, Liang J. Activation of the Nrf2 defense pathway contributes to neuroprotective effects of phloretin on oxidative stress injury after cerebral ischemia/reperfusion in rats. J Neurol Sci. 2015;351(1):88–92.
37. Jung M, Triebel S, Anke T, Richling E, Erkel G. Influence of apple polyphenols on inflammatory gene expression. Mol Nutr Food Res. 2009;53(10):1263–80.
38. Macdonald J, Galley H, Webster N. Oxidative stress and gene expression in sepsis. Br J Anaesth. 2003;90(2):221–32.
39. Huang W-C, Dai Y-W, Peng H-L, Kang C-W, Kuo C-Y, Liou C-J. Phloretin ameliorates chemokines and ICAM-1 expression via blocking of the NF-κB pathway in the TNF-α-induced HaCaT human keratinocytes. Int Immunopharmacol. 2015;27(1):32–7.
40. Çetiner M, Şener G. Demiralp. Metotreksat tedavisine bağlı ince barsakta oluşan oksidatif doku hasarında L-Karnitinin koruyucu etkisi. Turk J Haemato. 2004;21:97–100.

41. Özkan E, Akyüz C, Sehirli AÖ, Topaloglu Ü, Ercan F, Sener G. Montelukast, a selective cysteinyl leukotriene receptor 1 antagonist, reduces cerulein-induced pancreatic injury in rats. Pancreas. 2010;39(7):1041–6.

42. Galati G, Sabzevari O, Wilson JX, O'Brien PJ. Prooxidant activity and cellular effects of the phenoxyl radicals of dietary flavonoids and other polyphenolics. Toxicology. 2002;177(1):91–104.

43. Chlopicka J, Pasko P, Gorinstein S, Jedryas A, Zagrodzki P. Total phenolic and total flavonoid content, antioxidant activity and sensory evaluation of pseudocereal breads. LWT-Food Sci Technol. 2012;46(2):548–55.

44. Joven J, Rull A, Rodriguez-Gallego E, Camps J, Riera-Borrull M, Hernández-Aguilera A, et al. Multifunctional targets of dietary polyphenols in disease: a case for the chemokine network and energy metabolism. Food Chem Toxicol. 2013;51:267–79.

45. Scalbert A, Johnson IT, Saltmarsh M. Polyphenols: antioxidants and beyond. Am J Clin Nutr. 2005;81(1):215S–7S.

46. Pandey KB, Rizvi SI. Plant polyphenols as dietary antioxidants in human health and disease. Oxid Med Cell Longev. 2009;2(5):270–8.

47. Duthie GG, Duthie SJ, Kyle JA. Plant polyphenols in cancer and heart disease: implications as nutritional antioxidants. Nutr Res Rev. 2000;13(01):79–106.

48. Vita JA. Polyphenols and cardiovascular disease: effects on endothelial and platelet function. Am J Clin Nutr. 2005;81(1):292S–7S.

49. Covas M-I, Nyyssönen K, Poulsen HE, Kaikkonen J, Zunft H-JF, Kiesewetter H, et al. The effect of polyphenols in olive oil on heart disease risk factors: a randomized trial. Ann Intern Med. 2006;145(5):333–41.

50. Petti S, Scully C. Polyphenols, oral health and disease: a review. J Dent. 2009; 37(6):413–23.

51. Taguri T, Tanaka T, Kouno I. Antimicrobial activity of 10 different plant polyphenols against bacteria causing food-borne disease. Biol Pharm Bull. 2004;27(12):1965–9.

52. Arts IC, Hollman PC. Polyphenols and disease risk in epidemiologic studies. Am J Clin Nutr. 2005;81(1):317S–25S.

53. Zhang S, Morris ME. Effects of the flavonoids biochanin A, morin, phloretin, and silymarin on P-glycoprotein-mediated transport. J Pharmacol Exp The. 2003;304(3):1258–67.

54. Szabo S, Nagy L, Plebani M. Glutathione, protein sulfhydryls and cysteine proteases in gastric mucosal injury and protection. Clin Chim Acta. 1992; 206(1):95–105.

55. Nowakowska Z. A review of anti-infective and anti-inflammatory chalcones. Eur J Med Chem. 2007;42(2):125–37.

56. Cowan MM. Plant products as antimicrobial agents. Clin Microb Rev. 1999; 12(4):564–82.

57. Mahapatra DK, Bharti SK, Asati V. Chalcone scaffolds as anti-infective agents: Structural and molecular target perspectives. Eur J Med Chem. 2015;101: 496–524.

58. Cho H, Yun H, Lee C-S, Lee J. Apple flavonoid phloretin inhibits. Infect Immun. 2011;79(12):4819.

Permissions

All chapters in this book were first published in JPS, by BioMed Central; hereby published with permission under the Creative Commons Attribution License or equivalent. Every chapter published in this book has been scrutinized by our experts. Their significance has been extensively debated. The topics covered herein carry significant findings which will fuel the growth of the discipline. They may even be implemented as practical applications or may be referred to as a beginning point for another development.

The contributors of this book come from diverse backgrounds, making this book a truly international effort. This book will bring forth new frontiers with its revolutionizing research information and detailed analysis of the nascent developments around the world.

We would like to thank all the contributing authors for lending their expertise to make the book truly unique. They have played a crucial role in the development of this book. Without their invaluable contributions this book wouldn't have been possible. They have made vital efforts to compile up to date information on the varied aspects of this subject to make this book a valuable addition to the collection of many professionals and students.

This book was conceptualized with the vision of imparting up-to-date information and advanced data in this field. To ensure the same, a matchless editorial board was set up. Every individual on the board went through rigorous rounds of assessment to prove their worth. After which they invested a large part of their time researching and compiling the most relevant data for our readers.

The editorial board has been involved in producing this book since its inception. They have spent rigorous hours researching and exploring the diverse topics which have resulted in the successful publishing of this book. They have passed on their knowledge of decades through this book. To expedite this challenging task, the publisher supported the team at every step. A small team of assistant editors was also appointed to further simplify the editing procedure and attain best results for the readers.

Apart from the editorial board, the designing team has also invested a significant amount of their time in understanding the subject and creating the most relevant covers. They scrutinized every image to scout for the most suitable representation of the subject and create an appropriate cover for the book.

The publishing team has been an ardent support to the editorial, designing and production team. Their endless efforts to recruit the best for this project, has resulted in the accomplishment of this book. They are a veteran in the field of academics and their pool of knowledge is as vast as their experience in printing. Their expertise and guidance has proved useful at every step. Their uncompromising quality standards have made this book an exceptional effort. Their encouragement from time to time has been an inspiration for everyone.

The publisher and the editorial board hope that this book will prove to be a valuable piece of knowledge for researchers, students, practitioners and scholars across the globe.

List of Contributors

Dandigi M Panchaxari, Sowjanya Pampana and Anil Kumar Aravapalli
Department of Pharmaceutics, KLEU's college of Pharmacy, Nehru Nagar, Belgaum, Karnataka 590010, India

Tapas Pal and Bhavana Devabhaktuni
Research Scientist, R&D divison, Sparsha Pharma International Pvt. Ltd., Hyderabad, India

Marzieh Qaraaty and Mohsen Naseri
Traditional Medicine Clinical Trial Research Center, Shahed University, Tehran, Iran

Seyed Hamid Kamali
Department of Traditional Medicine, Faculty of Traditional Medicine, Shahid Beheshti University of Medical Sciences, Tehran, Iran

Fataneh Hashem Dabaghian
Research Institute for Islamic and Complementary Medicine, Iran University of Medical Sciences, Tehran, Iran

Nafiseh Zafarghandi
Department of Gynecology and Obstetrics, Faculty of Medical Sciences, Shahed University, Tehran, Iran

Roshanak Mokaberinejad
Department of Traditional Medicine, School of Traditional Medicine, Shahid Beheshti University of Medical Sciences, Tehran, Iran

Masumeh Mobli and Gholamreza Amin
Department of Traditional Pharmacy, Faculty of Traditional Medicine, Tehran University of Medical Sciences, Tehran, Iran

Mohammad Kamalinejad
Department of Pharmacognosy, School of Pharmacy Shahid Beheshti University of Medical Sciences, Tehran, Iran

Mohsen Amin
Department of Drug and Food control, Faculty of Pharmacy, Tehran University of Medical Sciences, Tehran, Iran

Azizeh Ghaseminejad
Department of Gynecology and Obstetrics, Tehran University of Medical Sciences, Tehran, Iran

Seyedeh jihan HosseiniKhabiri
Khatam Hospital, Tehran, Iran

Daryush Talei
Medicinal Plant Research Centre, Shahed University, Tehran, Iran

Subhabrata Paul and Rita Kundu
Department of Botany, University of Calcutta, 35, Ballygunge Circular Road, Kolkata 700019, India

Eskandar Alipour, Zinatsadat Mousavi and Zahra Safaei
Department of Chemistry, Islamic Azad University, Tehran-North Branch, Zafar St, Tehran, Iran

Mahboobeh Pordeli and Sussan Kabudanian Ardestani
Department of Biochemistry, Institute of Biochemistry and Biophysics, University of Tehran, Tehran, Iran

Maliheh Safavi
Biotechnology Department, Iranian Research Organization for Science and Technology, Tehran, Iran

Loghman Firoozpour
Drug Design and Development Research Center, Tehran University of Medicinal Sciences, Tehran, Iran

Negar Mohammadhosseini, Mina Saeedi, Abbas Shafiee and Alireza Foroumadi
Department of Medicinal Chemistry, Faculty of Pharmacy and Pharmaceutical Sciences Research Center, Tehran University of Medical Sciences, Tehran, Iran

Alireza Salehi
Research Center for Traditional Medicine and History of Medicine, Shiraz University of Medical Sciences, Shiraz, Iran

Mohammad Hashem Hashempur
Research Center for Traditional Medicine and History of Medicine, Shiraz University of Medical Sciences, Shiraz, Iran
Essence of Parsiyan Wisdom Institute, Traditional Medicine and Medicinal Plant Incubator, Shiraz University of Medical Sciences, Shiraz, Iran

Mojtaba Heydari
Essence of Parsiyan Wisdom Institute, Traditional Medicine and Medicinal Plant Incubator, Shiraz University of Medical Sciences, Shiraz, Iran

Alireza Ashraf
Shiraz Burn Research Center, Shiraz University of Medical Sciences, Shiraz, Iran
Department of Physical Medicine and Rehabilitation, Shiraz University of Medical Sciences, Shiraz, Iran

Kaynoosh Homayouni
Department of Physical Medicine and Rehabilitation, Shiraz University of Medical Sciences, Shiraz, Iran
Shiraz Geriatric Research Center, Shiraz University of Medical Sciences, Shiraz, Iran

Mohsen Taghizadeh
Research Center for Biochemistry and Nutrition in Metabolic Disease, Kashan University of Medical Sciences, Kashan, Iran

Abbas Kebriaeezadeh and Rassoul Dinarvand
Department of Pharmacoeconomics and Pharmaceutical Administration, Faculty of Pharmacy, Tehran University of Medical Sciences, Tehran, Iran

Shekoufeh Nikfar
Department of Pharmacoeconomics and Pharmaceutical Administration, Faculty of Pharmacy, Tehran University of Medical Sciences, Tehran, Iran
Food & Drug Organization, Ministry of Health & Medical Education, Tehran, Iran

Mohammad Abdollahi
Department of Pharmacoeconomics and Pharmaceutical Administration, Faculty of Pharmacy, Tehran University of Medical Sciences, Tehran, Iran
Faculty of Pharmacy, and Pharmaceutical Sciences Research Center, Tehran University of Medical Sciences, Tehran, Iran

Mohammad-Ali Sahraian
Department of Neurology, Sina Hospital, Tehran University of Medical Sciences, Tehran, Iran

David Henry
Institute for Clinical Evaluative Sciences, Toronto, Canada

Ali Akbari Sari
Department of Pharmacoeconomics and Pharmaceutical Administration, Faculty of Pharmacy, Tehran University of Medical Sciences, Tehran, Iran
Department of Health Management and Economics, School of Public Health, Tehran University of Medical Sciences, Tehran, Iran

Abolfazl Akbari, Gholam Reza Mobini and Fatemeh Shidfar
Department of Molecular Medicine, School of Advanced Medical Technologies, Tehran University of Medical Sciences, Tehran, Iran

Saeid Amanpour and Samad Muhammadnejad
Cancer Research Center, Cancer Institute of Iran, Tehran University of Medical Sciences, Tehran, Iran

Mohammad Hossein Ghahremani
Department of Molecular Medicine, School of Advanced Medical Technologies, Tehran University of Medical Sciences, Tehran, Iran
Department of Pharmacology and Toxicology, Faculty of Pharmacy, Tehran University of Medical Sciences, Tehran, Iran

Seyed Hamidollah Ghaffari
Hematology, Oncology and Stem Cell Transplantation Research Center, Shariati Hospital, Tehran University of Medical Sciences, Tehran, Iran

Ahmad Reza Dehpour
Department of Pharmacology, School of Medicine, Tehran University of Medical Sciences, Tehran, Iran

Mahdi Abastabar
Invasive Fungi Research Center, Department of Medical Mycology and Parasitology, School of Medicine, Mazandaran University of Medical Sciences, Sari, Iran

Ahad Khoshzaban
Stem Cells Preparation Uinte, Farabi Eye Hospital, Tehran University of Medical Sciences, Tehran, Iran

Mansour Heidari
Stem Cells Preparation Uinte, Farabi Eye Hospital, Tehran University of Medical Sciences, Tehran, Iran
Department of Medical Genetics, School of Medicine, Tehran University of Medical Sciences, Tehran, Iran

Ebrahim Faghihloo
Department of Virology, School of Public Health, Tehran University of Medical Sciences, Tehran, Iran

Abbas Karimi
Department of Molecular Medicine, Faculty of Advanced Technologies in Medicine (FATiM), Iran University of Medical Sciences, Tehran, Iran

Massoud Amanlou
Department of Medicinal Chemistry, Faculty of Pharmacy, Pharmaceutical Sciences Research Center, Tehran University of Medical Sciences, Tehran, Iran

Ali-akbar Saboury, Roya Bazl and Mohammad Reza Ganjali
Institute of Biochemistry and Biophysics, University of Tehran, Tehran, Iran

Shokoofeh Sheibani
Center of Excellence in Electrochemistry, Faculty of Chemistry, University of Tehran, Tehran, Iran

Mohammad Hossien Yazdi
Department of Pharmaceutical Biotechnology and Biotechnology Research Center, Faculty of Pharmacy, Tehran University of Medical Sciences, Tehran, Iran

Erfan Kheradmand
Department of Pharmaceutical Biotechnology and Biotechnology Research Center, Faculty of Pharmacy, Tehran University of Medical Sciences, Tehran, Iran
Science and Research Branch, Azad University, Tehran, Iran

Abas Akhavan Sepahi
Science and Research Branch, Azad University, Tehran, Iran

Fatemeh Rafii
Division of Microbiology, National Center for Toxicological Research, U.S. FDA, Jefferson, AR 72079, USA

Ahmad Reza Shahverdi
Department of Pharmaceutical Biotechnology and Biotechnology Research Center, Faculty of Pharmacy, Tehran University of Medical Sciences, Tehran, Iran
Department of Medical Biotechnology, School of Advanced Medical Technologies, Tehran University of Medical Sciences, Tehran, Iran

Mohammad Reza Oveisi
Department of Food and Drug Control, Faculty of Pharmacy, Tehran University of Medical Sciences, Tehran, Iran

Hossein Hosseinzadeh and Soghra Mehri
Pharmaceutical Research Center, Department of Pharmacodynamics and Toxicology, School of Pharmacy, Mashhad University of Medical Sciences, Mashhad, Iran

Ali Heshmati
School of Pharmacy, Mashhad University of Medical Sciences, Mashhad, Iran

Mohammad Ramezani
Pharmaceutical and Biotechnology Research Centers, School of Pharmacy, Mashhad University of Medical Sciences, Mashhad, Iran

Amirhossein Sahebkar
Biotechnology Research Center, Mashhad University of Medical Sciences, Mashhad, Iran

Khalil Abnous
Pharmaceutical Research Center, Department of MedicinalChemistry, School of Pharmacy, Mashhad University of Medical Sciences, 91775-1365 Mashhad, Iran

Muhammad Usman Minhas, Mahmood Ahmad, Liaqat Ali and Muhammad Sohail
Faculty of Pharmacy and Alternative Medicine, the Islamia University of Bahawalpur-63100, Punjab, Pakistan

Effat Souri, Amin Dastjani Farahani and Mohsen Amini
Department of Medicinal Chemistry, Faculty of Pharmacy and Drug Design and Development Research Center, Tehran University of Medical Sciences, Tehran 14155 6451, Iran

Reza Ahmadkhaniha
Department of Human Ecology, School of Public Health, Tehran University of Medical Sciences, Tehran 1417614411, Iran

Akbar Abdollahiasl, Mona Jaberidoost and Shekoufeh Nikfar
Department of Pharmacoeconomics and Pharmaceutical administration, Pharmaceutical policy research center and Faculty of Pharmacy, Tehran University of Medical Sciences (TUMS), Tehran, Iran

Abbas Kebriaeezadeh
Department of Pharmacoeconomics and Pharmaceutical administration, Pharmaceutical policy research center and Faculty of Pharmacy, Tehran University of Medical Sciences (TUMS), Tehran, Iran

Mohammad Abdollahi
Department of Toxicology and Pharmacology, Faculty of Pharmacy and Pharmaceutical Sciences Research Center, TUMS, Tehran, Iran

Rassoul Dinarvand
Department of Pharmaceutics, Faculty of Pharmacy, TUMS, Tehran, Iran

Abdol Majid Cheraghali
Food and Drug Organization, Ministry of Health and Medical Education, Tehran, Iran
Department of Pharmacology, University of Baqiyatallah Medical Sciences, Tehran, Iran

Arezou Lari
Students Research Committee, Faculty of Pharmacy, Kermanshah University of Medical Sciences, Kermanshah, Iran

Isaac Karimi
Laboratory of Molecular and Cellular Biology, School of Veterinary Medicine, Razi University, Kermanshah, Iran

Hadi Adibi and Alireza Aliabadi
Novel Drug Delivery Research Center, Faculty of Pharmacy, Kermanshah University of Medical Sciences, Kermanshah, Iran

Loghman Firoozpour and Loghman Firoozpour
Drug Design and Development Research Center, Tehran University of Medical Sciences, Tehran, Iran

Alireza Foroumadi
Drug Design and Development Research Center, Tehran University of Medical Sciences, Tehran, Iran
Neuroscience Research Center, Institute of Neuropharmacology, Kerman University of Medical Sciences, Kerman, Iran

Amir Gharib and Zohreh Faezizadeh
Department of Laboratory Sciences, Borujerd Branch, Islamic Azad University, Borujerd, Iran

Seyed Ali Reza Mesbah-Namin
Department of Clinical Biochemistry, Faculty of Medical Sciences, Tarbiat Modares University, Tehran, Iran

Ramin Saravani
Department of Biochemistry, School of Medicine, Zahedan University of Medical Sciences, Zahedan, Iran

Khalil Abnous
Pharmaceutical Research Center, School of Pharmacy, Mashhad University of Medical Sciences, Mashhad, Iran

Batoul Barati, Mohammad Reza Masboghi Farimani, Fatemeh Mohammadpour and Morteza Ghandadi
School of Pharmacy, Mashhad University of Medical Sciences, Mashhad, Iran

Soghra Mehri
Department of Pharmacodynamics and Toxicology, School of Pharmacy, Mashhad University of Medical Sciences, Mashhad, Iran

Farzin Hadizadeh and Mona Alibolandi
Biotechnology Research Center, School of Pharmacy, Mashhad University of Medical Sciences, P. O. Box 91775-1365, Mashhad, Iran

Seyedeh Sara Mirfazli and Abbas Shafiee
Department of Medicinal Chemistry, Faculty of Pharmacy and Pharmaceutical Sciences Research Center, Tehran University of Medical Sciences, Tehran, Iran

Marjan Esfahanizadeh and Kimia Tabib
Department of Medicinal Chemistry, School of Pharmacy, Shahid Beheshti University of Medical Sciences, Tehran, Iran

Farzad Kobarfard
Department of Medicinal Chemistry, School of Pharmacy, Shahid Beheshti University of Medical Sciences, Tehran, Iran
Phytochemistry Research Center, Shahid Beheshti University of Medical Sciences, Tehran, Iran

Loghman Firoozpour
Drug Design and Development Research Center, Tehran University of Medical Sciences, Tehran, Iran

Ali Asadipour
Neuroscience Research Center, Institute of Neuropharmacology, Kerman University of Medical Sciences, Kerman, Iran

Alireza Foroumadi
Department of Medicinal Chemistry, Faculty of Pharmacy and Pharmaceutical Sciences Research Center, Tehran University of Medical Sciences, Tehran, Iran
Neuroscience Research Center, Institute of Neuropharmacology, Kerman University of Medical Sciences, Kerman, Iran

Maryam Zahmatkesh
Department of Neuroscience, School of Advanced Technologies in medicine, Tehran University of Medical Sciences, Tehran, Iran

Tahmineh Mokhtari
Department of Anatomy, School of Medicine, Tehran University of Medical Sciences, Tehran, Iran

Gholamreza Hassanzadeh
Department of Neuroscience, School of Advanced Technologies in medicine, Tehran University of Medical Sciences, Tehran, Iran Department of Anatomy, School of Medicine, Tehran University of Medical Sciences, Tehran, Iran

Shahram Ejtemaei Mehr
Department of Pharmacology, School of Medicine, Tehran University of Medical Sciences, Tehran, Iran

Mohammad Sharifzadeh
Faculty of Pharmacy, and Pharmaceutical Sciences Research Center, Tehran University of Medical Sciences, Tehran, Iran

Fatemeh Attari and Hadi Aligholi
Department of Neuroscience, School of Advanced Technologies in medicine, Tehran University of Medical Sciences, Tehran, Iran Shefa Neuroscience Research Center, Khatamolanbia Hospital, Tehran, Iran

Mojtaba Khaksarian
Department of Physiology, Medical College, Lorestan University of Medical Sciences, Khorramabad, Iran

Ali Gorji
Shefa Neuroscience Research Center, Khatamolanbia Hospital, Tehran, Iran Epilepsy Research Center, WestfälischeWilhelms-UniversitätMünster, Münster, Germany

Mohammad Charehsaz, Hande Sipahi and Ahmet Aydın
Faculty of Pharmacy, Department of Toxicology, Yeditepe University, 34755 Atasehir, Istanbul, Turkey

Engin Celep and Erdem Yesilada
Faculty of Pharmacy, Department of Pharmacognosy, Yeditepe University, 34755 Atasehir, Istanbul, Turkey

Aylin Üstündağ, Özge Cemiloğlu Ülker and Yalçın Duydu
Faculty of Pharmacy, Department of Toxicology, Ankara University, 06100 Tandoğan, Ankara, Turkey

Bibi Marjan Razavi
Targeted Drug Delivery Research Center, Department of Pharmacodynamy and Toxicology, School of Pharmacy, Mashhad University of Medical Sciences, Mashhad, Iran

Hossein Hosseinzadeh
Pharmaceutical Research Center, Department of Pharmacodynamy and Toxicology, School of Pharmacy, Mashhad University of Medical Sciences, Mashhad, Iran

Hasan Fallah Huseini
Medicinal Plants Research Center, Institute of Medicinal Plants, ACECR, Karaj, Iran

Maryam Sotoudeh Anvari
Clinical and Surgical Pathology Department Tehran Heart Center, Tehran University of Medical Sciences, Tehran, Iran

Yaser Tajallizadeh khoob
Endocrinology and Metabolism Research Center, Endocrinology and Metabolism Clinical Sciences Institute, Tehran University of Medical Sciences, Tehran, Iran

Shahram Rabbani
Experimental Research Center, Tehran Heart Center, Tehran University of Medical Sciences, Tehran, Iran

Farshad Sharifi, Seyed Masoud Arzaghi and Hossein Fakhrzadeh
Elderly Health Research Center, Endocrinology and Metabolism Population Sciences Institute, Tehran University of Medical Sciences, 4th floor, No 4, Ostad Nejatollahi Street, Engelab Avenue, Tehran, Iran

Tatiane Teixeira Oliveira, Keina Maciele Campos, Ana Tereza Cerqueira-Lima, Tamires Cana Brasil Carneiro, Darizy Flávia Silva Amorim de Vasconcelos, Neuza Maria Alcântara-Neves and Camila Alexandrina Figueiredo
Instituto de Ciências da Saúde, Universidade Federal da Bahia, Salvador, Bahia, Brazil

Eudes da Silva Velozo
Faculdade de Farmácia, Universidade Federal da Bahia,Salvador, Bahia, Brazil

Ingrid Christie Alexandrino Ribeiro Melo, Eugênia Abrantes Figueiredo and Eduardo de Jesus Oliveira
Centro de Biotecnologia, Universidade Federal da Paraíba, João Pessoa, Paraíba, Brazil

Lain Carlos Pontes-de-Carvalho
Centro de Pesquisas Gonçalo Moniz, Fundação Oswaldo Cruz, Salvador, Bahia, Brazil

Shu-Ping You, Long Ma, Mukaram Tudimat, Shi-Lei Zhang and Tao Liu
Department of Toxicology, School of Public Health, Xinjiang Medical University, No. 393 Xinyi Road, Urumqi 830011Xinjiang Uyghur Autonomous Region, China

Jun Zhao
Key Laboratory for Uighur Medicine, Institute of Materia Medica of Xinjiang, Urumqi 830004, China
No. 140 Xinhua South Road, Tianshan District, Urumqi 830000Xinjiang Uyghur Autonomous Region, China
Mohsen Zeeb and Behrooz Mirza
Department of Applied Chemistry, Faculty of science, Islamic Azad University, South Tehran Branch, Tehran, Iran

Huiting Zeng, Ping Xue, Xiaochen Huang, Erxin Shang, Jianming Guo, Dawei Qian and Yuping Tang
Jiangsu Key Laboratory for High Technology Research of TCM Formulae, Nanjing University of Chinese Medicine, Nanjing 210023, China
Jiangsu Collaborative Innovation Center of Chinese Medicinal Resources Industrialization, Nanjing University of Chinese Medicine, Nanjing 210023, China
National and Local Collaborative Engineering Center of Chinese Medicinal Resources Industrialization and Formulae Innovative Medicine, Nanjing University of Chinese Medicine, Nanjing 210023, China

Shulan Su and Jin-ao Duan
Jiangsu Key Laboratory for High Technology Research of TCM Formulae, Nanjing University of Chinese Medicine, Nanjing 210023, China
Jiangsu Collaborative Innovation Center of Chinese Medicinal Resources Industrialization, Nanjing University of Chinese Medicine, Nanjing 210023, China
National and Local Collaborative Engineering Center of Chinese Medicinal Resources Industrialization and Formulae Innovative Medicine, Nanjing University of Chinese Medicine, Nanjing 210023, China
Jiangsu Key Laboratory for TCM Formulae Research, Nanjing University of Chinese Medicine, Nanjing 210046, People's Republic of China

Mehdi Aliomrani, Mohammad Reza Sepand and Ali Reza kazemi
Toxicology and Poisoning Research Centre, Tehran University of Medical Sciences, Tehran, Iran
Department of Pharmacology and Toxicology, Faculty of Pharmacy, Tehran University of Medical Sciences, P. O. Box, 1417614411, Tehran, Iran

Hamid Reza Mirzaei
Department of Immunology, Faculty of Medicine, Tehran University of Medical Sciences, Tehran, Iran

Saeid Nekonam
Department of Anatomy, Faculty of Medicine,
Tehran University of Medical Sciences,
Tehran, Iran

Omid Sabzevari
Department of Pharmacology and Toxicology,
Faculty of Pharmacy, Tehran University of
Medical Sciences, P. O. Box, 1417614411,
Tehran, Iran
Drug design and discovery Research Centre,
Tehran University of Medical Sciences,
Tehran, Iran

Index